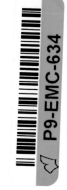
Ways of Living

Self-Care Strategies for Special Needs

2nd Edition

Charles Christiansen, EdD, OTR, OT(C), FAOTA, Editor

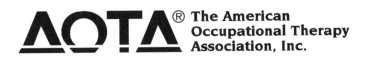
AOTA® **The American Occupational Therapy Association, Inc.**

The American Occupational Therapy Association, Inc.
4720 Montgomery Lane
PO Box 31220
Bethesda, Maryland 20824-1220
www.aota.org

Disclaimers

This publication is designed to provide accurate and authoritative information in regard to the subject matter covered. It is sold or distributed with the understanding that the publisher is not engaged in rendering legal, accounting, or other professional service. If legal advice or other expert assistance is required, the services of a competent professional person should be sought.

—From the Declaration of Principles jointly adopted by the American Bar Association and a Committee of Publishers and Associations.

It is the objective of The American Occupational Therapy Association to be a forum for free expression and interchange of ideas. The opinions expressed by the contributors to this work are their own and not necessarily those of either the editors or The American Occupational Therapy Association.

Cover illustration: Private Collection/Diana Ong/SuperStock
ISBN 1-56900-141-3

Printed in the United States of America.

This volume is dedicated to those special people who are able to exemplify the qualities of professionalism in their daily occupations. They put the needs of others first, demonstrate attitudes of attention and compassion, and honor their commitments. In short, they are ethical, competent, and caring. God bless them and keep them in good health. They are far too few in number.

Contents

Foreword

Our conception of man is that of an organism that maintains and balances itself in the world of reality and actuality by being in active life and active use. (Meyer, 1922)

Our profession was developed around the idea that people should be active in meaningful occupations. What happens when a person experiences limitations that make doing that difficult, if not impossible?

There is no more important freedom than the freedom of action. Occupational therapy practitioners must possess the knowledge and skills to help clients achieve their freedom of action (i.e., participate in the occupations of everyday life). We each have our own way of living: Making it possible for others to exercise their "way of living" is the hallmark of occupational therapy.

Occupational therapy practitioners must have knowledge and skills to help persons overcome the impairments and barriers that limit their potential for independent life. As well, we must have the knowledge and skills to preserve the person's identity as he or she learns compensatory and technologically supported strategies to continue his or her life. This book is not limited to physical strategies: It places major focus on how the client views the activities that are instrumental to his or her way of living.

For several decades many occupational therapy practitioners have found the emphasis on self-care defined by functional measures that have been limited to basic self-care. Studies of outcomes after stroke indicate that although persons can perform basic self-care, they are not returning to the meaningful tasks that they did as a spouse, a parent, or a worker nor are they returning to the leisure activities that brought pleasure to their lives (Niemi, Laakonson, Kotila, & Waltimo, 1988). Occupational therapy practitioners must define self-care needs from the perspective of the client and bring their best knowledge and skills to the planning of care. We must address the full scope of activities from basic to instrumental and, most importantly, address the issues that the client considers necessary to live his or her life.

This book gives the reader a conceptual framework for addressing the comprehensive needs of the clients we serve. In this second edition of *Ways of Living*, the reader will be given the context to help clients achieve their ways of living from a perspective that integrates self, meaning, capacity, impairment, and, most of all, the client's wishes. Dr. Christiansen has attracted very capable authors to this effort. Their perspectives need to be transmitted to students and practitioners, especially as the field takes a more active role in the community.

I want to tell you a story. My colleagues, Theresa Braford and Dorothy Edwards, started a program in St. Louis, Missouri. They had found a number of older adults who were experiencing physical and cognitive decline as well as social isolation. Most of these adults did not bother to get dressed every day. Some practitioners might have thought to focus on self-care, but Braford and Edwards decided to invite these elders to a weekly social and exercise program. The Area Agency on Aging agreed to provide transportation, and a staff member rode with the van driver to pick up the clients so that they would have the confidence to come. When the clients first began attending the group, they dressed in very simple, easy-to-put-on clothing, and their hair was often disheveled. Over time, the women started to wear their church clothes, did their hair, and put on makeup, and, now, most wear their hats. The men in the group also started grooming themselves and wearing nice pants and shirts. Did they have an activities in daily living problem, or did they not have anywhere to go or any reason to get dressed?

Society is struggling with issues faced by persons who have problems that limit their occupational performance. By making *doing* possible, the occupational therapy practitioner brings value not only to the client being served, but also to the society that must provide for persons who are vulnerable. Let us not put anyone in the vulnerable category who can be a productive and contributing member of society with help from an occupational therapy practitioner. This is a book central to the practice of occupational therapy.

M. Carolyn Baum, PhD, OTR/L, FAOTA
St. Louis, Missouri

References

Niemi, M. L., Laakonson, R., Kotila, M., & Waltimo, O. (1988). Quality of life four years after stroke. *Stroke, 19,* 1101–1107.

Meyer, A. (1922). The philosophy of occupation therapy. *Archives of Occupational Therapy, 1*(1), 1–10.

Preface

The great German philosopher and poet Johann Wolfgang von Goethe is credited with the following statement: "Things that matter most should never be at the mercy of things that matter least."

This is an important piece of wisdom for us all, both in our daily lives and in our practice as caregivers. Self-care tasks may seem mundane to those who take them for granted, but in many ways they occupy a central place in our overall efforts to maintain ourselves and to be accepted by others in the social world in which we live. In fact, self-care needs are so fundamental to who we are that our role in helping others meet them should be a source of continuing pride to all occupational therapy practitioners.

It is natural at the end of a century (or millennium) to think about changes and transitions. Occupational therapy has changed dramatically since the first edition of *Ways of Living* was developed. In revising the book, we considered the changes that have taken place in the field and, in the process, tried to listen carefully to the feedback provided by users of the initial volume. As a result, we added some chapters and modified some content in an attempt to make it more readable and useful. New chapters have been added on vision deficits, sexuality, and plans of care. We also added an important chapter on developmental disabilities in adults.

I am indebted to the support of some talented and dedicated workers in Galveston who contributed to my efforts to organize and complete the revision. These persons include Gina Van Wart, Charles Hayden, Natalie Sims, Patsy Marullo, Cindy L. Hammecker, and Donald W. Dietiker, PhD. Photographic support was provided by Eddie Hunter, for which I am grateful.

Charles Christiansen
Galveston, Texas

1

The Social Importance of Self-Care Intervention

Charles H. Christiansen

Charles H. Christiansen, EdD, OTR, OT(C), FAOTA, is Dean and George T. Bryan Distinguished Professor, School of Allied Health Sciences, University of Texas Medical Branch at Galveston, Texas.

Key Terms

activities of daily living (ADL)

competence

context

disability

disablement

identity

narrative

self-care occupations

self-maintenance

sick role

stigma

Objectives

On completing this chapter, the reader will be able to

1. Explain why occupations are social phenomena.

2. Define the term instrumental activities of daily living (IADL).

3. Explain how personal self-care activities relate to other categories of occupation.

4. Define stigma.

5. Identify ways in which persons achieve personal identity through self-care activities.

6. Illustrate how the situations or contexts create expectations for self-care.

In 1977, Dr. Tristram Englehardt, Jr., a physician and medical philosopher, wrote a paper in which he observed, "Humans are healthy or diseased in terms of the activities open to them or denied them" (p. 667). This quotation suggests that Dr. Englehardt has a good understanding of what makes life meaningful. Because of this understanding, he also appreciates the value of occupational therapy.

Englehardt's statement deserves further explanation to appreciate its meaning fully. Acute illnesses, such as the flu, are nuisances because of the pain and discomfort they cause. Persons with such illnesses may miss a day or two of their typical activities, but such inconveniences are temporary. In comparison, catastrophic illnesses and injuries, such as polio or traumatic brain injury, result in the permanent disruption of lives.

When such disastrous health problems occur, a person often does not understand what has happened to himself or herself. Medical diagnoses such as cerebral infarct or spinal cord lesion are not part of most people's everyday language. Therefore, the meaning of these terms is not readily understood. When presented with information involving such medical terminology, patients and family members typically want health care professionals to provide a functional translation. Thus, questions such as "Will I be able to ride my horse again?" or "Can I play the piano when I recover?" become the means for understanding the conditions. When such questions are raised, it becomes quite evident that it is what people do, not simply their physical conditions, that provides the meaning for their lives. In short, health and function are important because they enable meaningful living.

Yet it is interesting to observe that when a person is confronted with a disabling condition that will result in permanent disability, he or she seldom asks if they will be able to eat without assistance or go to the toilet. These ordinary acts of self-maintenance are taken for granted by able-bodied persons to such an extent that their basic place in everyday life is not apparent. It is only when their performance becomes difficult or impossible that the importance of these everyday requirements is evident. Indeed, persons with disabilities who write about their own experiences typically comment about the unexpected challenges presented by their inability to perform routine daily tasks such as dressing and bathing.

In *The Body Silent*, excerpted below, anthropologist Robert Murphy (1987) provided a personal account of the effects of a spinal tumor that progressively diminished his ability to live without assistance from others.

> I was quite self-sufficient back in that stage of my disability. I could dress my upper body, though I never did master pants and shoes, and I took care of most of my personal needs. I shaved, brushed my teeth, sponge bathed most of my body, and I used the toilet without assistance. Yolanda would go off to work every day, leaving lunch in the refrigerator, and I would fend for myself. I even managed to reheat coffee. The only time that I required help was in getting dressed in the morning and undressed at night. (p. 62)

The abnormal cells that caused Robert Murphy's tumor created gradual paralysis, which eventually cost him his life. Murphy experienced his gradual condition not as a series of biological events but rather as a progressive barrier that kept him from performing the daily tasks he had previously taken for granted. When his inability to walk and his lack of arm strength and coordination limited his ability to participate in everyday activities at home and in the community, he recognized that his very identity as a college professor, husband, and father was threatened.

Murphy was unique in the sense that he had unusual insight into his situation and was able to continue his career as a professor for many years. In another sense, however, his situation provides a typical example of the powerful consequences of having impaired function that interferes with the requirements of daily living. The ability to participate fully in everyday life activities is a quality of life issue that has a profound effect on a person's satisfaction and well-being. Being able to participate in the ordinary routines described in Murphy's excerpt assumes both practical and symbolic significance to those who take such tasks for granted.

Self-Care as a Category of Daily Living

Occupational therapy practitioners typically divide daily living activities into several broad categories. These are activities done to earn a living, those related to leisure and recreation, those related to resting or sleeping, and those related to personal care and self-maintenance.

Scientists studying occupation have been unable to agree on a useful method for classifying daily activities. It is difficult to categorize an activity without knowing more about where it is performed and for what purpose (Christiansen, 1994, 1997). For example, the game of golf can be "played" either by professional athletes who earn a living or by amateurs for recreation. Moreover, golf is often used as a means for promoting business transactions. Thus, is golf a play or leisure activity, a work activity, or both? The answer depends on the intended goals of the participants.

Self-Care and Self-Maintenance

Activities at home and in the community designed to enable basic survival and well-being are known as self-maintenance occupations. These are the duties and chores related to taking care of ourselves. Self-maintenance includes those tasks ranging from personal care (such as dressing and grooming) to using the telephone, managing medications, banking, and shopping for food. These tasks are sometimes referred to as activities of daily living or ADL.

The specific tasks that have been included under this heading vary. However, the term ADL nearly always includes toileting (bowel and bladder functions), bathing, dressing, eating, and grooming (including oral hygiene). These personal care tasks have come to be known collectively as basic "self-care." Table 1.1 identifies the tasks and explains all the activities involved in each task.

In the late 1960s, M. Powell Lawton, a gerontologist, recognized that living independently in the community required a level of competence that enabled the accomplishment of tasks beyond those of basic self-care. These more complex tasks were termed instrumental activities of daily living (IADL) and included use of the telephone, food preparation, housekeeping, doing laundry, shopping, money management, using transportation, and managing medication needs (Lawton, 1971). This overall set of basic self-care tasks and activities is viewed as a foundation for survival and for participation in the community. Research has shown that self-maintenance activities consume about 10% to 15% of the waking day of a person without disability (Szalai, 1972). Persons with disabilities require a slightly higher proportion of time to accomplish these self-maintenance activities (Lawton, 1990; Yelin, Lubeck, Holman, & Epstein, 1987).

The Social Significance of Self-Care Tasks

Clearly, the need of some self-care tasks cannot be denied, because if we are to continue living we must be able to take care of our bodily needs, including nourishment. Our survival requires the ability to acquire and prepare food as necessary and to eat. Beyond survival, however, daily living requires the ability to conform to societal expectations of hygiene, grooming, and dress, as well as to communicate effectively.

It is important to note that all tasks of daily living are embedded within a social framework, and life satisfaction and perceptions of well-being are related to our acceptance by others and our ability to participate in social activities (e.g., Cooper & Okamura, 1992; Ishii-Kuntz, 1990). Studies have shown that social factors are more important to life satisfaction and well-being than whether or not a person has a physical limitation or disability resulting from aging, injury, or disease (Affleck & Pfeiffer, 1988; Bowling & Edelmann, 1989; Rintala & Young, 1992).

Gaining access to locations where social activities take place and being accepted by the group are other important elements of a satisfactory lifestyle. For example, Fuhrer, Rintala, Hart, Clearman, and Young (1992) studied 640 persons with paralysis resulting from spinal cord injury who were living in the community. Their study hoped to explain the aspects of living that contributed to overall life satisfaction in these persons who were disabled as a result of their paralysis. The researchers found that participants who felt accepted and supported by the group, believed themselves to be in control of their lives, and were able to get around were more likely to be satisfied with their lives. In this study, no relationship was found between the extent of a participant's disability and his or her life satisfaction. Studies such as this make it clear that efforts in rehabilitation should be directed toward enabling persons to return to full participation within their communities.

Communities are not buildings and streets; rather, they are collections of people who share life experiences by doing things together. When persons engage in valued activities and occupations, they do so within contexts or situations. Contexts involve both the person and the environment, which typically includes other persons and physical objects, such as buildings, vehicles, and streets. To understand fully how health conditions affect person's

Table 1.1 AOTA-Recommended Terminology for Self-Maintenance Tasks
(Activities of Daily Living) (AOTA, 1994)

Task	Definition
Grooming	Obtainment and use of supplies; removal of body hair (use of razors, tweezers, lotions, etc.); application and removal of cosmetics; washing, drying, combing, styling, and brushing hair; caring for nails (hands and feet); caring for skin, eyes, and ears; application of deodorant.
Oral hygiene	Obtainment and use of supplies; cleaning mouth; brushing and flossing teeth, or removal, cleaning, and reinsertion of dental orthotics and prosthetics.
Bathing/showering	Obtainment and use of supplies; soaping, rinsing, and drying of body parts; maintaining bathing position; transferring to and from bathing position.
Toilet hygiene	Obtainment and use of supplies; clothing management; maintaining toileting position; transferring to and from toileting position; cleaning body; caring for menstrual and continence needs (including catheters, colostomies, and suppository management).
Personal device care	Cleaning and maintaining hearing aids, contact lenses, glasses, orthotics, prosthetics, adaptive equipment, and contraceptive and sexual devices.
Dressing	Selection of clothing and accessories appropriate to time of day, weather, and occasion; obtainment of clothing from storage area; dressing and undressing in a sequential fashion; fastening and adjusting clothing and shoes; application and removal of personal devices, prostheses, or orthoses.
Feeding and eating	Setting up food; selection and use of appropriate utensils and tableware; bringing food or drink to mouth; cleaning face, hands, and clothing (including management of alternative methods of nourishment). Performance of sucking, masticating, coughing, and swallowing.
Medication routine	Obtainment of medication; opening and closing containers; following prescribed schedules; taking correct quantities; reporting problems and adverse effects.
Socialization	Assessing opportunities and interacting with other people in appropriate contextual and cultural ways to meet emotional and physical needs.
Functional communication	Use of equipment or systems to send and receive information, such as writing equipment, telephones, typewriters, computers, communication boards, call lights, emergency systems, Braille writers, and augmentative communication systems.
Functional mobility	Movement from one position or place to another, such as in-bed mobility, wheelchair mobility, transfers (wheelchair, bed, car, tub, toilet, shower, chair, floor); performance of functional ambulation, driving, and transporting objects; obtainment of public and private transportation.
Emergency response	Recognition of sudden, unexpected hazardous situations, and initiation of action to reduce threat to health.
Sexual expression	Recognizing, communicating, and engaging in desired sexual activities.

lives, we must understand the situation or context and acknowledge that it is influenced by the person with the condition, as well as the environment in which he or she functions. Environments include other people (and their attitudes) and structures (which often create barriers to access).

To the extent that one or more self-maintenance tasks cannot be performed because of limitations imposed by the health condition or the environment, the ability of a person to become an active participant in community life is made more difficult. This means that life satisfaction is more difficult to achieve (Branholm & Fugl-Meyer, 1992). Thus, a clear and important relationship exists between meeting the essential requirements of daily living and well-being (Yerxa & Baum, 1986). A central theme of this book is that when rehabilitation providers direct their attention to the self-care and daily living requirements of their patients and clients, they enable social involvement and promote greater life satisfaction (Crisp, 1992).

Self-Care and Personality Theory

Psychologist Robert Hogan (Hogan, 1982; Hogan & Sloan, 1991) provided a basis for understanding the importance of daily self-maintenance activities in his theory of personality. He noted that humans evolved as group-living, culture-bearing, and symbol-using animals. Groups of people, whether in committees or communities, vary in terms of their acceptance by and influence within the group. We refer to this place in the group as our social standing. According to Hogan, these characteristics influence daily living in two fundamental ways. First, because we are social beings, it is necessary that we get along with others. Second, because social standing matters, much of our well-being requires an ability to compete successfully and to gain standing in the group.

The idea that human behavior may be influenced by a need for gaining social standing within groups is sometimes viewed as disturbing to persons who would prefer more tranquil, idealistic, and democratic views of the world. However, the existence of brothers and sisters who compete for attention, the need for second graders to "be first in line," and the presence of organizational charts are all examples of the influence of social standing on social behavior.

The ability to achieve and maintain standing in social groups requires a social identity, and Hogan noted that a good deal of time is spent developing, negotiating, repairing, enhancing, and defending who we are and who we would like to be. Identity is achieved mainly through our self-presentation, or how we are perceived by others during interactions.

Hogan claimed that the basis for social interaction occurs through roles, such as spouse, parent, friend, or colleague, each having different behavioral expectations as defined by the group (whether this group is a circle of friends, a family, a workplace, or a larger social organization). Because persons differ in the extent to which they can successfully fulfill their roles, these differences explain variations in influence and popularity that, over time, take on a more enduring quality known as reputation.

When persons are no longer able to perform their roles competently, both their social standing and their reputation can be threatened. Thus, chronic illness and disability can have a profound effect on social identity because they threaten the views others may hold of a person as well as that person's view of self, or self-identity.

Identity

Traditional views of identity suggest that a core self-concept comes from our interactions with others and through the successes or failures that we experience as we mature. Some developmental psychologists (e.g., Flavell, 1985; Kagan, 1989) believe that knowledge of the self and others occurs as our experiences reveal the characteristics that make people (including ourselves) unique. An important part of our development seems to be related to understanding that people differ from each other and that we are different from others. Other theorists (e.g., Cooley, 1902; Mead, 1934) have proposed that we develop our self-understanding by observing how others respond to us during social interactions.

According to Rogers (1982), an occupational therapist and gerontologist, if we are to view ourselves as competent persons who are able to overcome the challenges that confront us, we must have a sense of autonomy. Her view of autonomy requires freedom and self-reliance. Rogers suggested that autonomy is demonstrated through our ability to make choices and influence the world around us. Our sense of self, then, is profoundly influenced by our engagement in the everyday activities of the world in which we live and our ability to fulfill roles that are appreciated and valued by the social groups in which we claim membership.

Discussions of personal identity are not complete without a consideration of the importance of narrative. Narrative is a scientific term for personal or life-related stories. Recently, it has been proposed that persons understand themselves and their lives through stories. These accounts of events that involve us and are connected over time are described as self-narratives (Gergen & Gergen, 1988). According to Mancuso and Sarbin (1985), any slice of life, when carefully considered, is interpreted and experienced as part of a story. In speaking of the influence of narrative in self-identity, Polkinghorne (1988) wrote:

> We achieve our personal identities and self-concept through the use of [narrative], and make our existence into a whole by understanding it as an expression of a single unfolding and developing story. We are in the middle of our stories and cannot be sure how they will end; we are constantly having to revise the plot as new events are added to our lives. Self, then, is not a static thing or a substance, but a configuring of personal events into an historical unity which includes not only what one has been but also anticipations of what one will be. (p. 150)

Thus, our identity is based on our current views of the past and present, as well as our anticipation of the future. Because we interpret our lives as stories, we also live them as stories with many possible endings. The possible future chapters and endings for our stories involve many anticipated selves. These possible selves influence the choices we make and the behaviors we exhibit on a daily basis. Our behaviors are embedded within our striving to perform our roles in ways that enhance our views of self and the views others have of us.

In life, events happen that make some future chapters and story endings implausible. Thus, Robert Murphy, who had imagined himself as an active, highly mobile retiree, could no longer entertain that possibility after his spinal surgery. One view of his future self had suddenly become impossible. Moreover, a view he had of himself in the present had been compromised. In short, his self-identify was in transition.

Disability as a Threat to Identity

The work of occupational therapy practitioners brings them into daily contact with patients whose self-identities are in transition (Mattingly & Fleming, 1993). Many patients will not be able to return to their previous living situations and are in the process of trying to make new sense of who they are now and who they will become. Their identities are changing, and this is because their ability to perform as parent or spouse or worker may now be reduced.

Persons with spinal cord injuries offer dramatic examples of how abrupt role transitions are experienced. Patients with spinal cord injury are often young, active men in excellent physical condition who were skiing or swimming one instant and suddenly paralyzed for life moments later. During their rehabilitation, such persons encounter considerable anxiety regarding their roles as desirable marital partners, as productive members of the work force, and as accepted members of their peer groups (Zedjlik, 1992). See Box 1.1.

However, all persons, whether disabled or not, must confront transitions during their lives. The process of normal aging leads to a series of role

---

Box 1.1
Spinal Cord Injury: Sudden Life Transition

The contemporary American actor Christopher Reeve, who became famous in the movie *Superman*, is an example of a man who has experienced the traumatic life change of a spinal cord injury. His life changed dramatically in 1995 at the age of 42 after the horse he was riding in a competition balked at jumping a short fence. Because his hands were tangled in the reins, Reeve landed on his head, causing an injury to his spinal cord and permanent paralysis involving most of his body. Reeve remains active in various causes, including a drive to find a cure for paralysis. He has written a book titled *Still Me* (1998), in which he talks about the importance of social relationships in bringing meaning to his life. The following excerpt from his book illustrates this.

> When a catastrophe happens it's easy to feel so sorry for yourself that you can't even see anybody around you. But the way out is through your relationships. The way out of that misery or obsession is to focus more on what your little boy needs or what your teenagers need or what other people around you need. It's very hard to do, and often you have to force yourself. But that is the answer to the dilemma of being frozen—at least it's the answer I found. (p. 14)

changes at predictable stages in life. A person may move from being a parent responsible for rearing children to a grandparent who may increasingly rely on others for support. Often, as the capacity for self-reliance declines, persons are placed in situations where choice and control are limited, and where their sense of self as competent members of society becomes tragically diminished (Rosow, 1985).

During these life changes, acts that were previously viewed as ordinary or routine assume larger significance as symbols of competency. Thus, retaining or relearning the ability to perform tasks of self-maintenance (even with assistance), such as dressing without assistance, becomes a means of fostering self-identity. To permit others to perform self-care tasks for us may be interpreted symbolically as occupying a role of one who is dependent—as one who has assumed the "sick role."

As described by Parsons (1958, 1975), the *sick role* is a transitional state in which persons are exempted from typical role responsibilities during their recovery from an illness. Thus, for example, when we have the flu, people excuse us from our everyday obligations. We are permitted to miss work or school, and most deadlines are extended automatically. This exemption, however, requires that we take steps to facilitate our recovery, such as limiting our social activities and seeking medical attention if appropriate.

Unfortunately, when people become disabled, they are often viewed as sick. When viewed in this way, they are in danger of being assigned a permanently diminished standing by society because they are exempted from engaging in valued social roles. In the words of Goffman (1963), their identity has been spoiled, and they have become the victims of stigma.

Stigma

Stigma describes a social condition in which a person is devalued because he or she cannot meet expected "codes of behavior" in role performance. Goffman (1959) portrayed all interaction as consisting of crediting or discrediting role performances. A discrediting role performance can result from any number of behaviors that vary from those expected within a given situation.

For example, Goffman noted that behaviors such as yawning, stuttering, appearing nervous or self-conscious, problems with balance, losing muscular control, or losing one's temper can each diminish a person's creditability during a social encounter. Because persons with physical or emotional dis-

orders may be unable to control some behaviors that would be expected in a given situation, their performances can become discrediting. Thus, persons with obvious disabilities must learn to manage the impressions they convey during social interaction to avoid social stigma.

Disability may result in a changed body image that alters a person's view of self, as well as how he or she may be viewed by others. The following excerpt from the book *Able Lives* (Morris, 1988), written to document the experiences of women with spinal cord injuries, illustrates this reality:

> One of the hardest parts of becoming disabled is acceptance of, and living with, a changed body image. Our body shape and the aids we use (a wheelchair or crutches) are the visible signs of disability. Appearance plays a very important part in interaction with other people. What is more, women face an additional problem in that our physical attractiveness is generally the way our femininity and sexuality are measured by other people. (p. 160)

Thus, as the excerpt reveals, acceptance by others also requires maintaining expected standards of dress and appearance. People are expected to present themselves according to social norms, and the manner of their appearance and dress has been shown to influence perceptions of their status and competence. Thus, being able to manage basic self-care tasks is a fundamental prerequisite for successful social interaction for the able-bodied person, and it is no less important for the person with a disability. Learning to overcome stigma and regaining an acceptable social identity may be the most important challenge confronting someone with a disability.

Changing Social Attitudes Through Language

In recent years, persons with conditions that limit their participation in society, rehabilitation professionals, and social activists have banded together to influence legislation and language in an attempt to change prejudicial attitudes and influence social policy. Recognizing that language influences thought and attitudes, they have worked hard to introduce new terminology that does not perpetuate outdated views. The term *disablement* expresses a view that a person's ability to participate in society is based on a combination of factors. These factors include attitudes, social policies, and physical structures in the built environment, such as buildings, vehicles, and streets. The 1997 revision of the World Health

Organization's *International Classification of Impairments, Disabilities and Handicaps* (1980) reflects these changes. Levels of function previously classified as impairments, disabilities, and handicaps have been changed in the new volume, titled *International Classification of Impairments, Activities, and Participation: A Manual of Dimensions of Disablement and Functioning,* to avoid the use of terms that may perpetuate old views and attitudes (see Table 1.2).

Studies of Social Participation and Satisfactory Adjustment

Recent studies have confirmed the importance of overcoming stigma and becoming fully involved in social activities. Fuhrer and others (1992, 1993) found that depression among persons with spinal cord injury was not related to a person's degree of impairment or disability. Rather, depression tended to occur most often in persons who were unemployed or unable to participate in their usual social relationships. Persons who were able to find employ-ment, or who engaged in volunteer work or self-improvement activities, had higher overall morale.

These findings were similar to those reported by Rybarczyk and colleagues (1992), who found that depression among persons with leg amputations was less likely to occur when participants reported that they were comfortable with social contacts that involved acknowledgment of their amputation or prosthesis.

Other studies have shown that social support and the ability to feel competent are important factors in psychological adjustment and may be related to engagement in valued activities. Studies of adolescents with severe burns (Barnum, Snyder, Rapoff, Mani, & Thompson, 1998), of children and adolescents with spina bifida (Appleton et al., 1997), of persons with spinal cord injury (Elliott & Shewchuk, 1995; McColl & Skinner, 1995), and of men recovering from heart attacks (Sullivan, LaCroix, Russo, & Katon, 1998) have supported the importance of these factors in promoting adjustment and reducing depression.

Table 1.2 Changes in World Health Organization (WHO) Classifications

Classification Level	Body (body parts)	Person (person as a whole)	Society (relationships with society)	Situation (person and environment viewed together)
ICIDH (WHO, 1980)	Impairment (Loss or abnormality of psychological, physiological, or anatomical structure of function)	Disability (Restriction or lack [resulting from impairment] of ability to perform an activity in the manner or within the range considered normal)	Handicap (Disadvantage for a person resulting from impairment or disability that limits or prevents fulfillment of a role that is normal for that person	Not considered in this version
ICIDH-2 (Beta) (WHO, 1997)	Impairment (Loss or abnormality of a body structure or physiological or psychological function)	Activity (The extent of functioning at the level of the person. A person's daily activities)	Participation (Nature and extent of a person's involvement in life situations in relation to impairment, activities, health conditions, and contextual factors)	Contextual Factors (Features of the physical, social, and attitudinal world)

Summary

In this chapter, self-care tasks have been presented within a view that considers the importance of enabling the patient to maintain valued social roles. Maintaining the self in a manner that permits rewarding social interaction is fundamental to daily living and an important factor in life satisfaction.

Within the contexts of everyday life, bodily impairments and limitations in ability may interact with social attitudes and environmental barriers to restrict participation and diminish opportunities for the expression of personal identity. Occupational therapy practitioners can perform a valuable service by helping their patients explore and consider different views of self that are acceptable and offer reasonable prospects for personal fulfillment. Understanding how the patient is experiencing and interpreting the challenges of disablement will assist in this process. ◆

Study Questions

1. What are the main elements in a typical life situation or context?

2. How do the person and the context interact to limit social participation?

3. How do personal characteristics and personality influence social acceptance?

4. Define the tasks required for self-maintenance.

5. Define stigma. How do any personal experiences you have had with stigma make you feel? How can stigma be overcome?

6. Define narrative. What are the elements you would include when you are telling others about things in your life?

7. Define disablement. How do language and terms influence attitudes?

8. Why are social factors so important in the rehabilitation process?

References

Affleck, G., & Pfeiffer, C. A. (1988). Social support and psychosocial adjustment to rheumatoid arthritis: Quantitative and qualitative findings. *Arthritis Care and Research, 1*(2), 71–77.

American Occupational Therapy Association. (1994). Uniform terminology for occupational therapy— Third edition. *American Journal of Occupational Therapy, 48,* 1047–1054.

Appleton, P. L., Ellis, N. C., Minchom, P. E., Lawson, V., Boell, V., & Jones, P. (1997). Depressive symptoms and self concept in young people with spina bifida. *Journal of Pediatric Psychology, 22*(5), 707–722.

Barnum, D. D., Snyder, C. R., Rapoff, M. A., Mani, M. M., & Thompson, R. (1998). Hope and social support in the psychological adjustment of children who have survived burn injuries and their matched controls. *Children's Health Care, 27*(1), 15–30.

Bowling, A. P., & Edelmann, R. J. (1989). Loneliness, mobility, well-being and social support in a sample of over 85 year olds. *Personality and Individual Differences, 10,* 1189–1192.

Branholm, I. B., & Fugl-Meyer, A. R. (1992). Occupational role preferences and life satisfaction. *Occupational Therapy Journal of Research, 12,* 159–171.

Christiansen, C. H. (1994). Classification and study in occupation: A review and discussion of taxonomies. *Journal of Occupational Science, 1*(3), 3–17.

Christiansen, C. H. (1997). Understanding occupation definitions and concepts. In C. Christiansen & C. Baum (Eds.), *Occupational therapy: Enabling function and well-being* (pp. 3–25). Thorofare, NJ: Slack.

Cooley, H. C. (1902). *Human nature and the social order.* New York: Scribner.

Cooper, H., & Okamura, L. (1992). Social activity and subjective well-being. *Personality and Individual Differences, 13,* 573–583.

Crisp, R. (1992). The long term adjustment of 60 persons with spinal cord injury. *Australian Psychologist, 27*(1), 43–47.

Elliott, T. R. & Shewchuk, R. M. (1995). Social support and leisure activities following severe physical disability: Testing the mediating effects of depression. *Basic and Applied Social Psychology, 16*(4), 471–487.

Englehardt, H. T., Jr. (1977). Defining occupational therapy: The meaning of therapy and the virtues of occupation. *American Journal of Occupational Therapy, 31,* 666–672.

Flavell, J. (1985). *Cognitive development.* Englewood Cliffs, NJ: Prentice Hall.

Fuhrer, M. J., Rintala, D. H., Hart, K. A., Clearman, R., & Young, M. E. (1992). Relationship of life satisfaction to impairment, disability, and handicap among persons with spinal cord injury living in the community. *Archives of Physical Medicine and Rehabilitation, 73,* 552–557.

Fuhrer, M. J., Rintala, D. H., Hart, K. A., Clearman, R., & Young, M. E. (1993). Depressive symptomatology in persons with spinal cord injury who reside in the community. *Archives of Physical Medicine and Rehabilitation, 74,* 255–261.

Gergen, K. J., & Gergen, M. M. (1988). Narrative and the self as relationship. In L. Berkowitz (Ed.), *Advances in experimental and social psychology* (pp. 17–55). New York: Academic Press.

Goffman, E. (1959). *The presentation of self in everyday life.* New York: Doubleday.

Goffman, E. (1963). *Stigma: Notes on the management of a spoiled identity.* Englewood Cliffs, NJ: Prentice Hall.

Hogan, R. (1982). A socioanalytic theory of personality. *Nebraska Symposium on Motivation, 30,* 55–89.

Hogan, R., & Sloan, T. (1991). Socioanalytic foundations for personality psychology. *Perspectives in Personality, 3*(Part B), 1–15.

Ishii-Kuntz, M. (1990). Social interaction and psychological well being. *International Journal of Aging and Human Development, 30*(1), 15–36.

Kagan, J. (1989). *Unstable ideas: Temperament, cognition and self.* Cambridge, MA: Harvard University Press.

Lawton, M. P. (1971). The functional assessment of elderly people. *Journal of the American Geriatrics Society, 19,* 465–481.

Lawton, M. P. (1990). Age and the performance of home tasks. *Human Factors, 32,* 527–536.

Mancuso, J. C., & Sarbin, T. R. (1985). The self-narrative in the enactment of roles. In T. R. Sarbin & K. E. Scheibe (Eds.), *Studies in social identity* (pp. 233–253). New York: Praeger.

Mattingly, C., & Fleming, M. (1993). *Clinical reasoning: Forms of inquiry in a therapeutic practice.* Philadelphia: F. A. Davis.

McColl, M. A., & Skinner, H. (1995). Assessing inter- and intrapersonal resources: Social support and coping among adults with a disability. *Disability and Rehabilitation, 17*(1), 24–34.

Mead, G. H. (1934). *Mind, self, and society.* Chicago: University of Chicago Press.

Morris, J. (Ed.). (1988). *Able lives.* London: The Women's Press.

Murphy, R. F. (1987). *The body silent.* New York: Henry Holt.

Parsons, T. (1958). Definitions of health and illness in the light of American values and social structure. In E. G. Jaco (Ed.), *Patients, physicians, and illness* (pp. 165–187). New York: Free Press of Glencoe.

Parsons, T. (1975). The sick role and the role of the physician reconsidered. *Health and Society: Milbank Memorial Fund Quarterly, 53*(3), 257–278.

Polkinghorne, D. (1988). *Narrative knowing and the human sciences.* Albany, NY: State University of New York Press.

Reeve, C. (1998). *Still me.* New York: Random House.

Rintala, D., & Young, M. E. (1992). Social support and the well being of persons with spinal cord injury living in the community. *Rehabilitation Psychology, 37,* 158–163.

Rogers, J. (1982). The spirit of independence: The evolution of a philosophy. *American Journal of Occupational Therapy, 36,* 709–715.

Rosow, I. (1985). Status and role change through the life cycle. In R. H. Shanas & E. Shanas (Eds.), *Handbook of aging and the social sciences* (pp. 62–91). New York: Van Nostrand Reinhold.

Rybarczyk, B. D., Nyenhuis, D. L., Nicholas, J. J., Schulz, R., Alioto, R. J., & Blair, C. (1992). Social discomfort and depression in a sample of adults with leg amputations. *Archives of Physical Medicine and Rehabilitation, 73,* 1169–1173.

Sullivan, M. D., LaCroix, A. Z., Russo, J., & Katon, W. J. (1998). Self efficacy and reported functional status in coronary heart disease: A six month prospective study. *Psychosomatic Medicine, 60*(4), 473–478.

Szalai, A. (Ed.). (1972*). The use of time: Daily activities of urban and suburban populations in twelve countries.* The Hague, Netherlands: Mouton.

World Health Organization. (1980). *International classification of impairments, disabilities and handicaps: A manual of classification relating to consequences of disease.* Geneva, Switzerland: Author.

World Health Organization. (1997). *International classification of impairments, activities and participation: A manual of dimensions of disablement and functioning.* Geneva, Switzerland: Author.

Yelin, E., Lubeck, D., Holman, H., & Epstein, W. (1987). The impact of rheumatoid arthritis and osteoarthritis: The activities of patients with rheumatoid arthritis and osteoarthritis compared to controls. *Journal of Rheumatology, 14,* 710–717.

Yerxa, E. J., & Baum, S. (1986). Engagement in daily occupations and life satisfaction among people with spinal cord injuries. *Occupational Therapy Journal of Research, 40,* 271–283.

Zedjlik, C. (1992). *Management of spinal cord injury* (2nd ed.). Boston: Jones and Bartlett.

2

The Meaning of
Self-Care Occupations

Gelya Frank

Gelya Frank, PhD, is Associate Professor, Department of Occupational Science and Occupational Therapy, University of Southern California, Los Angeles, California.

Key Terms

aesthetic anxiety

compassion

disease

division of labor

existential anxiety

illness

infantilization

performance failure

reciprocity

sick role

stigma

stigma symbols

Objectives

On completing this chapter, the reader will be able to

1. Define illness and disability in terms of occupation (changes in what a person can or cannot do).

2. Describe some actual experiences of persons who need help with self-care.

3. Show how a person feels like "a different person" when his or her ability to perform familiar occupations changes.

4. Explain how needing help with self-care affects family and other personal relationships.

5. Explain how help with self-care is experienced by patients in hospitals and other institutions.

6. Show how eating, grooming, and using the toilet have important cultural and social meanings.

7. Discuss how occupational therapists can support patients to discover new and better ways to care for themselves.

Daily activities are laden with personal meaning, but when they are described in purely technical terms, they become impersonal. For example, words such as toileting, grooming, and feeding are used in health care delivery to refer to an area of occupational performance known as activities of daily living. This stark, impersonal, and technical language strips away the rich meanings that the body and its functions take on in our culture and offends the sensibilities of most occupational therapy practitioners.

Activities such as using the bathroom, combing hair, putting on clothes, and eating may be described objectively as a set of muscle movements. However, when a person suffers a stroke or a spinal cord injury, or becomes the parent of a child with a birth defect, he or she quickly discovers worlds of significance packed into even the simplest self-care activities. When occupational therapy practitioners speak to persons about their self-care, they need a language that fits their patients' experiences.

Defining Symptoms in Occupational Terms

Disease refers to a disorder as defined by medical science. Social scientists use *illness* to refer to the person's experience of that disorder or suffering (Eisenberg, 1977). Medical anthropologist Arthur Kleinman (1988) coined the term "illness problems" to refer to the practical problems that affect our ability to perform our usual daily activities as a result of disease.

> Illness problems are the principal difficulties that symptoms and disability create in our lives. For example, we may be unable to walk up our stairs to our bedroom. Or we may experience distracting low back pain while we sit at work. Headaches may make it impossible to focus on homework assignments or housework, leading to failure and frustration. Or there may be impotence that leads to divorce. (Kleinman, 1988, p. 4)

Kleinman (1988) suggested that health care providers have a better chance of giving meaningful care if first they gain an understanding of a patient's illness experience. Chronic illnesses, he noted, involve an experience of symptoms as sometimes better and sometimes worse. A sensitive health care provider can help the patient deal with feelings and practical problems that make the bad times worse. Thus, Kleinman said that medical care for persons with chronic illnesses should include, first, "empathic witnessing of the experience of suffering," and, second, "practical coping with the major psychosocial crises that occur from time to time" (p. 10). This is a prescription that occupational therapy practitioners should be well qualified professionally to carry out.

Self-Care Experiences— The Importance of "Self"

Personal accounts by adults of their own illnesses, or as parents of children with chronic illnesses and disabilities, show the personal side of self-care activities. The body's failure to perform activities once taken for granted poses threats to the person's sense of self (Corbin & Strauss, 1988).

For example, Agnes de Mille (1981), dancer and choreographer, first noticed symptoms of the stroke she suffered in 1975, in her seventies, when her hand didn't work to sign a contract. De Mille saw this performance failure as a threat to her lifetime identity. "Please do something fast," she told her doctor, "because I've got to be on the stage in one hour delivering a very difficult lecture and I've never been late for anything in the theater in my life" (pp. 21–22).

Persons who acquire a disability often say that their bodies become alien to them. Sometimes parts of their bodies even seem dead. "Half of me was imprisoned in the other half," wrote de Mille (1981, p. 57) about the weeks immediately after her stroke. Six months later she still felt as if her whole self was split in two.

> My right arm, my right leg, that whole side of my body gone. I was to be two bodies, one of them not my friend, alien. And must I drag this creature about with me, this Siamese horror, forever? Forever not my friend? Very likely. (p. 219)

Poet Audre Lorde (1980), 9 months after a modified radical mastectomy for breast cancer, also longed for a past self who could perform daily activities effortlessly.

> I must be content to see how really little I can do and still do it with an open heart. I can never accept this, like I can't accept that turning my life around is so hard, eating differently, sleeping differently, moving differently, being differently.... I want the old me, bad as before. (pp. 11–12)

In moments when the body performs effortlessly, the old sense of self may return. Like the women above, Robert F. Murphy (1987) believed that his personal history was "divided radically into two parts: pre-wheelchair and post-wheelchair," but his return to the lecture halls of Columbia University, even in a wheelchair, meant a return to his former self: "Hey, it's the same old me inside this body!" (p. 81).

It is rarely possible to recover the "same old me" without reevaluating one's identity. Social psychologists working with patients in rehabilitation suggest that "adjustment" to disability requires accentuating the positive—one's remaining assets—and turning away from the negatives—what is missing (Wright, 1983). Sociologists have called such efforts to reconstruct one's personal identity after chronic illness and disability *biographical work* (Corbin & Strauss, 1988). As Agnes de Mille (1981), who finally managed to get to the toilet in the night using a three-pronged cane, without falling or bumping herself, wrote: "My trip to the bathroom in privacy and decency meant more to me than a rave notice in the [New York] *Times*" (p. 167).

"Unspeakable Practices"— Toileting

Problems in using the toilet can have an effect on a person's sense of self. At Het Dorp, a planned independent living community for persons with physical disabilities in the Netherlands, sociologist Irving Kenneth Zola (1982) lived for a week as a participant observer. Zola, a spokesperson of the Independent Living Movement used a wheelchair for the first time in decades and reported how he handled the "unspeakable practices" of urinating and defecating from his new position. It was an experience that led him to reevaluate the part disability played in his overall identity.

Getting out of the wheelchair and onto the toilet, sitting on the toilet, and getting back into the wheelchair, Zola realized two things: First, the bathroom's barrier-free design made this work easier than he remembered it. Using the grab bar, he was able to raise himself from the toilet despite his weak stomach muscles and legs. He became aware of how unnecessary his previous difficulties in going to the bathroom had been. Second, Zola felt uncomfortable using the toilet from a seated position. He felt that a man of his age ought to urinate standing up. With his permission, readers may follow him into the bathroom on the morning of Friday, May 26, 1972.

Two difficulties did remain. For lack of a better term I call the first one "cultural" and the second "psychosocial." As a Western man I had been trained to urinate standing with both feet firmly planted on the ground. Thus, to sit and urinate took some getting used to. This did, however, provide a side benefit. Standing I had always needed one hand free to steady myself. Sitting at least made it a more relaxed activity. My second problem was more "psychosocial." Before leaving the bathroom I tried to think if I had "to go" again. Once more I was reduced to the status of a child as I recalled parental admonitions to the effect, "We are starting on a trip so you better use the toilet now." I did the same thing with my own children. What were the toilet facilities like elsewhere in the Village? Would they be as easy to negotiate as the one in my room? (1982, pp. 65–66)

Zola's story shows how the ability and willingness to adapt behavior—even in the most private situations—may hinge on unspoken cultural rules defining social identity. His ability to step back and observe how his reactions were shaped helped him. Such critical thinking can also help other persons with disabilities make choices about what works for them.

Architectural Barriers and Special Equipment

In Zola's case, barriers that he had previously experienced when manipulating a wheelchair were not present in a bathroom at Het Dorp. Robert F. Murphy (1987), writing about his progressive paralysis as a result of a spinal cord tumor, also talked about how the physical environment can affect the meaning of symptoms. The tumor made it difficult for him to climb the stairs, but his bedroom and study were on the second floor. Murphy became confined to the first floor of his two-story suburban home. He had considered getting a stairway lift, but the cost was so high that it would have been cheaper to buy a new home.

All discussion about how to get Murphy up to the second floor ended one day in 1977 when his son and his son's friend carried him upstairs. Murphy discovered that the bathrooms would have to be torn up to make them accessible. That was the last time he saw the second floor of his house. As it turned out, Murphy's paralysis soon worsened to the point where he would not have been able to transfer by himself to and from the lift and his wheelchairs anyway.

He moved permanently to the family room on the first floor, to which a half bathroom was added, and this action marked Murphy's change in status within the family. His choice of activities and the quality of his life were increasingly dictated by his self-care needs and limited by barriers in his environment. Losing his ability to move spontaneously meant losing aspects of his self.

> I could go nowhere without a driver, usually Yolanda [Murphy's wife] or Bob [his son], and every trip entailed logistics. If we wanted to eat at a restaurant or go to the movies, we had to call first to make sure there were no steps. And if we wanted to stay at a motel, we had to measure the width of the bathroom door, for my wheelchair is twenty-six inches wide. Whenever we traveled, we needed equipment. Aside from the wheelchair, we had to transport the walker, bedpan, urinal, and assorted accessories. As my condition worsened, the list grew longer. Gone were the days when we would give in to a sudden urge to go somewhere or do something. But gone also were the days when I could wander into the kitchen for a snack or outside for a breath of fresh air. This loss of spontaneity invaded my entire assessment of time. It rigidified my short-range perspectives and introduced a calculating quality into an existence that formerly had been pleasantly disordered. (1987, p. 76)

Home Care, Family Dynamics, and Rehabilitation Policy

When a person needs help with self-care activities, the meaning of self-care is affected by the attitude of his or her caregivers and by his or her level of finances and other resources. Within marriages, or with persons who live together, the couple typically works together to manage the disability (Corbin & Strauss, 1988). For example, a husband may help perform the self-care activities of his wife. Consequently, how the person with a chronic illness or disability experiences eating, dressing, and going to the bathroom is affected by the kind of help available.

Often the division of labor in the family becomes unbalanced when a spouse or children take care of another family member's basic needs. Feelings of exhaustion, depression, anxiety about money, self-pity, and resentment are common. Caregivers often feel guilty about having those reactions. In a study about couples managing chronic illness at home (Corbin & Strauss, 1988), one woman described her exhaustion over the physical work she did to help her husband.

> All night long he would say, "Get me water, put me on the commode." I would tell K., "Let me sleep; let me rest. I don't mind waiting on you hand and foot during the day, but at night let me sleep." . . . He got out of bed one night and urinated all over the floor. I had to get up and clean him up and put him back to bed. I didn't realize he was taking up so much of my energy. That twenty-four hour stuff was getting to me. . . . After he died, I was so exhausted. . . . I am still. . . . God was good to me in a way. Had [my husband] been sick any longer, it would have broken me physically and financially. (pp. 293–294)

Women, whether or not they work outside the home, are still responsible for most of the caring for family members with chronic illnesses and disabilities (Abel & Nelson, 1990). Studies show that wives more commonly remain married to and help with the self-care duties of their husbands with chronic illness or disability than the reverse (Asch & Fine, 1988), largely due to women's greater economic dependence on their spouse's income and benefits. The ability to give care effectively over time requires access to health insurance, rehabilitation services, quality nursing homes, home health services, attendants, and respite care—all matters of public policy (Fisher & Tronto, 1990; Strauss & Corbin, 1988).

As more men help their wife or children with self-care activities, they experience the same pressures as women have traditionally. More research is needed to show how men learn to provide care as they accept a more equal share of household tasks (Hochschild, 1989). An older man described his experience of being overwhelmed by the role of the role of caregiver for his wife.

> I am a bundle of nerves because I can't get out and play handball anymore. I have to give up my sex life. I am a healthy physical man. It is a toughie. You can't masturbate at seventy-three; it isn't going to do you any good. I'll be honest with you, there isn't a dame that I miss when I go out shopping or anywhere. . . . Sometimes I get impatient. She pushes me pretty hard in the morning: "I want my cereal. You didn't do this." I say, "Give me a chance. If you were in the hospital, you would have three or four attendants." I lift her out of the bed onto the commode. I have to make sure of the catheter. I say, "Honey, I only have two legs, two arms, and one mind." I can't afford to have someone living here full time. I would have to mortgage my house. Some of the bills I have received from the doctors are unbelievable. It has been a year now and I am still paying on some. . . . She gets

depressed and so do I. . . . Some of my friends are going to Reno on a bus. I wish I could climb on the bus and go with them. (Corbin & Strauss, 1988, p. 296)

A father of a child with emotional disabilities, Josh Greenfeld (1972), confessed his fear that he will always have to take care of his son Noah's bathroom problems.

What a night! Noah was up all of it. Two urinations, two b.m.'s, four diaper changes in all. And the period in between, he bounced and jumped and chirped. Obviously Noah isn't making much headway; he has become more and more lax in his toilet training. And when I project, all I see is a sleepy life of never-ending diaper-changing for us all. (pp. 106–107)

Too much responsibility on her shoulders as a parent caused Helen Featherstone's (1980) outrage when a practitioner suggested a small addition to her son Jody's home program. It was recommended that she brush Jody's teeth three times a day, for 5 minutes, with an electric toothbrush to counteract gum overgrowth caused by his antiseizure medication. Featherstone, mother of three children, was handling so many demands already that she exploded.

Jody, I thought, is blind, cerebral-palsied, and retarded. We do his physical therapy daily and work with him on sounds and communication. We feed him each meal on our laps, bottle him, change him, bathe him, dry him, put him in a body cast to sleep, launder his bed linens daily, and go through a variety of routines designed to minimize his miseries and enhance his joys and his development. (All this in addition to trying to care for and enjoy our other young children and making time for each other and our careers.) Now you tell me that I should spend fifteen minutes every day on something that Jody will hate, an activity that will not help him to walk or even defecate, but one that is directed at the health of his gums. This activity is not for a finite time but forever. It is not guaranteed to make the overgrowth go away but may retard it. Well, it's too much. Where is that fifteen minutes going to come from? What am I supposed to give up? Taking the kids to the park? Reading a bedtime story to my eldest? Washing the breakfast dishes? Sorting the laundry? Grading students' papers? Sleeping? Because there is no time in my life that hasn't been spoken for, and for every fifteen-minute activity that is added, one has to be taken away. (pp. 77–78)

Persons who receive their care at home often are highly aware of the sacrifices made for them by their family members and try to avoid demanding too much. While visiting the independent living community at Het Dorp, Irving Kenneth Zola (1982) found that the residents frequently mentioned how much freer they felt because of the availability of paid attendants. Such comments triggered a childhood memory for Zola. He remembered trying to avoid bothering his parents, partly because he disliked feeling guilty and childish because he could not take care of himself.

I recalled the experience of confinement at home after my accident. As much as my parents assured me of their love, I could not help but feel that I was a burden. So gradually I tried to adjust: to eat, to sleep, to defecate when it was convenient for them. They never asked for that adjustment, but I knew that if I made them stay up later, or get out of bed to fetch something, I would feel not only more like a little child, but guilty for making demands! (p. 126)

Irish author Christopher Nolan (1987) wrote about his "agony" as a 15-year-old schoolboy trying to sit through a science lesson and control his bowels after a dose of laxative. Born with cerebral palsy, he was used to asking for help except in going to the bathroom. "He knew he cast roles of responsibility on his fresh-faced friends, but bringing him to the toilet was a chore he would never ask them to do for him" (p. 117).

Hospitals and Institutional Care

The standard procedures of the hospital depersonalize patients. Hospital patients depend on strangers for their care. Routines dictate not only when to eat, when to comb hair or wash, but even when to go to the bathroom. In a real sense, hospitals are designed to be a factory for processing the sick, a "physician's workshop" (Rosenberg, 1987), rather than a place centered around *patients'* self-care needs and experiences. As Rober Murphy (1987) noted:

If dinner is scheduled for 4:30 p.m., as it was on a floor in which I once spent two months, then that's when you eat. And if your bowels don't move often enough to suit the nursing staff members, laxatives are the answer. The infamous routine that demands that all temperatures be taken at 6:00 a.m. is well known to all who have been patients. I even spent five weeks on one floor where I was bathed at 5:30 every morning because the daytime nurses were too busy to do it. (pp. 20–21)

Arnold Beisser (1989) was hospitalized for 3 years beginning in 1950 after becoming paralyzed by polio. His alienation from his own failed body ("more like a sack of flour than a human being" [p. 21]) grew worse because of depersonalized care. Beisser spent every moment of the first year and a half on his back in an iron lung. A young man in his mid-20s, who had been a national tennis champion and was a medical school graduate, he could no longer perform bladder and bowel functions that used to be automatic, even though he felt the urges. He had to depend on strangers to help him.

> Intermittently people would open one or another of the portholes of my new metal skin and invade my private space. They would enter the most personal and private parts of me as they reached inside to move a leg or arm, or insert a needle or a bedpan. There was not even the pretense that my new space belonged to me, and entry beneath my new metal skin was at the discretion of others. (p. 18)

Beisser's body boundary was now the iron lung. His head, which remained outside the machine, was the only part of him that was recognizably human. To Beisser, lying on his back, vulnerable, the persons who approached him seemed like attackers.

> I would often see their shadows before I saw them. They came at me from above like great condors, diving toward my exposed soft parts. People would capriciously and suddenly enter my most private spaces to do what was "best" for me. Since they did not ask my permission before doing things to me, they were like hostile invasions, and I felt violated. (1989, p. 23)

Beisser discovered that nurses and technicians treated his body as an object. He would become enraged to find that they had made judgments for him, assuming that they knew whether he felt hot or cold. But he quickly learned to smile patiently and to explain to his nurses why he might need the blanket despite their perception that he didn't. He dared not express his anger for fear of being punished by being ignored or handled roughly.

> You cannot get mad in hospitals. If you do, you may be in trouble. The next time you call for something, there may be a long delay in the nurses' response, or no response at all. There is always more than enough for the nurses to do in hospitals, so some things come first and some are left unattended. Angry patients come last. (1989, p. 19)

Persons who must depend on others for help with bowel and bladder functions are frequently treated like infants. Beisser realized that he was seen as a baby. Some of his caregivers were concerned with controlling an unruly child, others with nurturing a helpless infant.

> Nurses and attendants often talked to me as if I were a baby. If I became soiled through no fault of my own, they were likely to say, "Naughty, naughty," or "You've been a bad boy." Some people were so perplexed that they simply fled in despair. None of these attitudes helped clarify my confusion about how I thought of myself. (1989, p. 22)

Beisser's survival needs were "just a job" for some of his caregivers. Nurses or attendants might leave him suspended midair in a lift, or in some other awkward position, when the schedule called for them to go on a coffee break. Getting help while the nurses changed their work shift was impossible, no matter how urgent the problem. Beisser felt completely humiliated by these heartless helpers, who earned such nicknames as "Leona the Late," "Ed the Reluctant," and "Ivan the Terrible." He felt robbed of his sense of himself as a person and made to feel like "an undeserving outsider" (1989, p. 37).

However, Beisser (1989) had a completely different set of experiences with several helpers on the hospital staff who had compassion for his situation and treated his needs as more important than their own. With them, he learned about the life-enhancing effects of care that is generously given and felt "returned from exile" and "a pariah forgiven for his crime" (p. 38). It had been dehumanizing to have to worry about his basic needs. Simply knowing that compassionate and willing helpers were present made it possible for Beisser to relax and tolerate otherwise unbearable physical sensations.

> Getting enough air, being able to go to the bathroom when necessary, having enough food and rest are urgent needs, and I could do none of these elemental things for myself. When those needs were not met, I could not be compassionate to someone else. There is no opportunity for higher levels of human function when you are short of air, and all that you can think of is getting the next breath. I am not good for anything else unless these needs are met. But here is the remarkable thing. The urgency with which I experience my needs depends on the confidence I have that they can be met, whether they are or not. They are not so urgent when I am surrounded by people who willingly help me if called upon. (p. 39)

Feeding, Eating, and Dining

Eating is the most social of activities. Ideally, meals are shared. To partake of food together means to be involved in social relations, to be a recognizable member of the human community and of family life. Robert Murphy's (1987) inability to feed himself, a kind of performance failure, resulted in frustration and anger partly because the mess he made disgusted him.

> A paralytic may struggle to walk and become enraged when he cannot move his leg. Or a quadriplegic may pick up a cup of coffee with stiffened hands and drop it on his lap, precipitating an angry outburst. I had to give up spaghetti because I could no longer twirl it on my fork, and dinner would end for me in a sloppy mess. This would so upset me that I would lose my appetite. (pp. 106–107)

The body's failure to perform, barriers in the physical environment, the presence or lack of capable and compassionate helpers, and institutional routines consequently affect the meaning of eating.

Feeding Oneself—Shame and Pride

Diane DeVries, a woman born in 1950 without legs and with short arm stumps (Frank, 1999), suggests that persons with disabilities may experience deep shame about not being able to eat normally in public. Despite having no forearms or hands, DeVries applied strict standards of table behavior upon herself and others with disabilities similar to her own.

> Whatever I did, like feed myself, drink, I was able to do it without any sloppiness. You know, I've even seen a girl at camp with no arms that bent down and lapped her food up like a dog. . . . I knew her. And I went up to her and says: "Why in the hell do you do that?" And I said, "They asked if you wanted a feeder or your arms on. You could have done either one, but you had to do that." She said, "Well, it was easy for me." To me that was gross. She finally started wearing arms, and she started feeding herself. But that to me was just stupid, because people wouldn't even want to eat at the same table as her. (Frank, 1986, p. 209)

DeVries was proud of her own ability to eat and drink by herself without making a mess. Eating without help, like bowel and bladder control, is an important developmental milestone. Children with disabilities are more likely to develop a healthy sense of self and gain the acceptance of others if they find or are taught alternative ways of eating and going to the bathroom that are socially acceptable (Gliedman & Roth, 1980). DeVries' (1992) discovery of a way to feed herself, using her above-elbow

stumps, became an important foundation for developing a sense of herself as a competent person.

> I have been [feeding myself] for so long that I cannot recall when I took my first independent mouthful of food. According to Irene [Diane's mother], this memorable event occurred one morning when she left me sitting in my highchair before a bowl of cereal, as she went to prepare dishwater over at the sink. When she returned I was balancing a spoonful of food on the rim of the bowl, and by applying pressure to the spoon's handle, I was able to raise the food-laden spoon high enough for it and my mouth to meet. I was about three years old. (p. 112)

Food Choices—Preferences and Limitations

The problem of getting food into one's mouth, or adjusting to being fed by others, can be extremely upsetting. It can also be threatening to discover that a disability demands that you eat different food. A person developing a metabolic disorder, such as diabetes, may discover that the need to change his or her eating habits is a life and death struggle.

In fact, in a study of social factors contributing to the deaths of 40 patients on dialysis, researchers found that 11 deaths classified as due to cardiac arrest could be reclassified as due to eating restricted food, such as potato chips and beer, and ignoring restrictions on the intake of fluids (Plough, 1986; Plough & Salem, 1982). Some persons would rather risk dying than change their choice of comfort foods.

Hospitals and nursing homes schedule meals without considering when patients prefer to be served. Often the nutrition they provide comes in forms that cannot be eaten. Disability rights critic Anne Finger (1990) was dismayed and repelled by the routine institutional meal served to her in the hospital after the birth of her son.

> My breakfast tray arrives. Since I am on a liquid diet, I get a carton of milk—which I can't drink because I am lactose intolerant—a plastic container of reconstituted orange juice, a cup of beef broth and a square of red Jell-O on a white plastic plate. I drink the orange juice. (p. 123)

What we eat marks our social identity. In Western countries in the late 19th century, when capitalism was emerging, fleshy bodies signified wealth and health. But by the late 20th century, the ideal body type and food preferences had changed. Abstaining from food has become a marker of higher social status or class along with the slim, hard body

(Bordo, 1990). Popular media feature widespread eating disorders such as bulimia and anorexia—not that anorexia is new. It has been documented as early as the 17th century, but it has acquired new social meanings.

Food choices also mark personal identity and intentions. Pizza and beer on a date mean something different from ordering filet mignon and cabernet sauvignon. Sometimes the identification with the food we eat is so strong as to become a definition of the self in comparison with others present in the situation: "I am vegetarian" or "I am lactose intolerant" or "I am kosher." Persons may delight and take pride in eating spicy Szechewan, Indian, Thai, or Mexican food. They may need to eat Oreo cookies at least once a day.

Persons with disabilities, though, have less freedom than others in expressing their food preferences an needs because of low income, lack of mobility, and lack of public access. A Louis Harris (1986) survey indicated that Americans with disabilities shopped or ate out much less than other Americans. Persons with disabilities were three times more likely *never* to eat in restaurants than persons without disabilities. Up to 13% of persons with disabilities *never* shopped for groceries, as compared with only 2% of the population without disabilities.

Compared to most Americans, a disproportionate number of persons with disabilities and chronic illnesses are poor. They can't afford to eat at restaurants or buy a wide range of foods. Such conditions are especially severe for the homeless, the mentally ill population, many elderly and sometimes housebound women and men, and persons with developmental disabilities and mental illness in board and care facilities.

Meals as the Enactment of Social Relationships

Providing, preparing, and sharing food are important blocks in the foundation of social life. Every society distinguishes between foods that are edible and inedible and defines proper eating behavior. Birthdays, coming of age ceremonies, and anniversaries are celebrated by sharing food across households. Almost all holidays, secular and religious, involve some kind of feasting or fasting. In religious life, food often symbolizes the holiest of states, whether eaten in communion with or offered as a sacrifice to God or the ancestors.

Food is necessary to survival, but the act of dining means more than consumption of calories.

"The dining room is concerned, of course, with food," wrote Agnes de Mille (1981), "and therefore had been the focal point of my life as a child. It was the place of family interchanges" (p. 197). She goes on to talk about neither bread and soup, nor pheasant and souffles, but about the faces, manners, and emotions associated with the changing roles of the family members who have sat in the various seats.

For de Mille's 32nd wedding anniversary, 1 month after her stroke, her husband Walter brought together a party at the hospital of the people she loved, including her son Jonathan. It brought back memories of many happy celebrations in the past and gave de Mille the sense that she could overcome her disability. Evidently, the food provided at the party was there more for symbolic purposes than its nutritional value.

> The celebration was topped by the hospital's present, a great big beautiful wedding cake, very rich and delicious. (The wedding cake Walter and Jonathan had brought was later given to the nurses.) And I knew that my friends and Walter were glad that I was alive, glad for me, glad for Walter. Glad for what I was beginning to be able to do. And there was happiness there because I was going to live. And we had toasts, many of them. They did. I had only a thimbleful of the champagne. (de Mille, 1981, p. 79)

The celebration strengthened de Mille's determination to recover. At 8:00 she found herself in bed; her husband leaned over the pillow. "I'm going to live," she whispered. "I'm going to make it. I'll be out of here soon" (1981, p. 80).

Robert Murphy, Diane DeVries, and others who have spoken above, have told us how important eating independently is to their sense of dignity, but having an enjoyable family meal sometimes means giving up the goal of independent self-feeding that occupational therapy practitioners encourage in their patients. This mother of a small child who is blind continued to spoon-feed her child to preserve quality of life for the family.

> Rosalyn Gibson ... told the group that she still spoon-fed her blind three-year-old because the alternatives created such chaos. Meanwhile, the teachers encouraged Nancy to feed herself at school and urged Rosalyn to follow their lead. ... they spoke of time saved in the long run. Rosalyn thought about the family meals ruined by flying food and recrimination, and the long hours of clean-up. (Featherstone, 1980, p. 29)

In another case, reported by occupational therapist Esther Huecker, getting a patient 2 years of age to eat required engaging him in a social relationship. Timmy, who had Hirschsprung disease, was totally dependent on intravenous feeding. The occupational therapist's task was to get Timmy to enjoy food despite his unfamiliarity with hunger and reluctance to put objects in his mouth. After months of treatment, a successful meal became like "a dance" between them.

> His mother had saved his food tray so that we could have dinner together. We began our usual rituals. He brushed his teeth, washed his face, opened all of the containers, and began to smell and name what was on his plate. Timmy picked up a green bean and dipped it into the gravy to lick. I talked about putting gravy on his potatoes, but there was no hole to keep it from spilling. He gingerly poked a hole with his finger and licked the potatoes. He helped to mince some chicken in a grinder and then took small tastes from a spoon. The meal felt like a well-choreographed dance. I could anticipate his needs and prepare him for his risk-taking actions. His success generated more risk taking. After exploring and tasting everything on his tray several times, Timmy announced he was "all done." Picking him up from the high chair, I felt exhilarated that the experience had been so satisfying. Timmy put his arms around my neck and gave me a kiss, something that had never occurred in a spontaneous moment. (Frank, Huecker, Segal, Forwell, & Bagatell, 1991, p. 258)

When persons cannot reciprocate by giving something of equal value to their helpers, anthropologist Murphy (1987) wrote, they often are made to feel less valuable than others. He described two young women living together in a wheelchair-adapted apartment in a retirement housing project, whose creative solution to feeding problems challenged that potential devaluation.

> One is a spinal cord-damaged quadriplegic with good upper body strength, although she has considerable atrophy of the hands. The other has cerebral palsy; she has moderate speech impairment and very limited arm and hand use. Both women use wheelchairs. Nevertheless, they both completed college, where they lived in dorms, and now were sharing an apartment. Each had a van, and the two did their own cooking and shopping, taking care of all their needs. The woman with cerebral palsy was unable to hold and use eating implements, so she was hand-fed by the other. (pp. 201–202)

In the mutual relationship of these two women, one helping the other takes place within a larger context of give and take. Together they ap-

pear to transform one's "feeding" the other into dining together. In occupational therapy, even when the treatment goal is focused narrowly on helping a person get food to his or her mouth with built-up utensils, eating remains an expression of social membership, cultural values, and personal preferences.

Grooming and Dressing as Self-Expression

Grooming and dressing are often affected by chronic illness or disability. Yet clothing, hairstyle, figure, jewelry, and cosmetics are important markers of a person's social identity, tending to display a person's gender, age or stage in life, occupation, status, ethnicity, and class (Storm, 1987). Changes in personal appearance send a message that the person's place in society has changed.

Hospital gowns, pajamas or nightgown, and slippers worn as regular daytime attire, and wheelchairs or other adaptive equipment announce: "Here is a sick person!" Uncombed hair and strong body odors, at least in mainstream North American culture, mark a person as an outsider, someone on the margins of society. They are examples of "stigma symbols" (Goffman, 1963), which suggest that the person is not competent to participate in society.

The term *stigma* refers to negative judgments about (a) minority ethnic and racial groups, (b) morally disapproved behaviors, or (c) physical differences caused by chronic illnesses or disabilities (Goffman, 1963). To escape from being stigmatized, immigrants might hide their strangeness by learning the language of the new country. In the same way, persons with chronic illnesses or disabilities may often hide or cover up aspects of their appearance that could be discredited and try to "pass" as normal.

Chronic illnesses and disabilities are likely to stigmatize a person only when they become obvious to others. (See Figure 2.1.) Grooming and dressing not only reveal information about one's social identity but can also conceal information that would be socially damaging. Gaining control over and maintaining one's appearance can help to redefine a disability for oneself and others.

Stigma and Deviance Disavowal

Young persons learn to view themselves in terms of the reactions they get from others (Mead, 1934). Horrified glances from family members or members of the community can damage a child's self-image,

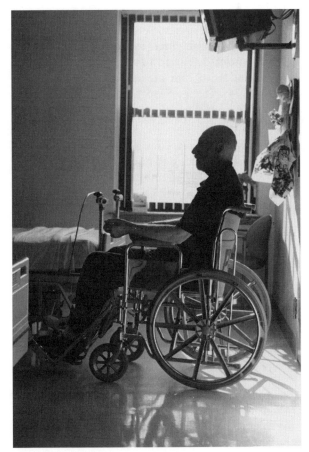

Figure 2.1 Often, the presence of a disability can result in stigma, creating feelings of isolation and social rejection. (Image © Photodisc, Inc.)

morbid self-hatred from festering in her mind. She could, at least inwardly, hold her head high. (Leibowitz, 1989, p. 119)

When persons with disabilities experience negative judgments, they don't have to accept them. Instead, they can act strategically to influence how they are seen and treated. For example, they may vigorously reject the sick role (Parsons, 1951), which excuses them from work—but at the price of reduced social status and control over their situation until declared well by a doctor. The sick role threatens to become a permanent trap for persons with disabilities or chronic illnesses because they never will be cured.

Some members of the Independent Living and Disability Rights Movement (ILDRM) resist this trap by becoming militant. They make a point of showing off their stigma symbols to protest stereotypes of social inferiority and to combat discrimination. Landmark changes in laws, policies, and social awareness such as the Rehabilitation Act of 1973 and the American With Disabilities Act of 1990 have been achieved in part by activists' courageous displays of their disabilities in public (Berkowitz, 1987).

A nonmilitant approach is the clever use of fashion to avoid being stigmatized. Clothing, makeup, and hair styles create a language or cultural code that persons use to communicate information about themselves (Barthes, 1967; Sahlins, 1976; see Figure 2.2.). Persons with disabilities can use clothing and cosmetics to (a) conceal a defect, (b) distract attention away from it, or (c) compensate for it (Kaiser, Freeman, & Wingate, 1990). Agnes de Mille (1981) used all three of these strategies after her stroke.

> I bought Chinese suits with long coats and the brace was hidden in my pants [concealment] and I was told I looked very smart. . . . indulging myself with the loveliest tunics and Indian Benares silk pants of contrasting or complementary tones and little colored slippers [deflecting attention]. The more decrepit my body, the more dashing my dress [compensation]—plain but très gai, très daring. Another flag went up the mast to signal my recovering and making my new life a happy one. (p. 223)

Poet and essayist Nancy Mairs (1987, 1989) also described selecting clothes because she could manage to button them. Diagnosed with multiple sclerosis at about age 30, Mairs lost some of her ability to groom and dress herself.

> With only one usable hand, I have to select my clothing with care not so much for style as for ease of ingress and egress, and even so, dressing can be laborious. I can no longer do fine stitch-

but even children with an obvious disability can be amazingly resilient if at least one key person has been an advocate of his or her intrinsic value as a person. The autobiography of Jane Addams, a leader of the settlement movement during the Progressive Era (ca. 1890–1920) and co-founder of Hull House in Chicago, where one of the first occupational therapy courses was taught, provides a famous example. Although Addams was born with a spinal deformity, her father's supportive view helped the girl to develop a sense of self-worth.

> As a child, Jane Addams imagined herself to be a grotesque outsider: "I prayed with all my heart that the ugly, pigeon-toed little girl, whose crooked back obliged her to walk with her head held very much upon one side, would never be pointed out to the visitors as the daughter of this fine man." The tender gallantry of Mr. Addams bowing to his little girl and tipping his "high and shining silk hat" in public recognition, a charming fairy-tale picture the older autobiographer remembers with abiding gratitude, prevents a

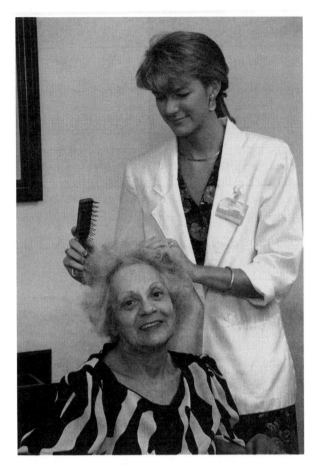

Figure 2.2 For many persons with chronic illnesses, grooming and dressing are an important means of self-expression. (Image © Photodisc, Inc.)

ery, pick up babies, play the piano, braid my hair. (p. 121)

But she also managed to dress in a way that created an impression of her as a woman in the mainstream of society. The photo of Mairs on the dust jacket of her memoir *Remembering the Bone House* (1989) shows an attractive woman dressed in a simple shift. Her straight hair cut to chin length and the tilt of her shoulders draw attention to Mair's incisive yet kind dark eyes and generous mouth. A touch of cosmetics (nail polish and lipstick) and a bit of jewelry (long earrings, a wide bangle bracelet, a glimpse of narrow gold chains about her neck and wrist, plain gold wedding ring) add to the effect of sensuality and elegance (rather than plainness or disability) in this portrait.

Not all persons want to or can invest themselves or their resources in grooming and dress. But grooming and dress serve expressive functions, as in the case of Billy, who was born with multiple handicaps, dependent on a ventilator, and fed through a gastrostomy tube (Pierce & Frank, 1992). Occupational therapist Doris Pierce wrote: "When Billy was dressed in his first baby outfit, his oldest brother, who had refused to see Billy since his first visit, stayed with him all day" (Pierce & Frank, 1992, p. 974). In her field notes, Pierce recorded Billy's oldest brother's comment, "He looks like a real baby!"

Finally, there are circumstances in which the display of stigmatizing behaviors may serve a purpose by keeping others away. Anthropologist Paul Koegel (1987) wrote about homeless, mentally ill women in Los Angeles.

> Were they chronically mentally ill or were they simply reacting very sanely to the enormous stress of an insane situation? Was the fact that they wore four pairs of pants during the summer a reflection of an inability to properly identify weather-appropriate clothing or was it a highly conscious strategy aimed at frustrating potential rapists? . . . Was their poor hygiene the result of poor self-management skills or their restricted access to sinks and showers? (p. 30)

Similarly, occupational therapist Sandra Greene (1992), who studied a day shelter for women in the Los Angeles area, found a wide range of strategies related to grooming and dress among its homeless clients. A few were able to maintain a normal appearance, taking pride in their personal cleanliness and dress. Some rented storage spaces to protect their clothing from theft. They were aware that carrying suitcases or bundles of possessions marked them as homeless. For others, just taking a shower was important, even when they made no attempt in their dress to conceal their homelessness.

> For women who value passing as a non-homeless woman, the availability of a place to keep clean is extremely important so that they don't "look like one of these filthy women." For some women who do not seem to take steps to pass as a non-homeless woman, this service is still considered important and is often mentioned as one of the services they like to use at the shelter. (p. 168)

Resisting Cultural Stereotypes of Beauty, Fashion, and Sexuality

Stigma is always relative to the dominant values of a particular culture. Anthropologist Nora Groce (1985) studied the population on Martha's Vineyard, where there had been, since the early 17th century, a high incidence of hereditary deafness resulting from the small gene pool and frequent intermarriage of families on the island. She discovered that hearing impairments were not stigmatized there.

> I thought to ask Gale what the hearing people in town had thought of the deaf people.
>
> "Oh," he said, "they didn't think anything about them, they were just like everyone else."
>
> "But how did people communicate with them—by writing everything down?"
>
> "No," said Gale, surprised that I should ask such an obvious question. "You see, everyone here spoke sign language."
>
> "You mean the deaf people's families and such?" I inquired.
>
> "Sure," Gale replied, as he wandered into the kitchen to refill his glass and find some more matches, "and everybody else in town too—I used to speak it, my mother did, everybody." (pp. 2–3)

Writers in the Disabilities Rights Movement are challenging mainstream stereotypes of beauty and sexuality in society. Research shows that people tend to attribute positive personal characteristics to those who are physically attractive and negative characteristics to those who are seen as abnormal or different (Kaiser et al., 1990). Negative stereotypes of men and women with disabilities have been perpetuated in television, films, fiction, and drama (Kent, 1987; Longmore, 1987).

Political scientist Harlan Hahn (1988), a polio survivor, posed the question, "Can disability be beautiful?" Hahn suggested that, when confronted with disability, able-bodied people tend to experience an "existential" anxiety (the projected threat of the loss of physical capabilities) and an "aesthetic" anxiety (fear of others whose traits are perceived as disturbing or unpleasant). His historical research indicates, however, that Western cultures have eroticized as well as stigmatized persons with physical differences. Although it is rarely openly acknowledged, Hahn argued, persons with disabilities in art and literature often have been portrayed with a certain sexual appeal.

Hahn urged persons with disabilities to speak out as cultural critics of rigid, conformist ideals of the body beautiful. The culturally shared "language" of grooming and dress provides a vocabulary to do so. Some students with disabilities, for example, wear T-shirts with disability rights mottos and humorous slogans that display their social uniqueness and suggest a desire for more attention from society. Examples include: "I'm no quad; I'm just tired of walking," "High level quads do it with a 'joy stick'," "I'm accessible," and "If I prove I'm

better, will you admit I'm equal?" (Kaiser et al., 1990, p. 42).

Growing up without legs and arms except for above-elbow stumps, Diane DeVries has made choices since childhood about her grooming and dress (Frank, 1999). She accepted certain cultural ideals of attractiveness while also challenging negative stereotypes about persons with disabilities. As a child, DeVries wore shift dresses over a three-wheeled scooter used with a crutch. During puberty, she decided that the scooter was strange-looking and decided to use an electric wheelchair instead.

While any piece of adaptive equipment may be a stigma symbol, a wheelchair was more appropriate for DeVries than her three-wheeled scooter, especially at the county rehabilitation facility where she then lived among teenagers and young adults with disabilities. In a peer culture of disability, DeVries modeled herself after a young woman with a spinal cord injury who encouraged her to use her female assets to look "together." For DeVries, looking together has meant:

> To go around in whatever you're in, your wheelchair, or your braces, or whatever, and not look clumsy. It's not looking "self-assured" either. I keep wanting to say that, but I don't think that's the word. I mean, people are already looking at you. You know, any crip's going to be looked at. But at least if they look at you, at least they'll say: "Wow, look at that person in the wheelchair. Hey, but you know, not too bad!" (Frank, 1986, p. 208)

Some persons with amputations deal with stigma by choosing to wear long sleeves or full skirts to cover their missing limb or limbs.

> I get a different response from people when I wear short sleeves so I very seldom wear short sleeves. It camouflages my disability (missing arm) when I wear long sleeves.
>
> Because of my amputation at the hip, I prefer dresses without a waist or gathering at the bodice of the dress. Dresses that flare out more at the tail are more attractive. (Kaiser et al., 1990, p. 39)

DeVries prefers, however, to wear close-fitting clothes that accentuate her assets. Displaying what she does have has been a better strategy for her than attempting to conceal her multiple limb deficiencies.

> Like when I was a kid, I hated wearing skirts and dresses, because with a skirt you could notice even more that there are legs missing than when you wore shorts and a top. Shorts and a

top fitted your body and that made the fact that no legs were there not look so bad. (Frank, 1986, p. 209)

Overcoming Barriers to Self-Expression

These choices that persons with disabilities make to show who they are do not always win the approval of the helpers—family members, professionals, and attendants—they depend on. There is a fine line between help and control. Diane DeVries liked dresses with narrow straps that she could slip into by herself and that allowed her the greatest freedom of movement. Some members of her rehabilitation team criticized her for this as indicated in the chart notes of a meeting held when DeVries was entering adolescence.

> Diane prefers wearing spaghetti strap or other low cut sun dresses because she feels less encumbered and can also undress more easily. Those present felt that this is somewhat unattractive and possibly disturbing. It has been suggested to the family that she wear unbuttoned bolero jackets over the dresses but this has not been carried through. The subject of Diane's appearance to those present and to those around her was discussed at length. This seems to be a definite problem. Some felt that the cart [which Diane uses for mobility] is disturbing to behold. Some felt that they prefer seeing her with the prosthesis and others dissented. This area might be explored further as this seems to be a somewhat problematic area. (Frank, 1986, p. 207)

Interviewed later as an adult, DeVries suggested that persons with handicaps learn to say "no" and to stay in control of their grooming and dress when helped by another.

> Like me, I would never wear a skirt, a long skirt, like they used to. I've even seen some people with no arms wearing long sleeves pinned up or rolled clumsily so they're this fat. You can find a lot of clothes that fit you. It's not hard. If they have someone take care of them, they won't tell them: "No. I want my hair this way." They'll just let them do it. That's dumb. It's your body. They're helping you out. (Frank, 1986, p. 210)

At conventions of Little People of America (LPA), a self-help organization for persons of profound short stature, one of the best-attended events is the annual fashion show (Ablon, 1984). Although most little people can wear children's clothing, with minor alterations, and children's shoes, children's styles are inappropriate for mature persons. The fashion show displays clothing made by the models themselves or made for them and adult-size clothing adapted with major alterations. Women model elegant suits, dresses, and sports clothes, while men usually model formal suits. LPA members also attend sewing workshops and patronize representatives of tailoring firms who fit them and take custom orders. Women sometimes order shoes from Hong Kong, where average sizes are smaller than in the United States.

Claiming control over one's appearance, self-expression, and social identity can be a very positive experience. Ernestine Amani Patterson (1985) had an intense desire to wear her hair braided in cornrows, African-style, with colorful beads and tinkling bells, but her blindness limited her from doing them herself. After beauticians and others discouraged her, a woman from Liberia, owner of "a most exotic African artifacts shop," finally gratified her desire. By insisting on cornrows Patterson rejected the isolating stigma of blindness and claimed her identity as a Black sister.

> Of course, people are still the same—inevitable and specific in their cruelty "Your hair is pretty," or "Your dress is pretty." The lines between womanhood and blindness are never supposed to meet. And with Blackness on top of that, what must people be seeing! And although I seldom hear: "You are looking nice," I am not the same, even if they are. Since that Saturday in the shop with the wooden floor and squeaky steps, where the heater had to be turned on against the chilly morning, I have always looked forward to the bus ride and short walk there. Mrs. Younger [her Liberian friend] has not only increased her clientele, other girlfriends of hers from Africa help out with the hair. So it's lovely talking to all of them. And since most of these women are used to me now, we relate as Black sisters. And though this was not a first step in my growth, mine is actually a case wherein the style of my hair altered the shape of my head within. How many women can say that with satisfaction about any beauty treatment they try? (p. 243)

Conclusion

Self-care is not simply an objective routine. Every disability affects not only the body parts that have been impaired but the entire person in relation to family members, friends, and helpers, health care practitioners, and the wider society. The narratives of persons with chronic illnesses and disabilities show that, once survival needs are met, the key problems caused by impairments are *occupational*. Performance failures of the body prevent persons from engaging in the customary activities that fill their lives and give them meaning. Personal identity and social relations are at stake in even the simplest activities of self-care, which result in basic self-esteem or profound shame.

Occupational therapy practitioners can help persons with disabilities by recognizing that self-care occupations are deeply meaningful. Persons must cope with feelings of frustration when their ability to perform daily activities breaks down. They experience anger and depression over loss of control. They suffer feelings about being helpless and dependent on others. They feel distress and guilt about the added family responsibilities that their illness may cause and their inability to reciprocate as fully as they would like.

Persons with chronic illnesses and disabilities need access to basic health care through adequate insurance, rehabilitation services, attendant care, respite care, adaptive equipment, employment opportunities, and income supports. In addition, compassionate caregivers can make an important difference in the quality of life for the person with a chronic illness or disability.

Persons adapt to disability over time. Their attitudes toward their disabilities—the meanings they attach to them—depend partly on where they stand on the rehabilitation path, because attitudes change. Caregivers' attitudes can change, too. The ability to reevaluate cultural rules about "the right way" to do things can make impairments less handicapping and less stigmatizing. As the stories by persons with disabilities show, self-care occupations can be approached in ways that enhance, rather than limit, personal and social identity. Occupational therapy practitioners who pay attention to the meaning of self-care occupations will have a chance to help patients make the changes that matter most. ◆

Study Questions

1. Why is it important for occupational therapists to pay attention to the difference between a patient's "illness" and "disease"?

2. How do the body's performance failures affect a person's sense of self?

3. How does the setting in which a person needs help with self-care affect its meaning? Within the family? In hospitals and other institutions?

4. What are some of the meanings associated with toileting? Feeding? Grooming? Why are such terms by themselves inadequate to describe these occupations?

5. Describe some ways in which persons with chronic illnesses and disabilities can avoid or resist stigmatization.

6. What can occupational therapists do to help persons with chronic illnesses and disabilities to discover new and more satisfying ways of accomplishing self-care occupations?

References

Abel, E. K., & Nelson, M. (1990). Circles of care: An introductory essay. In E. K. Abel & M. K. Nelson (Eds.), *Circles of care: Work and identity in women's lives* (pp. 4–34). Albany, NY: State University of New York Press.

Ablon, J. (1984). *Little people in America: The social dimensions of dwarfism.* New York: Praeger.

Asch, A., & Fine, M. (1988). Introduction: Beyond pedestals. In M. Fine & A. Asch (Eds.), *Women with disabilities: Essays in psychology, culture, and politics* (pp. 1–37). Philadelphia: Temple University Press.

Barthes, R. (1967). *Système de la mode.* Paris: Seuil.

Beisser, A. R. (1989). *Flying without wings: Personal reflections on being disabled.* New York: Doubleday.

Bell, R. (1985). *Holy anorexia.* Chicago: University of Chicago Press.

Berkowitz, E. D. (1987). *Disabled policy: America's programs for the handicapped.* New York: Cambridge University Press.

Bordo, S. (1990). Reading the slender body. In M. Jacobus, E. F. Keller, & S. Shuttleworth (Eds.), *Body/politics: Women and the discourses of science* (pp. 83–112). New York: Routledge & Kegan Paul.

Corbin, J. M., & Strauss, A. (1988). *Unending work and care: Managing chronic illness at home.* San Francisco: Jossey-Bass.

de Mille, A. (1981). *Reprieve: A memoir.* New York: Doubleday.

DeVries, D. (1992). *Autobiography.* Unpublished manuscript.

Eisenberg, L. (1977). Disease and illness: Distinctions between professional and popular ideas of sickness. *Culture, Medicine, and Psychiatry, 1,* 9–23.

Featherstone, H. (1980). *A difference in the family: Living with a disabled child.* New York: Penguin.

Finger, A. (1990). *Past due: A story of disability, pregnancy and birth.* Seattle, WA: Seal Press.

Fisher, B., & Tronto, J. (1990). Toward a feminist theory of caring. In E. K. Abel & M. K. Nelson (Eds.), *Circles of care: Work and identity in women's lives* (pp. 35–62). Albany, NY: State University of New York Press.

Frank, G. (1986). On embodiment: A case study of congenital limb deficiency in American culture. *Culture, Medicine and Psychiatry, 10,* 189–219.

Frank, G. (1999). *Venus on wheels: Two decades of dialogue on disability, biography, and being female in America.* Berkeley, CA: University of California Press.

Frank, G., Huecker, E., Segal, R., Forwell, S., & Bagatell, N. (1991). Assessment and treatment of a pediatric patient in chronic care: Ethnographic methods applied to occupational therapy practice. *American Journal of Occupational Therapy, 45,* 252–263.

Gliedman, J., & Roth, W. (1980). *The unexpected minority: Handicapped children in America.* New York: Harcourt Brace Jovanovich.

Goffman, E. (1963). *Stigma: Notes on the management of spoiled identity.* Englewood Cliffs, NJ: Prentice Hall.

Greene, S. L. (1992). *An ethnographic study of homeless mentally ill women: Adaptive strategies, needs and services.* Unpublished master's thesis, University of Southern California, Los Angeles.

Greenfeld, J. (1972). *A child called Noah.* New York: Holt, Rinehart & Winston.

Groce, N. E. (1985). *Everyone here spoke sign language: Hereditary deafness on Martha's Vineyard.* Cambridge, MA: Harvard University Press.

Hahn, H. (1988). Can disability be beautiful? *Social Policy, 18,* 26–32.

Harris, L., & Associates. (1986). *The ICD survey of disabled Americans: Bringing disabled Americans into the mainstream.* New York: International Center for the Disabled.

Hochschild, A. (1989). *The second shift: Working parents and the revolution at home.* New York: Viking.

Kaiser, S. B., Freeman, C. M., & Wingate, S. B. (1990). Stigmata and negotiated outcomes: Management of appearance by persons with physical disabilities. In M. Nagler (Ed.), *Perspectives on disability* (pp. 33–45). Palo Alto, CA: Health Markets Research. (Reprinted from *Deviant Behavior, 6,* 205–224).

Kent, D. (1987). Disabled women: Portraits in fiction and drama. In A. Gartner & T. Joe (Eds.), *Images of the disabled, disabling images* (pp. 47–63). New York: Praeger.

Kleinman, A. (1988). *The illness narratives: Suffering, healing, and the human condition.* New York: Basic Books.

Koegel, P. (1987). Ethnographic perspectives on homeless and homeless mentally ill women. In P. Koegel (Ed.), *Proceedings of a two-day workshop sponsored by the Division of Education and Service Systems Liaison.* Bethesda, MD: National Institute of Mental Health.

Leibowitz, H. (1989). The sheltering self: Jane Addams's *Twenty Years at Hull-House.* In *Fabricating lives: Explorations in American autobiography* (pp. 115–156). New York: Knopf.

Longmore, P. K. (1987). Screening stereotypes: Images of disabled people in television and motion pictures. In A. Gartner & T. Joe (Eds.), *Images of the disabled, disabling images* (pp. 65–78). New York: Praeger.

Lorde, A. (1980). *The cancer journals.* San Francisco: Spinsters Ink.

Mairs, N. (1987). On being a cripple. In M. Saxton & F. Howe (Eds.), *With wings: An anthology of literature by and about women with disabilities* (pp. 118–127). New York: The Feminist Press.

Mairs, N. (1989). *Remembering the bone house: An erotics of place and space.* New York: Harper & Row.

Mead, G. H. (1934). *Mind, self, and society: From the standpoint of a social behaviorist.* Chicago: The University of Chicago Press.

Murphy, R. F. (1987). *The body silent.* New York: Henry Holt.

Nolan, C. (1987). *Under the eye of the clock: The life story of Christopher Nolan.* New York: St. Martin's Press.

Parsons, T. (1951). Illness and the role of the physician: A sociological perspective. *American Journal of Orthopsychiatry, 21,* 452–460.

Patterson, E. A. (1985). Glimpse into transformation. In S. E. Browne, D. Connors, & N. Stern (Eds.), *With the power of each breath: A disabled women's anthology* (pp. 240–243). Pittsburgh, PA: Cleis Press.

Pierce, D., & Frank, G. (1992). A mother's work: Feminist perspectives on family-centered care. *American Journal of Occupational Therapy, 46,* 972–980.

Plough, A. L. (1986). *Borrowed time: Artificial organs and the politics of extending lives.* Philadelphia: Temple University Press.

Plough, A. L., & Salem, S. R. (1982). Social and contextual factors in the analysis of mortality in end-stage renal disease patients. *American Journal of Public Health, 72,* 1293–1295.

Rosenberg, C. E. (1987). *The care of strangers: The rise of America's hospital system.* New York: Basic Books.

Sahlins, M. (1976). La pensée bourgeoise: Western society as culture. In *Culture and practical reasons* (pp. 166–204). Chicago: University of Chicago Press.

Strauss, A., & Corbin, J. M. (1988). *Shaping a new health care system: The explosion of chronic illness as a catalyst for change.* San Francisco: Jossey-Bass.

Storm, P. (1987). *Functions of dress: Tool of culture and the individual.* Englewood Cliffs, NJ: Prentice Hall.

Wright, B. A. (1983). *Physical disability—A psychosocial approach* (2nd ed.). New York: Harper & Row.

Zola, I. K. (1982). *Missing pieces: A chronicle of living with a disability.* Philadelphia: Temple University Press.

3

Assessment of Self-Care Performance

Catherine Backman
Charles H. Christiansen

Catherine Backman, MS, OT(C), is Senior Instructor and Head, Division of Occupational Therapy, School of Rehabilitation Sciences, and PhD Candidate, Department of Health Care and Epidemiology, Faculty of Medicine, University of British Columbia, Canada.

Charles H. Christiansen, EdD, OTR, OT(C), FAOTA, is Dean and George T. Bryan Distinguished Professor, School of Allied Health Sciences, University of Texas Medical Branch at Galveston, Texas.

Key Terms

assessment

correlation

evaluation

feasibility

reliability

stability

standardized

validity

Objectives

On completing this chapter, the reader will be able to

1. Describe the basic purposes of self-care assessment.

2. Understand the meaning of performance contexts.

3. Describe the relationship between self-care performance and performance components.

4. Describe factors that contribute to our confidence in self-care assessment instruments.

5. Identify important characteristics of self-care instruments.

6. Appreciate the importance of involving the client in determining self-care skills that should be assessed.

7. Describe the purposes and characteristics of several widely used self-care assessment instruments, including many developed by occupational therapy practitioners.

8. Understand the inadequacies of using assessment instruments that have not been validated.

This chapter identifies and discusses ways of assessing self-care skills. It also outlines the basic process for considering assessment information and determining appropriate options for treatment. Because many terms related to self-care are used in the assessment literature, readers are encouraged to review the meanings of these terms by referring to the key words at the beginning of the chapter and to the glossary.

Self-Care Assessment

Many instruments and recommendations for evaluating self-care skills and activities of daily living (ADL) are available in the literature (Law & Letts, 1989). The challenge for therapy personnel is to develop effective strategies for determining the self-care ability of their clients by selecting the most appropriate instrument(s). Some instruments are standardized, whereas many others are not; some are diagnosis specific; few are based in theory (McDowell & Newell, 1987) or are adequately validated (Law & Usher, 1988). In recent years, therapy personnel have come to appreciate the importance of using instruments with known validity or reliability and avoiding the use of "home-grown instruments" (Fisher, 1992b, p. 278).

Purposes of Self-Care Assessment

There are at least four reasons for assessing self-care ability (Christiansen & Ottenbacher, 1998).

1. *To describe self-care status.* An objective description of a client's self-care ability at a given time can be useful to identify problems, goals, and plans for therapy. It will identify if, or how much, personal assistance is required to complete self-care tasks and assist in discharge planning. A description of status may be required to determine compensation in the case of clients who have sustained temporary or permanent injuries attributed to the negligence of others.

2. *To measure change and monitor progress.* Periodic assessment will help monitor the effects of therapy by detecting improvement or changes in performance that can guide further intervention.

3. *To facilitate communication and decision making.* The results of a self-care assessment will enhance communication between the therapist and client, as well as among team members, family members, and others involved in providing treatment or assistance in self-care tasks. Assessment results can also guide the client's decision making, especially when it comes to prioritizing goals for therapy or choosing between independence and personal assistance in managing self-care.

4. *To evaluate programs and conduct research.* The use of standardized instruments helps promote comparability in research or evaluation of outcomes attributed to therapeutic programs. This is particularly important, given the emphasis on evidenced-based practice.

Several factors influence our confidence in self-care assessments. They include basing the assessment on the patient's or client's needs and circumstances, understanding the relationship between performance of self-care and performance components (or skill constituents), and appreciating the difference between assessments based on self-report versus those based on an observation of the person's actual performance. Each of these factors is discussed in the following sections.

Performance Contexts and Client-Centered Assessment

Performance contexts are factors that can influence the feasibility and appropriateness of treatment goals. They include physical, social, and cultural factors that affect the setting in which a person performs daily occupations, as well as the client's age, developmental level, life cycle, and health or disability status. Client-centered assessment is particularly focused on performance contexts in making intervention choices relevant.

Client-centered assessment is an approach in which the client's roles, values, and priorities guide the assessment process. During a typical day, people sleep, participate in leisure and play activities, engage in productive or work occupations, and maintain themselves and their environments. Self-care, as one of these main areas of daily occupation, is rarely assessed in isolation. Whereas self-care skills are fundamental to a person's daily life, they represent only a part of the repertoire of behaviors required to lead a meaningful life (Keith, 1984, p. 75).

The need to determine those tasks that are most important to the client is a vital step in the assessment process. Various sources (Canadian Association of Occupational Therapists, 1997; Christiansen &

Ottenbacher, 1998; Law, Baptiste, et al. 1994) agree that assessment should focus on activities that match the client's personal goals. This is because the relative importance of independence in self-care varies with the person.

Consider a person who accepts assistance with personal hygiene or dressing because this enables him or her to spend more time at work (Alexander & Fuhrer, 1984, p. 54). This does not imply that the occupational therapist should withhold an informed opinion that could modify client goals, but it does suggest that communication among the health care providers, client, and family members will direct the assessment and intervention plans in an informed manner that takes into account the relevance of goals to the person. An assessment will be more meaningful if the process is collaborative and the client has the opportunity to choose the tasks that require evaluation (Fisher, 1992a).

This philosophy reveals a limitation of standardized self-care instruments. Standardized instruments, by their nature, do not have items that represent all situations. Moreover, the normative data they provide may have little meaning within specific contexts. On the other hand, a lengthy list of self-care tasks would be impractical and would make it difficult to compare the efficacy of treatment approaches across large numbers of patients. Thus, both standardized and nonstandardized instruments have a place in assessing function.

Ideally, clients should be assessed in environments that represent their everyday living situations (Rogers & Holm, 1994). The demands of the environment and the interaction between the client and environment need to be considered as part of the self-care assessment. Effective assessments are always individualized and capture the uniqueness of the client, whether standardized instruments are used in the process or not.

A number of important decisions are made based on a person's ability to independently perform self-care tasks. When a person cannot eat, bathe, or dress independently, some type of personal assistance is required. The person's previous occupational roles and social and physical environments may change. After an evaluation of self-care activities, it is possible to determine whether, and how much, care or assistance is necessary. This information contributes to decision making regarding discharge from acute and rehabilitation facilities back to the pre-admission environment or into long-term care, nursing, and supported home care environments.

Self-Care Performance and Performance Components

A person's ability to perform daily occupations is supported by performance components. These components fall into three major categories: sensorimotor, cognitive, and psychosocial and psychological. Thus, a person's general health and physical abilities, mental and emotional states, and relationships with others can influence the performance of tasks in the area of self-care. It is important to understand the relative influence of these factors on a person's performance. This enables the therapist to consider all the barriers to function during intervention planning.

Although standardized assessments may be useful in identifying who is in need of therapeutic services, they give little information on how to focus intervention (Fisher, 1992b). They may provide information on those self-care tasks a person cannot do (e.g., dress, eat), but do not provide much information about the reasons why these tasks cannot be done (e.g., limited dexterity, memory loss, apraxia). Nor do they typically provide information on the importance of the task to the client. The existence of pathology does not automatically mean that a person cannot complete a task that he or she could have completed before an illness or injury. For example, decreased hand strength resulting from arthritis may or may not influence the person's ability to open a can of tomatoes (Lawton, 1990, p.528). Understanding the relationship between performance areas and performance components or constituent skills will help occupational therapy personnel choose interventions based on the needs of individual clients.

Self-Report Versus Observation of Actual Performance

Approaches to self-care assessment may use interviews, written questionnaires, or direct observation of performance to obtain data. Data may consist of numerical scores intended to quantify the client's performance, or they may be used to prepare written descriptions. Interviews and questionnaires may use self-report, whereby the client responds to the questions, or proxy report, in which a family member or caregiver provides the information. Some instruments are designed for use by either interview or observation, or a combination of both. Advantages of self-report instruments include their low cost and relative speed of administration (Jette, 1987).

However, their reliability and validity are of major concern—is it really valid to judge performance based on a person's recollection of what he or she can do rather than on actually observing that person do a task?

Studies of self-report instruments have shown that what patients or their family members say that a client can do does not always match the person's actual day-to-day performance (Edwards, 1990). A client may be capable of doing a defined task under certain circumstances, or on an occasional basis, but is unable to do so on a regular basis. When it comes to daily self-care tasks, it is important to determine a person's consistent level of function. This can be done reliably and validly only in the environment in which persons experience their day-to-day living (Alexander & Fuhrer, 1984). This means that, ideally, therapy personnel should select measures that assess actual performance.

Assessing Self-Care Abilities

The following is a proposed strategy for assessing a person's performance in self-care. It assumes that an assessment will be client-centered and will make use of direct observation of performance where appropriate. It also assumes that the assessment will proceed from the general to the specific (otherwise known as the "top down" assessment approach). This is a logical approach for two reasons. First, occupational therapy personnel are concerned with functional performance in daily living. If a patient or client can satisfactorily perform tasks of daily living, the presence of some underlying impairment has no functional consequence. If performance is not satisfactory, however, then a further determination of the cause of the dysfunction is warranted. In this case, the therapist may be interested in identifying problems within the specific performance components that support task completion. This type of approach to assessment helps the therapist and the client focus on the goals of intervention and therefore may help to motivate the client and assist him or her in understanding the reasons for therapy.

Identify Client Priorities

Identify the client's priorities and proceed with a self-care evaluation only if it is relevant to that client. One instrument based on this orientation is the Canadian Occupational Performance Measure (COPM; Law, Baptiste, et al., 1994). The COPM is designed to assess clients' perceptions of their occupational performance. Although it is not limited to the evaluation of self-care, it is a tool that can help determine whether self-care is problematic and should be evaluated in more detail. The COPM is a semistructured interview that focuses on a client's activities in the areas of self-care, productivity, and leisure. Because the COPM involves the client in identifying key occupational performance problems, it is an ideal initial assessment tool. If the client identifies one or more self-care problems as priorities, specific evaluation tools can be selected to collect additional data. For example, if the client identifies dressing and bathing as problems, an observational assessment of these self-care activities would be a logical second step.

Select Instruments

Select one or more instruments based on their purpose and on the priorities established with the client in step one. The assessment is most often required to identify problems, establish goals for intervention, and measure its effects. Practitioners should select assessment tools that will not only measure change but will also measure change within their own domain of practice. Limiting the number of scales used can enhance communication among team members and help practitioners determine their efficacy among clients with different types of problems (Law & Letts, 1989).

Validate and Communicate Results

Share with the client the data obtained with the self-care instruments and validate the interpretation of findings with him or her. It is also important to document and communicate the findings with others who need to know, such as family members, team members, or referral sources. Simple graphic displays of data that summarize narrative comments often have a better effect than narrative or numbers alone and are especially useful for indicating problem areas and illustrating change over time.

Select Instruments for Assessing Self-Care Skills and Environments

Numerous characteristics should be considered in selecting an instrument to measure any aspect of functional performance, including self-care. Several authors have described some of the desirable characteristics and ways that instruments may vary. These characteristics include the following.

- *The scope of the tasks addressed by the instrument.* Some instruments cover a broad range of functional tasks; others are limited to a few self-care tasks. The extent to which instruments address each self-care task or the level of function assessed will also vary. For example, dressing may be evaluated by a single item referring to the complete task, or it may be broken down into component parts, such as putting on socks, fastening shirt buttons, and so forth.

- *The instrument's sensitivity to change in a client.* Sensitivity is of particular importance in measuring the effect of intervention. An instrument that lacks sensitivity will not indicate small gains in the client ability to perform self-care tasks.

- *The reliability of the test procedures.* The procedures should be clearly stated in the test manual or protocol. The scores or descriptors obtained with an instrument should be consistent from one test period to another and between different test administrators. (See Figure 3.1.)

- *The validity of the instrument.* Validity relates to the behaviors that the assessment instrument measures and how well it does so. A test that is valid in one situation may not be valid under changed circumstances. For example, a test of mobility that was developed for ambulatory participants may not be suitable for wheelchair users. In this example, the content validity is not precisely determined by a statistical calculation; rather, it is a judgment call on the part of the potential test user. How well a test measures what it purports to measure may be more precisely determined by comparing performance on the test with another instrument that is considered to be an accurate indicator of the behavior of interest. This is often expressed as a correlation coefficient, indicating the extent of the relationship between two instruments. If two tests are measuring the same thing, a person's performance using the first measure should relate to his or her performance on the second. (See Figure 3.2.)

- *The nature of the resulting data.* Once the assessment is completed, an assessment instrument may provide a detailed profile describing the client's self-care ability, or it may result in a single code or numerical value that represents a measure of overall function. Instruments may be descriptive or evaluative, and the purpose will direct the type of data collected. Useful evaluative instruments quantify function, based on the assumption that the numerical score will change as the participant's performance changes. However, a single overall score for something as complex as self-care is misleading (Fisher, 1992b), so caution is advised when interpreting a global score resulting from the sum of several subtests. Most instruments for adults are designed to yield scores that allow practitioners to measure change or to compare performance to normative data. Some tests will have a developmental focus, so that the resulting data will indicate the participant's performance in relation to a developmental continuum.

- *Feasibility.* The time required to administer the test, special training, and special equipment required all influence the usefulness of the instrument in any given setting.

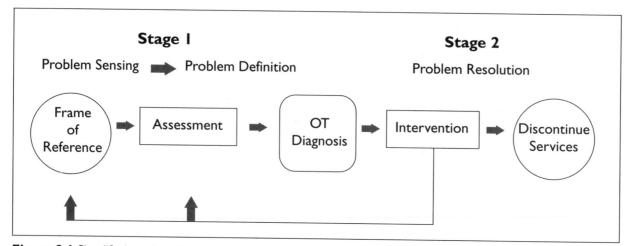

Figure 3.1 Simplified model of the occupational therapy process. *Note.* From "Occupational Therapy Diagnostic Reasoning: A Component of Clinical Reasoning," by J. C. Rogers and M. B. Holm, 1991, *American Journal of Occupational Therapy, 45,* p. 1046. Copyright © 1991 by The American Occupational Therapy Association. OT = occupational therapy.

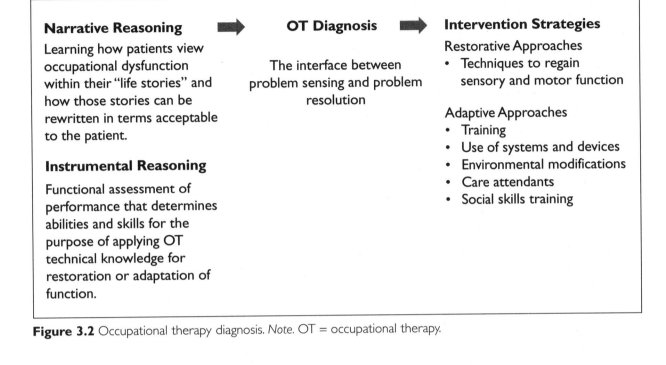

Narrative Reasoning

Learning how patients view occupational dysfunction within their "life stories" and how those stories can be rewritten in terms acceptable to the patient.

Instrumental Reasoning

Functional assessment of performance that determines abilities and skills for the purpose of applying OT technical knowledge for restoration or adaptation of function.

OT Diagnosis

The interface between problem sensing and problem resolution

Intervention Strategies

Restorative Approaches
• Techniques to regain sensory and motor function

Adaptive Approaches
• Training
• Use of systems and devices
• Environmental modifications
• Care attendants
• Social skills training

Figure 3.2 Occupational therapy diagnosis. *Note.* OT = occupational therapy.

Assessment instruments suitable for program evaluation and research purposes have similar desirable characteristics. Comprehensiveness, accuracy, sensitivity to change, and feasibility are just some of the characteristics to be considered before making a choice (Bombardier & Tugwell, 1987).

Widely Used Self-Care Instruments

This section contains a brief description of five widely used instruments for assessing self-care. The instruments are discussed in the order of their development. For ease of comparison, two tables are provided. Table 3.1 summarizes the characteristics of the instruments, including the presence of reliability, validity, and sensitivity data; the sample populations tested; and means by which the data may be obtained (e.g., observed performance, interview, written self-report).

Katz Index of ADL

The Katz Index of ADL (Katz, Downs, Cash, & Grotz, 1970; Katz, Ford, Moskowitz, Jackson, & Jaffe, 1963) was developed to measure function in chronically ill and aging populations. It summarizes self-care ability in six areas: bathing, dressing, going to the toilet, transferring, continence, and feeding. Performance can be observed, or questions

can be asked of the client. The rater then checks one of three descriptors for each of the six areas: independent, some assistance required, or dependent. The criteria for each of the three ratings are defined for each of the six areas. The ratings are then transformed into a global score represented by letters:

A = independent in all six functions
B = independent in any five functions
C = independent in all but bathing and one other
D = independent in all but bathing, dressing, and one other
E = independent in all but bathing, dressing, going to the toilet, and one other
F = independent in all but bathing, dressing, going to the toilet, transfers, and one other
G = dependent
Other = cannot be classified in A through G, dependent on two or more functions.

The letter scores represent a hierarchy of returning function during rehabilitation that closely resembles a developmental sequence. The authors noted that feeding and continence tended to return earlier than did the transferring and toileting ability, which returned before dressing and bathing skills. Thus, a person able to perform a given activity independently should also be able to perform all activities performed by persons graded

Table 3.1 Summary of Characteristics of Instruments Reviewed

Instrument	Reliability	Validity	Reported Use	Method(s)
Assessment of Motor and Process Skills (AMPS)	95% interrater reliability using Rasch analysis	Validity testing ongoing Concurrent validity established	Adults with variety of disabling conditions	Observation
Arnadottir OT-ADL Neurobehavioral Evaluation (A-ONE)	Interrater = .84 Stability = .85 Internal = .18–.78	Content validity Comparison of A-ONE with neuroimaging	Cortical CNS damage from CVA, Alzheimer's disease, Pick disease, TBI	Observation
Barthel Index	Stability = .89 Interrater = .95	Criterion = .89 Detects change in parallel with Katz	Hospitalized seniors Adults after stroke	Interview Observation Chart review
Canadian Occupational Performance Measure (COPM)	Stability = .63–.84	Sensitive to changes in perceptions of performance	Adults with range of disabilities at a variety of sites	Interview
Functional Independence Measure (FIM™)	Interrater = .86–.95	Criterion = .62–.84 (with level of help required)	Hospitalized adults Adults in rehabilitation settings	Interview Observation
Home Occupation Environment Assessment (HOEA)	Interrater = .95	Content through expert opinion Factor analysis	Patients with senile dementia	Observation
Katz Index of ADL	Scalability = .74–.88	Criterion = discharge score predicts need for personal assistance	Adults who are chronically ill Adults after stroke Adults with hip fractures	Observation
Klein-Bell ADL Scale	Interrater = 92%	Criterion = .86 (with hours of personal care required)	Adults with disabilities Children with cerebral palsy	Observation
Kitchen Task Assessment (KTA)	Interrater = .87–.96	Correlation between scores on KTA and clinical diagnostics	Adults with senile dementia (Alzheimer's disease)	Observation
Milwaukee Evaluation of Daily Living Skills (MEDLS)	Interrater = .80	Content validity determined by expert panel	Adults in long-term psychiatric settings	Observation Interview
Pediatric Evaluation of Disability Inventory (PEDI)	Interrater reliability = .96–.99 Internal consistency = .95–.99	Expert panel content Scores correlate with age; and WeeFIM™ and Battelle Scores (.62–.97)	Children with trauma, spina bifida, cerebral palsy, TBI, developmental delay	Interview Observation
Performance Assessment of Self-Care Skills (PASS)	Interrater agreement = 96%–99%	Content based on established scales	Adults with various medical and psychiatric diagnoses including dementia and depression	Observation

(continued)

Table 3.1 (*continued*)

Instrument	Reliability	Validity	Reported Use	Method(s)
Safety Assessment of Function and the Environment for Rehabilitation (SAFER) Tool	Interrater = .80 Internal = .83	Expert panel Scores correlated with cognitive impairment	Seniors living in home environments, both well and with disabilities of both physical and mental types	Observation
Functional Independence Measure for Children (WeeFIM™)	Interrater = >.90 Stability = .83–.99	Scores predict amount of caregiver assistance needed	Children with brain injuries, brain tumors	Interview Observation

Note. ADL = activities of daily living, CNS = central nervous system, CVA = cerebral vascular accident, TBI = traumatic brain injury.

at lower levels in the scale. This makes the Katz Index of ADL a true Guttman scale and allows it to correctly classify the functional ability of clients 86% of the time.

Barthel Index

The Barthel Index (Mahoney & Barthel, 1965) was designed to measure independence before and after intervention and to indicate the amount of personal care required. It consists of 10 items: feeding, transferring between wheelchair and bed, personal toileting, transferring on and off the toilet, bathing, walking on level ground, climbing stairs, dressing, bowel control, and bladder control. Items within the index have varied weighting toward the total score. A score of 100 represents a person who is continent, eats, bathes, and dresses independently; is able to rise from the bed, chair, and toilet; walks at least a block; and can go up and down stairs. The authors point out that such a person is not necessarily able to live alone, as the Barthel Index is limited to self-care, but a person scoring 100 would not require a personal attendant. The Barthel Index has been used as a direct observation tool and as a guide for scoring self-care based on interviews or a review of medical charts. It has good stability over time (.89) and interrater reliability (.95).

At least five versions of the Barthel Index have been used in the literature. These versions have different levels, scoring, and sensitivity. Many studies published in the literature support the validity of the Barthel Index. These studies have shown that it is sensitive to change, that it is a significant predictor of rehabilitation outcome, and that it correlates significantly with other measures of patient status (cf. Christiansen & Ottenbacher, 1998).

Functional Independence Measure

The Functional Independence Measure (FIM™) evolved from a task force of rehabilitation providers that met to develop a reliable and valid instrument that could be used to document the severity of disability, as well as the outcomes of rehabilitation. The conceptual basis for the FIM is that the level of disability should indicate a burden of care (Heineman et al., 1991). There are 18 items in six categories. *Self-care* includes eating, grooming, bathing, dressing upper body, dressing lower body, and toileting. *Sphincter control* includes bladder management and bowel management. *Mobility* addresses three transferring skills: bed/chair/ wheelchair, toilet, and tub/shower. *Locomotion* refers to either walking or using a wheelchair and using stairs. *Communication* includes comprehension and expression. The final category, *social cognition*, includes social interaction, problem solving, and memory. Items are weighted equally, and each item is scored on a 7-point scale, where 7 and 6 indicate the absence of a helper and 5 through 1 represent increasing levels of assistance from a helper. A score of 7 is complete independence that is judged to be timely and safe, while 6 indicates independence with the use of one or more devices. Scores for the 18 items are summed to obtain a total FIM score.

Since 1983, the FIM has been studied extensively in many countries. It has satisfactory interrater reliability and stability and has been shown to be a valid predictor of assistance required by persons with a disability for many types of conditions. It correlates well with other measures of functional performance and also predicts the general satisfaction of clients with their overall condition. Studies using the FIM have shown that the burden of care for a person with a disability reflects both motor and cognitive dimensions. Studies using the FIM with amputees showed that it was better able to predict outcome for clients who scored in the upper quartiles at admission. Because of the growing number of facilities that use the FIM as part of a large rehabilitation database project (the Uniform Data System), use of the FIM is widespread in North America and growing throughout the world. Table 3.2 lists the components of the FIM, as well as the levels of scoring.

Measuring Self-Care in Children

Although some of the instruments cited above have been used with children, there are two instruments specifically designed to measure functional performance in younger clients—the Functional Independence Measure for Children (WeeFIM™) and the Pediatric Evaluation of Disability Inventory (PEDI). They are described below.

WeeFIM™

In 1987 the FIM was adapted to measure the severity of disability in children in a developmental context. Each of the 18 items of the FIM is considered in relation to chronological age, developmental norms, and appropriate expectations for children from 6 months to 7 years of age. The WeeFIM is meant to give clinicians an overall view of the child's actual daily performance in six areas: self-care, mobility, locomotion, sphincter control, communication, and social cognition. The WeeFIM uses the same 7-point ordinal scale to assess level of function as does its parent instrument, the FIM.

The WeeFIM has been standardized for specific age groups, so measures of disability are age appropriate (State University of New York at Buffalo, 1994). Studies have shown that tasks included in the WeeFIM demonstrate a developmental sequence and that it has acceptable reliability and validity in tracking the effect of developmental disability in children of preschool and middle childhood (Msall, DiGaudio, & Duffy, 1993). It has been used to document the outcomes of rehabilitation in children after brain injury and after inter-

Table 3.2 Components of the Functional Independence Measure (FIM™)

Motor Items

Self-Care
- A. Eating
- B. Grooming
- C. Bathing
- D. Dressing Upper Body
- E. Dressing Lower Body
- F. Toileting

Sphincter Control
- G. Bladder management
- H. Bowel management

Transfer
- I. Bed, chair, wheelchair
- J. Toilet
- K. Tub, shower

Locomotion
- L. Walk, wheelchair
- M. Stairs

Cognitive Items

Communication
- N. Comprehension
- O. Expression

Social Cognition
- P. Social interaction
- Q. Problem solving
- R. Memory

Levels of Scoring

Independence
- 7 = Complete independence (Timely, safely)
- 6 = Modified independence (device)

Modified Independence
- 5 = Supervision
- 4 = Minimal assistance (Participant 75%+)
- 3 = Moderate assistance (participant 50%+)

Complete Dependence
- 2 = Maximal assistance (participant 25%+)
- 1 = Total assistance (participant 0%+)

ventions for primary brain tumors and in other populations (Msall, Monti, Duffy, & LaForest, 1992). Scores on the WeeFIM™ have predicted the amount of caregiver assistance necessary to complete ADL (Msall et al., 1993). Because the WeeFIM™ was designed to provide a minimal essential data set, it is not meant to replace more comprehensive assessments of motor, cognitive, or developmental status.

PEDI

The PEDI was developed to assess children between the ages of 6 months and 7.5 years of age. The scale was designed to be a discriminative device to identify functional deficits, as well as an evaluative instrument to measure progress in rehabilitation intervention. The PEDI measures functional status along three dimensions: functional skill level, caregiver assistance, and modifications of adaptive equipment (Haley, Coster, & Fass, 1991). The PEDI has 197 functional skills items and 20 complex functional items for which caregiver assistance and modification are assessed across three content domains—self-care, mobility, and social function. Administration time ranges from 45 to 90 minutes and may be completed by a structured interview with the parent, teacher, or another caregiver familiar with the child. The child may also be observed performing individual items. Examples of skill areas in the self-care domain include use of utensils, use of drinking containers, brushing the hair, and washing the body and face (Reid, Boschen, & Wright, 1993). Studies of the PEDI have demonstrated that it has concurrent validity and successfully documents outcomes after various rehabilitation interventions (Coster, Haley, & Baryza, 1994; Dudgeon et al., 1994; Hinderer & Gupta, 1996; Ziviani & Wright, 1995).

Other Self-Care Scales Developed for Occupational Therapy Practice

This section describes four functional assessment approaches developed by occupational therapy personnel. The list of scales presented is not intended to be exhaustive; however, the scales cited were chosen because of their specific focus, scoring methods, or unique characteristics.

Arnadottir OT-ADL Neurobehavioral Evaluation (A-One)

The A-One (Arnadottir, 1990) is a two-part assessment designed specifically for persons with central nervous system deficits who are 16 years of age and older. Part one consists of two subscales: the first provides a score of functional independence and the second quantifies specific neurobehavioral impairments, such as apraxia, abnormal muscle tone, unilateral neglect, perseveration, agnosia, and organization and sequencing for each of the ADL do-

mains. Domains assessed include dressing, grooming and hygiene, transfers and mobility, feeding, and communication. Part two of the assessment, which is optional, is used to relate the findings of part one to help localize the site of lesions and processing functions.

Reliability and validity data are provided by the author, with average interrater reliability coefficients (kappa) reported for all items of all scales at .84. All but five items attained statistical significance in agreement between raters. Stability coefficients for 1 week were reported at .85 or higher. More research needs to be done using this specialized scale with other populations, since many of the validation and standardization studies have been limited to Iceland.

Assessment of Motor and Process Skills

The Assessment of Motor and Process Skills (AMPS) is an observational evaluation used to examine the abilities of persons to perform instrumental activities of daily living (IADL) tasks (Fisher, 1994). The AMPS requires a clinician to observe a person performing an IADL task as that person would ordinarily perform it. The person selects several familiar tasks from among more than 50 possible tasks, which include options such as sweeping the floor, folding laundry, or making a bed. After the observation, the clinician rates the person's performance in two skill areas: motor (movement) and process (cognition) on a 4-point scale. Motor items represent an observable taxonomy of actions used to move the body, while process (cognitive) skills reflect the organization and execution of a series of actions over time aimed at completing a task.

The raw score ratings by the observer are analyzed using a mathematical procedure (Rasch analysis) that adjusts the final score for the difficulty of the item, the simplicity of the task, and the leniency of the person doing the rating. Because of this process, the resulting estimates of ability can be compared between persons rated, even if they elect to perform different tasks.

The AMPS has been used in a series of studies with persons who have psychiatric, orthopedic, neurologic, cognitive, and developmental disabilities, as well as with healthy community-dwelling adults (Fisher, 1993). These studies have established the preliminary reliability and validity of the instrument. Because it uses a nontraditional approach and requires the use of mathematical analysis unfamiliar to many therapy personnel, the AMPS has not achieved widespread use. However, it represents an important development in the evolution of functional assessment instruments.

COPM

The COPM (Law, Baptiste, et al., 1994) is a scale designed for use by occupational therapy personnel to assess clients' perception of their occupational performance. It is not limited to the evaluation of self-care, but it is a tool that will help determine whether self-care is problematic and important to evaluate in more detail. The COPM is administered in a five-step process using a semistructured interview. First, problems are defined jointly with the client and appropriate caregivers. The client is then asked to rate the importance of each activity on a scale of 1 to 10. The client (or caregiver) is also required to rate his or her ability to perform the specified activities and his or her satisfaction with the performance on the same 10-point scale. These scores are then compared across time. Two scores are given—one for performance and one for satisfaction. Administration time averages between 30 and 40 minutes.

Studies using the COPM have been conducted in several countries (Law, Polatajko, et al., 1994). Data from these studies indicate that the change scores were sensitive to perceived changes in the clients' performance. Because of its interview format, the approach is deemed unsuitable for use with clients having significant cognitive impairment.

Because the COPM involves the client in identifying key occupational performance problems, it is a useful initial assessment tool (Toomey, Nicholson, & Carswell, 1995). If the client identifies one or more self-care problems as priorities, specific evaluation tools can be selected to collect additional data. For example, if the client identifies dressing and bathing as problems, an observational assessment of these self-care activities would be a logical second step.

Kitchen Task Assessment

The Kitchen Task Assessment (KTA) is a specialized assessment developed to assess the capabilities of a person with dementia to perform tasks of daily living (Baum & Edwards, 1993). The goal in developing the KTA was to obtain a sample of the person's behavior in a simple measure that captures the person's current capacity to perform a task. Validation studies on the instrument are being done under the auspices of the memory and aging project of the Alzheimer Research Center at Washington University, School of Medicine, in St. Louis.

The KTA provides for the direct observation of a client making pudding. A 4-point scale (0–3) permits therapy personnel to rate performance on various dimensions of the task as independently competent, requires verbal cue, requires physical assistance, or totally incapable. The dimensions of task performance rated are initiation, organization, performance of all steps, sequencing, judgment and safety, and completion. Scores can range from 0 to 18, with lower scores indicating higher performance. Procedures and necessary kitchen tools and supplies have been standardized, along with criteria for the various dimensions and ratings.

Studies have compared performance scores on the pudding task, along with a clinical diagnostic rating (CDR). The CDR assessed memory, orientation, judgment and problem solving, community affairs, home and hobbies, and personal care. These studies have demonstrated that scores on the KTA decline as cognitive function declines. Statistical analysis has shown that the KTA measures cognitive function and that this performance component explains 84% of the variation of the scores on the test (Baum & Edwards, 1993). The scale is designed to be sensitive to changes in performance over time, as well as to provide useful information about the level of cognitive support (i.e., verbal cues or physical assistance) necessary to optimize the performance of persons with cognitive loss or impairment. Reliability for the patient samples grouped according to severity of their dementia ranges from .87 to .96.

Klein-Bell ADL Scale

The Klein-Bell ADL Scale (Klein & Bell, 1982) is composed of easily observable components of ADL in all persons, regardless of diagnosis or disability. It consists of 170 items that are scored as "achieved" or "failed," and full credit is given for independence with the use of assistive devices. Items are assigned a point value corresponding to their level of difficulty, as determined by a group of 10 occupational therapy practitioners, physical therapists, and nurses experienced in rehabilitation. The more difficult items are worth 3 points, less difficult items 2 points, and the easiest items 1 point. If the person achieves the item, full points are given; no points are given for failed items. The scores are summed for an overall independence score.

An interrater reliability study using occupational therapy practitioners and nurses as raters achieved 92% agreement overall. Predictive validity was assessed by first contacting former patients and inquiring about the number of hours per week of assistance that was required to complete ADL and then comparing this number with the predischarge Klein-Bell ADL scores. The resulting correlation showed that the Klein-Bell scores explained 74% of the variation in assistance after discharge. The Klein-Bell ADL appears to have greater sensitivity to change than the Katz Index or the Barthel Index. However, the larger number of items contained in the scale may account for this finding.

Milwaukee Evaluation of Daily Living Skills

The Milwaukee Evaluation of Daily Living Skills (MEDLS) (Leonardelli, 1988a; 1988b) was designed to measure the performance of long-term psychiatric clients. A broad range of self-care tasks are assessed in 20 subtests. The self-care areas included in the MEDLS were based on a survey of professionals working with clients with chronic mental illness (Leonardelli, 1989). The subtests may be used individually or in any combination, and a screening form is provided in the manual to assist in selecting the subtests applicable to any one client. It takes approximately 80 minutes to administer 18 subtests at one time. Tasks are observed by the occupational therapist and are preferably done at the time and place that are part of the client's routine. There is no cumulative score; each subtest is scored separately based on performance in that area. The manual provides a description of the method, a skill list, and key words for observing each skill, as well as scoring criteria for each subtest.

Initial interrater reliability has been assessed with residents in a psychiatric facility; the assessment resulted in moderate to good results, depending on the subtest ($r = .40$ for shaving, which was not significant; other subtests ranged from .60–1.00 and were significant at $p < .001$). Other studies have shown that the MEDLS correlates well with other established and developing instruments designed to document patient performance (Margolis, Harrison, Robinson, & Jayaram, 1996). An interesting recent study showed that the MEDLS correlated highly with the Hopkins Competency Assessment Test, a measure of a patient's competency to consent to treatment (Jones, Jayaram, Samuels, & Robinson, 1998).

Performance Assessment of Self-Care Skills

The Performance Assessment of Self-Care Skills (PASS) (version 3.1) is a criterion-referenced instrument designed to evaluate independent living capacity in adults, both healthy and those who are impaired (Rogers & Holm, 1994). The PASS has been used for planning intervention as well as for documenting change over time.

There are 26 items in the scale, addressing functional mobility, personal care, and home management. Each of three areas of information relating to performance (independence, safety, and outcome) is scored on a 4-point scale (ranging from 0 = dysfunction to 3 = function) for each task. Each task is broken down into subtasks, which allows the evaluator to pinpoint the specific aspect of the performance that is problematic. The scale also documents the amount of assistance needed to complete the tasks, thus providing a guide to the need for caregiving support necessary for the client.

The PASS is based on four established functional assessment tools for seniors and has been used on groups with various psychiatric and medical conditions. Its psychometric properties suggest satisfactory reliability and validity.

Instruments To Assess the Performance Environment

All self-care activities take place within an environmental context. For assessments conducted outside a rehabilitation hospital or skilled care facility, it is appropriate and relevant to determine the safety and adequacy of the setting and the extent to which it supports performance. Two assessment instruments that are used to evaluate this aspect of self-care performance will be briefly reviewed. They include the Safety Assessment of Function and the Environment for Rehabilitation (SAFER) Tool and The Home Occupation Environment Assessment (HOEA).

SAFER Tool

The SAFER tool was designed to identify risk factors in the living setting of seniors that can result in injury and to permit recommendations regarding safety (Letts & Marshall, 1995). The SAFER tool has 97 items grouped into the domains of living situation, mobility, kitchen, fire hazards, eating, household, dressing, grooming, bathroom, medication, communication, wandering, memory aids, and general. The SAFER was developed to address the need for an "acceptable, standardized instrument focusing on safety and function within the home environment" (Letts & Marshall, 1995, p. 53).

Relevant items to be assessed within a particular living environment are listed adjacent to three columns (addressed, not applicable, and problem), which are checked by the evaluator as observations are made. Some items (e.g., elevators) are not relevant for given settings and are marked not applicable.

An interesting attribute of the SAFER tool is the choice of items that reflect a transactional relationship between the person interacting with the environment. A panel of clinicians and seniors systematically selected the items for inclusion in the tool, and some items were discarded after analysis of content and construct validity. This process also provided the basis for guidelines to assist practitioners in using the tool, which is organized in the form of questions to consider when completing an environmental assessment.

This descriptive environmental assessment demonstrates acceptable reliability and validity as an assessment of a person's ability to function safely within a home environment. A recent study of the SAFER tool demonstrated that environments with greater safety risks correlated with cognitive impairment (Letts, Scott, Burtney, Marshall, & McKean, 1998), suggesting that a relationship exists between level of independence and safety.

HOEA

The HOEA (Baum, Edwards, Bradford, & Lane, 1995) is an assessment developed specifically for clients with dementia. The assessment addresses behavioral and environmental items that suggest the client's ability to live safely in a given environment. Items on the scale were initially developed based on expert opinion and then were factor analyzed to determine those item clusters that correlate with high risk. A checklist allows the therapist to indicate whether or not a given item was assessed and to provide a score on a 4-point scale (no problem observed, requires monitoring, requires attention, or high-risk situation).

Behavioral items include impaired judgment, disheveled appearance, possible abuse or neglect, depressed mood, difficulties with finance, difficulties with managing medications, awareness of surroundings, understands questions, slurred speech, slow response, difficult to understand, hearing problem, smell, and vision. Environmental items include the following categories: accessibility within the home, sanitation, food storage, and general safety issues.

Because the HOEA is a new scale, it has not yet been validated or studied extensively, and research continues. Further study is needed with this instrument aimed at persons with cognitive deficits.

Conclusion

Effective assessment of function is essential to planning and modifying intervention strategies and making informed choices about safe environments for patients. The choice of an instrument for assessing self-care ability will depend on the characteristics of the setting, the characteristics of the patient or client, and the purpose of the assessment. No one "gold standard" for self-care assessment is ideally suited for each of the purposes outlined at the beginning of the chapter.

Although past reviews of ADL scales in the literature have made recommendations in support of specific scales (Law & Letts, 1989), these reviews become less useful as new scales are developed. Familiarity with the scales reviewed in this chapter should give the therapist a basis for making an informed decision. The use of well-validated scales is important because intervention decisions must be based on valid information.

There is a great need for more clinician reports of how existing scales perform in varied settings and with different populations. Are they sensitive to change? Do they predict future occupational performance at home? Can existing interview and self-report instruments be modified to include observation of performance rather than reported performance? Studies that support the development and validation of existing scales are needed. The use of ad hoc or "homemade" evaluations is not acceptable. Because occupational therapy personnel have expertise in performance evaluation, they should be at the forefront of the development of performance-based assessments (Fisher, 1992b). ◆

Study Questions

1. What two assessment instruments are suitable for determining the self-care skills of children?

2. The SAFER Tool is an instrument for measuring

   a) Self-care for persons with dementia.
   b) Self-care for adults with neurological impairment.
   c) IADL skills.
   d) Environmental and performance issues relating to safety.
   e) C & D above.

3. True or False: All self-care scales measure mobility.

4. True or False: Stability is a measure of the consistency of an instrument over time.

5. What three scales were designed especially for a population with cognitive deficits?

References

Alexander, J. L., & Fuhrer, M. J. (1984). Functional assessment of individuals with physical impairments. In A. S. Halpern & M. J. Fuhrer (Eds.), *Functional assessment in rehabilitation*. Baltimore: Paul H. Brooks.

Arnadottir, G. (1990). *The brain and behavior. Assessing cortical dysfunction through activities of daily living*. St. Louis, MO: Mosby.

Baum, C., & Edwards, D. F. (1993). Cognitive performance in senile dementia of the Alzheimer's type: The Kitchen Task Assessment. *American Journal of Occupational Therapy, 47*, 431–436.

Baum, C. M., Edwards, D. F., Bradford, T., & Lane, R. (1995). *Home Occupation-Environment Assessment (HOEA)*. St. Louis, MO: Occupational Therapy Program, Washington University.

Bombardier, C., & Tugwell, P. (1987). Methodological considerations in functional assessment. *Journal of Rheumatology, 14*(Suppl. 15), 6–10.

Canadian Association of Occupational Therapists and Health Services Directorate, Health and Welfare Canada. (1997). *Enabling occupation: An occupational therapy perspective*. Ottawa, ON: Canadian Association of Occupational Therapists.

Christiansen, C. H., & Ottenbacher, K. J. (1998). Evaluation and management of daily self care requirements. In J. DeLisa & Bruce M. Gans (Eds.), *Rehabilitation medicine: Principles and practice* (pp. 137–165). Philadelphia: Lippincott-Raven.

Coster, W. J., Haley, S., & Baryza, M. J. (1994). Functional performance of young children after traumatic brain injury: A 6-month follow-up study. *American Journal of Occupational Therapy, 48*, 211–218.

Dudgeon, B. J., Libby, A. K., McLaughlin J. F., Hays, R. M., Bjornson, K. F., & Roberts, T. S. (1994). Prospective measurement of functional changes after selective dorsal rhizotomy. *Archives of Physical Medicine and Rehabilitation, 75*(1), 46–53.

Edwards, M. M. (1990). The reliability and validity of self-report activities of daily living scales. *Canadian Journal of Occupational Therapy, 57*, 273–278.

Fisher, A. G. (1992a). Functional measures, part I: What is function, what should we measure and how should we measure it? *American Journal of Occupational Therapy, 46*, 183–185.

Fisher, A. G. (1992b). Functional measures, part II: Selecting the right test, minimizing the limitations. *American Journal of Occupational Therapy, 46*, 278–281.

Fisher, A. G. (1993). The assessment of IADL motor skill: An application of the many-faceted Rasch analysis. *American Journal of Occupational Therapy, 47*, 319–329.

Fisher, A. G. (1994). *Assessment of motor and process skills* (Research ed. 7.0). Fort Collins, CO: Department of Occupational Therapy, Colorado State University.

Haley, S. M., Coster, W. J., & Fass, R. M. (1991). A content validity study of the *Pediatric Evaluation of Disability Inventory. Pediatric Physical Therapy, 3*, 177–184.

Heineman, A. W., Hamilton, B. B., Wright, B. D., Betts, H. B., Aguda, B., & Mamott, B. D. (1991). *Rating scale analysis of functional assessment measures* (Final Report to the National Institute on Disability and Rehabilitation Research). Chicago: Rehabilitation Institute of Chicago.

Hinderer, S. R., & Gupta, S. (1996). Functional outcome measures to assess interventions for spasticity. *Archives of Physical Medicine and Rehabilitation, 77*(10), 1083–1089.

Jette, A. M. (1987). The functional status index: Reliability and validity of a self-report functional disability measure. *Journal of Rheumatology, 14* (Suppl. 15), 15–19.

Jones, B. N., Jayaram, G., Samuels, J., & Robinson, H. (1998). Relating competency status to functional status at discharge in patients with chronic mental illness. *Journal of the American Academy of Psychiatry and the Law, 26*(1), 49–55.

Katz, S., Downs, T. D., Cash, H. R., & Grotz, R. C. (1970). Progress in development of an index of ADL. *Gerontologist, 10*, 20–30.

Katz, S., Ford, A. B., Moskowitz, R. W., Jackson, B. A., & Jaffe, M. W. (1963). Studies of illness in the aged. The index of ADL: A standardized measure of biological and psychosocial function. *Journal of the American Medical Association, 185*, 914–919.

Keith, R. A. (1984). Functional assessment measures in medical rehabilitation: Current status. *Archives of Physical Medicine and Rehabilitation, 65*, 74–78.

Klein, R. M., & Bell, B. (1982). Self-care skills: Behavioral measurement with Klein-Bell ADL scale. *Archives of Physical Medicine and Rehabilitation, 63*, 335–338.

Law, M., Baptiste, S., Carswell, A., McColl, M. A., Polatajko, H., & Pollock, N. (1994). *Canadian occupational performance measure* (2nd ed.). Toronto, Ontario: Canadian Association of Occupational Therapists Publications.

Law, M., & Letts, L. (1989). A critical review of scales of activities of daily living. *American Journal of Occupational Therapy, 43*, 522–528.

Law, M., Polotajko, H., Pollock, N., McColl, M., Carswell, A., & Baptiste, S. (1994). Pilot testing of the Canadian Occupational Performance Measure: Clinical and measurement issues. *Canadian Journal of Occupational Therapy, 61,* 191–197.

Law, M., & Usher, P. (1988). Validation of the Klein-Bell activities of daily living scale for children. *Canadian Journal of Occupational Therapy, 55,* 63–68.

Lawton, M. P. (1990). Aging and performance of home tasks. *Human Factors, 32,* 527–536.

Leonardelli, C. A. (1988a). *The Milwaukee evaluation of daily living skills: Evaluation in long-term psychiatric care.* Thorofare, NJ: Slack.

Leonardelli, C. A. (1988b). The Milwaukee evaluation of daily living skills (MEDLS). In B. J. Hemphill (Ed.), *Mental health assessment in occupational therapy: An integrative approach to the evaluative process.* Thorofare, NJ: Slack.

Leonardelli, C. A. (1989). Specification of daily living skills for persons with chronic mental illness. *Occupational Therapy Journal of Research, 9,* 323–333.

Letts, L., & Marshall, L. (1995). Evaluating the validity and consistency of the SAFER Tool. *Physical and Occupational Therapy in Geriatrics, 13*(4), 49–66.

Letts, L., Scott, S., Burtney, J., Marshall, L., & McKean, M. (1998). The reliability and validity of the safety assessment of function and the environment for rehabilitation (SAFER Tool). *British Journal of Occupational Therapy, 61*(3), 127–132.

Mahoney, F. I., & Barthel, D. W. (1965). Functional evaluation: The Barthel index. *Maryland State Medical Journal, 14,* 61–65.

Margolis, R. L., Harrison, S. A., Robinson, H. J., & Jayaram, G. (1996). Occupational therapy task observation scale (OTTOS): A rapid method for rating task group function of psychiatric patients. *American Journal of Occupational Therapy, 50,* 380–385.

McDowell, I., & Newell, C. (1987). *Measuring health: A guide to rating scales and questionnaires.* New York: Oxford University Press.

Msall, M. E, DiGaudio, K. M., & Duffy, L. C. (1993). Use of functional assessment in children with developmental disability. *Physical Medicine and Rehabilitation Clinics of North America, 4,* 517–527.

Msall, M. E., Monti, D., Duffy, L. C., & LaForrest, S. (1992). Measuring functional independence in children with spina bifida [Abstract]. *Pediatric Research, 31,* 12A.

Reid, D. T., Boschen, K., & Wright, V. (1993). Critique of the Pediatric Evaluation of Disability Inventory. *Physical and Occupational Therapy in Pediatrics, 13*(4), 57–87.

Rogers, J. C., & Holm, M. B. (1994). *Performance Assessment of Self-Care Skills (PASS)* (Version 3.1). Unpublished functional performance test. Pittsburgh, PA: University of Pittsburgh.

State University of New York at Buffalo. (1994). *Functional Independence Measure for Children (WeeFIM™)* (Outpatient Version 1.0). Buffalo, NY: State University of New York at Buffalo.

Toomey, M., Nicholson, D., & Carswell, A. (1995). The clinical utility of the Canadian Occupational Performance Measure. *Canadian Journal of Occupational Therapy, 62,* 242–249.

Ziviani, J., & Wright S. (1995). Pediatric Evaluation of Disability Inventory: Review and applications. *New Zealand Journal of Occupational Therapy, 46*(1), 15–18.

4

Planning Intervention for Self-Care Needs

Charles H. Christiansen

Charles H. Christiansen, EdD, OTR, OT(C), FAOTA, is Dean and George T. Bryan Distinguished Professor, School of Allied Health Sciences, University of Texas Medical Branch at Galveston, Texas.

Key Terms

compensation

disability prevention

health promotion

ICIDH-2

narrative

occupational therapy diagnosis

plan of care

remediation

Objectives

On completing this chapter, the reader will be able to

1. Appreciate the difference between independence and interdependence.

2. Understand that intervention planning requires ethical decision making.

3. List the steps in the occupational therapy intervention process.

4. Understand the difference between procedural and narrative reasoning.

5. Identify and understand the distinction among the four principal categories of intervention: remediation, compensation, disability prevention, and health promotion.

6. Appreciate the social considerations necessary in determining intervention goals and options.

7. Define social impression management and understand the importance of the patient's social identity as a factor in selecting among intervention options.

8. Appreciate that intervention decisions have important ethical considerations.

All goal-directed actions take place twice. They begin as thoughts about what actions might be taken and are followed by the actions themselves in physical space. This sequence also describes the process for intervention. A plan of care is thought out and documented by a caregiver *after* an organized process of gathering, analyzing, and interpreting information. The plan of care serves as a bridge between the stages of evaluation and intervention (Rogers & Holm, 1991, 1997).

This complex process of diagnostic and clinical reasoning considers information from many sources and includes both subjective and objective types of information. Once this information has been considered, the practitioner must choose from among several categories of intervention. The purpose of this chapter is to describe these sources of information and to describe the process of planning intervention for self-care.

Analyzing Performance Information

Evaluation is a process of gaining an understanding of the patient to make clinical decisions. Understanding of the patient comes from observation, interaction, and assessment using formalized measurement of performance. The quality of decision making is directly related to the type, amount, and quality of information provided to the practitioner. Because self-care is the focus, the occupational therapy practitioner is interested in determining how well the patient is able to accomplish the very necessary tasks and functions of self-care. This more technical type of assessment requires objective and accurate methods.

Practitioners are interested in learning as much about the patient's history, lifestyle, and personal characteristics as well. Thus, when it comes time to select from among intervention options, choices will be made that provide the *right* fit for *this* particular patient at *this* particular time. This aspect of evaluation, often portrayed as understanding the patient's "story," is more subjective and has ethical implications. Thus, effective treatment planning has correct choices from a technical standpoint and right choices from an ethical perspective. This planning requires the practitioner to base decisions on information from different domains of knowledge. These domains include those from the procedural realm as well as those of narrative realm.

The procedural realm of information includes the practitioner's conceptual frame of reference and the objective data obtained from standardized instruments. While procedural reasoning provides insight into a broad range of general situations, it alone is not sufficient for occupational therapy practice. When practitioners rely exclusively on procedural reasoning, they are likely to focus their treatment on performance components rather than on life tasks (Mattingly, 1991; Mattingly & Fleming, 1993).

The second type of data is from the narrative realm. Using this type of information, practitioners guide their intervention by imagining where the patient is now and where this patient might be at some future point after discharge. The practitioner tries to understand the larger picture of the patient's story. This contemplation gives the practitioner a richer basis for organizing goals and intervention strategies.

The information available to therapy personnel can be organized using various hierarchies, each of which represents a systems approach. In the United States, a hierarchy developed by the National Center for Medical Rehabilitation Research has gained popularity in recent years. This hierarchy is contrasted with the framework now under development by the World Health Organization (1998) as shown in Table 4.1.

Regardless of the hierarchy chosen, each shows that task performance in daily living can be viewed at different levels and that each level has influences on performance. Typically, therapy personnel are interested in performance components (such as motor, sensory, cognitive, psychosocial, or perceptual) to the extent that one or more of these components interfere with carrying out desired tasks. For example, a stroke or cerebral vascular accident (CVA) can result in neurological problems that interfere with motor planning and coordinated movement. It can also create perceptual difficulties that make task performance difficult.

As a result of these deficits, a person may not be able to perform the activities necessary for self-care. For example, a woman may be unable to dress or groom herself because of left hemiparesis. As observed in chapter 1, dressing and grooming are important in a social world, and, thus, the strategy for achieving satisfactory grooming is instrumental to daily living.

Table 4.1 Comparison of NCMRR (1993) and WHO (1998) Classifications

NCMRR Classification	**WHO Classification (ICIDH-2)**

Term
  Definition
Pathophysiology
  The interruption of normal structures
Impairments
  Loss or abnormality or both of cognitive, communicative, physical, emotional, psychological, or anatomical structure or function
Functional Limitation
  Any restriction or lack of ability to perform an action in the manner consistent with the purpose of an organ or organ system
Disability
  An inability or limitation in performing tasks, activities, and roles
Societal Limitation
  Restrictions caused by structural or attitudinal barriers that limit fulfillment of roles or deny access to services and opportunities
	Term
	  Definition in the context of a health condition
	Impairment
	  Loss or abnormality of body structure or of a physiological or psychological function (e.g., loss of limb, loss of vision)
	Activity
	  The nature and extent of functioning at the level of the person. Activities may be limited in nature, duration, and quality (e.g., taking care of oneself, maintaining a job).
	Participation
	  The nature and extent of a person's involvement in life situations in relation to impairment, activities, health conditions, and contextual factors

Formulating an Occupational Therapy Diagnosis

What intervention options are available for the patient and which should be chosen? Rogers and Holm (1997) have identified the occupational therapy diagnosis as a problem statement that succinctly describes the occupational status of a person and identifies the problems that are amenable to intervention. The process for formulating an occupational therapy diagnosis involves the development of a descriptive problem statement.

As described by Rogers and Holm (1997), the descriptive problem statement has four elements that represent each of the elements that ought to be considered by the practitioner in determining treatment options. The first part of the statement describes the patient's occupational performance problem. The second part explains the reasons underlying the problem in terms of the applicable performance components. The third element considers details of sensorimotor, cognitive, and social-emotional function drawn from observation and assessment. This third element in organizing diagnostic information relevant to occupational therapy clinical reasoning is called *explanatory evidence*. The fourth element of relevance to the practitioner in formulating a plan of care concerns the diagnostic

information available from the physician about the patient's medical condition.

Consider the following information pertinent to CVAs or strokes. A left hemiplegia is caused by a CVA in the brain's right hemisphere. After a stroke, patients are sometimes depressed; depression can influence motivation to engage in treatment activities. CVAs may occur in persons with other medical problems, such as obesity, hypertension, and macular degeneration. These medical problems are examples of diagnostic factors that influence decisions relevant to diagnostic reasoning and planning intervention for a person who has suffered a stroke.

In developing an informed plan of care, the practitioner must consider several factors that include both subjective and objective data (or cues). These data include the patient's medical or psychiatric diagnosis, the reason for referral, the patient's goals and preferences, the probable or desired discharge environment, the patient's demographic characteristics, the setting in which intervention is to be delivered, the limitations on therapy (such as reimbursement restrictions), and the practitioner's frame of reference for practice (Rogers & Holm, 1997, Holm, Rogers, & James, 1998).

The process of effective clinical reasoning is complex. Experienced clinicians are able to analyze the information available to them and discern patterns that lead quickly to tentative hypotheses about the most important problems and their underlying causes. Thus, diagnostic formulations result from careful attention to information, from the confirmation of hypotheses, and from previous experience. Together, these elements suggest realistic possibilities for intervention.

Formulating the Plan of Care

An analysis of the results of evaluation, which occurs during diagnostic reasoning, leads to development of the plan of care. Typically, a plan of care includes an explicit statement of the functional goals (long term as well as short term); the intervention procedures to be used; the type, the frequency, and the duration of intervention; and recommendations (e.g., referrals to other professionals).

For certain types of funding in the United States, levels of function must be explicitly stated in documentation according to criteria and definitions provided by funding agencies. Table 4.2 lists the definitions of levels of function provided by the Health Care Financing Administration.

Intervention Goals

Goals must indicate expected changes in functional performance as a result of intervention. Frequently, the goals of intervention cannot be achieved during a patient's length of stay within a care facility. In this case, important short-term goals are identified that can be achieved in either functional tasks or their underlying performance components. Expected outcomes are always carefully delineated along with the factors that impede the person's functional performance (e.g., limited attention span or restricted range of motion). Table 4.3 gives a sample of self-care goals and intervention strategies.

Selecting Intervention Options

The range of intervention options available to therapy personnel falls into the following four principal categories: (a) remediation, (b) compensation, (c) disability prevention, and (d) health promotion. The presence of categories does not imply that the occupational therapy practitioner selects one approach. Rather, intervention approaches from several categories are often used in an integrated fashion. Moreover, the emphasis on a particular type of intervention is likely to shift during the course of intervention. Figure 4.1 shows the process for occupational therapy intervention.

Remediation

Remediation strategies focus on performance components and, therefore, have an influence on biological, physiological, or neurological processes. For example, the practitioner may incorporate motor or sensory techniques to fully or partially develop or restore sufficient voluntary control or movement to enable task accomplishment. Techniques derived from theories of neuroscience, biomechanics, and motor control are included among remediative approaches. The objective is to recover sufficient sensation, cognition, and voluntary movement to enable task performance in a safe and effective manner.

Trombly (1993) has emphasized that the performance components typically assessed by occupational therapy practitioners (such as sensorimotor control of the upper extremity) only partially predict task performance. Nearly 40% of such performance is explained by other factors, such as level of motivation or environmental conditions. Therefore, the practitioner must consider many factors during the assessment process, ensuring that the assessment begins with a thorough understanding of the unique context that characterizes each patient. When choosing therapeutic options that address performance components, such as balance or sensation, the practitioner must explain to the patient the relationship between those abilities and the safe performance of relevant tasks (such as bathing).

Sometimes remediative intervention requires training, and this training can be habilitative or adaptive in nature. Habilitative training approaches are used when, as in the case of congenital or developmental disorders, skills are being learned for the first time. Typically, the acquisition of self-care skills takes place over extended periods and involves the careful structuring of tasks, frequent monitoring to correct performance errors, and feedback. Behavior modification techniques, through which desirable behaviors are rewarded through positive reinforcement and undesirable behaviors are ignored and extinguished, are often useful. Such operant conditioning, often provided through token reward systems, allows successive approximations toward each goal through an incremental process known as shaping. Practice occurs as needed. (See Box 4.1.)

Adaptive training is based on the recognition that skills can be successfully accomplished in many ways, and the successful completion of the task is the primary goal. In this approach, training is frequently combined with compensatory strategies, such as the use of orthoses, prostheses, or other types of assistive or adaptive devices or systems. For

Table 4.2 Definitions of Levels of Functional Performance

Level	Definition
Total assistance	The need for 100% assistance by one or more persons to perform all physical activities or cognitive assistance or both to elicit a functional response to an external stimulation.
Maximum assistance	The need for 75% assistance by one person to physically perform any part of a functional activity or cognitive assistance or both to perform gross-motor actions in response to direction.
Moderate assistance	The need for 50% assistance by one person to perform physical activities or provide cognitive assistance to perform gross-motor actions in response to direction.
Minimum assistance	The need for 25% assistance by one person for physical activities or to provide cognitive assistance to perform functional activities safely.
Standby assistance	The need for supervision by one person for the patient to perform new activity procedures that were adapted by the therapist for safe and effective performance. A patient requires standby assistance when errors and the need for safety precautions are not always anticipated by the patient.
Independent status	No physical or cognitive assistance is required to perform functional activities. Patients at this level are able to implement the selected courses of action, to consider potential errors, and to anticipate safety hazards in familiar and new situations.

Note: From Health Care Financing Administration. (n.d.). *Medicare Intermediary Manual* (Publication 13. Section 390-6.4, pp. 20–21). Washington, DC: U.S. Government Printing Office.

Table 4.3 Sample Self-Care Goals and Intervention Strategies

Evaluation Data	Diagnoses	Goals	Intervention Strategies

History/Narrative
  Client is male, 67 years old, retired school administrator
  Active premorbidly in volunteer work and outdoor hobbies
Sensorimotor
  Proprioception intact
  Grade 3 (fair) muscle strength in left wrist, elbow, and shoulder flexors and extensors
  No visual field cut
  2-point discrimination absent on right digits
Cognitive
  Follows simple directions
Affective
  No interest in activities
	Medical
	  Right CVA
	  Depression
	Occupational therapy diagnosis
	  Performance
	    Unable to initiate or complete dressing or bathing tasks without verbal cues and physical assistance
	Performance components
	  Left hemiparesis
	  Apathy
		Client will demonstrate improved upper-extremity endurance and strength so that with task modifications and assistive devices he is able to dress independently in less than 30 minutes.
		Client will shower independently using adaptive equipment and safe practices.
			Remediation
			  Neuromotor techniques to facilitate normal tone and to improve strength and coordination
			Compensation
			  Train in use of dressing skills by introducing dressing aids (stocking aid, zipper pull, hook-and-loop fasteners)
			  Train family members
			Disability prevention
			  Grab bars in tub and shower
			  Nonslip surfaces

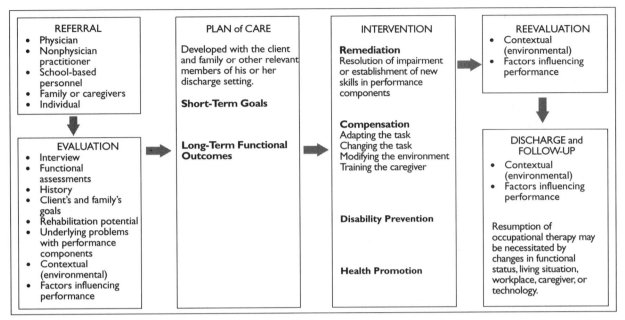

Figure 4.1 Occupational therapy intervention for self-care.

Box 4.1
Remediating Social Skills

Social skills training recognizes that competence in dealing with others involves several dimensions. To be socially competent, persons must have the ability and the skill to understand situations and social expectations, to initiate sociable behaviors, and to demonstrate those characteristics related to presentation of self that influence positively how a person is viewed by others.

Training programs often focus on understanding roles and motives of others, on thinking through problem situations, and on understanding moral dilemmas. Specific social skills that can be practiced include showing confidence and enthusiasm, using assertive behaviors when appropriate, and demonstrating good grooming. Persons can be taught to initiate interaction, to respond with sensitivity to others, and to understand expectations in social situations.

Some social skills training has been used effectively as a primary intervention tool in treatment of persons with mental impairments and emotional problems, as well as in other populations. Typically, these programs use group-oriented approaches that include role-playing and modeling of behaviors that allow practicing social behaviors under various circumstances. Assertiveness training is often a part of such programming. The assumption behind these approaches is that the most difficult aspects of some illnesses are behaviors that are viewed as socially maladaptive and unacceptable. The goal is to improve social behaviors and, thereby, reduce the alienation and rejection so often experienced by persons who have difficulties interacting with others.

example, the person with only one functional arm can continue to don and button a shirt, using substitute motions and a device to pull the button through the buttonhole. When remediative approaches are unlikely to be successful or are too costly in terms of time, energy, or expense, compensatory or adaptive approaches are necessary (Trombly, 1993).

Compensatory Strategies

In compensatory strategies, the objective is to identify new ways to accomplish the required task within remaining performance capabilities. Before any strategies are selected, it is useful for the practitioner and patient to examine together and to prioritize the array of tasks to be performed. Often, the task environment or context can be modified or adapted to enable successful performance. Thus, compensatory strategies may focus on modifying the task, the context, or both.

Many strategies can be used to adapt a task and the task environment to enable one to meet self-care objectives satisfactorily. First, the person can be taught to perform a task within his or her capabilities. Second, the environment can be modified to permit accomplishment of the task despite limitations in ability or skill. Third, systems or devices can be designed or acquired to enable performance, despite limited cognition, strength, or sensory ability. Another compensatory strategy involves having an agent or caregiver assist with task requirements or perform them entirely. Home health personnel, family members, or personal care assistants can help accomplish self-care tasks according to the needs of the person receiving assistance. Each of these categories of compensatory approaches is described in more detail below.

Use of adaptive systems and devices. Occupational therapy practitioners often use the broad term assistive technology to refer to the systems and devices designed to help persons compensate for lost or diminished functions. During recent years, a dramatic increase has been made in the number of such devices and systems available to practitioners and their patients. Sadly, some studies have shown that because of the difficulty experienced by the average rehabilitation provider in keeping up with the latest assistive technology, some useful devices and systems are never considered or recommended to persons who could benefit from them (Newrick & Langton-Hewer, 1984).

Devices range from those described as low technology, which include such items as special utensils with built-up handles and shoelaces that can be tied with one hand, to high-technology devices, which include electronic remote control devices that activate appliances and speech synthesizers that store and speak words and sentences. Smith (1991) has noted that patients are too often provided with more technology than is necessary and that practitioners should be mindful that the best solution is often the simplest. Often, patients may need equipment at one phase of their rehabilitation but not at another, particularly if they find they can manage without them (Haworth, 1983). In other cases, experience after discharge from a rehabilitation setting may result in a change of strategies based on reordering priorities because of time and energy.

Cosmetic (appearance-related) considerations may also limit the use of prostheses and adaptive devices. Stein and Walley (1983) reported that 60% of the persons with an upper-extremity amputation they studied preferred myoelectric prostheses over conventional devices, even though usage decreased with the myoelectric protheses and they were slower than the conventional devices. Concern with acceptable appearance (cosmesis) was felt to influence this choice. That is, patients preferred the device that was viewed as having a better appearance even though it may not have provided functional benefits that were as good as the less visually appealing conventional prostheses. Clearly, the most important criterion in evaluating an assistive device is whether or not it meets the needs of the consumer.

It appears that during the first 3 months after discharge, newly established routines and habits determine whether or not a specific device or strategy is going to be used consistently. Studies of the use of devices after discharge confirm that adaptive strategies may change depending on the situation (Garber & Gregorio, 1990; Gitlin, Levine, & Geiger, 1993). Moreover, the social acceptability of a given strategy may change depending on the setting or even depending on the context within the same setting.

Environmental modifications. Environmental modifications can vary from the rearrangement of furniture to major alterations in the design of rooms or dwellings. Common examples include widening doorways, building ramps, and converting family rooms into bedrooms for facilitating wheelchair access. Within bathrooms, the addition of grab bars, special toilet seats, and other safety equipment can dramatically improve the completion of self-care tasks by persons with limitations.

The Americans With Disabilities Act (ADA) in the United States, as well as efforts by advocacy groups in other countries, have made apparent the need to design environments and to make other accommodations so that persons with functional limitations are not deprived of societal access or participation. Unfortunately, persons with disabilities often encounter bureaucratic obstacles that preclude timely completion of necessary environmental modifications or the acquisition of devices to facilitate adaptation. As societal attitudes reflect improved awareness of environmental barriers, buildings, playgrounds, and access areas will incorporate the curb cuts, ramps, and signage that permit their use by persons with motor and sensory deficits.

Use of family members and personal care attendants. Another strategy available to the patient involves the use of family members or other personal care attendants or caregivers to assist in the performance of various self-maintenance tasks. Family members or friends may voluntarily provide assistance without compensation. However, it may be necessary, or even preferable, to find paid assistance. A study by Nosek (1993) found that inadequate personal care assistance affects the long-term health and well-being of persons who are discharged from rehabilitation facilities and concluded that a much better system for providing caregivers is needed. Her study found that burnout, fatigue, and other factors typically compromise the quality of care provided by family members. However, because outside attendants are often unavailable or economically infeasible, the study recommended that rehabilitation facilities do a much better job of training family members to provide such services. The study also recommended that rehabilitation facilities ensure that patients are trained to manage personal care attendants adequately.

One of the most important and difficult requirements for the patient will be to define all of the activities for which assistance is required. Some self-care tasks, such as dressing, grooming, and oral hygiene, are performed daily. Others, such as washing the hair, doing the laundry, or changing the bed, may be done less frequently. The list of activities must be categorized according to those requiring no assistance, those requiring some assistance, and those that the personal care attendant must perform for the patient. Practitioners can assist in the formulation of these lists by helping the patient gain a realistic and thorough understanding of his or her strengths and limitations related to self-care.

Disability Prevention

As a primary category of intervention, disability prevention includes those parts of the plan of care that promote safety or prevent health problems.

Disability prevention seeks to identify risk factors before an accident occurs to improve safety and to reduce the risk of injury, hospitalization, chronic disability, and death.

Self-care tasks are not only important foundations for engaging in a social world, but they also include tasks that promote nutrition, hygiene, and, in certain cases, prevent specific health problems, such as taking medication to control diabetes, HIV, or epilepsy. Thus, by enabling the person to complete self-care tasks, disability prevention is taking place. Always, it is important for the practitioner to emphasize safety in the performance of tasks. For persons with visual difficulties, sensory deficits, balance disorders, or other conditions that place them at risk for personal injury, attention must be paid to object placement, environmental design (lighting, nonslip surfaces), safety apparatus (e.g., grab bars), and safe-task methods. To assist in determining appropriate preventive strategies within environments, several checklists and tools are available to therapy personnel. These checklists and tools are identified in the chapter on assessment.

Health Promotion

A fourth intervention approach involves strategies directed at health promotion. Because the time and energy available for task performance may be limited, teaching patients how to manage and conserve these resources is an important part of helping them successfully adapt to their disability or unique life circumstances. Moreover, by learning how to structure one's daily routine, unnecessary stress and its physical consequences can be avoided.

In many cases, while strategies are available to enable completion of certain tasks, the cost in terms of time and energy of doing so without assistance in the face of competing demands makes it necessary and more logical to have others complete them. For many aspects of self-care, what matters most may be the outcome, not the means by which it was achieved. Thousands of hair salons would be out of business if the general public did not hold a similar view. Moreover, many find that using personal care services enhances their quality of life by promoting relaxation and by reducing tension and perceived stress. The study by Nosek (1993) described earlier, reporting the health promoting qualities of personal assistance, is applicable here. Respite care may also be viewed as a form of health promotion for both family members and patients.

Strategies to meet the goal of health promotion cannot be considered complete if adequate consideration has not been given to the patient's sense of life satisfaction and well-being. Lifestyles that include goal-directed occupations that reflect competence, that are viewed as less stressful, and that permit meaning and the adequate expression of personal identity are likely to result in greater levels of life satisfaction (Christiansen, Backman, Little, & Nguyen, 1999). This is true regardless of disability status, employment, or age.

Weaving Strategies Into a Successful Plan of Care

Often, the care plan for a given person may involve a combination of strategies. For example, persons with a spinal cord injury at level C-6 may learn to use their remaining wrist movement to produce tenodesis action that extends and flexes the fingers sufficiently to permit grasp with the use of a wrist-driven flexor hinge splint. The movement made possible by the splint allows objects, such as a cup, to be grasped. However, these objects may need special modifications: A cup may have adapted handles or a rim designed to prevent spilling. In other instances, the addition of a flexible straw and lid may improve cup efficiency. When dining in a restaurant, the person may prefer the assistance of a family member or caregiver and avoid using the splint and adapted cup altogether. Each possible strategy for assisting with the performance of self-care tasks must be evaluated in terms of its simplicity, cost in time and energy, and perceived benefit to promoting an enhanced quality of life from the standpoint of a particular patient (Weingarden & Martin, 1989).

Because there are many ways to accomplish a given task, several strategies should be identified and used depending on individual preferences and the varied situational contexts in which valued roles must be performed. The context of the rehabilitation setting, including the physical environment, the persons involved, and the daily routines, varies from that of the patient's home and community. Thus, a self-care strategy appropriate for the clinical setting may not be appropriate for the home or community. Family members or other caregivers are often present in the postdischarge living environment to assist with self-care tasks, and devices may seem awkward, inefficient, or out of place. (See Box 4.2.)

Summary

The mainstay of occupational therapy practice consists of using strategies that enable persons to engage in daily occupations. In this chapter, the

---

Box 4.2

Independent or Interdependence?

What does independence mean? Certainly, it means more than simply doing something on your own. A person can be considered independent while performing tasks that require the use of adapted devices or environments, or while overseeing others to meet various needs. In truth, few persons in the modern world can claim that they are entirely self-reliant. Most of us depend on others extensively as we manage the affairs of our daily lives. We depend on others for practical reasons—on those who transport goods to the market, on those who manufacture and sell goods, and on those who work in service occupations, such as police officers, hair stylists, butchers, mechanics, bus drivers, and employees of public utilities.

We also depend on others for emotional support and for providing behavioral models and expectations that guide and influence our behavior. Our very understanding of the events in our daily lives is derived from shared interpretations of the world around us. Therefore, it can be claimed we are dependent on others for providing the very structure that gives us our sense that the reality of daily life has stability and continuity.

Many have argued that independence as a principal goal in occupational therapy is a misleading and potentially damaging concept as a means of viewing recovery or therapy outcome. Adopting a recovery model that recognizes and values interdependence will improve therapy and more accurately reflect the realities of our social existence. Perhaps, an interdependent view of outcomes in rehabilitation can provide a broader, more socially appropriate set of options for the therapist in planning self-care management strategies.

---

process of planning intervention was described. Planning is a process that bridges evaluation and intervention and that requires a careful analytical process that we call diagnostic and clinical reasoning. Both procedural (specific functional assessments and medical information) as well as narrative (the patient's story) types of information are considered in this clinical reasoning process.

During the evaluation phase, therapy personnel consider and analyze information from interviews, the patient's history, observations, and specific assessment instruments. After considering the established goals and evaluation data, an occupational therapy diagnosis is made. This occupational therapy diagnosis serves as a basis for planning intervention that is documented in a plan of care.

Therapy personnel have several possibilities for intervention, including the remediation of underlying impairments and the use of compensation strategies involving tasks, environments, and caregivers. Strategies to prevent disability and to promote health may also be included in the plan of care. Skilled, effective intervention weaves together an appropriate mix of many types of strategies as intervention progresses and the needs of the patient change. The art of therapeutic practice is to select the types of intervention that are most appropriate for a given patient. ◆

Study Questions

1. What are the elements in determining an occupational therapy diagnosis?

2. What is the difference between independence and interdependence?

3. What are the four major categories of intervention?

4. Define remediation.

5. Outline the steps in the occupational therapy intervention process.

6. What is the definition of cosmesis and why is it an important consideration in intervention?

References

Christiansen, C., Backman, C., Little, B. R., & Nguyen, A. (1999). Occupations and well-being: A study of personal projects. *American Journal of Occupational Therapy, 53,* 91–100.

Garber, S. L., & Gregorio, T. L. (1990). Upper extremity devices: Assessment of use by spinal cord injured patients with quadriplegia. *American Journal of Occupational Therapy, 44,* 126–131.

Gitlin, L. N., Levine, R., & Geiger, C. (1993). Adaptive device use by older adults with mixed disabilities. *Archives of Physical Medicine and Rehabilitation, 74,* 149–152.

Haworth, R. J. (1983). Use of aids during the first three months after total hip replacement. *British Journal of Rheumatology, 22,* 29–35.

Health Care Financing Administration. (n.d.). *Medicare Intermediary Manual* (Publication 13. Section 390-6.4, pp. 20–21). Washington, DC: U.S. Government Printing Office.

Holm, M. B., Rogers, J. C., & James, A. B. (1998). Treatment of activities of daily living. In M. E. Neistadt & E. B. Crepeau (Eds.), *Willard and Spackman's occupational therapy* (9th ed., pp. 323–364). Philadelphia: Lippincott.

Mattingly, C. (1991). The narrative nature of clinical reasoning. *American Journal of Occupational Therapy, 45,* 998–1005.

Mattingly, C., & Fleming, M. (1993). *Clinical reasoning: Forms of inquiry in a therapeutic practice.* Philadelphia: F. A. Davis.

National Center for Medical Rehabilitation Research. (1993). *Research plan for the National Center for Medical Rehabilitation Research.* Washington, DC: National Institutes of Health.

Newrick, R., & Langton-Hewer, R. (1984). Motor neuron disease: Can we do better? A study of 42 patients. *British Medical Journal, 289,* 539–542.

Nosek, M. A. (1993). Personal assistance: Its effect on the long term health of a rehabilitation hospital population. *Archives of Physical Medicine and Rehabilitation, 74,* 127–132.

Rogers, J. C., & Holm, M. B. (1991). Occupational therapy diagnostic reasoning: A component of clinical reasoning. *American Journal of Occupational Therapy, 45,* 1045–1053.

Rogers, J. C., & Holm, M. B. (1997). Diagnostic reasoning: The process of problem identification. In C. H. Christiansen & C. M. Baum (Eds.), *Occupational therapy: Enabling function and well-being* (pp. 138–156). Thorofare, NJ: Slack.

Smith, R. O. (1991). Technological approaches to performance enhancement. In C. Christiansen & C. Baum (Eds.), *Occupational therapy: Overcoming human performance deficits* (pp. 747–788). Thorofare, NJ: Slack.

Stein, R. B., & Walley, M. (1983). Functional comparison of upper extremity amputees using myoelectric and conventional prostheses. *Archives of Physical Medicine and Rehabilitation, 64,* 243–248.

Trombly, C. A. (1993). Anticipating the future: Assessment of occupational function. *American Journal of Occupational Therapy, 47,* 253–257.

Weingarden, S. I., & Martin, M. C. (1989). Independent dressing after spinal cord injury: A functional time evaluation. *Archives of Physical Medicine and Rehabilitation, 70,* 518–519.

World Health Organization. (1998). *International classification of impairments, activities, and participation (ICIDH-2)* (beta field release version). Geneva, Switzerland: Author.

5

Methods for Teaching Self-Care Skills

Martha E. Snell
Laura K. Vogtle

Martha E. Snell, PhD, is Professor of Education, Curry School of Education, University of Virginia, Charlottesville, Virginia

Laura K. Vogtle, PhD, is Assistant Professor, Division of Occupational Therapy, and Director, MasterUs Program, University of Alabama, Birmingham, Alabama.

The authors are grateful to Amy Evans and Jan Rowe for their careful reading of this manuscript and suggestions for revision.

Key Terms

acquisition

antecedents

baseline data

consequences

fluency

functional skills

generalization

graduated guidance

maintenance

partial participation

probe data

response latency

response prompts

stages of learning

stimulus prompts

system of least prompts

time delay

training data

Objectives

On completing this chapter, the reader will be able to

1. Discuss the need for age appropriate and functional guidelines/goals for future clients in their care.

2. Describe and detail the stages of learning that are part of skill development and relate them to age appropriate and functional guidelines or goals.

3. Discuss the importance of task analysis to the process used in teaching self-care skills.

4. Know the different components of teaching strategies, including the use of prompts and feedback and different kinds of antecedents and consequences, available for use when teaching self-care skills.

5. Understand the need for systematic evaluation to support the need for continuing or changing teaching strategies used in self-care training.

6. Understand the importance of careful documentation and graphing of baseline and training data to document progress and to support reimbursement requests.

R egardless of what tasks are being taught to whom, some general principles and methods of good instruction should be used during intervention. When the person being taught has cognitive limitations, several other guidelines should be reflected in teaching, and additional methods should be considered. The purpose of this chapter is to describe these principles and methods for occupational therapy practitioners. The chapter is organized into four sections: (a) initial planning of instruction, (b) direct assessment of performance, (c) teaching strategies to be used in treatment, and (d) evaluation of learning and teaching achieved during intervention.

Initial Planning of Instruction

Guiding Principles

Age appropriate and functional. Select teaching goals that

- are suited to the person's chronological age;

- are needed by that person now and later in life;

- are valued by the person, by his or her family members, and by peers;

- are likely to be achieved with or without task modifications;

- will contribute meaningfully to the person's independence; and

- may improve the person's positive self-image.

Perhaps the most important aspect of occupational therapy intervention involves decisions about setting appropriate goals. While it is possible to devise methods to develop just about any skilled behavior, if unneeded or inappropriate tasks are the focus of therapy, the learner's time (patient, client, or student) and the practitioner's time are wasted. For example, when modifications such as hook-and-loop fastening shoes or elastic laces are available and preferred by the learner, teaching shoe tying can be an inappropriate goal. Practitioners should consider several principles when selecting therapy goals in self-care.

1. Tasks chosen for intervention need to suit a person's chronological age.

2. Selected goals should be useful to the person in both current and future life settings.

3. Goals should be ones the person or the family members or both have chosen and deem important.

4. Goals should enable the person to achieve normalized outcomes seen in the typical population, such as self-management, mobility, leisure, employment, and so forth.

5. Even if partial participation rather than independent function is the goal, objectives that are realistic for the learner and suited to his or her life setting should be selected.

With persons who have cognitive disabilities, one often develops skills suitable for persons younger than the person to whom the skills are being taught. This approach violates the first principle. Sometimes the task targeted is valid (useful and age appropriate), but the activities, materials, or methods used to teach the skills are not. For example, teenagers with apraxia may be asked to toss beanbags into a wooden frog's mouth to improve eye-hand coordination, when an adapted pool game or a TV computer game would be more typical of activities chosen by this age group.

The second through the fifth principles address different aspects of skill functionality; that is, skills selected for instruction have meaning for the person being treated, can be used on a routine basis in familiar settings, and, if not learned, will need to be performed by someone else. Functional or useful goals are likely to be used, not forgotten through disuse, and will promote less dependence on others. Functional skills have purpose and, thus, are valued by others. Learning to perform skills that are valued by persons in the client's environment improves the way a person is viewed by others and by himself or herself. Selecting goals that have little value or purpose to the person means that the skills taught will not be used once learned.

For many persons, it is more appropriate to learn part of a task rather than to attempt the entire skill or to perform the skill in typical ways. This practice is known as partial participation (Baumgart et al., 1982) and includes

- help from others on difficult steps (e.g., the practitioner brushes Anne's teeth, but Anne learns to open her mouth, hold it open, and close it) (Snell, Lewis, & Houghton, 1989),

- changing the order of the task performance (e.g., John puts his bathing suit on before getting to the pool),

- changing the rules (e.g., Elliott bats for Tim, then pushes him in his wheelchair to the bases), or

• adding adaptations (e.g., Carla uses the computer by operating a large joystick switch).

Goals that include partial participation should be carefully planned so they will be functional in a persons's life settings and thus used. Reassessment at later times is important, because the person may be able to learn more or all of the task and, therefore, may need modifications or adjustments (Ferguson & Baumgart, 1991).

Functional skills often involve part of a daily schedule or routine and, thus, may include more extensive or independent activities of daily living. Brown and her colleagues (Brown, Evans, Weed, & Owen, 1987) described two types of related abilities that can help occupational therapy practitioners build a core activities of daily living (ADL) task to become part of a larger routine or role: extension and enrichment abilities. *Extension skills* include the ability to initiate a routine, prepare for the task, monitor the speed and quality of the task, problem-solve, and terminate the task or clean up when done. *Enrichment skills* involve expressive communication (through nonsymbolic or symbolic means), social behavior, and choice-making. The first column in Table 5.1 illustrates how this component model is applied to the task of grooming one's nails. (The remaining columns illustrate component analysis and will be discussed later in this chapter.)

When ADL skills are viewed in this comprehensive manner, practitioners need to work actively as part of a team and avoid "dividing up" the client into parts that reflect each team member's professional territory. Pooling talents will strengthen teaching strategies. Depending on the setting, a variety of persons (staff members, peers, family members) may contribute to teaching a self-care task. Professionals will pay closer attention to teaching the motor and cognitive learning requirements involved. However, all who assist in teaching or supervising task performance should be alert to the variety of extension skills (initiate, prepare, monitor tempo, etc.) and expansion skills (communication, choice-making, and social behavior) that are embedded within ADL tasks.

Ecological inventories. How does one determine which tasks are functional for a particular person? The most important source of this information is the client. If at all able to give information through interview or direct assessment, the person who will be the focus of intervention needs to contribute to the initial assessment. Skill checklists, such as ADL inventories, are often used to assess current abilities and to identify target goals. They can be particularly

valuable for those clients who are unable to contribute to interviews. Although ADL checklists can help determine if a person has the obvious prerequisite skills, they may lead practitioners to focus on skills that are not needed or that are less needed than others. Sometimes the sequencing nature of a checklist causes clinicians to regard tasks appearing earlier on the list as prerequisites to later skills, when they may not be. This assumption is particularly true for early childhood assessments, such as the Denver II (Frankenburg, Dodds, Archer, Shapiro, & Bresnick, 1992). To avoid this problem and to develop a more comprehensive picture of the client in his or her routine environments, practitioners can interview those who know most about the person's current performance needs, such as parents and family members, past teachers, peers, and practitioners; and those who would be familiar with upcoming skill needs, such as the next teacher or practitioner, peers, job coaches, and so forth.

Some examples of these indirect methods of functional assessment are the Pediatric Evaluation of Disability Inventory (Haley, Ludlow, & Coster, 1993), the Functional Independence Measure (Hamilton, Laughlin, Fiedler, & Granger, 1994), and the Functional Independence Measure for Children (McCabe & Granger, 1990). These assessment tools are described elsewhere in this book. Comparable assessments exist in special education and are called ecological inventories and environmental assessments (Brown & Snell, in press; Ford et al., 1989; Giangreco, Cloninger, & Iverson, 1993). By using these kinds of tools, references for goals are assessed through direct interview or by observation. "Informants" who know the client or who know settings client will use in the future are asked questions, such as the following:

• What skills do you think are important for _____ to learn?

• What skills are required of _____ that he or she does not know or that others must perform regularly?

• Are there some skills critical to _____'s safety and health that he or she might learn partially or totally?

• What skills are expected of _____'s peers in the same activities and places?

• Could _____ learn to assist with this skill (partial participation) or to perform the skill with adaptations? Without adaptations?

The client may be asked a variety of questions (or may be observed with input from those who know

Methods for Teaching Self-Care Skills

Table 5.1 Task Analysis Illustrating the Sensorimotor Task Component Model Used for Treatment Planning

Task Step	Task Component	Sensory Component	Motor Component	Grasp Component
Inspects nails to see if dirty or jagged	Initiation of task	Vision, light touch	Finger extension, wrist extension, forearm supination and pronation	N/A
Finds and selects materials	Preparation for task	Vision, light touch, pressure discrimination	Finger flexion and extension, wrist extension, elbow flexion and extension, possible shoulder action	Radial digital grasp, lateral tip pinch, pad-to-pad pinch
Cleans and trims nails	Core steps of task	Vision, pain, light touch, pressure discrimination	MCP and IP flexion, extension, and abduction for all digits, including the thumb; wrist flexion and extension; ulnar and radial deviation; isolated finger control	Lateral tip pinch, pad-to-pad pinch, possible gross grasp
Checks nails for cleanliness and neatness	Quality monitoring	Vision	MCP and IP flexion and wrist extension, possible shoulder action	N/A
Grooms nails within an acceptable amount of time	Tempo monitoring	Rapid motor response to sensory input	Use of feedforward and feedback mechanisms to ensure motor efficiency, finger flexion and extension, possible shoulder action	Rapid change of grasp patterns as required by the task
Resolves problems that arise (such as locating materials)	Problem solving	Variable	Variable	Variable
Puts trimming supplies away	Termination of task	Vision, light touch, pressure discrimination	Finger flexion and extension, wrist extension, elbow flexion and extension, possible shoulder action	Radial digital grasp, lateral tip pinch, pad-to-pad pinch
Communicates about any aspect of nail grooming (such as length of nails, hang nail)	Communication	Variable	Variable	N/A
Makes choices within task (such as to polish or not)	Choice-making	Variable	Variable	Variable
Performs routine at appropriate time and location	Social aspect of task	Variable	Variable	Variable

Note. IP = interphalangeal; MCP = metacarpophalangeal; N/A = not applicable.

61

him or her to deduce the answers), such as "What skills do you want to learn? What part of this skill is hard for you? What part of this skill is easy for you?"

Therapy personnel also may examine program entry requirements or may visit programs, desired places of employment, or future residences to understand what skills are needed for the person to participate and to consider creative accommodations. Once complete information is obtained, practitioners work with the client's team to set priorities. They consider assessment information from all team members at this time. The skills that seem most needed and functional for the person typically become intervention objectives or habitation targets.

Stage of Learning

Learning is often viewed as occurring in stages or phases, from initial instruction or acquisition to expanded instruction or generalized skills (Snell & Brown, in press). During the initial phase of teaching, learners receive assistance and more feedback (reinforcement and error correction) as they progress to the stage of self-regulated, developed skills. *Prompting* refers to the assistance provided to move a learner from initial learning to mastery of a skill. Others call this assistance *scaffolding* (Wood, Bruner, & Ross, 1976). Regardless of the term, most agree that some assistance should be provided initially to decrease a learner's frustration with new or difficult tasks and to facilitate success while reducing errors. What type of assistance to provide and how much depends on the learner's cognitive and motor abilities and personal preferences. As the learner's competence increases, assistance is reduced. Figure 5.1 illustrates the relationship among the four stages of learning (Snell & Brown, in press).

1. *Acquisition learning* concerns initial learning of a skill. In this stage, learners may not be able to perform the target skill at all or may perform with limited competence (performance accuracy ranges from 0%–60%).

2. *Maintenance learning* concerns the routine use of a skill and improving its accuracy under fairly stable and familiar conditions. At this stage, learners perform the target skill with limited competence but do not initiate the task during typical daily routine (roughly 60% accuracy or better during maintenance).

3. *Fluency or proficiency learning* concerns improving the accuracy, quality, and speed of performance. At this stage, learners perform the skill with limited competence in that they may be too slow,

sloppy, or inattentive to detail (roughly 60% accuracy or better).

4. *Generalization learning* concerns performance under changing conditions (location, materials, time, task variation, etc.). At this stage, learners perform the skill with limited competence in that they fail to initiate or are unable to complete the task when the performance context changes in some way (roughly 60% or better accuracy).

On the basis of these brief descriptions, it becomes clear that teaching approaches and criteria should vary somewhat to match the different stages of learning. When therapy personnel view learning in these four stages, they are more likely to adjust their teaching methods as they shift their teaching focus from one stage to another; to avoid an overemphasis on new skills; and to broaden their teaching focus so maintenance, fluency, and skill generalization are equally valued with acquisition or beginning performance of new skills.

While skills proceed from acquisition to later stages, instruction can focus concurrently on stages 2 through 4 if practitioners are clear about their goals, if instruction does not get too complex, and if task performance data are kept to evaluate whether learning is occurring. The following case may help clarify this process.

After a head injury, 13-year-old April wanted to learn to put her shoes, socks, and ankle-foot orthoses on fast enough so that she could put them on every day before school rather than having her parents do it for her. This project was undertaken in June with hopes for proficiency in the task by early September. The final goal of 10 to 15 minutes for putting the items on was decided on with input from the parents. In the acquisition learning phase, the therapist worked with her on accuracy: getting shoes and socks on over her heels and putting the orthoses on correctly. Once she achieved correct performance about two thirds of the time on these difficult steps, the focus shifted to maintenance. Her parents agreed she could perform the task by herself on weekends, and they would simply check out whether items were on correctly when she was done and document her performance speed. April was working on independent maintenance of her skills. Her parents agreed to purchase Velcro®-fastening shoes to eliminate lacing and tying that could improve her speed from her initial efforts of 40 minutes. Throughout the summer, she worked hard and used a clock to time herself. April's efforts to use shoes with Velcro® fasteners and her daily monitoring of performance time represents a focus on flu-

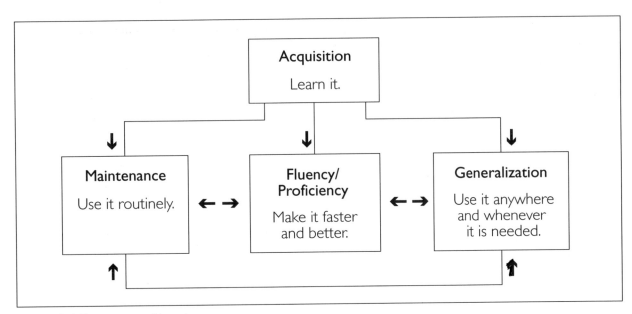

Figure 5.1 Four stages of learning.

ency learning. By mid-July, she was able to get the orthoses on tight enough that her family members no longer worried about blisters. Her time was reduced to 25 minutes—good but still short of her goal. April and her parents made several additional task improvements that were aimed at improving fluency even more, that is, better timing while still getting her orthoses on tight enough. First, April would get up early enough to put her shoes on before her parents left for work. With this arrangement, she usually managed to get up 4 to 5 days a week to work on speed. Second, the therapist made improvements in the orthoses' Velcro® fasteners, which made the task easier. By the start of school, April was able to get all items on in 15 minutes and was willing to get up early enough to put them on by herself each day. Once back in school, April requested that she work on generalizing the skill from home to school. At the end of October, she was able to change her shoes for physical education in 10 minutes without help.

Maintenance and generalization are promoted even during initial learning (acquisition) when practitioners select skills that are functional, needed, or valued by others, because these skills will be routinely required over multiple settings. By targeting tasks suited to the person's age, he or she may be more inclined to use them, and peers, family members, or practitioners will tend to encourage appropriate skills more than they would skills or behaviors that stigmatize the person in some way. Additionally, when skills are not fluent or proficient, other persons

are not likely to encourage their use. For example, consider the following.

- A fifth grade boy who writes so slowly that the parents always do his assigned homework
- Caregivers for a woman who recently had a stroke often perform many of her ADL tasks because the client forgets to care for her affected side
- A young woman who knows how to make up beds but cannot be hired for motel housekeeping because sheets and blankets are draped unevenly and none of the wrinkles are smoothed

These examples are problems in fluency and generalization; and unless the therapeutic process addresses them, instruction does not result in skills that others will value. Stated another way, those skills that cannot be performed at a reasonable speed with required accuracy and quality or cannot be used regardless of changes in materials and location are not socially valid skills.

During the acquisition stage of learning, practitioners can build some elements into the intervention plan that will promote generalization from early on. Ways to do this include

- teaching under natural or as close to natural conditions as possible;
- using real, not simulated, materials that are appropriate to the task (e.g., real shoes to teach dressing and shoe tying; real clothes to teach dressing and buttoning, not button boards or dolls, although larger clothes may be used during early instruction);

- involving multiple teaching examples (staff members, locations, materials, etc.); and
- selecting the multiple examples carefully, starting with those that best sample the range of variation (e.g., a turtleneck, tank top, and T-shirt are taught first because they best sample the range of variations in collar, sleeve length, fit, and fabric from a group of eight pull-over shirts) (Day & Horner, 1986).

This practice of teaching the general case teaches persons a generalized skill that is durable across commonly expected changes in stimulus conditions and response requirements.

Target objectives or goals must specify the behavior, the criterion for performance, and the conditions or context under which the behavior or skill will be performed. The conditions for performing a skill concern issues of when and where the task is performed, who is present, what materials are involved, and what assistance or adaptations are allowed or possible. A general rule to follow is to let the individual learner's reality dictate the conditions for learning. If the person shows little or no learning under natural conditions, then the conditions may be simplified; for example, with fewer variations in materials, location, times, and practitioners; with less noise and distraction, and so forth. Eventually, however, the person must learn to perform the skill under natural conditions or the skill will not be useful.

The occupational therapy practitioner collaborates with other team members to rewrite selected teaching goals as instructional objectives. Using April's case from earlier in the chapter, we illustrate the objective her team wrote for the skill of putting on shoes and socks.

Target objective: April will be able to put her Velcro®-fastening shoes, socks, and ankle–foot orthoses on in 10 minutes each morning at home before school without assistance from her parents.

Behavior: Putting on Velcro®-fastening shoes, socks, and orthoses

Performance criterion: In 10 minutes

Conditions or context:

  When: Each morning before school

  Where: At home

  Who is present: No one

  Materials: Shoes, socks, and ankle–foot orthoses

  Assistance: None, by herself

  Modifications: Velcro® fasteners

Direct Assessment of Skills

Often we have referred to assessment and data collection as an evil necessity. We use the evil label for several reasons.

- Persons seldom learn during evaluation, so it seems like wasted time.
- Many practitioners find assessment or data collection tedious and time-consuming, especially when time with a client is restricted by reimbursement or case-load size.
- Many practitioners are less experienced in using the data gathered and, thus, cannot justify the effort it takes.

But some performance data are necessary, because only information relevant to the performance of the target behavior can provide the objective information required to judge the success of therapy. For instruction during therapy to be efficient and effective, practitioners need to gather and analyze performance data related to the identified goals. When data indicate minimal or slower progress than expected, the therapy approach or conditions can be changed. Likewise, if the data indicate that the goal has been met, then instruction can be directed toward a different stage of learning for the same skill or toward other skills.

> Ron, an adolescent with a spinal cord injury, has learned to perform several wheelchair push-ups every 15 minutes with 60% accuracy over an 8-hour day. On the basis of these data, his therapist might direct therapy toward additional improvement in his accuracy while also shifting the focus of instruction toward several new goals. These goals might include (a) promoting his routine and spontaneous use of the skill in all the situations where training has occurred (maintenance), (b) improving his consistency of performing push-ups (fluency), and (c) extending the expectation for unprompted push-ups to the home or school setting (generalization).

Assessment Data

Observational data. There are many kinds of data pertinent to teaching skills. This discussion primarily addresses *client performance data;* that is, data that measure some aspect of skill performance relevant to the goals set by the practitioner, client, and family members. These data are mainly collected through direct observation of the client or patient during performance of the skill. However, valuable data can be collected *after* the skill has been performed. There are at least three different ways to do this.

1. Measure the permanent products resulting from the performance (e.g., checking to see if Josh fastens all his pajama buttons correctly after bathing; estimating the spillage on the table and floor after Sam finishes eating).

2. Socially validate the client's performance by seeking the opinions of peers or caregivers on the success of instruction of a skill they regularly see (e.g., Is Sam's eating neat enough?).

3. Socially validate the client's performance outcomes by comparing the client's performance with peers for the same skill (e.g., How fast and how neatly do Sam's peers eat?).

Peer comparisons to validate program outcomes socially can be made in two ways: (a) obtain the subjective opinions of peers (e.g., in sensitive ways, ask peers to help by suggesting how Sam could "fit in" better at lunch) and (b) compare the client's performance to the peers' performance (e.g., note the spillage by Sam's place in contrast to his peers or observe to see if peers and Sam clear their trash).

Test and training data. Observational data on performance are collected under either training or test conditions. Both types of data (training and test) can be useful to practitioners. *Training data* reflect student performance during training or treatment sessions (e.g., when assistance, corrective feedback, and reinforcement are provided according to the therapy plan). *Test data* reflect performance during nontraining conditions (also referred to as criterion conditions) when little or no assistance or feedback is available other than that naturally occurring in the environment. Test data often show lower performance than do training data.

Types of Tasks

Discrete and chained behaviors. Target behaviors can be thought of as being either *discrete behaviors* (individually distinctive behaviors that stand alone) or *chained behaviors* (a routine or skill involving a sequence of discrete behaviors). Practitioners target many types of discrete behaviors, including lip closure, steps taken during walking, type of grasp used during household chores, and time taken to get dressed. Discrete behavior targets are typically defined in observable terms, then counted during a fixed period of time or over a set number of opportunities. For example, a practitioner defines what constitutes the form of grasping that is targeted for Muriel who is a 5-year-old with cerebral palsy. The targeted grasp is the correct response and other

inappropriate versions of picking up and holding toys and objects are incorrect responses. Then the daily activities during which grasping occurs and which can be measured are identified, along with the length of the observation period. Data gathered might be rate of performance, such as the number of correct and error grasps Muriel makes during 10 minutes of toy and block play with peers in kindergarten. Because this example might be highly variable because of changing opportunities during play, a better measurement procedure might be to count her correct (and error) grasps during the first 10 opportunities to grasp during playtime.

Chained behaviors are those involving a sequence of behaviors that constitute a skill or that complete a task. The sequence of behaviors often is identified as steps in a task analysis of the skill. Examples include dressing tasks; standing and transfer tasks; some vocational skills; and most grooming, housekeeping, and cooking tasks. Frequently, task analyses serve as the guide for teaching and testing because they list the behaviors and the sequence involved in performing target skills.

Preparing task analyses. Task analysis can be broadly defined as the process of scrutinizing and breaking down routines or relationships between sequenced chains of behavior. Often what practitioners teach is analyzed into smaller steps or component behaviors (Watson, 1997). Commercially available task analyses may seem to be time-savers, but we do not recommend them, because they fail to individualize the task to the context: person, location, and materials. Instead, to develop good task analyses, several steps are important as follows:

• Spend time observing the person and others performing the task.

• Develop the best approaches for completing the task.

• Ask others' opinions about the task performance (including the person who will learn it or family members who will support it).

• Field-test the task analyses and revise them with needed improvements.

To promote skill generalization, develop a task analysis that is relatively generic or suits a number of situations where the learner will need to perform the skill (see Table 5.2).

The task analysis in Table 5.2 breaks eating, drinking, and wiping with a napkin into response steps and identifies the relevant stimuli (discriminative stimuli) for each response. While there are many

Table 5.2 Task Analysis for Teaching Spoon, Cup, and Napkin Use

Behavior	Discriminative Stimuli	Response
Spoon	"Eat"	Grasp spoon
	Spoon in hand	Scoop food
	Food in spoon	Raise spoon to lips
	Spoon touching lips	Open mouth
	Mouth open	Put spoon in mouth
	Food in mouth	Remove spoon
	Spoon out of mouth	Lower spoon
	Spoon on table	Release grasp
Cup	"Drink"	Grasp cup
	Cup in hand	Raise cup to lips
	Cup touches lips	Tilt cup to mouth
	Liquid in mouth	Close mouth and drink
	Liquid swallowed	Lower cup to table
	Cup on table	Release grasp
Napkin	"Wipe"	Grasp napkin
	Napkin in hand	Raise hand to face
	Napkin touching face	Wipe face
	Face wiped	Lower napkin
	Napkin on table	Release grasp

Note. From "Using Constant Time Delay to Teach Self-Feeding to Young Students With Severe/Profound Handicaps: Evidence of Limited Effectiveness" by B. C. Collins, D. L. Gast, M. Wolery, A. Holcombe, and J. Letherby, 1991. *Journal of Developmental and Physical Difficulties, 3,* p. 163. Copyright© 1991 by Plenum Publishing. Reprinted by permission.

ways to analyze tasks, the approach illustrated earlier in Table 5.1 focuses on component analysis or an analysis of the sensory, motor, and grasp components in addition to the behavior chain involved in the skill or activity. What task analysis methods have in common is the delineation of sequenced, observable behaviors that lead to the accomplishment of a given task. The kind of task analysis used will depend on the needs of the child, the user (therapy practitioner, teacher, or parent), and the nature of the therapeutic goals.

We have found the following guidelines valuable in the development of task analyses.

1. Use steps of fairly even size

2. Be sure each step is observable and results in a visible change in behavior

3. Order the steps in a logical sequence, but indicate when the sequence is optional

4. Distinguish any steps requiring another person's assistance and those parts of the task performed by persons other than the student or client

5. Write the task steps in second-person singular (so they can be used as verbal prompts)

6. Use language meaningful to the student or client with whom it will be used and place in parentheses any additional information that may be difficult for the client to understand but needed for the observer (e.g., using a pincer grasp)

7. Place the steps on a task analytic data sheet that allows one to record step-by-step data over a number of days (see Figure 5.2) (Snell & Brown, in press)

Conducting task analytic assessments. Once a good task analysis is prepared, the therapy practitioner uses it as a guide for observing and measuring the client's performance and for teaching the skill or task. The client or student is asked to perform the skill, then each behavior or step in the task analysis is observed and scored as correct or incorrect. For example, Figure 5.2 contains the teaching objective and task analysis for the routine tasks Chris needs to gain independence in sitting down on a chair.

Chris is a boy 3½ years of age who attends a preschool 5 mornings a week. His therapy is integrated into daily activities to address func-

Name: Chris
Instructor: Maura
Instructional Cue: "Find you chair"
Program: Sitting
Method: Least to Most/4-second latency

Objective: Given a natural opportunity or a request to sit in a preschool cube chair for an activity and a response latency of 4 second, Chris will perform correctly on at least 88% (7 of 8 steps) of the task analysis without assistance for 3 consecutive training opportunities and one probe.

Step	2/27*	3/4*	3/5*	3/6*	3/7*	3/18	3/19	3/20	3/21	3/22	3/25	4/8	4/11	4/12	4/16	4/17	4/18	4/22	4/23	4/26	4/29	4/30	5/1	5/2*
		Baseline*									Training													Probe
1. Face cube chair	—	—	—	—	—	P	P	P	P	P	V	+	+	+	+	+	+	+	+	+	+	+	+	+
2. Bend forward	—	—	—	—	—	P	P	P	P	P	V	+	+	+	+	+	+	+	+	+	+	+	+	+
3. Grip arm handles	—	—	—	—	—	G	+	G	G	G	V	+	+	+	+	+	+	V	+	+	+	+	+	+
4. Shift right arm to left arm handle	—	—	—	—	—	P	P	P	P	P	P	+	+	+	+	+	G	+	+	+	+	+	+	+
5. Twist trunk and hips	—	—	—	—	—	P	P	P	+	+	V	+	+	V	V	+	+	+	+	+	+	+	+	+
6. Lower bottom to chair	—	—	—	—	+	+	+	+	+	+	+	+	+	+	+	+	+	+	+	+	+	+	+	+
7. Reposition hands and feet	+	—	+	+	+	+	+	+	+	+	+	+	+	+	+	+	+	+	+	P	+	+	+	+
8. Push bottom to back of chair using feet and hands	+	+	+	+	+	+	+	+	+	+	+	+	+	+	+	+	+	+	+	P	+	+	+	+
	25	13	25	25	38	58	50	38	50	50	38	100	100	88	88	100	88	88	100	75	100	100	100	100*

Key:

Baseline*
(+) independent
(—) error

Training
(+) independent
(V) verbal prompt
(G) gestural prompt
(P) physical prompt

Figure 5.2 Task analysis data sheet for Chris's objective of sitting down in a chair. Created by Maura Burke. Used by permission.

tional skill needs and to improve the likelihood that he will generalize his learning to the daily routine. Before being taught this skill, Chris waited for help to sit down and to stand up from a chair, as his balance was unsteady and he sometimes fell when not assisted. His therapy practitioners and teachers planned to use a total-task approach to develop the ability to both sit in and stand up from a chair, so that whenever training and practice occurred, each step would be performed in order, with the needed assistance provided. His teachers used the task analysis to guide their observation of his performance on each step.

Two general methods of task analytic observation can be used: single opportunity and multiple opportunity. With single-opportunity task analytic assessment, the learner is asked to perform the task. Testing stops after the first error, with all remaining steps scored as errors. Errors include performing the wrong step, making a mistake on a step, taking too long (if time is important), or not performing. With multiple-opportunity task analytic assessment, the learner is asked to perform the task. Each step is observed. Whenever an error occurs, it is recorded, and the tester positions the student for the next step. Positioning for testing a step is done without comment or instruction because this is a testing context not a teaching one.

Chris's teacher and therapist decided to use a multiple-opportunity task analytic assessment approach so they could observe his performance on all steps during each test. His baseline performance over 5 days of assessment was collected and graphed (Figures 5.2 and 5.3). He consistently missed the first 5 steps, but was successful on the last 3, though inconsistently and with slightly improving performance over the 5 days. His baseline performance seems to indicate that Chris did not know the skill and that selecting the task as a goal was appropriate. His parents and teacher also indicated independent sitting and standing as much-needed skills for many daily activities at home and at school.

When enrichment goals (communication, choice-making, social behavior) are addressed at the same time as the original or core skills, these goals can simply be placed on the task analysis sheet. For example, if the teacher and therapist want to include making a choice about which chair to sit in or about verbalizing his success ("Sit!" as Chris sometimes says when he is successful), these choice-making and communication goals could go directly into the task sequence (if that can be predicted). Or, they could simply be listed at the end of the

task analysis with frequency count entered for each observation. If it is helpful for practitioners to keep a record of significant problem behaviors that occur (e.g., having tantrums, falling down, or legs giving out), these behaviors can be defined and added to the end of the task steps as well.

The graph of Chris's performance data (Figure 5.3) is summarized in percentage form; that is, the percent of 8 task steps performed correctly during each observation. Because Chris is still in the acquisition stage of learning (< 60% correct), his team decided to include only core behaviors in the task analysis and not to include extension skills (initiate, prepare, problem-solve, monitor tempo and quality, and terminate). These extension skills might be added later along with enrichment skills (communication, choice-making, social behavior). However, if enrichment behaviors are added to a task analysis, they are graphed separately from the core skill steps or from the core steps plus extension skills. Any problem behaviors added to the bottom of the task analysis need to be analyzed separately, because the intended goal is to decrease their frequency by replacing them with more appropriate behaviors. The use of data and graphing is discussed further in the last section of this chapter.

Teaching Strategies

Before discussing general teaching strategies, it might be helpful to review Table 5.3 that illustrates the events that may take place before and after the targeted self-care behavior. *Antecedent events* are those things that occur before the target behavior; some events are intentionally arranged while other antecedents may not be under the practitioner's control.

> Just before learning spoon, cup, and napkin use at lunch (see the task analysis in Table 5.2), Sam is hungry. Hunger serves as a powerful internal antecedent stimulus. The school bell ringing at lunchtime and classmates rushing to their backpacks to get packed lunches are also stimuli that set the occasion for lunchtime. Once the children are seated in the lunchroom, more specific stimuli are present, such as the therapist's request to Sam "Let's eat," and also task discriminative stimuli created by performing each response in the chain of taking a spoonful of food.

As shown in Table 5.2, performance of each response (right-hand column) creates an antecedent discriminative stimulus (middle column) relevant to the next or upcoming response in the chain.

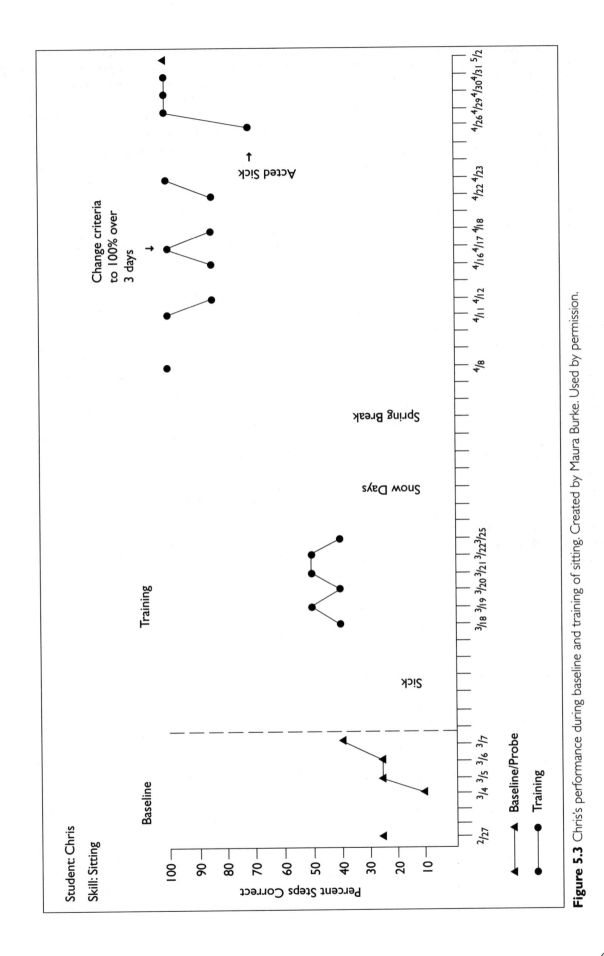

Figure 5.3 Chris's performance during baseline and training of sitting. Created by Maura Burke. Used by permission.

Table 5.3 Possible Antecedent and Consequence Events That May Precede and Follow the Target Response

Antecedent Events			
New Stimuli "To Be Learned"	**Controlling Stimuli or Prompts**	**Response**	**Consequence**
Teacher's request	Response prompts	Correct response	Confirmation reinforcement
Task materials	Verbal instructions	Approximation	Self-reinforcement
Time of day	Pictorial prompts	Incorrect response	Praise and approval
Location	Gestures/pointing	Error	Choice
Persons present	Modeling	No response	Preferred activity
Internal stimuli	Physical assistance Partial Full	Inappropriate behavior	Tangible reinforcer
			Error feedback
	Stimulus prompts Color coding Stimulus fading		Pause for self-correction
			Ignore and no positive reinforcement
			Correction

[handwritten note: Why pt. does activity]

To teach Sam the three targeted mealtime skills, his practitioners decided to use physical prompts, such as hand-over-hand assists, or planned antecedent events; they used only as much hand-over-hand assistance as was needed to get him to demonstrate each behavior in the three targeted chains. The physical prompt worked for Sam; that is, the physical assistance prompts controlled his behavior, but the discriminative stimuli that resulted from performing each step of the task did not yet control the responses that they preceded. When the therapist placed the spoon in Sam's hand, he seemed to know he needed to scoop some food, but he did not yet respond in a way that got food on the spoon. One major goal of instruction was to fade out the controlling antecedents that were provided by teachers or practitioners (i.e., requests to "eat" and physical prompts). At the same time, Sam was taught to attend to the relevant antecedent stimuli (i.e., food on his plate with a spoon, napkin, and filled glass beside it; spoon in hand, food on spoon, spoon touching lips, etc.).

Also portrayed in Table 5.3 are *consequences*, or the events (planned or unplanned) that may be used after a target response. During treatment sessions, consequences include

- comments or information given about the accuracy of the response (confirmation of accuracy—"that's right");

- feedback about an error ("You forgot to hold the bottom of the zipper" while pointing to the end of the zipper);

- reinforcement (approval, praise, activity choice, tangibles);

- correction;

- extinction or waiting for self-correction, ignoring errors, withholding comments when performance is not "up to par"; and

- punishing consequences (withholding reinforcement, giving sharp criticism, requiring excessive practice after an error, time out).

Let us offer a few comments on punishing consequences. Much of the early special education research on self-care instruction of persons with developmental disabilities employed punishing consequences or intensive teaching practices or both (e.g., excessively lengthy training sessions) (Farlow & Snell, in press). Now, however, punishing consequences are regarded as socially invalid practices. We know that for most learners punishment does not contribute to creating good learning conditions. First, punishment does not teach skills nor does it always reduce problem behaviors. Second, the practitioner is put into a position of "me against you" control, emphasizing the negative aspects of a teaching relationship, which may hinder the practitioner's effectiveness as a teacher. Third, punitive methods often are socially invalid or unacceptable to professionals, peers, or care providers and may violate the learner's basic rights. When a problem behavior exists that is not serious, it is best to ignore it and focus on teaching needed skills or alternate replacement skills. If the problem behavior harms the learner, others, or task materials, a careful study of the situation is called for with the possible development of a behavior support plan. This chapter cannot deal adequately with this important topic, and the reader is referred to a variety of useful references on problem behavior (Carr et al., 1994; Durand, 1990; Meyer & Evans, 1989; Zirpoli & Melloy, 1993).

Artificial and Natural Prompts and Feedback

Antecedents and consequences can be naturally occurring or intentionally arranged by a practitioner. They can either help or hinder learning. As clients advance into different stages of learning, artificial antecedents and consequences should be faded out, leaving only those consequences that are natural, because these are the stimuli that clients must attend to and perform around. The teaching task becomes one of directing learners to attend to things in the environment that assist them in performing skills. In many cases, natural cues should be emphasized as prompts from the very beginning of learning.

> Sam, who is learning to use a spoon and napkin, will benefit from having his teachers call attention to his peers, who sit nearby and can remind him to wipe his face clean.

> Rose, an older woman described in chapter 8 who has recently had a stroke, is relearning many of the daily living skills she once performed with ease. The practitioner's verbal, gestural, and physical assists will be helpful, as will the confirmations about her performance and the help with her errors. However, Rose must learn to pay attention to the visual and tactile cues from the left side of her body and the cues of material placement. This attention will permit her to self-regulate and recognize whether or not her body is moving as it should be while she is dressing or helping her daughter with meal preparation (e.g., patting lettuce dry, putting salad in a bowl). In place of the practitioner's consequences, the comments and reactions of others that naturally occur will become the corrective and reinforcing consequences.

For many children, adolescent, and adult clients, the natural antecedents of peer modeling and the

consequences of peer approval provide important means for learners to judge their own performance.

Antecedents: Instructional Cues

An *instructional cue* can be a request to perform a target skill ("Get your lunch" or "Find your chair"), or it may be other stimuli that alert the learner to perform the task without a request.

> Sam follows his peers to the cafeteria line; their actions of lining up, getting a tray, taking a spoon and fork, moving down the line, and so forth cue him to begin the task of moving through the line to get his lunch.

> Chris hears his teacher call "circle time" and watches his peers move to their cube chairs.

One common error of therapy personnel and teachers is saying too much. When the instructional cue is a request, it should be stated once in a way that the client understands. Instructional cues should not be questions ("Do you want to tie you shoes?") unless the client is being given an option to do the task. To make cues understandable, the practitioner must be familiar with the client's level of comprehension. Spoken instructional cues may be accompanied by gestures if symbolic communication is less meaningful or by signs or picture symbols if the learner uses these symbols to augment or replace verbal communication. When the person does not make the desired response, assistance or prompts are given to encourage his or her performance rather than just repeating the cue.

The best conditions for teaching most people involve embedding instruction within the activity or routine, thus providing many natural cues for the learner (e.g., location, task materials, time of day, others performing a similar task, and the need for the task to be completed).

> For Chris, who is learning to sit and stand by himself during preschool activities, the natural cues include his peers getting cube chairs, the teacher calling for circle time, and others taking a seat. Chris's performance after several weeks of training was good enough for his therapist to replace the instructional cue, "Find your chair" with directing his attention to natural cues. Whenever Chris failed to perform the first task step, then the teacher and therapist will use one of three prompts given in order of increasing assistance, and only as needed.

Antecedents: Prompts

Types of prompts. As shown in Table 5.3, there are two general types of prompts (response prompts and stimulus prompts). Stimulus prompts (also called stimulus modification procedures by Wolery, Ault, & Doyle, 1992) require a gradual change from easy to hard. This is exemplified by fading out color coding to teach a child to discriminate her grooming items from those of her classmates and family members or by teaching a person to write his or her name by fading the stimulus prompts from tracing letters, to thickly dotted letters, to thinly dotted letters, and finally to no dotted guidelines.

By comparison, response prompts encompass various types of teacher assistance that are directed toward the learner's responding. In an order of increasing assistance, they include

- specific verbal instructions ("open the shampoo");
- pictorial or two-dimensional prompts, such as showing the learner photos of task steps;
- gestures, such as pointing to needed materials or gesturing toward children's seats when it is time to begin class;
- the provision of models or demonstrations of the target response; and
- physical assistance, either partial (nudging a client's hand toward the toothpaste) or full assistance (using hand-over-hand assistance to get the client to pick up the toothpaste) (Wolery et al., 1992).

We will limit our detailed discussion to response prompts, as they are both more versatile for self-care tasks but also require less effort to use.

Prompts can be given individually (e.g., verbal request to pick up the soap in a hand-washing task or demonstrating the first step in a job task), in combinations (e.g., verbal request plus pointing to the soap; therapist gestures toward the fourth photo in an instruction book that illustrates 8 steps involved in shaving), or as part of a planned hierarchy of prompts given one at a time as needed.

Latency. With many prompts, a short *latency* or period of time is given before prompting a client to initiate the task step without help. The latency may be as short as 3 seconds or as long as 15 seconds, but it needs to be determined on an individualized basis depending on the client's natural response latency on known tasks (i.e., how long it takes the client to initiate a fairly familiar task step). Response latency will be slower when muscle tone is atypical and movement is less volitional or when vision is limited.

Selection of prompts. Prompts must be selected to fit the client, the situation, and the task. For exam-

ple, some students or clients with cerebral palsy or other neurological conditions may understand the task and the order of its steps but need to learn to manage their tone, to develop muscle control, and to grade movement. For these learners, prompts of deep pressure on the required muscles may be far more effective than verbal or model prompts.

> In a three-step task analysis of standing up from sitting written for Chris, the therapist provides support at the knees after Chris scoots to the edge of the chair and then positions his hands on the arm rests. At this point, Chris can push up to stand.

Some prompts depend on the learner having certain kinds of component skills before they can be used; if the learner does not have these skills, the prompt is not a controlling stimulus for a given response.

> Rose's therapist has made some task-step photos to prompt her completion of daily living tasks; but because Rose has very limited vision and does not readily associate pictured items with three-dimensional items, the photos will not prompt the required response. Her therapist will need to select another prompt that "works" for Rose or enlarge the photos and teach her to associate them with objects first.

Some kinds of assistance may be more permanently added to the task for steps clients cannot master independently (permanent assistance or partial participation). This version of partial participation may involve prolonged personal assistance in that it may include various inhibitive or facilitative therapy techniques, such as tone reduction during a movement, support at a point of control (the hips, elbow, etc.), or even the performance of one or several entire steps.

> Roberta, an occupational therapist, applies a tone-reduction technique, such as firm vibration at the forearm and wrist whenever working with John on dressing skills. This personal assistance or permanent prompt is continued (rather than faded out) because it allows John to move his arm forward. In the same dressing task, the therapist completes several very difficult non-target steps (place the shirt over John's head and hold one sleeve out) but teaches the remaining task steps.

Fading. Many ways exist to prompt someone who does not know the steps in a particular task. Because all prompts will need to be faded out for the person to achieve complete independence, prompts must be added to instruction with care. Unneeded or overly excessive assistance will only create more dependency on the practitioner. In the sections that follow, we describe five effective prompting procedures. These prompting procedures are listed in a rough order of increasing intrusiveness and difficulty: observation learning or modeling, simultaneous prompting, time delay, system of least prompts, and graduated guidance. The last three approaches incorporate fading strategies. Practitioners can simply apply prompts singly or in combination without any organized approach for eliminating them; however, prompts need to be faded eventually, and abrupt fading may result in performance set-backs for many learners with developmental disabilities.

Observation learning or modeling. A series of recent studies support the use of modeling or learning by watching another perform a target task in part or in full. This ordinary approach to teaching has been referred to as observation learning (Wolery et al., 1992) and passive observation (Biederman, Fairhall, Raven, & Davey, 1998) and has been effective with a wide range of clients who have disabilities and a wide range of functional tasks. Because modeling is a fairly nonintrusive, natural approach that has a good success record, it might be used as a prompting method before other more complex methods are chosen.

Learning through observation of models or demonstrations requires focused attention, memory, and the ability to imitate. Some have referred to this type of learning as a "see-then-do" method. When clients are missing some of these prerequisite abilities, this approach can be simplified and coupled with reinforcement for improved attending or imitating. Also model prompts may be repeated, exaggerated, or given partially, and model prompts may be paired with other prompts (gesturing or partial physical prompts). However, researchers have shown that uncomplicated modeling of entire tasks can also be effective. For example, modeling or passive observation of the whole task without verbal prompting was more successful in teaching a range of dressing, eating, and grooming tasks to school-aged students who had Down syndrome than was hand-over-hand guidance with verbal prompts across task steps (Biederman et al., 1998).

Wolery and his colleagues (1992) have repeatedly demonstrated the success of observational learning in small groups of students with the same targeted tasks. Instruction was directed to one student for all or half of a task while one or two others watched; instruction then moved to another in the group while others observed. Even when no praise was provided for observing, students learned skills they had observed being taught to peers but were never directly taught them. With observational learning, students may be praised (or prompted if necessary) for attending to the model, as they must see a model before they can learn by this method.

Simultaneous prompting. Simultaneous prompting involves the provision of both teaching trials and testing (probe) trials during daily self-care routines. Prompts are not gradually faded but simply present during teaching trials and absent during probe trials. This method has been applied more often to academic tasks but less often in teaching self-care (Sewell, Collins, Hemmeter, & Schuster, 1998). Because it is simple to use and has support, we are presenting it here. To use simultaneous prompting, on teaching trials the practitioner gives the controlling prompt (one that is known) at the same time that the target stimulus (one that is not known) is being taught. In the following activity-based example with a preschooler, physical prompts are the controlling stimuli or prompt, while the target stimulus is putting on a pullover that involved 10 steps.

> Lynn, who is almost 3 years old and developmentally delayed, chooses dress-up play and selects a green pullover shirt from the clothing box. The practitioner points to it, saying, "Put on your shirt." At the command, the practitioner immediately places her hands over Lynn's and physically guides her through each step in the task until the shirt is on. The practitioner explains what is happening as the task is performed and delivers praise after each task step as long as Lynn allows her guidance. When done, the practitioner offers Lynn an activity-based choice while holding up materials: "Do you want to cook something or should we sweep?"

During intermittently given probe trials, practitioners simply withhold prompts or physical assistance, give 5 seconds for the client to initiate the task step, allow 25 seconds to complete a step, and praise when the step is completed. Errors and failures to respond are ignored, but the practitioner performs the task step and repeats the task direction, giving the client an opportunity to perform each task step in sequence. Criterion is reached when clients perform the task completely during several consecutive probes.

> After Lynn could complete all dressing steps during three probe trials in a row, her team regarded her performance as meeting criterion, and the skill became one to maintain and to generalize to home.

Time delay. Another approach for giving and fading assistance is to pause or add a delay period before giving a prompt. During delay periods, the learner may either wait for assistance or try the response on his or her own. If the learner tries, the response may be correct or incorrect.

> Sam is learning some basic self-eating skills (Table 5.2). His practitioners decide that a physical prompt is best for him and plan to fade the prompt using time delay. They start teaching each skill using a no-delay period (zero seconds) between the discriminative stimulus and the prompt, so Sam gets physical prompts continuously through each spoon, napkin, and cup cycle for several meals. Then his therapist inserts a 4-second pause between each discriminative stimulus and the prompt, allowing Sam time to attempt the response without help. For some steps in the tasks, Sam waits for assistance (prompted correct responses); for others, he completes the steps (independent responses). On a few steps, he tries on his own and makes errors, and the therapist immediately repeats that step with help. Because Sam can eat faster when he tries on his own rather than waiting out the delay for help, time delay seems to motivate him to initiate without help. Because help is forthcoming at the end of a delay period, uncertain learners can simply wait.

Practitioners using time delay more often adopt the simpler *constant-delay* approach (e.g., no delay or 0-second delay followed by delays of 4 seconds). They also may use *progressive-delay* trials in which a delay is gradually increased from 0 to 6 or 8 seconds or longer, depending on the learner's natural response latency (e.g., 0, 2, 4, 6, or 8 seconds) (Schuster & Griffen, 1990; Snell & Brown, in press). Time delay has been found effective across many academic tasks as well as daily living tasks (preparing snacks, making beds, etc.) and self-care tasks like eating and drinking (Collins, Gast, Wolery, Holcombe, & Letherby, 1991; Snell, 1982; Wolery, Ault, Gast, Doyle, & Griffen, 1991) and dressing (Hughes, Schuster, & Nelson, 1993). Progressive time delay is more complicated to use than constant delay, while applying either time delay approach to a chained task like eating or dressing is more complicated than applying it to a discrete or isolated responses like lip closure and grasping or repeated responses like stepping. Balancing the effectiveness of a teaching approach with the staff requirements is something teams will need to consider in their choice of prompting methods. The principle of parsimony, to seek the simplest but still effective method, is one that

teams should heed as they make these choices (Etzel & LeBlanc, 1979).

When using either delay approach, the practitioner needs to select a single (e.g., model) or a combined prompt (e.g., verbal plus physical) rather than a hierarchy of prompts and should plan how or when to increase the delay. The best guide is to increase the delay only after a period of several sessions or trials of successful waiting responses (the learner does not make an error but allows himself or herself to be prompted) or correct responses (the learner makes the response during the delay without help). If the learner makes errors before the prompt, the delay might be shortened for several trials. If the learner makes an error after the prompt, the prompt may not work for that person. If this happens repeatedly, another prompt should be considered. The delay should not be increased after errors; instead, the practitioner should determine what type of error has occurred and address it accordingly. These decisions rely on the team's thinking about the task, the client, and the client's performance.

System of least prompts. A *system of least-intrusive prompts*, also called least prompts for short, involves selecting a hierarchy of prompts that work both for the learner and for the task. These prompts are used one at a time, starting with less assistance and moving to more assistance. Practitioners select a latency period or a short time when no assistance is given and the student initiates the response with no help or with no additional help.

> Chris, the preschooler learning to sit in and to stand up from a chair, did not readily perform the steps in these tasks. His therapist planned to use a prompting procedure and discussed the options with his team. Because he could follow some verbal-gestural directions and often imitated models, they chose a prompting procedure with a "built-in" means for fading: a system of least prompts.
>
> Chris has some high tone as a result of cerebral palsy. With Chris's preschool teachers, his therapist decides to use a slightly long latency of 5 seconds. Thus, his therapist will pause for 5 seconds after her instructional cue to let him initiate the first step in the target task and before giving any assistance (unless he begins making an error, at which point she will interrupt the error with the least intrusive level of assistance). She will pause for the latency (5 seconds) after giving any type of assistance or prompt to allow him to initiate the step with a certain amount of assistance.

Typically, three levels of prompts are used (though only two may be used): verbal instructions (simple statements for each task step); verbal instructions plus a model or gesture (depending on the step, the practitioner will point to the materials needed; for other tasks a brief, partial model or demonstration of the movement required may be used); and verbal instructions plus physical assistance (the practitioner provides only as much guidance as is needed, placing a hand on the person's hand, wrist, forearm, or elbow, or at control points such as the knees, shoulders, waist, or hips).

> The practitioner starts with the least-intrusive prompt but proceeds to more-intrusive prompts if Chris cannot complete a particular step of the task or if he makes an error and needs more help. For each step of the task, the practitioner will initially wait for Chris's initiation during the latency before giving any help; then if he does not initiate (or makes an error), she will offer a verbal prompt and wait. If he does not initiate the response (or makes an error), she will provide a verbal prompt and gesture and wait during the latency again. Finally, if Chris does not complete the step within 4 seconds following the gesture, the practitioner will move to the most-intrusive prompt and physically help him to complete the step.

A least-prompts system is adaptable to many tasks and persons; it has been demonstrated to be effective for persons with mental retardation and other disabilities across many daily living tasks (Snell, 1997). On the negative side, this system is initially a bit complex for practitioners to learn. It employs artificial, instructor prompts rather than natural ones, and it can appear to be quite intrusive to learners. An example would include physically helping a person move through the step of grasping a box of cereal in the grocery store. A least-prompt system that uses modeling and physical prompts is better during the acquisition phase of learning, while more subtle prompts are better during later stages of learning. Examples of subtle prompts include an initial nod to confirm a hesitant student to keep going, followed by a nonspecific verbal prompt of "What's next?", followed finally, if needed, by gestures toward relevant stimuli cues.

Some persons are tactilely defensive and do not like to be touched; others cannot use certain prompts because of skill limitations (e.g., not everyone can imitate a model prompt or follow verbal instructions). Therefore, the practitioner needs to select prompts that work with a particular person, or, like simple verbal instructions, that could be learned after being associated with meaningful prompts. Least-prompts systems require that at least two levels of prompts be selected, that they be arranged in a hierarchy from least to most intrusive, and that prompts be preceded by a latency period. The later or more-intrusive prompts in the hierarchy might be more consistently effective than the earlier or less-intrusive prompts. This hierarchy is all right as long as all the selected prompts are at least partially effective with a client. Given these basic characteristics, the least-prompts system can be adapted to suit many different learners and tasks.

Prompt systems, especially least prompts and time delay, offer several advantages; they have a built-in plan for fading out assistance, result in fewer errors than most teaching methods, and have a research basis of demonstrated effectiveness. When practitioners rely only on consequences to teach new skills, students may become discouraged by their errors and fail to make progress. The combined use of antecedent-prompt strategies with planned consequences is the best teaching approach.

Graduated guidance. Therapy personnel using *graduated guidance* apply more intrusive physical prompts first, then fade them out. Several variations of graduated guidance have been applied when teaching self-care procedures to persons with disabilities. In the hand-to-shoulder approach, practitioners initially provide full hand-over-hand guidance throughout the task but give only the amount of assistance that is needed for the learner to complete the task. This requirement—to give only as much help as is needed—means that practitioners must become highly sensitive to the pressure cues learners give back as they are being assisted. If the learner's hands move in the desired direction during a dressing task, the practitioner tries to back off and give less guidance. But if the student stops forward movement before he or she should, the practitioner provides the movement. The general order of fading assistance is from the learner's hands upward to the shoulder and then to omit physical assistance altogether. This approach has been used to teach eating and dressing skills (Azrin & Armstrong, 1973; Azrin, Schaeffer, & Wesolowski, 1976; Richman, Sonderby, & Kahn, 1980).

One difficulty with graduated guidance is deciding when to reduce assistance. The best approach is to try reducing assistance periodically while encouraging the student or client to perform with less assistance. The learner's own movements are the best guides to when less assistance is needed. Another approach is to use a brief waiting period before physically assisting each step (or some steps) in the task, thus giving the student opportunities to initiate each step before being prompted. Watching the student perform without any help (or test performance) can also help determine what steps may need less assistance.

A second general graduated-guidance approach involves using three different levels of physical assistance, varying again from more assistance to less assistance during training. The levels of physical assistance are full hand-over-hand assist, two-finger assist, and "shadowing" the person's hand from about 1 to 2 inches.

This approach has been used with dressing skills (Reese & Snell, 1991), to teach adults leisure skills (Demchak, 1989), and with exercising in physical education (Moon, Renzaglia, Ruth, & Talarico, 1981). In both graduated-guidance approaches, if the learner resists the prompted movement, the practitioner may maintain contact with the learner but simply wait until there is no resistance before continuing to assist. When the practitioner has successfully reduced assistance, praise for the learner's increased effort should be increased. When the learner seems to require more assistance, more assistance can be given. Graduated guidance allows the learner to "get the feel" of the movement required by a skill and gradually to take more responsibility for making the movement without the practitioner's guidance. This method does not work for persons who are tactilely defensive, do not like to be guided, or chose to move very quickly, nor will it work for those who become dependent on physical assistance. Often unnaturally intensive training and punitive correction methods have been coupled with graduated guidance; these strategies are ones we do not recommend using. Graduated guidance may be appropriate when it is suited to the learner and if less-intrusive prompting has not been successful.

Reinforcing Consequences After Correct or Approximate Responses

Table 5.3 shows some of the consequences that adults and peers can offer to a learner after a target response. The following practices for using positive consequences are recommended for most learners.

Reinforcement schedule. During early learning or acquisition, reinforcement after correct and approximate responses (even when they were prompted) facilitates learning. The reinforcement will occur more frequently during acquisition than during later stages of learning but should be reduced to an intermittent frequency so the student learns to perform without continuous reinforcement from others. If continuous schedules are not reduced over time, students may fail to use the skill under natural conditions when little reinforcement is forthcoming.

Appropriate to learner. Reinforcing consequences should suit the learner's chronological age, preferences, level of understanding, and the learning situation. Some learners find simple confirmation reinforcing ("That's right"), while others like and benefit more from task-specific praise ("Good job sweeping in the corner"). For some students, tangibles (toys, stickers, food) or preferred activities can be provided at the end of a relatively long task during the acquisition stage, but it is best to let the learner have a choice about the consequence rather than trying to anticipate what the person might find enjoyable.

Natural reinforcers. During later stages of learning, it is good to teach the learner to self-monitor his or her performance by asking and answering, "How well did I do this time?" It is also helpful to teach learners to look to more natural forms of self-reinforcement, such as taking a midmorning break at the completion of cleanup tasks or participating in the next activity once seated in circle at preschool.

Consequences are also part of prompt systems. For least prompts and graduated guidance and when single prompts are used (with time delay or simply with a fixed latency), praise is the typical consequence given for completing a step. Only if more concrete reinforcers are needed should they be added, and then they should meet the appropriateness criteria. Early in learning, praise can be given after the completion of every step whether or not the step was prompted. As learning progresses, the reinforcing consequences need to be decreased, so praise (and other reinforcing consequences) is reserved for progress made on more difficult steps and is not given for steps completed with the most intrusive prompts.

Consequences After Errors

When clients or patients make errors, there are many different ways to respond. The stage of learning and the type of error made will influence the consequence, as will many of the learner's characteristics (e.g., age, disabilities, skills). Consider Chris, the preschooler who is learning to sit and to stand up from sitting.

Before Chris has learned these tasks to about 60% accuracy, the therapist will need to correct any errors (e.g., "Grab the chair right here," while pointing to the chair arms) by showing Chris how to respond.

Corrections typically involve assistance given after mistakes. Some prompt systems provide clear ways to respond to errors. For example, in a least-prompts approach the therapist interrupts any mistakes with the next prompt in the hierarchy. However, if the incorrect response is simply a failure to respond, then the next prompt in the hierarchy is given after the latency. In graduated guidance, the teacher also responds to errors by giving more assistance but typically more physical assistance.

> If Linda, who is learning to brush her teeth, fails to remove the cap before squeezing the tube of toothpaste, the therapist may move her guiding hand away from Linda's elbow (a point of less assistance) to the wrist or hand (both points of greater assistance) and ask Linda to repeat the missed step.
>
> Once Linda has learned more of the tooth-brushing task, the therapist might ask her, "What's next?" (nonspecific verbal prompt) when Linda hesitates on a step she has done before without help. Alternately, the therapist may simply wait longer, giving Linda time to self-correct.

Both of these approaches encourage more self-correction and independence by the client, something that is especially desirable during the later stages of learning. Persons in these stages of learning a skill may simply check with the practitioner when they have completed the task; if it has not been done adequately, the practitioner might withhold approval or ask them to try again. As we have noted earlier, the use of punitive consequences for errors is inappropriate.

Evaluation of Learning and Teaching

This section contains procedures for evaluating outcomes of therapeutic intervention. Clinicians may not always have the opportunity to follow up on training recommendations. This lack of evaluation happens, for instance, when return visits to occupational therapy are not approved by reimbursement agencies, or in early intervention or school system settings in which practitioners commonly treat children once a week for short periods of time. Under these circumstances, opportunities for evaluation of intervention outcomes may be restricted by time constraints or may not be possible at all. These situations are unfortunate realities in the current practice environment. It is our recommendation that practitioners take time to read the following sections and consider ways to modify the evaluation methods to suit individual settings and needs. For instance, when the practitioner is not routinely present in a classroom setting, the teacher or aide may be able to collect information. Some families are good at such detail as well.

Client performance data (from testing and training) are used in a number of ways. Test data help teachers and practitioners to make decisions about what learning areas to target, depending on the learner's *baseline data* (performance before instruction begins) and to judge progress once training has begun by monitoring the learner's progress using criterion or test conditions. This practice is referred to as *probing* or collecting *probe performance data*. Whenever possible, probes taken in the setting where the goal behavior is used is best as it gives a realistic picture of learning. A third way is to make decisions about program changes, such as hospital discharge or transition to another unit or service.

Baseline and Probe Data

Baseline data should be collected over at least two sessions or until it seems fairly stable, not varying by 40% or more in either direction (Farlow & Snell, 1994). If only one assessment is possible, practitioners might ask family members, the client, or others who are familiar with the client's performance how well the client currently performs the task and estimate if performance is stable. When these data are relatively representative of the learner's performance, then instruction can begin with baseline performance serving as a comparative guide for judging progress made during training.

> Chris's baseline performance (Figure 5.3) was measured over a week and indicated some improvement. Probe data involved repeating the test observation after teaching has begun.

Many of us have found that probe observations need not be taken more than once every 5 training days (when training or therapy is daily) unless progress is poor. Even then, training data, rather than probe data, are more useful when analyzing the reasons for lack of progress (see Farlow & Snell, 1994). Test data (both baseline and probe) typically are recorded using symbols for correct and incorrect responses (see Figure 5.2). Test data may be summarized as the percent or number correct out of the total opportunities. It is useful to record these data on the same graph as training data but to use different symbols to distinguish between them (see Figures 5.2 and 5.3). Furthermore, the ungraphed or step-by-step task analytic data should be saved and dated because this record shows which steps were correct and which were missed. Chris's trial-by-trial data are shown in Figure 5.2 and his percent correct performance is graphed in Figure 5.3.

Training Data

Training data are collected during the training session. Typically, learners perform a given skill better during training than during test conditions. This difference can be painfully obvious to clinicians who treat in one-on-one intervention sessions, then find task performance plummets in natural settings. When recording training data, use symbols for correct responses and for the types and amounts of assistance needed by the learner to complete the behavior or step in the task. Thus, steps in the three tasks in Table 5.2 (spoon, cup, and napkin use) could either be rated "correct" or noted with a "P" to indicate that a physical prompt was given (see Figure 5.2). If several prompts are possible, different symbols may indicate which prompt obtained the response (e.g., "V" for verbal, "G" for gestural, "M" for model, "P" for physical assist).

If parents, caregivers, teachers, or spouses will be collecting data, remember to take time to teach them how to record correctly. Training data provide the practitioner with objective information about how the learner responds to the therapy program and can be used to support requests from reimbursement sources for further sessions. Like test data, training data should be both preserved in an ungraphed form (so the information on individual steps is not lost) and graphed using the percent correct or the number of steps correct. Note that in Figure 5.2, Chris's baseline and probe data are indicated with an asterisk.

Using Data

Besides simply scanning graphs for the trend in progress and for variability, teachers or practitioners can examine raw or ungraphed (step-by-step) data for specific error patterns or problem areas that provide clues to needed changes if progress is poor. Dated anecdotal records about student behavior, interfering circumstances, and illnesses will also help resolve why progress may be inadequate. These kinds of data are particularly helpful in clients with complex problems, such as sensory disturbances.

Chris's data (Figure 5.2) indicate steady progress with less and less assistance on the first 5 steps of the task during March and April. On April 26, he did require some physical assistance on steps he usually got correct, and the teacher noted on the graph that he did not appear to feel well that day. Because his performance was soon back to its higher level, the teachers made no changes in the program.

Farlow and Snell (1994) provided a detailed method for using data effectively; Brown and Snell (in press) also give some guidelines for this approach. Ottenbacher's book *Evaluating Clinical Change: Strategies for Occupational and Physical Therapists* (1986) gives similar information. Several general steps are involved in analyzing data to improve treatment programming.

1. *Collect data relevant to the treatment goals.* Collect training data whenever the client is seen (several times a week is optimal but is not usual in most therapy settings). Collect probe data in other settings periodically or have others involved in the client's life do so.

2. *Preserve step-by-step data and graph data.* Indicate on the graph dates and types of data: baseline, intervention, test, and training data. In addition, note (and date) any relevant anecdotal comments pertinent to the performance data on the back or front of the graph. Use graphs that show all attendance dates so absences, vacations, and other missed days are clear (see Figure 5.3). Connect data that are from continuous periods of time.

3. *Determine trend if unclear.* If the data seem to be reliable and representative of the client's performance, determine the trend after graphing 6 to 8 data points. Trends will be ascending, flat, or descending. If the data are not representative (i.e., the learner has been sick) or not reliable (e.g., for 3 of the data points the aide recalled the performance rather than recording the data during the performance), examine the trend after more data have been collected.

   Chris's initial flat progress in March was followed after spring break by perfect performance during training. This higher-than-criterion performance caused the therapist and teacher to increase the criterion to 100% (Figure 5.3).

4. *Ascending trends.* If the trend is ascending, continue the program unless the criterion goal has been met, whereupon the goal needs to be changed.

5. *Flat or descending trends.* If the trend is flat or descending, work with the client or the learner's team or both depending on the setting to deter-

mine the possible reason(s) for the lack of progress. Is there a cyclical variability related to time; that is, some days or sessions are worse because of a weekend, the therapist or certified occupational therapy assistant, a prescribed medication, or other changing factors? Are test data better than training data? If so, what are the differences between the two situations? Does the client have difficulty with the same step(s) across sessions? What are the reasons for errors? Is it a specific step? Are the errors setting, time, or staff specific? Are they a result of the learner not attempting the task or performing it incorrectly? Is the learner reinforced after making errors?

6. *Make comparisons.* Compare performance on other tasks and behaviors with this performance. Are the errors similar? Does the target behavior interact with other behaviors (e.g., interfering behavior)? Are problem behaviors increasing? Does the program prevent access to other interactions and activities?

7. *Develop a possible explanation.* Working with the client or learner's team, develops a feasible explanation(s) for the lack of progress.

8. *Plan program improvements.* As a team, decide on programmatic changes that will address the potential reasons for the behavior. If more than one explanation is developed, determine which one(s) should dictate program change, perhaps by making more observations.

> Millie is an adolescent who is working on improving her use of a power wheelchair at school. Millie's lack of progress on driving seems cyclical or related to sessions that isolate her from peers, but she is improving during training sessions held during physical education class with peers and at lunchtime in the cafeteria. Anecdotal records state that Millie often refuses to try driving during these sessions where no progress is being made and has cried several times. Two potential explanations could be developed. First, during these time periods when there is progress, Millie's trainers are doing something different (and more effective) than are her trainers at other times. Second, Millie enjoys instruction in the context of her peers, perhaps it's the cheering they sometimes give her when she tries harder at driving.
>
> The first explanation was ruled out after team members realized that instructors during physical education and lunch were rotated and not specific to those times. Millie's team then decided to focus on the second explanation. They asked Millie if she might prefer to have a peer volunteer help during the times of the day when peers had not been present. When Millie indicated she would like this, they recruited volunteers and included them in all training sessions where little progress was occurring. Data collected after this change indicated that her progress showed ascending trends in all sessions.

In current practice settings, ongoing evaluation is usually required by reimbursement sources. Practitioners gather and examine student performance data to address these 8 program evaluation steps. Relevant data include probes or intermittent test data (during baseline and probes of training progress) and training data that are supplemented with anecdotal notes about the client's performance and social validation of the progress attained. To validate clients' progress socially, one can query learners themselves, their peers or family members, and their teachers and practitioners to obtain subjective opinions about progress or can compare learners' performance to their peers' performance.

Though learning evaluation is never simple, it need not be overly complex to provide information pertinent to the effectiveness of a therapy program. The evaluation process should be *ongoing*, not applied at the conclusion of a program or a school year in those settings when ongoing access to the client is possible. Ongoing evaluation means that if the data indicate the client's progress is below expectations, the data are analyzed to clarify the reasons and to design the needed program changes. The data are then used to monitor whether program changes actually lead to performance improvements.

Summary

The goal of most occupational therapy intervention strategies is to teach persons in ways that promote learning and that encourage their normalized performance. To accomplish these ends, practitioners need to target goals that will be useful to an individual learner, to use methods that are both relatively uncomplicated but also effective and respect the learner, and to evaluate the client's progress on an ongoing basis. ◆

Study Questions

1. What is the rationale for setting goals appropriate to chronological age that are commonly used in daily routines?

2. How can persons who may learn to do part of a task initially become independent in that task over time?

3. How do you see the stages of learning fitting into occupational therapy goal setting?

4. Why do you think multiple sources of data are important in planning self-care treatment?

5. What consideration should an occupational therapist give to antecedent events and consequences used in treatment? Why are they important?

6. What is the difference between baseline and training data, and how could an occupational therapist, who may see a patient only once a week, collect information on this kind of data?

7. How can graphed information be valuable to an occupational therapist; that is, what influence can such information have on setting goals and treatment?

References

Azrin, N. H., & Armstrong, P. M. (1973). The "mini-meal": A method for teaching eating skills to the profoundly retarded. *Mental Retardation, 11*(1), 9–11.

Azrin, N. H., Schaeffer, R. M., & Wesolowski, M. D. (1976). A rapid method of teaching profoundly retarded persons to dress by a reinforcement-guidance method. *Mental Retardation, 14*(6), 29–33.

Baumgart, D., Brown, L., Pumpian, I., Nisbet, J., Ford, A., Sweet, M., Messina, R., & Schroeder, J. (1982). Principle of partial participation and individualized adaptations in educational programs for severely handicapped students. *Journal of the Association for the Severely Handicapped, 7*, 17–27.

Biederman, G. B., Fairhall, J. L., Raven, K. A., & Davey, V. A. (1998). Verbal prompting, hand-over-hand instruction, and passive observation in teaching children with developmental disabilities. *Exceptional Children, 64*, 503–511.

Brown, F., Evans, I., Weed, K., & Owen, V. (1987). Delineating functional competency: A component model. *Journal of the Association for Persons with Severe Handicaps, 12*, 117–124.

Brown, F., & Snell, M. E. (in press). Meaningful assessment. In M. E. Snell & F. Brown (Eds.), *Instruction of students with severe disabilities* (5th ed.). Columbus, OH: Merrill.

Carr, E. G., Levin, L., McConnachie, G., Carlson, J. I., Kemp, D. C., & Smith, C. E. (1994). *Communication-based intervention for problem behavior: A user's guide for producing positive change.* Baltimore: Paul H. Brookes.

Collins, B. C., Gast, D. L., Wolery, M., Holcombe, A., & Letherby, J. (1991). Using constant time delay to teach self-feeding to young students with severe/profound handicaps: Evidence of limited effectiveness. *Journal of Developmental and Physical Disabilities, 3*, 157–179.

Day, H. H., & Horner, R. H. (1986). Response variation and the generalization of a dressing skill: Comparison of single instance and general case instruction. *Applied Research in Mental Retardation, 7*, 189–202.

Demchak, M. A. (1989). A comparison of graduated guidance and increasing assistance in teaching adults with severe handicaps leisure skills. *Education and Training in Mental Retardation, 24*, 45–55.

Durand, V. M. (1990). *Severe behavior problems: A functional communication training approach.* New York: Guilford.

Etzel, B. C., & LeBlanc, J. M. (1979). The simplest treatment alternative: Appropriate instructional control and errorless learning procedures for the difficult-to-teach child. *Journal of Autism and Developmental Disorders, 9*, 361–382.

Farlow, L. J., & Snell, M. E. (1994). *Making the most of student performance data* (Research to Practice Series). Washington, DC: American Association on Mental Retardation.

Farlow, L., & Snell, M. E. (in press). Teaching self care skills. In M. E. Snell & F. Brown (Eds.), *Instruction of students with severe disabilities* (5th ed.). Columbus, OH: Merrill.

Ferguson, D. L., & Baumgart, D. (1991). Partial participation revisited. *Journal of the Association for Persons with Severe Handicaps, 16*, 218–227.

Ford, A., Schnorr, R., Meyer, L., Davern, L., Black, J., & Dempsey, P. (1989). *The Syracuse community-referenced curriculum guide for students with moderate and severe disabilities.* Baltimore: Paul H. Brookes.

Frankenburg, W. K., Dodds, J., Archer, P., Shapiro, H., & Bresnick, B. (1992). The Denver II: A major revision and re-standardization of the Denver Developmental Screening Test. *Pediatrics, 89*(1), 91–96.

Giangreco, M. F., Cloninger, C. J., & Iverson, V. S. (1993). *C.O.A.C.H.: Choosing options and accommodations for children.* Baltimore: Paul H. Brookes.

Haley, S. M., Ludlow, L. H., & Coster, W. J. (1993). Pediatric evaluation of disability inventory: Clinical interpretation of summary scores using Rasch rating scale methodology. *Physical Medicine and Rehabilitation Clinics of North America, 4*, 529–540.

Hamilton, B. L., Laughlin, J. A., Fiedler, R. C., & Granger, C. V. (1994). Interrater reliability of the 7-level Functional Independence Measure (FIM). *Scandinavian Journal of Rehabilitation Medicine, 26*, 115–116.

Hughes, M. W., Schuster, J. W., & Nelson, C. M. (1993). The acquisition of independent dressing skills by students with multiple disabilities. *Journal of Developmental and Physical Disabilities, 5*, 233–295.

McCabe, M. A., & Granger, C. V. (1990). Content validity of a pediatric Functional Independence Measure. *Applied Nursing Research, 3*(3), 120–122.

Meyer, L. H., & Evans, I. H. (1989). *Nonaversive intervention for behavior problems: A manual for home and community.* Baltimore: Paul H. Brookes.

Moon, S., Renzaglia, A., Ruth, B., & Talarico, D. (1981). *Increasing the physical fitness of the severely mentally retarded: A comparison of graduated guidance and hierarchy of prompts.* Unpublished manuscript, University of Virginia.

Ottenbacher, K. J. (1986). *Evaluating clinical change: Strategies for occupational and physical therapists.* Baltimore: Williams & Wilkins.

Reese, G. M., & Snell, M. E. (1991). Putting on and removing coats and jackets: The acquisition and maintenance of skills by children with severe multiple disabilities. *Education and Training in Mental Retardation, 26,* 398–410.

Richman, J. S., Sonderby, T., & Kahn, J. V. (1980). Prerequisite vs. in vivo acquisition of self-feeding skill. *Behaviour Research and Therapy, 18,* 327–332.

Schuster, J. W., & Griffen, A. K. (1990). Using time delay with task analyses. *Teaching Exceptional Children, 22*(4), 49–53.

Sewell, T. J., Collins, B. C., Hemmeter, M. L., & Schuster, J. W. (1998). Using simultaneous prompting within an activity-based format to teach dressing skills to preschoolers with developmental delays. *Journal of Early Intervention, 21,* 132–145.

Snell, M. E. (1982). Analysis of time delay procedures in teaching daily living skills to retarded adults. *Analysis*

and Intervention in Developmental Disabilities, 2, 139–155.

Snell, M. E. (1997). Teaching children and young adults with mental retardation in school programs: Current research. *Behaviour Change, 14,* 73–105.

Snell, M. E., & Brown, F. (in press). Instructional planning and implementation. In M. E. Snell & F. Brown (Eds.), *Instruction of students with severe disabilities* (5th ed.). Columbus, OH: Merrill.

Snell, M. E., Lewis, A. P., & Houghton, A. (1989). Acquisition and maintenance of toothbrushing skills by students with cerebral palsy and mental retardation. *Journal of the Association for Persons with Severe Handicaps, 14,* 216–226.

Watson, D. E. (1997). *Task analysis: An occupational performance approach.* Bethesda, MD: American Occupational Therapy Association.

Wolery, M., Ault, M. J., & Doyle, P. M. (1992). *Teaching students with moderate to severe disabilities.* White Plains, NY: Longman.

Wolery, M., Ault, M. J., Gast, D. L., Doyle, P. M., & Griffen, A. K. (1991). Teaching chained tasks in Dyads: Acquisition of target and observational behaviors. *Journal of Special Education, 25,* 198–220.

Wood, D. J., Bruner, J. S., & Ross, G. (1976). The role of tutoring in problem-solving. *Journal of Child Psychology and Psychiatry, 17*(2), 89–100.

Zirpoli, T. J., & Melloy, K. J. (1993). *Behavior management: Application for teachers and parents.* New York: Macmillan.

6

Self-Care Strategies for Children With Developmental Disabilities

Jane Case-Smith

Jane Case-Smith, EdD, OT/L, BCP, FAOTA, is Associate Professor, Division of Occupational Therapy, The Ohio State University, Columbus, Ohio.

Key Terms

cerebral palsy

developmental disabilities

functional mobility

powered mobility

Objectives

On completing this chapter, the reader will be able to

1. Apply the Person–Environment–Occupation Model to self-care intervention for children with developmental disabilities.

2. Describe the sequence of development of feeding, bathing, dressing, communication, and mobility.

3. Define variables that influence acquisition of feeding skills.

4. Describe and apply intervention strategies to improve feeding in children with primary motor, sensory, and behavioral impairments.

5. Describe the variables that influence acquisition of dressing skills.

6. Identify and apply intervention strategies to improve dressing skills in children with primary motor and sensory problems.

7. Describe the variables that influence acquisition of bathing skills.

8. Explain intervention strategies to improve bathing skills in children with primary motor and sensory problems.

9. Identify and describe the variables that influence ability to use augmentative communication systems.

10. Describe selection of and intervention to promote use of augmentative communication systems.

11. Describe the variables that influence use of mobility devices.

12. Describe mobility devices, selection of devices, and intervention to promote the child's independence in mobility.

Addressing the self-care needs of children requires knowledge of normal development within a systems context. The child's skills and functional limitations must be viewed in the context of the family and the child's living setting and surroundings. Figure 6.1 lists the factors determining the child's level of independence in self. These factors include his or her motor, sensory, and behavioral abilities; the family's structure, culture, and values; and the home and child-care environments. Children learn self-care skills as a part of everyday family life. Thus, the child's self-care skills cannot be considered outside this context.

For example, in many Far Eastern cultures, the mother feeds children until age 5 or 6. This custom is because feeding the child is an important demonstration of the mother's affection and caring. Teaching a child from a family within this culture to self-feed at 2 or 3 years of age would be inappropriate because it would interfere with this act of motherly love. Other mealtime rituals differ among ethnic groups and according to the family's values. For example, some families do not have established mealtimes, whereas others reserve the family's evening meal as the most important time of the day. Table 6.1 provides examples of family variables that highly influence a child's self-care development.

In this chapter, the Person–Environment–Occupation Model is used to help understand how five specific self-care skills are acquired by children

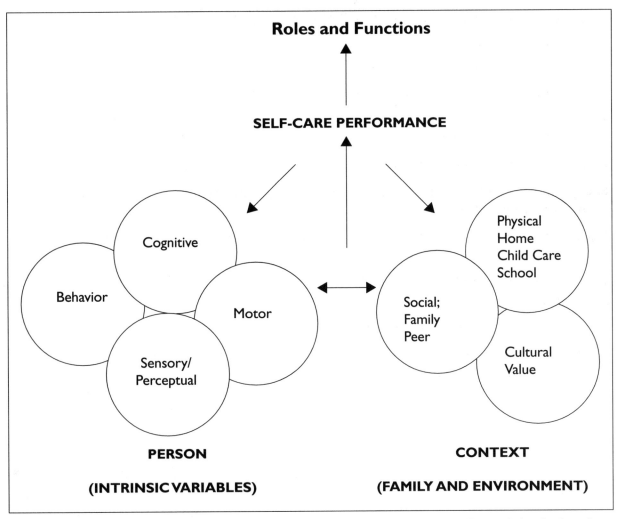

Figure 6.1 Roles and functions of self-care performance. *Note.* From "Motor Behavior Research: Implications for Therapeutic Approaches to Central Nervous System Dysfunction," by V. Mathiowetz & J. B. Haugen, 1994, *American Journal of Occupational Therapy, 48,* pp. 733–745. Copyright 1994 by the American Occupational Therapy Association. Adapted with permission.

Table 6.1 Family Variables That Influence a Child's Development of Self-Care Skills

Variable	Influence on Self-Care Development
Culture	Does the family value self-care independence? What foods are accepted? What clothing is appropriate? Is assistive technology accepted? What family traditions and rituals must be respected in designing intervention?
Time	Are family members able to extend the time required in care of the child? When in the family's daily routine, can self-care skills be practiced?
Commitment	Are the parents committed to the effort needed to promote self-care independence? Can family members apply the self-care interventions with consistency and regularity?
Communication	Do family members communicate daily problems and successes with each other?
Adaptability and flexibility	Can family roles adapt to changes in routines? Can family members share caregiving responsibilities?

with developmental disabilities. The five self-care tasks to be considered are feeding, dressing, bathing, functional communication, and mobility.

For each task, the influence of specific sensory, motor, and behavioral problems on self-care skill development is considered. The sequence of typical self-care development is also described as a way of thinking about how the child's performance on that task can be evaluated.

Next, the influences of the child's personality and abilities (intrinsic variables) and context (family and environment) most applicable to the task are considered. Then, on the basis of an analysis of the child and his or her context, intervention strategies are defined. Wherever possible, case studies are used to illustrate the principles.

Feeding

Development of Oral Feeding and Self-Feeding Skills

Oral Feeding. The full-term infant is born with the ability to consume nutrition, thereby sustaining life and growth. He or she first accomplishes feeding using rooting to find the nipple and sucking to express liquid from a nipple. A gag reflex and automatic cough are also present to prevent aspiration of liquids, ensuring that the liquid taken in moves through the correct passageway to the stomach and digestive system. These early reflexes are integrated at 2 to 3 months of age, and the infant develops rhythmic sucking movement. From basic sucking at 4 months, the development of oral feeding proceeds quite rapidly, and by 2 years, a child is proficient in drinking, chewing, and biting. Typical development of oral feeding is presented in Table 6.2.

Self-Feeding. Although all children do *not* follow a typical sequence of development, it is helpful to identify a typical sequence (without focusing on age) to provide general guidelines about the expected order in which skills develop. The infant practices self-feeding for many months before he or she accomplishes independence at mealtime. Hand to mouth is one of the first motor behaviors that the infant demonstrates, and he or she may hold a bottle by 6 months of age. Finger feeding a cracker or soft cookie is generally accomplished by 8 months of age. By 7 to 8 months of age, the child usually sits in a high chair with the family at the dinner table. While observing the other family members, he or she engages in food play or finger feeding. The infant may play with a spoon by banging it on the high chair tray. Dried cereal or small bits of soft foods provide entertainment and multiple opportu-

Table 6.2 Typical Development of Oral Feeding

Age	Feeding Skill	Type of Food and Utensil
Neonate	Oral reflexes of rooting and sucking; sucking is strong and rhythmic	Breast or bottle
1 month	Suckling: Rhythmic back-and-forth tongue movement with jaw opening and closing	Breast or bottle
4 months	Strong sucking: Tongue moves up and down, good lip seal	Breast or bottle
6 months	Efficient sucking, good jaw stability, and lip seal	Breast or bottle, may introduce the cup, may begin pureed foods
9 months	Long sequence of continuous sucking; jaw stability improves on cup; uses a munching pattern with purred foods; beginning of diagonal jaw movements; lateral tongue movements	Pureed and soft foods, bottle or breast, cup
12 months	Rotary chewing movements; active upper lip in removing food; licking present	Soft foods, some table foods, bottle or breast, cup
18 months	Well-coordinated rotary chewing; controlled and sustained biting; mobile tongue, including tongue elevation	Table foods, soft meat
2 years	Well-graded and sustained bite; circular rotary jaw movements; tongue reaches lips and all gum surfaces; good lip closure; good jaw stabilization on cup	Most meats and soft vegetables; cup without lid

(handwritten annotation: Gag Reflex   Cough Reflex)

nities to practice pincer grasp and finger skills. The selection of finger foods should match the child's oral motor skills. Nuts, hard candy, popcorn, grapes, and hot dogs cut width-wise are not recommended because these foods can totally occlude the airway if aspirated. Soft foods that dissolve in the mouth or require minimal chewing and are not as large as the airway are appropriate for first finger feeding. To develop independent spoon feeding, the infant must understand the use of a tool and must have control of midrange elbow and wrist movements, including supination and pronation. Spoon feeding often develops between 15 and 18 months of age. At this time, shoulder and wrist stability are adequate for holding the spoon to scoop the food and bring it to the mouth with minimal spillage. The child holds the spoon in a pronated gross grasp and brings the spoon to the mouth using exaggerated shoulder and elbow movements. This movement works best with foods that stick to the spoon.

By 24 months of age, the child uses a supinated grasp of the spoon, holding it in the radial fingers. The subtle movements at the wrist and forearm needed to obtain the food and efficiently enter the spoon into the mouth also emerge at this age. With this increased control, the child may begin to use a fork and to eat foods that are more difficult to handle (e.g., peas, corn, rice, cold cereal).

Between 12 and 18 months of age, the child learns cup drinking, initially with a cup that has a lid and a spout. Some children can best manage a cup with handles; others prefer a small plastic cup without handles. A child tends to spill from a cup until 24 months of age, when jaw stability and hand control increase (Case-Smith & Humphry, 1996; Morris & Klein, 1987).

Individual (Child-Related) Factors That Influence Feeding

Motor Impairment. Feeding requires advanced motor skills. The child must use a versatile sequence of oral movements in which tongue, cheek, jaw, and lip movements are coordinated. Children with significant motor impairments (e. g., cerebral palsy or trisomy 21) often have difficulty in coordinating the sequence of oral movements necessary for successful feeding. Children with cerebral palsy frequently exhibit low muscle tone (hypotonia) in the face, neck, and trunk that results in instability of the head and trunk. This postural instability may cause poor postural alignment; the child may fall into trunk and cervical flexion unless properly positioned. The child may also demonstrate hyperextension of the neck, thereby placing him or her at risk for aspiration because of improper alignment of the pharynx.

The child's jaw often moves in wide excursions, completely open or closed, without controlled mid-range movement. This child lacks the graded jaw movement needed for chewing and cup drinking. With very low facial muscle tone, the child's mouth is often open, which makes swallowing difficult and may result in drooling.

In the child with hypotonia, the tongue may be inactive, moving primarily with movement of the lower jaw. The tongue may exhibit primitive back-and-forth movements rather than up-and-down or lateral movement. Extreme movements of the jaw and tongue can disrupt coordination of the suck, swallow, and breathe pattern. The extreme movement of the tongue may relate to poor neck and jaw stability because the tongue does not have a sufficient base of stability for controlled movement. Hypotonia may also involve the lips so that they become inactive. As a result, the child's ability to seal the lips on the bottle's nipple, the cup's rim, or the spoon is inadequate and results in food loss or air intake. Hypotonic cheeks result in less suction of the nipple and difficulty maintaining food in the tongue's center.

Alternately, a child can demonstrate hypertonicity or fluctuating muscle tone in the face and oral area. The child with muscle tone that is too high (spasticity) may exhibit tonic oral reflexes or abnormal motor patterns that are not observed in a child who is typically developing. These patterns are highly disruptive to the feeding process and should be inhibited using therapeutic techniques. Table 6.3 lists some of the functional problems associated with developmental disabilities.

Sensory Processing Impairment. The sensory systems also contribute to the development of feeding skills. A child with sensory defensiveness of the face and oral areas demonstrates aversion to touch on or in the mouth and to textured foods inside the mouth. This child demonstrates spitting, choking, or gagging when food is placed in the mouth, particularly if the food's texture is unfamiliar. Introduction of new textures usually results in aversive responses in any young infant. However, when the child has hypersensitivity of oral touch, these responses continue well beyond the time usually required of children to develop tolerance. Tactile hypersensitivity can limit the child's amount of nutritional intake and the variety of foods that are accepted. It also can result in negative behaviors at mealtime.

Behavioral Problems. Feeding difficulties are usually accompanied by behavioral problems because the child with sensory processing impairment may experience feeding as uncomfortable and stressful. Parents often misunderstand the child's negative responses, and they become anxious about the child's limited nutritional intake and negative behaviors. The parents' increased attention is rewarding to the child, and, therefore, the negative behavior is repeated to gain the attention and emotional response of the parent.

Avoidance behaviors can result from inappropriate feeding methods (Morris & Klein, 1987). When the child is fed textures or amounts that exceed oral capabilities or both, he or she may respond with negative behavior (e.g., spitting, crying) to indicate displeasure. These behaviors most often result when the parent is insensitive to the child's cues. For example, the child indicates satiation or discomfort to a food texture, and the parent does not respond. The child then exhibits more obvious negative behaviors that generally disrupt the feeding interaction.

Behavior problems are prevalent during feeding for several reasons. First, for the child with severe impairments and minimal motor control, feeding may be the only opportunity to exercise control over the social environment. The goals and schedules of the caregivers generally determine the child's daily activities. However, feeding differs in that no one can force the child to eat. Furthermore, refusal to eat almost always causes a reaction in the caregiver or feeder, allowing the child to feel some control over his or her environment.

Second, the child quickly becomes aware that the parent is concerned and anxious about the refusal to eat. Generating this emotional response reinforces the behavior. The child quickly learns that negative behaviors at mealtime draw increased attention.

For the child with sensory processing problems, feeding is associated with genuine discomfort. Children with autism or pervasive developmental disabilities may experience this discomfort and have no method of communicating their dislike other than through negative or disruptive behaviors (such as spitting, screaming, running away) (Klein & Delaney, 1994).

Table 6.3 Functional Problems in Feeding Associated With Developmental Disabilities

Condition	Associated Feeding Problems
Cerebral palsy	Primitive sucking and chewing Hypertonia or hypotonia Difficulty sequencing suck, swallow, breathe Difficulty coordinating lip, tongue, and jaw mobility Postural instability
Sensory processing dysfunction	Poor tolerance of tactile input Limited chewing and biting skills Oral motor planning problems Sensory defensiveness
Autism or pervasive development disorder	Sensory defensiveness Poor tolerance of specific tastes Difficulty in communicating about feeding Fetishes about feeding (i.e., only eats certain foods)
Respiratory or cardiac problems	Poor endurance Difficulty coordinating between swallowing and breathing Purposely limits intake to limit workload of eating and digestion
Severe sensorimotor disabilities	Poor stability and mobility of oral structures Limited control of chewing and drinking Swallowing problems and risk of aspiration Nutritionally at risk because of oral motor and communication problems
Failure to thrive	Negative interactions between feeder or caregiver and child Behavioral problems associated with feeding

Context Variables That Influence Feeding

Caregivers. Feeding almost always involves interaction with others. Initially, feeding is an intimate experience between mother and child (Humphry, 1991; Humphry & Rourk, 1991). The feelings evoked during feeding contribute to the attachment that develops between parent and child. Early in development, the parent establishes a rhythm with feeding, making sustained eye contact and initiating first communications (e.g., when infant signals hunger and satiation). Therefore, feeding is an initial time for responsive give-and-take between parent and child (Barnard & Kelly, 1990). Holding the child close to the body, patting and stroking, and maintaining eye contact are important elements of feeding.

When the child is not responded to, he or she may become passive, no longer initiating communication. In infants with failure to thrive, the parent may not respond to the infant's signals or may not read the infant's cues (Box 6.1).

Family Structure, Culture, and Values. The family structure affects the child's development of feeding skills (Humphry & Case-Smith, 1996). In families of a single parent or when one parent is frequently away from home, feeding responsibilities may fall onto one person. For the child who must be fed four to five meals a day, each requiring 1 hour of time, this responsibility can be overwhelming. One mother explained:

I am the only one who can feed him. The staff at the child-care center try to feed him, but

Box 6.1
Failure To Thrive

Failure to thrive (FTT) is the abnormal retardation of growth and development of an infant that results from conditions that interfere with normal metabolism, appetite, and activity. The resulting prolonged nutritional deficiency may result in permanent, irreversible retardation of physical, mental, and social development.

FTT can be caused by a multitude of birth defects and genetic problems that leave babies unable to suck or swallow or to process the food they have eaten. It has also been linked to psychosocial causes, such as severe maternal deprivation. Many infants with feeding problems are very sensitive to their environment. They may not sleep well and respond poorly to changes in their schedules. They startle easily at bright lights and noises, and they never cry or fuss because they are hungry. Many children with FTT have exceptionally sensitive oral reflexes that cause them to reject or gag on pureed or solid foods.

Because FTT is such an elusive medical problem that can strike children from any social or ethnic background, many families struggle for months before they get adequate medical guidance. Parents who believe that their child is not thriving and have not been informed of medical or developmental problems should ask their physician or occupational therapist for a referral to a pediatric gastroenterologist or a nutritionist. Getting help early is important because retardation in growth and mental development at a young age is generally irreversible.

niques should be taught to multiple family members and child-care providers so that this responsibility can be shared.

Cultural background highly influences the eating routine, the amounts and types of food given to the child, how the foods are served, and how much independence is valued. In certain cultures, large amounts of food are served, which can be overwhelming to a young child who struggles to eat. Although every culture has certain foods that are easier to masticate (e.g., rice, curry, cornmeal, yogurt), standard food items may consist of fatty meats or foods that are difficult to chew (Box 6.2).

Family Life Cycle. The parent–child interaction during early feeding soon becomes family mealtime. Family mealtimes can help the child build skills as he or she now has multiple role models and is usually highly motivated to become a full participant in the family meal. This social environment can reinforce the child's efforts to eat, but it can also compound his or her frustrations about eating, resulting in disruptive, acting-out behaviors.

Most families establish a system that allows the child to participate in the family mealtime. This approach maintains the social benefits of family gatherings and promotes the child's feeding skills. If the child requires supportive seating, the wheelchair can be placed near to the table. When specific handling techniques are required, the child may be fed before the mealtime and be allowed to play with food on his tray while the family eats. Establishing eating as a social event is an important goal for every child, even when oral motor skills are limited.

Home and Child-Care Context. The home and child-care environments may promote or inhibit the development of feeding skills. Sensory aspects of the environment, such as noise levels and lighting, can interfere with the child's ability to eat. Thus, quiet, nonstimulating and calming environments can allow the child to concentrate and perform at optimal levels. Music can promote a level of arousal that is optimal for eating. For example, calming music that has 1 beat per second can promote sucking (Morris & Klein, 1987).

The physical arrangement of the home can promote or deter development of feeding skills. Tables and chairs should be modified to meet the needs of young children. A comfortable and adaptable arrangement for feeding is needed, particularly when a young child requires physical support and adapted equipment for success in feeding.

they worry when he chokes, and they do not know how to hold him and place the spoon so that he can swallow. He is starving when he comes home from the child care, so I feed him a small meal then and dinner later. Since his birth 4 years ago, I have fed him almost every meal.

Given the stressful requirements of a child who requires specific handling techniques, feeding tech-

Box 6.2
Cultural Differences Influence Mealtime Habits

One aspect of eating that varies among cultures is the amount of independence that is expected of young children. The following examples illustrate how these cultural differences and personality differences influence the feeding experiences of the child.

Elise is of Hispanic–American background and her 18-month-old son, Juan, who demonstrates athetoid cerebral palsy, is learning to finger feed. Juan mashes the food in his fingers and usually smears it on his high chair before bringing it to his mouth. Because his movement is poorly controlled, he also smears it on his face and in his hair as he aims for his mouth. Elise is thrilled that he is demonstrating an interest in self-feeding and can accomplish it with finger foods and a cup with a lid. She encourages him and believes that this sign of independence is a step toward gaining his manhood.

Timika, of Japanese descent, has a 2-year-old daughter, Kita, who has problems in motor control similar to Juan. Timika is a neat woman, who maintains a clean and orderly home at all times. She feeds Kita with a small spoon and has a cloth nearby to immediately wipe food that falls from her mouth. Timika has never allowed Kita to finger feed or attempt to use the cup. In her culture, children are fed by their parents for many years, so she sees no value in promoting self-feeding and has indicated to the occupational therapist that self-feeding is not one of her goals for Kita.

Oral Feeding Intervention

Evaluation. Evaluation of feeding and other self-care skills generally has four components. The first involves the chart, file, or report review. Information about child's medications, developmental course, prognosis, and systemic or metabolic problems is essential before making recommendations about feeding. The second evaluation component is the interview of the parent or caregiver. The perspective of the parent is crucial for establishing the concerns

and priorities. The caregiver's description of feeding the child (covering the complete 24-hour daily cycle) enables the therapist to understand the problem from an insider's perspective. The therapist asks questions, such as those presented in Table 6.4, to begin to make goals and plans with the family.

After gaining extensive information about what the child eats and how he or she is fed, the practitioner observes the infant eating in the third step of the evaluation. The parent is asked to feed the child foods that he or she typically eats at home. The goal is to demonstrate feeding as it typically occurs. Parent-child interaction is observed, oral skills are documented, swallowing problems are noted, and behaviors are analyzed. The parent and child's communication during feeding is important, and the pace of feeding as well as the amount of food should be guided by the child.

In the fourth step of the evaluation, the practitioner further observes and analyzes the child's feeding skills, using hands-on feeding. This evaluation allows the practitioner to observe oral motor and sensory skills more closely. The therapist tries specific handling techniques to observe their effects in order to determine their potential use in promoting the child's feeding skills. Different textures are given to the child to assess his or her sensory tolerance. A variety of food textures (e.g., viscous and chewy, crunchy, mixed) are used to facilitate the child's highest levels of oral motor skills.

When self-feeding is evaluated, the child is placed in supportive seating and observed while using fingers, utensils, cups, and straws to eat and drink. Use of a variety of foods is also important to evaluation of self-feeding. The parents are interviewed about how, where, and what the child eats at home. The practitioner must respect cultural differences in how food is eaten, including use of a bottle well beyond the first year and use of utensils that are culturally specific.

Consultation with the physician and nutritionist is important to designing intervention, particularly when the child has a failure-to-thrive condition, is on medications, or has a history of metabolic problems. Modifications to the child's feeding methods or diet should not be made without frequent communication with the other health care professionals who are caring for the child. In all feeding interventions, the nutritional status of the child is of highest priority and cannot be compromised, particularly in children with related health concerns. With this in mind, interventions for children with (a) primary motor dysfunction, (b) primary sensory processing problems, and (c) behavior problems are described.

Table 6.4 Practitioner's Interview With Caregiver Regarding Child's Feeding

Requested Information	Probes
Describe feeding of your child.	Who feeds him or her? How does your child respond to feeding?
Describe your child's feeding problems	Does she or he have difficulty sucking, drinking, biting, chewing? Does your child cough or choke?
How much help does your child need with feeding?	What are ways that you help your child eat?
How do you know when your child is hungry?	What are different behaviors that indicate that your child is hungry?
How do you know when your child has had enough?	When and why do you think your child stops eating (endurance can be an issue)?
When and how often is your child fed?	How long does a meal take?
Describe your child's diet.	Include formula, milk, all foods.
Describe where your child is fed.	In highchair, lap, at table, wheelchair. Describe child's position.
What equipment is used in feeding?	Describe bottles, nipples, spoon, adapted equipment.
Describe your child's response to feeding.	When does he or she most enjoy feeding?
How does your child react to new foods, foods with different textures or tastes?	Does his or her response vary according to the time or day? According to the place?
Describe the environment during feeding.	Who is present? What is the activity level, noise level?
What recommendations have been given to you regarding feeding?	How have these recommendations worked?

Motor Impairment

Positioning. During eating, postural alignment and stability must be adequate to support oral motor control. Full external support is required when postural stability is low. For example, a high-back chair with lateral supports and straps may be recommended for a child with spastic quadriparesis. The goal of the feeding positioning device is to provide an optimal level of head and trunk support that will allow the child to demonstrate his or her highest level of oral motor control.

For the child who has not developed head control, lateral head supports are beneficial. Slightly reclining the chair while maintaining 90° of hip flexion assists the child in head control and facilitates oral movements for feeding. A slightly reclined position (30°) also enables the child to use gravity to assist in the suck-swallow sequence (Morris & Klein, 1987). Whether the chair is tilted backward or is upright, neck alignment in neutral (with head directly over shoulders) or in slight flexion is critical so that

the throat structures are in optimal alignment for efficient swallowing. A slightly forward position of the head appears to facilitate swallowing by bringing the throat structures closer together and by making closure of the trachea easier. Therefore, this position of slight flexion should be considered for children with swallowing problems. If the child is at risk for aspiration, a videofluoroscopic study can reveal the head and neck position that results in optimal swallow.

Handling techniques before feeding. Children with hypotonicity of the oral musculature may benefit from techniques to improve muscle tone. Tapping or quick stretch of cheeks and lips provides sensory input that can activate tone for improved lip closure (Glass & Wolf, 1997). When tapping is applied symmetrically and rhythmically, it also promotes organized responses in the child. Quick stretch to the masseter and buccinator muscles before feeding can increase muscle tone and enhance lip closure (Glass & Wolf, 1997). Deep pressure applied slowly can inhibit muscle tone in the child with hypertonicity. Vibration is a strong stimulus that can increase or decrease tone by flooding sensory receptors. The child's response to this stimulus should be carefully observed at times other than mealtime to evaluate its effect.

Handling during feeding. With the head well supported, the practitioner's or parent's fingers, or cupped hand, can be placed under or around the child's chin to enhance jaw stability. One finger places pressure through the front of the chin to promote chin tuck and another finger provides support under the jaw (see Figure 6.2). The goal of this support is to assist in jaw stability and to provide support for the tongue's movement. This technique of jaw support has evidence of effectiveness with premature infants (Einarisson-Backes, Deitz, Price, Glass, & Hays, 1994) and with children who have cerebral palsy (Gisel, Applegate-Ferrante, Benson, & Bosma, 1995). Jaw support seems to work best with infants who have not yet learned abnormal motor patterns.

When spoon feeding, downward pressure on the tongue with the bowl of the spoon can inhibit tongue retraction or protraction and facilitate sucking. This

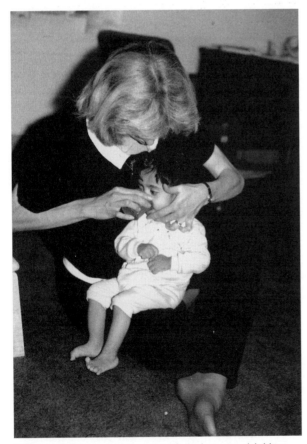

Figure 6.2 Use of jaw control during cup drinking.

gentle pressure with a spoon promotes a cupped tongue and an organized suck-swallow pattern.

When the practitioner determines a technique to be effective, he or she recommends that the technique be implemented on a regular basis. Instruction to parents and other caregivers is essential and should be reinforced with modeling, pictures, or feedback as the caregiver tries the techniques. Continual monitoring of the child's response to handling techniques (ideally including observation in the child's natural environment) is critical to assist in problem solving and to help the caregiver adapt the techniques when needed.

Sensory aspects of food. Altering the sensory qualities of food is another way to improve oral motor skills (Case-Smith & Humphry, 1996). A child's tongue movement is guided by the texture of food or drink and responds to the sensory stimulus in the mouth. Foods that are smooth and stick together can facilitate organized tongue responses. Thick, heavy, and cohesive foods (e.g., oatmeal, puddings) tend to facilitate an efficient suck-swallow pattern. Highly textured foods result in increased tongue movements. Foods that break apart and fill the mouth with sensory input can cause disorganized responses, coughing, or choking.

To promote more mature oral movements, the occupational therapy practitioner carefully selects appropriate textures to use in therapy and to recommend to the family. The practitioner selects food textures for the child on the basis of the child's level of oral motor skill and his or her sensory tolerance. Some guidelines for texture selection are provided in Table 6.5. A combination of the strategies can be more successful than selecting any one method. Foods that are contraindicated for a child with severe oral motor problems are those that break apart into small pieces that are difficult to manage (e.g., raw carrots, crisp cookies) and those that are tough and require a grinding motion to masticate.

Case Study
Trevor: A Child With Oral Motor Dysfunction

History

Trevor had a history of neonatal asphyxia. Initially, he was extremely hypotonic and moved very little. He was given liquids through an oral–gastric tube, but his oral sucking was adequate for oral feeding by 3 weeks of age. During bottle-feeding, he was positioned upright with head well supported; jaw support was applied;

Table 6.5 Guidelines for Selection of Food Texture

Developmental Level	Recommendation
Child demonstrates a munching pattern and does not have lateral tongue movements.	Use pureed, smooth foods.
Child has poor tongue control and an inefficient suck–swallow pattern.	Avoid thin liquids and thicken liquids when possible.
Child is demonstrating beginning chewing skills.	Use soft foods that have cohesion (e.g., cheeses, chicken, well-cooked vegetables with no skins). Graham crackers, butter cookies, and some cereals good foods for chewing because they dissolve quickly once inside the mouth, presenting less risk of choking.
Child maintains a munching or sucking pattern for an extended period.	A food grinder is an excellent method for varying the texture of food and allowing the child to eat a variety of foods despite low-level oral motor skills.
Child demonstrates beginning chewing skills but tends to mash foods between the tongue and upper pallet.	Grainy breads and crackers are better than soft white breads or white crackers, which tend to stick to the upper pallet.
Child demonstrates some lateral movement of the tongue.	Add foods with texture (e.g., peas, beans) to smooth and cohesive foods (e.g., mashed potatoes). Thicker foods tend to stay in the mouth longer and increase the work of the tongue, and they are easier to control. Peanut butter is an example of a food that is generally too thick when consumed by itself.
Child needs additional muscle tone and strength for effective biting and chewing.	Some foods can increase muscle tone for improved chewing. Viscous foods such as Fruit Roll-Ups® promote rotary chewing and graded jaw movements. Some dried fruits (e.g., apricots, apples) can be used to increase chewing. Tough or fibrous meats are contra-indicated in children without basic chewing skills.
Child with beginning chewing skills has not yet developed controlled bite.	The therapist holds a long piece of vegetable or meat between the side teeth to promote graded biting. Strips of cheese or lunch meat can be used. Soft cookies and crackers placed to the side can also promote controlled biting. Pretzels and apple slices require more jaw strength and can be tried as a next step in biting skill.

and a soft preemie nipple was used. This method was slow, but his growth was adequate with nutritional supplements.

Current Feeding Problem

He was bottle-fed until 10 months of age when the mother expressed interest in attempting pureed foods. At this point, several problems had to be overcome. At 10 months, he exhibited a pattern of spastic quadriparesis. He demonstrated extreme hypersensitivity because he had not experienced texture in his mouth. When textures were attempted, he spit them out and turned his head. His head and trunk control remained poor. He required full support to sit.

When a spoon was introduced, he demonstrated wide jaw excursions, his mouth opened to its full range then clamped shut on the spoon in a tonic bite. His tongue moved in extension-retraction and was not effective in taking the food from the spoon. Lateral tongue movement was poorly controlled. He gagged easily if the spoon was placed in the center of his tongue. His suck–swallow pattern was disorganized, and he often coughed when given small amounts of food.

Intervention

Positioning. Trevor required full head and trunk support for feeding. A feeder chair was used because it provided complete support, had a strapping system, and helped to maintain a position of 90° hip flexion. He tended to arch in all positions; therefore, additional support was provided at the anterior upper trunk to maintain his alignment. Backward pressure on the front of his chest helped to maintain a position of chin tuck, important for an efficient suck-swallow response. Although the strapping helped with his postural alignment, he attempted to arch and hyperextend his head. A small pad was placed behind his head to prevent hyperextension and to promote child tuck. The feeding chair was placed at a 60° angle so that gravity assisted his oral movements and swallow. This angle also prevented food loss from his mouth.

Handling. To decrease his sensory defensiveness before feeding, Trevor's mother gently stroked the area around his mouth and his lips with a warm washcloth. She also stroked his gums and rubbed his tongue. Trevor liked this input and would frequently bite the washcloth and smile.

During feeding, the mother was instructed to use jaw control. She placed her hand around Trevor's jaw, with her third finger under his mandible, her index finger along his cheek, and her thumb on his front mandible to reinforce his chin tuck. Her hand prevented his wide jaw movement and gave support to his tongue to move the food back in his mouth for swallow. She placed the spoon in the center of his tongue and pressed down gently to facilitate a suck–swallow response. Smooth pureed foods were used; textured food was avoided until his suck-swallow response became more reliable.

Family variables. The mother generally fed Trevor. She frequently asked the practitioner whether she was applying the techniques correctly. The practitioner reassured her often that her gentle touches and careful attention to his responses were important to the success of the feeding efforts. She was always responsive to his cues and waited patiently for his responses. Although her hesitancy established a comfortable pace for Trevor, the time required for a meal

was not realistic in the family's busy daily schedule. The practitioner encouraged her to place slightly more food on the spoon and to establish a somewhat quicker pace. This was possible after Trevor's initial hypersensitivity was reduced. The practitioner reassured the mother that Trevor would indicate whether the amount or pace exceeded his capability. With practice she became more comfortable, and feeding became more efficient.

The practitioner discussed with the mother who else could be trained to feed Trevor and who might give her respite from this responsibility. She identified her mother as someone else who could help and the best candidate to learn the techniques.

These methods worked fairly well, although Trevor could only take in small amounts of food on the spoon and his suck-swallow response was slow and inefficient, thereby requiring several attempts. He required 15 minutes to eat a bowl of pureed food. This level of oral feeding was acceptable because his primary nutritional source was formula from the bottle. The mother's goal in the following 6 months was to increase the amount of food he could take by mouth and to increase the textures that were acceptable to him. The grandmother attended the subsequent therapy sessions and learned how to position and handle Trevor for feeding. One day a week she helped to care for Trevor, allowing his mother a day of respite. ■

Sensory Processing Impairment. When a child has difficulty tolerating tactile input, often the face and oral areas are particularly sensitive. Sensory defensiveness of the oral area may be a result of an extended period of nonoral feeding or from lack of appropriate oral experiences. Sensory defensiveness can be identified through observation and parent interview. The practitioner asks about food textures that can be tolerated by the child. During the observation, the child should be offered a variety of textures. Aversive responses, choking, gagging, or expressions of discomfort all can indicate sensory processing problems.

Intervention. When the child has oral tactile defensiveness, sensory input at times other than the mealtime is important. Oral play with rubber toys and a warm, wet washcloth can be helpful. Children generally enjoy these textures. In particular, rubber toys promote tongue and jaw movements and are an acceptable method of desensitizing the oral area. Brushing with a regular or Nuk® toothbrush helps to desensitize the child's mouth (see Figure 6.3). Children often begin to chew on these brushes on their own. Asking the parent to brush the child's

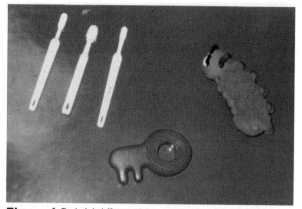

Figure 6.3 A Nuk® toothbrush set and rubber toys. These items help desensitize the mouth, and children often enjoy chewing them.

teeth and gums three times a day may easily fit into the family's daily routine; however, routines vary and parents may select more playful methods of oral stimulation.

An optimal time to desensitize the oral area is immediately before eating. Sensory preparation at this time can improve acceptance and tolerance of the meal. The amount and type of sensory input must rely on the child's responses to touch. Many times, the child can tolerate self-stimulation more than application by another. In children with severe tactile hypersensitivity, the practitioner should begin with application of deep pressure around the mouth and then entering the mouth, rubbing the child's gums and upper palette. Stroking and rubbing can be done with the finger or a washcloth. Toothbrushing, with extra input to the gums and sides of the tongue, can help prepare the child for feeding. Rhythmic deep stroking is often more accepted by the child. If the parent or practitioner establishes the same routine for desensitization each time (e.g., begins around the mouth and then rubs along the gum line), the child generally demonstrates more tolerance of the stimulation.

Guidelines for introducing food textures to the child with sensory processing problems are presented in Table 6.6. Among the most difficult textures to tolerate are small, discrete bits of food, such as small pieces of meat, corn, or raisins. With some children, hiding textured food in smooth-food substances like pudding or applesauce makes the texture tolerable. In other children, any discrete bit of food is expelled from the mouth.

Understanding the basis of the child's oral defensiveness is important when planning an intervention program. Sensory processing problems that

relate to a neurological impairment are often among the most difficult to overcome. When sensory intolerance appears related to lack of oral sensory experience, such as in the child fed with a gastrostomy tube, the sensory defensiveness is easier to overcome. This child generally improves rapidly when given graded sensory input. Although the guidelines in Table 6.6 apply to many children, every child is unique and has individual preferences for oral sensory experience, food textures, and tastes.

Behavioral Problems. Behavioral problems during feeding are not easily solved. Usually, the child's behavior reflects a greater issue of negative interactions and a history of problems in feeding. The following are some guidelines for occupational therapy practitioners to improve the child's behaviors during feeding.

1. Perform a functional analysis of the problem. What initiates the negative behaviors? Often, the behavior is a form of communication. What is the child attempting to communicate by his or her behaviors?

2. When the source of the disruptive behaviors is identified, discuss with the parent how that situation can be avoided or how it can be modified so that the disruptive behavior is not needed.

3. Assist the parent in reading the child's cues. Often, these problems occur when a child's gestures and speech are difficult to understand and cues are subtle. Help the parent or caregiver increase sensitivity to the child's gestures or facial expressions that indicate discomfort, satiation, or dislike of a food.

4. Recommend that the feeders give the child choices during feeding so that he or she participates in the meal. Giving the child simple choices at mealtime can promote the child's feeling of control. The child can select which food to eat or indicate when a bite is desired. The child should direct the pace and sequence of the meal, for example, choosing a drink versus solid food, or meat versus a vegetable.

5. The child who struggles to eat or has oral hypersensitivity needs consistent praise and positive touches. Positive interaction between the child and parent or other family members can be as important as the amount of nutritional intake. Each influences the other.

6. Behavioral management techniques can be helpful when behaviors become highly disruptive to the family mealtime. Consultation with a psychol-

Table 6.6 Food Texture Progression

Recommendations	Examples	Nutritional Value	Precautions
1. To facilitate sucking and swallowing, use pureed or soft foods.	Gelatin	High sugar Limited protein value	Avoid gelatin with fruit pieces.
	Pureed meats and vegetables	Good variety of vitamins and protein	Avoid using baby foods for extended periods.
	Pudding or custard	High carbohydrates; milk provides calcium and protein	Tapioca pudding can be very offensive to hyper-sensitive children and may provide extra stimulus to hyposensitive children.
	Applesauce	Low calorie; high fluid content	
2. To facilitate sucking and swallowing, use a heavy food that easily forms a bolus and gives proprioceptive input.	Mashed potatoes (excellent consistency for providing proprioceptive input)	High carbohydrate; adding margarine provides calo-ries; adding powdered milk adds protein and calcium	Mixing firm bits of food with mashed potatoes may not be tolerated by sensitive children; incon-sistency in texture may cause choking.
	Oatmeal	High carbohydrate; milk adds calcium and protein	
3. Liquids may need to be thickened to improve and facilitate swallowing.	Liquids may be thickened with yogurt, wheat germ, gelatin, cereal, carrageen	Yogurt: protein and calcium Wheat germ: carbohydrates and fiber Gelatin: see above Cereal: carbohydrates, vitamins (depends on the type of cereal)	Avoid high carbohydrates to thicken liquids; when food pools in the back of mouth, alternate with thinner liquids; avoid cornstarch.
4. To promote chewing initially, use chewy or gummy foods that hold together to make a bolus.	Bananas; cheese; progress to chicken, lunch meat, marshmallows, soft vegeta-bles, crackers, dried fruit, apples, zwieback toast, graham crackers	Fruits: carbohydrates and vitamins Cheese: protein and calcium Meat: protein Vegetables: vitamins and complex carbohydrates	Avoid foods and meats that break apart; avoid vegetables with skins unless well cooked.
5. To promote chewing when jaw is more sta-ble but movement is primitive, use crispy or harder solids.	Crackers, graham crackers, dried fruit	Crackers: complex carbohydrates Graham crackers: complex carbohydrates and fiber Dried fruit: high-calorie carbohydrates	If you use carrots or beef jerky, avoid allowing child to bite off pieces. Use of tough meat may increase abnormal postures.

(continued)

Table 6.6 (*continued*)

Recommendations	Examples	Nutritional Value	Precautions
6. To desensitize the mouth, grade the texture of the food; use a blender, if possible, to make small variations in texture.	Begin with pureed, then progress to soft foods, then lumpy or solid.	Different nutrients can be provided in a variety of textures.	Do not begin with lumpy foods—a hypersensitive child will be intolerant of these. When blending foods, avoid mixing all foods together.
Use a variety of tastes, textures, and temperatures.	Be creative, given the above guidelines.	Variety should improve the nutritional balance.	Consult nutritionist and occupational or speech therapist for advice.

ogist may be helpful. A regime can be established in which limits to the child's behavior are defined, and specific consequences result when the child exceeds the limits. When the discipline technique is consistently applied, the child learns which behaviors are allowed and which are not. Generally, "time out" or elimination of something desired is an effective consequence of disruptive behaviors.

Intervention for Self-Feeding

When children have motor limitations such as cerebral palsy that interfere with self-feeding, a variety of therapeutic interventions may be needed to increase their skills. Positioning, handling, and adaptive interventions are described in the following sections.

Positioning. Correct alignment and adequate support for stable trunk and head are essential for demonstration of eye–hand coordination in self-feeding. The midrange movement of the hand and arm through space require either well-developed trunk stability or sufficient external support so that the trunk is aligned and stable. Smooth, graded movement of the arms at midline requires adequate postural stability as a base of support. The child must feel secure and relaxed during self-feeding to use the strength, control, and endurance needed to eat an entire meal. Positioning with head, neck, and trunk in correct alignment (the chin tucked, shoulders depressed and slightly forward, and the pelvis in neutral alignment) allows the child to use both hands at midline and in midspace for spoon to mouth and cup drinking. This position can be maintained in a wheelchair or feeder chair with pelvic and hip abductor straps. Lateral trunk supports may also be helpful. When the child tends to retract his or her shoulders, padded humeral "wings" attached to the back of the chair can help to maintain the child's arms in a forward shoulder protracted position. These wings help to maintain a scapular position that allows for neutral shoulder rotation and forearm supination (Danella & Vogtle, 1992).

When the shoulder is unstable, an external support to the upper arm or elbow can help the child accommodate to control a hand-to-mouth pattern. The child can stabilize his arm on a small, short bolster placed under his or her arm. The bolster separates the child's elbow from the trunk, maintaining a position of some shoulder abduction. Then, by stabilizing the elbow on a tray or table, the child scoops food and reaches his or her mouth with minimal movement of the shoulder and elbow. The bolster, in combination with the tray surface, serves as a lever from which the child can effectively move hand to mouth.

Simply raising the tray or table surface can also assist the child whose hand-to-mouth pattern is unstable. With the child bearing weight on his elbows, raising the height of the wheelchair tray promotes upright sitting and humeral abduction (Bergen & Colangelo, 1985). This postural help can improve hand-to-mouth control as the child stabilizes his or her elbow on the tray and then uses simple elbow flexion and extension to feed. Positioning with an elevated, well-fitting tray enables the child with cerebral palsy to gain the postural control needed to self-feed independently when given easily managed foods (see Figure 6.4).

Handling Techniques. For the child with athetoid cerebral palsy and limited control of arms in space, handling during feeding should emphasize postural stability and proximal support of the arms (Boehme,

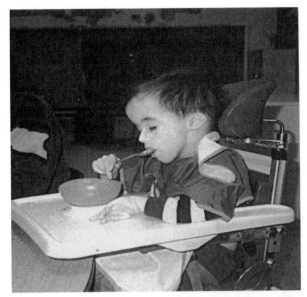

Figure 6.4 A boy feeds himself, with his elbow resting on an elevated tray.

1988). An aide, parent, therapist, or assistant can hold the child during self-feeding from behind to promote shoulder depression and protraction and scapular stability. Support and guidance of the upper arm may be needed to establish a smooth hand-to-mouth pattern. This support should help the child stabilize his or her arm in space rather than move it through the range. Hand-over-hand methods tend to make the child a passive rather than an active participant in the feeding process. Therefore, the least amount of support should be given that allows the child to successfully use a spoon, fork, and cup.

To provide subtle guidance of the spoon to mouth, the practitioner holds the spoon handle in between his or her own extended index and third fingers. The practitioner slips these fingers holding the handle into the child's palm and places his or her thumb on the dorsum of the child's hand. Using a gross grasp, the child holds onto the practitioner's fingers that align the spoon handle, and the practitioner then facilitates a self-feeding pattern by subtly guiding the hand-to-mouth pattern. This technique is particularly successful with a child who has developed a basic hand-to-mouth pattern but spills frequently. The practitioner's or parent's fingers inside the child's hand support the small movements of hand and wrist needed to enter the spoon in the mouth and to reduce spillage.

One disadvantage of these handling techniques is that they require the teacher or parent to be seated behind the child. Therefore, face-to-face communication is limited. The position required to use these techniques makes implementation during family mealtime difficult. They can be successful when used for snacks at school or at home. When providing these techniques, the caregiver should work to decrease the amount of physical assistance so that the child continually makes small gains in independence during the meal.

Adaptive Equipment. Adaptive equipment for feeding is readily available and is often helpful in enabling the child to be more independent in self-feeding. Parents have frequently remarked that adapted utensils, plates, and cups with handles and lids help to increase the child's ability to self-feed and to decrease spillage and frustration. Helpful feeding equipment includes built-up handles, plates with high curved rims, and nonskid pads (Scherzer & Tscharnuter, 1991) (see Figure 6.5). Morris and Klein (1987) provide numerous examples of utensils, cups, and bowls that enable the child to self-feed successfully. Plates or bowls with raised edges and resistive surfaces give the child a stable surface for obtaining the food.

Characteristics of spoons that assist the child in self-feeding are enlarged handles, latex-covered spoon bowls, and angled handles. Cups with lids reduce spillage. Lids without spouts may be helpful when the child exhibits suckling (in and out) tongue movement. Straws can promote the child's ability to suck and can allow the child to drink without lifting the cup from the table surface. More sophisticated adapted equipment, such as the electric feeder, may enable a child to self-feed without using his or her arms. Criteria for selecting adaptive equipment to improve the child's independence in self-feeding include durability, ease of cleaning and use, and developmental appropriateness.

Family Variables. Cultural values highly influence the timing and degree of self-feeding desired by the family. When both parents are working, the child's self-sufficiency in feeding may be highly desirable. Working parents may not have the time to work with the child in promoting self-feeding. Inevitably, helping a child through the steps of self-feeding requires more time than simply feeding the child. Therefore, parents must balance the time required for learning self-feeding with the time saved by the outcome of a child who can independently self-feed.

In many cultures, feeding a child is a highly valued interaction that the parent wants to preserve and

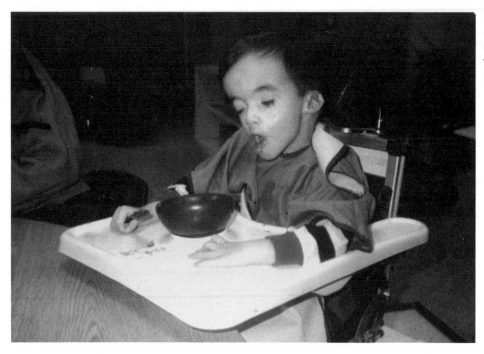

Figure 6.5 A bowl with a high rim and suction cup at its base enables the child to eat independently.

continue until middle childhood. This parent would be disinterested in techniques to help the child become more independent in feeding. The parent's desire to continue feeding the child should be respected.

Dressing

Dressing skills in children without disabilities develop over a 4- to 5-year period, within the first 6 years of life. The emergence of these skills depends on the child's interest and self-initiative and the value that family members place on dressing independence.

Typical Development

The child first begins to participate in dressing at about 12 months of age. It is not until 5 or 6 years of age that the child can accomplish the most difficult fasteners. Table 6.7 provides some guidelines about the sequence and typical ages that specific dressing skills are accomplished.

Variables That Influence Dressing

Motor Dysfunction. Dressing requires basic and complex motor skills. Balance and postural stability are needed to reach one's feet and body parts. Strength may be needed to fit tight clothing over body parts. Dexterity and eye–hand coordination are needed to close and open fastenings and to button and tie.

For the young child with cerebral palsy, dressing may be difficult. Postural support may be needed as the child shifts weight reaching overhead or when bending to reach for his or her feet. Problems in dexterity and two-hand coordination may interfere with ability to fasten and properly arrange clothing.

Sensory or Perceptual Impairments. A child must first be able to tolerate and accept the feel of clothing next to his or her skin. Although almost all children tolerate touch, some children do not tolerate certain textures. Infants' clothing is typically soft, but clothing for older children can be stiff or rough. Children must learn to accept increasing texture and variety in clothing materials. Body awareness and body image are inherent in the task of dressing. A child learns to match body parts to clothing pieces and in the process learns the important perceptual concepts of front, back, right, and left. Visual perception and kinesthesia are important to recognizing clothing characteristics and how those fit his or her body (Shepherd, Coley, & Proctor, 1996).

Children with sensory processing problems may not tolerate certain types of materials or clothing. They may become irritable when dressed or may resist dressing. As an infant, the act of dressing may be particularly distressing because it involves multi-

Table 6.7 Sequence of Typical Development of Dressing

Age (in years)	Self-Dressing Skills
1	Cooperates with dressing (holds out arms and feet) Pulls off shoes, removes socks Pushes arms through sleeves and legs through pants
2	Removes unfastened coat Removes shoes if laces are untied Helps pull down pants Finds armholes in over-the-head shirt
2½	Removes pull-down pants with elastic waist Assists in pulling on socks Puts on front-button coat, shirt Unbuttons large buttons
3	Puts on over-the-head shirt with minimal assistance Puts on shoes without fasteners (may be on wrong foot) Puts on socks (may be with heel on top) Independent in pulling down pants Zips and unzips jacket once on track Needs assistance to remove over-the-head shirt Buttons large front buttons
3½	Finds front of clothing Snaps or hooks front fastener Unzips front zipper on jacket, separating zipper Puts on mittens Buttons series of three or four buttons Unbuckles shoe or belt Dresses with supervision (help with front and back)
4	Removes pullover garment independently Buckles shoes or belt Zips jacket zipper Puts on socks correctly Puts on shoes with assistance in tying laces Laces shoes Consistently identifies the front and back of garments
4½	Puts belt in loops
5	Ties and unties knots Dresses unsupervised
6	Closes back zipper Ties bow knot Buttons back buttons Snaps back snaps

Note. From *Pre-Dressing Skills*, by M. D. Klein, 1988, Tucson, AZ: Therapy Skill Builders. Copyright 1988 by Therapy Skill Builders. Adapted with permission.

ple light touches of body parts seldom touched. This child may later insist on only wearing certain clothes on the basis of his or her preferred texture (e.g., the child may wear the same dress day after day).

Children with sensory problems are often limited in their perceptual development, and their awareness of body scheme and body image may be inadequate. This child may have difficulty distinguishing right and left sides of the body and, therefore, have difficulty identifying which leg goes with which pant leg or which sleeve goes with which arm. The child with visual-perceptual problems will have difficulty learning to button and lace and tie shoelaces. Motor planning and bilateral integration problems also interfere with performing these skills.

Cognition. Children with cognitive delays may also have difficulty learning body parts, right and left sides, and the steps required to tie or buckle. Learning to dress often requires more time, but because dressing is repeated on a daily basis, it may become an area of independence for children with cognitive impairment. Appropriate dressing with clothing neatly arranged requires that the child can self-assess his or her appearance. This skill may be inadequately developed when cognition is impaired.

Family System, Culture, and Values. The family's overall function is less important to dressing than feeding primarily because dressing requires less time; that is, it is performed generally twice a day. Expectations for the child's independence should be applied consistently and held constant across caregivers (Kellegrew, 1998), and the techniques used to promote dressing (e.g., backward chaining) should be applied consistently. Communication among family members about the child's skills in dressing helps to facilitate consistency in expectations as these skills develop.

Cultural values influence dressing traditions and the type of clothes worn. Persons from Middle Eastern cultures prefer to cover almost all body parts, including the head. Children may be required to wear multiple layers of clothing or can wear very simple, one-piece clothing. As in feeding, parents of different cultures may not value independence in their children. Mothers may expect and want to dress their children until school age (i.e., 6 years) (Chan, 1992). Parents of a child with disabilities often highly value their child's physical appearance. They may want their child to appear as normal or attractive as possible to reduce the stigma they may experience and to increase others' acceptance.

Case Study
Megan: An Illustration of Family Values and Dressing

Megan was a beautiful 7-year-old girl who had cerebral palsy, and her mother always dressed her in the styles that were most fashionable. This included blue jeans overalls that have multiple fasteners at the shoulder and waist as well as shorts, pants, and dresses with tiny buttons placed in awkward positions. These outfits made it impossible for Megan to manage her clothing for independent toileting. The teaching staff members at school were frustrated because she remained dependent in dressing tasks when she could be independent if she wore simpler, easy-to-manage clothes.

The occupational therapist suggested that Megan wear sweat shirts and sweat pants with an elastic waist to school so that she could be independent in toileting. This suggestion angered the parents because they highly valued Megan's appearance in the latest fashions and beautifully tailored clothes. They valued how others at school perceived her appearance much more than how independently she was able to function at school. The occupational therapist made alternate suggestions for clothing that was both fashionable and easy to manage; however, the parents continued to primarily use clothing that created the image that they held of their daughter as a beautiful, meticulously dressed child. The school-based team decided that respect for the parents' priorities was most important; therefore, throughout the school year, the teachers continued to help Megan with toileting and dressing. ■

Intervention for Dressing

Motor Impairment

Activities to improve performance. When the child is introduced to self-dressing, the activity should take place cooperatively between parent and child. The child begins to participate more in dressing, and the parent allows the child to attempt the movements required to dress and undress. For example, the young child with poor trunk control can be dressed in a supported sitting position. The child can sit between the parent's legs with the pelvis and lower trunk supported. Seated behind the child, the parent guides the infant's movements as he or she pushes the arms and legs through sleeves and pant legs. This activity allows the child to practice bilateral movement needed to don shirts and pants. To pull on pants, the child can move into a quadruped position over the parent's thigh and then back into sitting.

When a child has limited control of movement, dressing intervention often requires special handling and positioning techniques as well as appropriate clothing and adapted equipment. Through motor analysis of each task, the practitioner identifies which components of movement interfere with accomplishing dressing independence (see Table 6.8). Those skills that are emerging but require physical assistance from another person become the focus of therapy. If reduced active range of motion is a problem, the practitioner provides activities to enhance shoulder strength and controlled mobility. Weight-bearing activities in a hands-and-knees position or in sitting can promote active range supported by adequate co-contraction of the shoulder. Reaching activities that include some resistance (involve pushing with hands at shoulder height) are examples of how practitioners

design intervention to improve missing components of dressing performance.

Dressing practice is integrated into therapy sessions. The motor components identified as missing or deficit are facilitated using therapeutic positioning or handling. Practice on a low bench with the practitioner sitting behind the child can allow for a dynamic interplay between the practitioner and child during a dressing activity. The low bench enables the child to work on balance with feet supported. The firm and small surface of the bench allows the practitioner to assist the child at the trunk or proximal arm and easily synchronize his or her body movements with those of the child. He or she can use trunk and legs to support and guide the child's trunk in the equilibrium reactions required during dressing.

The practitioner's goals in handling during an upper-body dressing activity include enhancing pos-

Table 6.8 Motor Analysis for Donning a T-Shirt

Donning a T-Shirt	Observe
Reach for shirt	Shoulder stability in directed reach Trunk control in forward weight shift Quality of reach—smooth and directed Symmetry of bilateral reach
Grasp of shirt	Hand opening Grasping pattern and control Use of two hands together Isolated distal finger prehension
Bring T-shirt over head	Use of two hands together Ability to maintain grasp during active movement of shoulder and elbow Adequate shoulder range for bringing shirt over top of head Smooth bilateral shoulder flexion with elbow flexion Maintenance of head and trunk stability Resistive grasp and arm flexion during forceful movement of shirt opening over head
Right arm through sleeve	Ability to locate arm opening (using visual or tactile perception or both) Ability to stabilize shirt with left hand Shoulder extension with elbow flexion to position arm Shoulder abduction with elbow extension to push arm through sleeve
Left arm through sleeve	Same, location of the sleeve is usually easier May require slightly greater arm strength to push through sleeve if the T-shirt fits tightly

tural stability and symmetry, bilateral coordination, controlled reach (including reach overhead and across midline), and use of hands in space. Lower-body dressing requires well-developed trunk control and sitting equilibrium. To place feet through pant's legs, the child must reach forward and across the midline with the arms extended; this skill is quite difficult for the child with cerebral palsy because it involves a combination of shoulder flexion and elbow extension with shoulder mobility and elbow stability. Assisting the child by supporting his or her trunk or scapula can help him or her develop these movements. Supporting the child at the pelvis can reinforce neutral pelvic alignment, backward weight shift, and trunk rotation required to reach for his or her feet.

Therapeutic activities that elicit the child's balance in the sit-to-stand transition are emphasized. As the child prepares to stand to pull up pants, forward weight shift and trunk and hip extension are facilitated. A goal of therapy becomes adequate standing balance such that the child can lean forward and pull his or her pants over the buttocks. Although therapy sessions may emphasize these individual performance components, it is important that the child also have opportunities to integrate the performance components into functional dressing activities. In addition to therapy designed to improve performance, adapted techniques, adapted equipment, and appropriate clothing are methods to increase independence in dressing.

Adapted techniques. A primary method of adapting the dressing activity so that a young child becomes independent is to provide supportive positioning. When the child is unstable in sitting and lacks the balance needed to reach forward and to the sides, seating should be provided that is supportive to the trunk—including pelvis and shoulders. Some children dress in their wheelchair so that they can shift their weight side to side using the armrests for support. The child may dress in the corner of a room, so that his or her trunk is supported in side-to-side movements (Shepherd et al., 1996).

Adapted techniques have been developed to simplify the hand and arm movements required during dressing. Children are taught to don their coats by laying the coat on the floor upside down, pushing both hands through their sleeves while lifting the coat overhead. This technique requires over-the-head arm movement but eliminates crossing the midline and reaching behind the trunk. One-hand tying techniques can be used. Often, children must first learn to tie their shoes using the "bunny ear"

method that requires symmetrical hand movement rather than asymmetrical movements that include crossing the midline.

Adapted equipment. Buttonhooks, long shoe horns, long-reach zipper aids, and adapted shoe ties are examples of equipment that can increase the child's dressing independence (Klein, 1988; Shepherd et al., 1996). Metal rings can be placed on the zipper. A dressing stick can aid in donning socks when range of motion is limited in the shoulder or the lower extremity. These devices are inexpensive and can be quite helpful, especially when the child approaches adolescence and independence in dressing becomes more important.

Appropriate clothing. Clothing for children with movement impairments should be easy to don and doff. Pullover garments should have easy, wide openings with necklines that can stretch. Flexible, elasticized waistbands and large sleeve openings are helpful. Garments that enable the child to dress independently are loose fitting, with stretchy (knit) fabrics, elastic waistbands, and few (or no) fastenings. Velcro® fastenings can replace buttons, zippers, and shoelaces. Examples of clothing easy to don and doff are sweatshirts and pants, oversized T-shirts, and elastic-waist shorts and skirts. Often, these types of clothing are available in attractive styles, and many children enjoy wearing oversized clothing. However, practitioners should be sensitive to the parents' and child's preferences. Clothing selection is the family's choice and is based on their likes and dislikes, their cultural background, how much they value style, and the resources available to invest in clothing.

Sensory or Perceptual Impairments. Children with hypersensitivity to touch may benefit from preparation for dressing. Joint compression, brushing, or deep-pressure techniques can help to calm or organize the child's sensory system before dressing. These techniques are designed to raise the threshold of sensory receptors so that the multiple, light touches involved in dressing do not disorganize the sensory system. If the parent is helping the child dress, firm touch and secure holding can help the child tolerate the tactile input of the material to his or her skin because sensation can be overwhelming. Using a routine in dressing (e.g., always the pants first and the shirt last) can help to prepare the child. Verbal cueing about the dressing activity can also help the child know what touch inputs to expect.

Children with perceptual impairments may have difficulty with spatial awareness, figure-ground awareness, or motor planning. The child may experience a combination of perceptual problems that create limitations in dressing. In addition to working on these individual components during therapy sessions, the practitioner can suggest teaching strategies, adapted techniques, and appropriate clothing to increase the child's independence and success in dressing.

Teaching strategies. The child with motor planning problems benefits from practice. The steps of the dressing task can be reinforced with verbal cues (e.g., regarding what comes next) or with visual cues (e.g., pointing). Positive reinforcement is helpful with recognition that dressing requires effort and concentration of the child. Backward chaining methods can be effective in teaching a child to dress. In this technique, the parent or caregiver performs most of the dressing task, allowing the child to complete the final steps. The parent systematically performs fewer of the beginning steps, allowing the child greater participation in completing the task (Klein, 1988). This technique results in a sense of accomplishment. When applied appropriately on the basis of the child's level of skill, this method is often highly successful with children who have motor planning problems.

The parent who observes the child dressing can give verbal cues when the child seems confused or is approaching the task incorrectly. Timing of the verbal prompts and gesture is critical for success. Verbal cues should be given before the child makes an error, thereby avoiding frustration and the need to correct dressing steps. Positive reinforcement is important to helping the child become independent in dressing. In addition to making positive remarks, the parent might suggest that the child stand before a full-length mirror to admire his or her appearance.

Adapted techniques and appropriate clothing. Adapted techniques and selected clothing can increase independence and success in dressing tasks. The child may benefit from learning the methods for donning a coat and tying shoes that involve symmetrical movements rather than asymmetrical movements and that avoid crossing the midline. Velcro fasteners are helpful, or fasteners should be avoided when possible. Easy to don (put on) clothes should be recommended. The parents can help the child organize the task by laying out clothes in the order that they should be donned. Parents should give the child sufficient time to work on dressing without rushing.

For children who have difficulty identifying the front and back or right and left sides of garments, tags can be sewn inside the garment to help with correct orientation for donning. Sometimes garments can be marked inside with colors for right and left. Clothing in which the front and back and right and left can be easily distinguished should be purchased. A selection of T-shirts and sweatshirts with designs on the front is recommended for this purpose. For the child with tactile hypersensitivity, clothes should "feel good." Soft, knit fabrics are generally easier to tolerate than stiff cotton or wool. However, children vary in their response to the texture of clothing, and, given the great variety of synthetic blends available on the market, children should be allowed to feel and select their clothes before purchase.

Bathing Skills

Bathing is a relaxing and pleasurable activity for most children and parents. Bath time generally includes playful interaction and learning about one's body in addition to hygiene. It is important that children with disabilities experience bathing as a relaxing, enjoyable experience in which they are comfortable and safe.

Typical Development of Bathing Skills

A child is interested in participating in washing himself or herself by 2 years of age. By 4 years, a child may wash and dry with supervision. Complete independence in bathing cannot be expected until 8 years of age. At this time, the child can wash all body parts and prepare the bath and shower water.

Variables That Influence Bathing Skills

Motor impairments. Postural stability and sitting balance are required for the child to sit in the bathtub. Because the tub's surface is slippery and hard, falls can easily cause injury, making postural stability an important issue in the bathing activity. To use a washcloth or soap, the child must maintain his or her grasp during active range of the shoulder and arm. This combination of mobility of the shoulder and elbow and stability of the hand (to maintain grasp) is difficult for children with cerebral palsy who tend to move their arms in synergistic patterns. Range-of-motion limitations can create problems in bathing, particularly in reaching back and buttocks. Children with coordination problems may become independent in bathing but may not achieve the same level of cleanliness as other children.

Sensory and perceptual impairments. Children with sensitivity to touch may have a low tolerance for bathing. With hypersensitivity, reactions to bathing vary. Some children appear more comfortable in the water than in other environments, others respond negatively to the bathing experience. Frequently, parents of children with tactile sensitivities report that their children have temper tantrums at bathtime. Because it is heavy and slightly textured, the feel of a wet washcloth is often acceptable to children who demonstrate aversive responses to other types of touch. Children with body scheme delays may have difficulty understanding the parent's verbal cues about washing specific body parts. They may ignore certain body parts. Table 6.9 presents issues in bathing for children with different conditions.

Family values and cultural background. Cultural values influence how the family defines bathing, how often bathing is performed, and the importance of hygiene. In many cultures, bathing once a week is the norm, and daily bathing is considered excessive. Parents may continue sponge bathing outside a bathtub for the first 3 to 4 years of the child's life. Often, parents have rituals about bathing (e.g., regularity of hair washing) that are highly ingrained. Sensitive questioning about their traditions or habits related to bathing allows the practitioner to understand this routine and offer the most helpful recommendations for improving the child's independence in this activity of daily living.

Intervention for Bathing

Motor Impairment

Activities to improve performance. Through a motor analysis of the bathing tasks, specific motor skills are identified to become a focus of intervention activities. Often, the movements that limit bathing independence are reaching to the feet, back, and head. Intervention activities that improve reach to various body parts are directed toward improving range of motion, strength, and postural stability.

In the child with cerebral palsy, the ability to reach his or her feet may be limited by tight hamstrings and postural instability. In coordination with physical therapy, activities to increase range of motion at the hips are implemented. Reaching to the top of the head and the back are also difficult for the child with cerebral palsy. Postural stability with scapular stability and mobility are emphasized in intervention activities. The child should be given opportunities to practice grasping an object while moving his or her upper arm, including motions of internal and external rotation. Practice of these movements helps the child develop the active range and arm–hand control needed to manage a washcloth. Activities that involve reaching overhead and behind can build the motor skills required for washing the back and head.

Table 6.9 Issues in Bathing for Child With Different Diagnosed Conditions

Diagnosis	Potential Problems
Cerebral palsy	Sitting balance in tub Easy startle Range-of-motion limitation affecting reach to all body parts Reaching and washing hair Transferring in and out of tub Poor control of the soap and washcloth in hands
Spina bifida	Sitting balance Sensation in legs Motor planning Tactile defensiveness
Hypersensitivities	Aversion to bathing; may have a tantrum at bath time Does not bathe thoroughly because uncomfortable
Cognitive delays	Has difficulty sequencing the bathing task Does not thoroughly complete task Limited dexterity and delayed fine motor skills

Adapted techniques and adapted equipment. Safety becomes a focus for children whose sitting balance and motor control are delayed. The practitioner recommends methods for lifting the child into the tub and achieving sitting stability once in the tub. The child should be held symmetrically in slight trunk and neck flexion. This method of securely holding reduces the possibility of the child exhibiting a startle response and falling backward or to the side.

Nonslip bath mats or rubber appliqués are helpful, although most tub surfaces are now nonslip quality. If a bath mat is not available, a temporary solution is to seat the child on a towel or large washcloth.

A variety of bath chairs are commercially available. Hammock chairs made of plastic netting stretched over polyvinyl chloride (PVC) piping support the child's head and trunk in a semireclined position. The hammock chairs, which are commercially available or can be fabricated, offer the child stability and safety and raise the position of the child in the tub to ease the bathing task for the parent. When the child develops head control and sitting balance is emerging, commercially available bathtub rings increase the sense of security in the tub (Shepherd et al., 1996).

A handheld shower helps to direct water to different body parts without body movement and shifts in posture. For the child with limitations in balance and motor control, a handheld shower helps the child or parent easily to reach all body parts and to rinse without submersion in the water (e.g., for the child in a tub chair).

Options for adapted equipment or assistive technologies change as the child grows to adult size. Many of these options are described in detail elsewhere in this book. As the child with cerebral palsy approaches school age and continues to require assistance in bathing, use of a shower chair with locking wheels should be considered. The chair provides back support and comfort during the shower. It requires a shower stall accessible to a chair on wheels and an adjustable showerhead. When the family does not have an accessible shower, the bathtub can be adapted to increase the child's independence in self-bathing. Grab bars should be installed to assist the child entering the tub, and bathtub benches with back support to the trunk allow the child with limited postural stability to transfer into the tub. Tub benches provide both comfort and safety during the bath, allowing the child to focus on good hygiene.

Sensory or Perceptual Impairments. When sensory or perceptual impairments are present, the occupational therapy practitioner first helps the parent understand that the child's aversive response to bathing is a sensory processing problem. When the child's negative behaviors are understood as an aversive response, parents can more readily adopt a positive, confident approach and use verbal cueing and reassurance.

The child can be given deep pressure before the bath to raise his or her threshold for tactile input. Here, the practitioner may recommend that the washcloth and towel be used with deep pressure in rhythmic, organized strokes. The extremities and back should be washed before the stomach and face. After bathing, the child can be wrapped tightly in a towel and held snugly in the mother's lap. This procedure can be followed by deep rubbing of arms and legs using lotion or oils. Drying and applying lotions after bathing are natural and enjoyable methods of helping the child adjust to stimuli perceived as unpleasant and of developing more tolerance toward bathing.

For the child with perceptual problems and limitations in body scheme development, bathing is an important learning opportunity. The child can learn about his or her body by naming parts while touching and visualizing. Bathing offers a natural multisensory method for learning about the body.

Functional Communication

Communication skill is essential to living in social groups. It begins with the eye contact of parent and neonate and develops throughout childhood. General milestones in oral and gestural communication are presented in Table 6.10. The variables that contribute to written and oral communication are complex and multifaceted. Augmentative communication systems are available to increase a person's conversational skills or to improve graphic communication skills. When augmentative communication is considered as a viable alternative for a child, the occupational therapist is one of the professional team members who assists in selecting, positioning for, training in, and using augmentative communication.

Variables That Influence Use of Augmentative Communication Systems

Motor Performance. In children with moderate to severe cerebral palsy, oral motor delays often interfere with speech production, and alternative communication methods must be considered. When a child has relatively high cognitive level and severe

Table 6.10 Milestones in the Development of Communication

Age (in months)	Communication Skills
3	Quiets to voice Looks at person who is talking Reacts to tone of voice Smiles to person who is talking
6	Repeats sounds that are imitated by a caregiver Imitates inflection Turns head when name is called Stops activity when name is called Begins to listen Requests a toy with a gesture
9	Imitates familiar two-syllable words (baba, dada) Makes gestures for "up" and "bye-bye" Responds to "no" Uses eye gaze during communication
12	Imitates two-syllable words (different sounds) Identifies three objects Responds to "give me" Takes turns
15	Imitates new two-syllable words Follows simple commands Identifies most common objects when they are named Appropriately indicates "yes" or "no" in response to questions Identifies two body parts Uses words to express wants
18	Imitates environment sounds during play Retrieves objects on verbal request Uses inflection Greets familiar persons with an appropriate vocalization
21	Identifies at least four animals Identifies 15 or more pictures of common objects Uses inflection patterns Experiments with two-word utterances
24	Imitates three-syllable words Follows three-part commands Uses greetings and farewells appropriately Says "no" Uses words in play Uses words to describe remote events Uses words to request action Answers simple questions with a verbal response

Note. From *The Carolina Curriculum for Infants and Toddlers with Special Needs,* by N. Johnson-Martin, K. G. Jens, S. Attermeier, & B. Hacker, 1996, Baltimore: Brookes. Copyright 1996 by Paul H. Brookes, Co. Adapted with permission.

motor problems, simple communication by gesture is inadequate, and a communication method that simulates speech becomes a priority. When considering an augmentative communication system, it is important that posture, mobility, and manipulation are evaluated to determine the appropriate type of augmentative communication device and the method of alternative access.

To access augmentative communication, the child needs to be in a position that optimizes his or her ability to control the device. If the trunk or head or both are unstable, external support is crucial. In evaluating the child's posture, these questions should be asked:

- Is the child's head stable and in a position that allows complete viewing of the keyboard? Is the head sufficiently stable that he or she can control eye movements to scan the keys or track the cursor?
- Is trunk and shoulder stability sufficient for controlled arm movement and adequate active range of arms?
- Is trunk control adequate to maintain a midline position during arm and hand movements?
- Is trunk stability sufficient that the child can maintain upright posture through a communication exchange?

When postural alignment is adequate for upright posture for short periods, but endurance is limited, external support is recommended so that the child is not fatigued and can concentrate on his or her communication efforts rather than on maintaining upright posture.

Generally, the control of the device is through the child's arm and hand. The child's motor control of arms and hands determines the type and size of keyboard that can be used. When hand movements are poorly controlled, the keys can be enlarged or a keyguard can be used with the device. When hand strength is weak, a membrane keyboard can enable the child to make item selections with minimal pressure. Keyboards have been designed that accommodate limited range of arm movement and excessive arm movement. A primary concern in establishing an augmentative communication system is the accuracy of arm movement for selecting the keys. Accuracy in using an augmentative communication device requires both eye–hand coordination (hitting the correct key) and timing (particularly when a scanning method is used and the child must hit a switch when the cursor signals the correct letter). It is also important to evaluate

speed of movement to determine the most efficient method of communication. If the child's movements are delayed, then methods of selecting individual letters to spell words become impractical for producing conversational speech.

If the point of access is the head or eyes rather than the hands, range, speed, and accuracy of head and eye movements must be evaluated. Generally, methods of access using the head and eyes require visual scanning. Therefore, timing and accuracy are critical to establishing the most practical method of communication.

Cognitive Performance. Cognition is highly related to a person's communication interests and needs. Operation of an augmentative communication device can require only basic skills or can require highly sophisticated skills. The basic skills needed to successfully operate augmentative communication devices include (a) alertness, (b) attention span, (c) vigilance, (d) understanding of cause and effect, (e) ability to express preferences, (f) ability to make choices, (g) understanding of object or pictorial permanence, and (h) symbolic representation skills.

Cognitive skills that directly relate to choice of an augmentative communication system include categorization, sequencing, matching, and sorting (Cook & Hussey, 1995). Memory is important because the keyboard must be stored in memory, and many of the new devices require multiple steps to enter into the system and select the topic of conversation. When an encoded or symbol system is used, and most augmentative communication languages involve encoding, the child must remember what each symbol stands for and how combination of symbols means different words.

Evaluation of cognition and language should include both receptive and expressive language, level of problem solving, and memory, with an emphasis on the child's ability to understand and remember symbols. Children with severe cognitive disabilities may have extreme limitations in the abilities listed above, but they can benefit from augmentative communication. Systems appropriate for these children are ones that enable the child to communicate basic needs and make simple decisions (McNaughton & Light, 1989).

Visual Perception Performance. Augmentative communication devices require adequate visual acuity and perceptual skills. In addition, the child must be able to scan and track to follow the sequence of letters or symbols on the device. If the child has difficulty visually scanning, the number of keys and the placement of keys must be considered. Increasing the size of the keys, increasing the contrast between the key and the background, and increasing the spacing between the keys can accommodate problems in visual acuity. Various foreground–background combinations can be tried to improve the contrast. The issues of greatest concern in visual perception are spatial relationships, form recognition and constancy, and figure–ground discrimination (Cook & Hussey, 1995). Each of these areas of visual perception has specific implications for the layout of keys and the system's configuration.

Family Variables. The family's acceptance of technology determines whether an augmentative communication device will work for the child. When a family has interest in technology, a sophisticated device can be considered. For families who seem perplexed by technology or avoid technology as much as possible, a simple device or simple method of augmenting communication is recommended. All devices require training to use, problem solving when they do not work, and tolerance for learning new programs and systems. All require patience to operate, and most involve some programming to upgrade and appropriately meet the child's needs.

Families that are disorganized may have difficulty maintaining the device in accessible places and keeping up with needed changes in vocabulary and required maintenance. Most often, the barriers to using augmentative communication are barriers of knowledge because most families are unfamiliar with the equipment and need to learn how to operate it and to problem solve when the device malfunctions.

Home and School Environments. Aspects of the environment that are important to consider when evaluating for augmentative communication include how the device will be transported and how the child will be assured of immediate access to the device at all times. If the child is mobile, a method for transporting the device is needed. The device always needs to be handled with care (e.g., should not have liquids spilled on it). Often, it is placed on the wheelchair tray; however, if the child is ambulatory, carrying the device is not always a viable option. A system for carrying the device may include placement in a book bag or hanging it on a wheeled walker. The environments in which the child will use the device may include the playground and the cafeteria, and provisions for use across environments must be made.

Social Environments. Other children initially respond with interest to the novelty of an augmentative com-

munication device. However, after the children have acclimated to its presence, they may grow impatient with the delays required to deliver a communication message using the device. Human communication occurs very rapidly (about 150 to 175 words per minute). A child with a disability may only produce 10 to 12 words per minute with an augmentative communication device. For children using scanning, the rate may be 3 to 5 words per minute (Cook & Hussey, 1995). Great patience is required to maintain a conversation with another person who is speaking at a rate of 5 to 10 words per minute. Practitioners find that often the conversation partner finishes sentences for the child or speaks for the child without waiting for the child to initiate the communication.

Intervention Strategies To Improve Functional Communication

Designing and Selecting an Augmentative Communication System. Occupational therapy practitioners are part of the team that helps the family select an augmentative communication system. When designing an effective augmentative communication system, the therapeutic team must make the following decisions:

- What type of system will adequately meet the child's current communication needs?
- What system will be capable of growing with the child to meet future communication goals?
- How will the child access the system, including what selection method is most appropriate and what control interface is needed?
- What skills need to be supported or developed for the child to use the system successfully?

A range of devices is available, and the most sophisticated is not always the best choice. Nonelectric devices, such as picture boards and books, may be most appropriate for a new user (Musselwhite & St. Louis, 1988). In general, the advantages of non-electric devices are that they are (a) low cost, (b) easily transported, (c) easily changed and adapted, and (d) nonthreatening and comfortable for the communication partners to use. The child may use a head pointer, mouth stick, or hand to select the pictures. Some disadvantages of these systems are that they do not provide an audible or visible message (e.g., on screen) and that expansion of vocabulary is limited.

A variety of electronic devices are currently available to meet the growing needs of children who have limited speech. The advantage of the current technology is that it is versatile and flexible;

therefore, it is meant to grow with the child. Typically, newer devices are easier to program and reprogram on a regular basis. These features allow the vocabulary and messages available to the child to be updated regularly by a parent or teacher. In making a decision about which device to use and how to introduce it to the child, the device's features need to be considered. The team must ask the following questions:

- How will the child access the device? Will direct selection or scanning be used?
- What vocabulary is needed? What prestored messages should be used? How much versatility in vocabulary is needed?
- What type of output does the device provide? Is the speech synthesized or digitized? Is written output provided?
- How portable is the device? Can the device be easily transported? Can it be used on a wheelchair or on other surfaces?
- Does the device include environmental controls (e.g., can be used to operate the television or radio)?

Children can access electronic communication devices with direct selection or scanning.

Direct selection. In direct selection, a user points directly to the key or symbol. The child targets his or her choice and then selects it by pointing or pressing. Although hands are most often used, the head can be used with a head pointer. Examples of devices that use direct selection are a computer keyboard, the Unicorn Expander® keyboard, and touch talker.

If the child appears to have the potential for a direct selection device but is not completely reliable, adaptations may be made to improve accuracy and endurance. Increasing the child's postural support, adjusting the height or angle of the device, or using a variety of tools for access (e.g., head stick, hand stick) may enable the child to use this method successfully.

Indirect selection. In scanning, the child is presented with a display that is sequentially scanned by a cursor or light. He or she selects a symbol or key by hitting a switch or clicking the mouse when the cursor or light reaches it. Various scanning methods are available, depending on the number of symbols that the child requires for everyday communication. In item-by-item scanning, the cursor moves to all possible symbol choices one at a time. Item-by-item methods are simple but are slow; therefore, this method is not feasible when many choices are

available. To increase the rate of selection, row–column scanning and group–item scanning methods can be used. In row–column scanning, the rows are lighted sequentially, and the child selects the row with the desired item in it. Then the cursor scans the columns sequentially, and the child selects the item when the cursor reaches it. Group–item scanning is similar in that the cursor scans groups of several items. After the child selects a group, the cursor scans individual items within the group, and the child selects the desired item when it is reached. Most new devices make available both direct selection and scanning, and, often, both the scanning method and speed can be programmed.

Although scanning can be accomplished with minimal motor skill, it requires controlled visual tracking skills, attention skills, and an understanding of sequencing (Cook & Hussey, 1995). Scanning requires more time than direct selection but gives the user more options for access. In designing the system, a range of switches can be used to make selections, with a goal of optimal accuracy and speed. The features that should be considered in selecting a switch for a child include

- the type and size of activating surface,
- the force and pressure required to activate the switch,
- the range of motion required,
- the alternatives in positioning the device, and
- the sensory feedback the switch provides.

Examples of switches that can be used with augmentative communication systems are sip-and-puff, joystick, infrared, light sensitive, and movement or sound-activated (Brandenburg & Vanderheiden, 1987; Smith, 1991). Figure 6.6 shows a dual press switch. Innovations in scanning allow the child to make selections with wireless infrared pointing systems that can be attached to the head. Switch selection should be based on what the child can use reliably with a minimal effort for long periods.

Positioning the Device and the Child. After a device has been selected, the occupational therapy practitioner offers recommendations about how the device can be accessed throughout the day (see Figure 6.7). If the child spends much of the day in a wheelchair that has a tray, it may be appropriate to mount the device and switch, if needed, on the tray or wheelchair. The mounting of the device can determine whether the child is able to use it efficiently or independently. The mounting can include

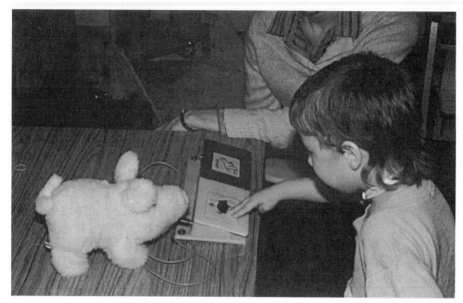

Figure 6.6 A dual switch can be introduced to facilitate decision making and turn taking.

hardware such as clamps or flexible mounting systems (gooseneck arms with clamps). The device should be mounted so that the child has adequate range of motion, strength, visual field, and motor control to operate it. Most powered wheelchairs allow for an adjustable, swing-away mount that holds an augmentative communication device that can easily be adjusted and positioned for optimal viewing and access. Mounting the device at an angle is usually ideal for viewing and for hand control. It is important that the child's wheelchair is considered at the time of ordering an augmentative communication device so that an integrated system can be developed that considers device interface with environmental control units, the wheelchair, and computers.

Positioning should consider the child's optimal posture for head, arm, and hand control and should consider issues in endurance and effort. An optimal seating position offers maximum postural stability and alignment. The feet should be flat, with the hips flexed at 90° and good alignment of the trunk. This correct postural alignment can be maintained with straps, trays, and footrests.

Enhancing the Child's Performance To Use a Device

The skills needed to access the device are developed in a number of contexts that support and challenge the child's ability to communicate using the device. Because most augmentative communication devices can be adapted to meet the child's current skill level, training for optimal use incorporates

the device itself. Most devices offer different overlays with a range of keys—as few as 4 and as many as 128 (at any one time).

In addition to adapting the device itself, optimal access for the child should be explored using low technology. Sometimes a hand or head pointer can improve accuracy, and a keyguard is helpful with children who have difficulty with control or hand stability. The variety of switches that can be used for scanning is almost endless, and these switches can be mounted at various angles and positions to improve the child accuracy and speed.

Therapy sessions can focus on improving the child's switch access and fine motor control. In addition, visual attention, visual perception, and cognitive skills can limit device use and can become goals of the occupational therapy practitioner to improve the child's use of the augmentative communication system. Sustained attention, figure–ground perception, and visual scanning skills are areas to address in preparing a child to use a device. These skills can be developed in tandem with use of the device in daily communication because, often, the most rewarding activity is successful communication with peers and family.

Case Study
Amy's First Augmentative Communication System

Amy was 4 years old when an augmentative device was considered. She had multiple disabilities, including total blindness, cerebral palsy, and cognitive delays. She was fed via a gastro-

making, although she became highly resistant when handled or when held in a sitting position. She had approximately six signs that she used with family members, "love," "mom," "dad," "sis," "bye-bye,"and "no." Her parents were highly supportive of and motivated for her to communicate with them and with her peers.

After an evaluation by an augmentative communication team, an Introtalker® with four programmed messages was introduced. The keys were identified by different textures—corduroy, a coin, and velvet—that she was known to tolerate. Quickly, Amy became consistent in locating the message keys. Because she lacked sitting balance and had poor tolerance for being in her wheelchair, the Introtalker was placed on the floor, and she rolled to it, accessing it in a sidelying position. She had greater control in her left arm and hand and was able to locate the keys quickly through systematically touching the device with that hand. Within a month of providing the device, she began to request it with grunts. Her use of the messages was appropriate to the situation. Within several months, the device was adapted to include 12 spaces covered with 12 different textures. She indicated "want," "down," "stop," "want music," "want mom," " want up," "love," and "want sis." The classroom staff members were so excited that they could now communicate with Amy that they made every opportunity for her to use her device. After 2 years of almost no communication, Amy was able to indicate what she wanted and to make simple choices in play and daily activities.

Amy became a different child with her new communication ability, and she was more willing to participate in other classroom activities. She maintained a more positive affect and began to seek interaction. She began to laugh and giggle in the classroom and to participate more in circle and group time. The communication device was always by her side, as she learned to roll holding onto the device, and her peers became interested in using it with her. By the time Amy entered school, she was using her device with more than 30 messages programmed on different overlays. ∎

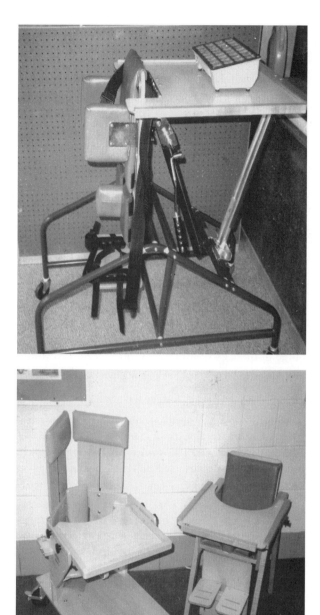

Figure 6.7 Options for positioning when using an augmentative device include (counterclockwise from top) (a) a prone stander, (b) a corner chair, and (c) a Rifton child's chair.

stomy tube and used only three or four sounds to indicate pleasure or displeasure. She did not sustain interaction with any of the preschool staff members. She rolled from place to place, primarily away from those who attempted to hold her because she had extreme hypersensitivity to touch. She had no opportunities for decision

Integrating the Augmentative Communication System Into the Home and Classroom. An augmentative communication device is fully integrated into the child's daily life, only if it is accepted in all environments and understood by all communication partners. Because communication needs are constant, the device should always be in proximity to the child. Extended downtime and repair time is unacceptable to the child and his or her communication partners. Therefore, good quality devices with integrity of parts should be obtained.

One important focus of the occupational therapy practitioner's intervention is to assist in integrating use of the device into the child's daily life (see Figure 6.8). All of the child's communication partners need to support the child's use of the system. The practitioner helps parents, teachers, and aides learn to operate and program the device. One goal is that all communication partners can solve problems so that they are able to prevent device failure and periods of disuse. The practitioner should provide initial instruction and ongoing consultation so that all caregivers and teachers understand the child's skill level, how the device operates, the child's working vocabulary, and the optimal setup for using the device. The daily caregivers are crucial to ensuring that the child has immediate access to the device and that assistance is provided as needed. Because even the most proficient user produces communication that is slower than normal speech, the partners must adapt the pace and rhythm of a natural turn-taking interaction. Patience and attentiveness beyond that required in normal conversation are necessary. It may be tempting to speak for the child rather than allowing him or her to use the device.

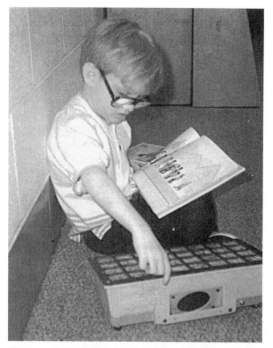

Figure 6.8 The Introtalker® communication device uses direct selection (the child touches the appropriate cell, and the device emits a word or phrase). *Note.* For more information, contact Prentki-Romich, Wooster, OH 44691.

Knowing the child's vocabulary and communication skills allows the practitioner and teacher to provide an optimal amount of assistance and support without communicating for the child.

As much as possible, the child's skills should be developed in natural communication experiences with peers or family members. It is important that the communication experiences are meaningful and that ongoing efforts are made to create a vocabulary and a system that enables the child to communicate at a level that matches his or her cognitive skills. The case study about Amy illustrates the types of outcomes that can be realized when augmentative communication is successfully implemented.

Functional Mobility

All children who are nonambulatory are candidates for mobility devices. Although the wheelchair is the most common solution to mobility limitation, a range of devices should be considered for the young child. Play toys on wheels (e.g., carts, scooter boards) and strollers may be the first transportation devices for the child (Swinth, 1997). Powered mobility is considered when a child is unable to self-propel a wheelchair manually, or it can be an appropriate additional chair when a person must independently propel long distances, as in changing classrooms in high school or college.

The occupational therapy practitioner is a member of the educational or health care team that makes recommendations about which mobility device appears optimal to improve the everyday function in the child. Practitioners provide specific recommendations regarding (a) seating and positioning to support the child's optimal function, (b) adapting the environment to accommodate the device, and (c) integrating the wheelchair into the child's daily life. The third objective may involve assisting the child in developing transfer and self-propulsion skills and in directing the chair in his or her environment.

Typical Development of Mobility

Children become mobile at an early age. Purposeful rolling often begins at 5 months of age, and crawling or pivoting on the abdomen begins by 6 months of age. Mobility milestones of the first 5 years are listed in Table 6.11. With these first forms of mobility, the child learns about his or her environment and begins to understand perceptual concepts such as depth, direction, space, and body scheme. As children become mobile, they learn about the properties of space and develop rules about exploring

Table 6.11 Typical Development of Mobility

Age (in months)	Mobility Milestone
3–4	Rolls accidentally
6–7	Rolls in both directions Rolls sequentially and segmentally
7	Crawls forward on belly
8–9	Creeps on hands and knees Cruises sideways
11	Walks with one hand held Cruises in either direction
15	Walks independently, stopping and starting Creeps up stairs
18	Walks independently, seldom falls Runs stiffly Walks up stairs while holding on Walks down stairs while holding on
24	Runs well Walks up stairs without support Jumps down from step

their environments. Studies have demonstrated that the development of mobility is related to the development of cognitive and social skills (Butler, 1986). Specific goals that can seem to be acquired through mobility include spatial awareness, speed, distance, directionality, and independence (Chiulli, Corradi-Scalise, & Donatelli-Schultheiss, 1988). The development of independent mobility seems to provide the infant with a sense of mastery over the environment that is critical to self-esteem and self-image.

Variables That Influence Mobility

Mobility Impairment. Children who have motor disabilities often require devices to achieve independent mobility. Wheelchair mobility should be considered for children with limitations in strength (muscular dystrophy, myotonia), paralysis (myelomeningocele), or poor motor control (cerebral palsy). The child with limited lower-extremity strength or control and adequate upper-extremity strength and control may be a candidate for a self-propelled chair. When a child lacks postural and arm control, a transport chair or stroller or powered mobility needs to

be considered. In all types of wheelchairs, seating for optimal postural alignment and control are critical. Seating components (e.g., adapted cushions, lateral and head supports, strapping) ensure that the child is comfortable, is in good alignment for seeing the environment and functioning within it, and has an even distribution of weight. Children with severe or multiple disabilities or limited strength almost always need seating components that assist in postural stabilization and alignment. Appropriate seating generally allows for optimal control of arms and eyes as well as good respiration and skin integrity.

Visual Impairment. Candidates for self-propelled or powered mobility devices must have visiual acuity sufficient to direct the chair. Poor visual acuity and visual perception dysfunction can significantly limit a child's ability to control and direct the wheelchair. A child with visual-perceptual problems may not be a candidate for powered mobility.

Cognitive Impairment. If children are to move purposefully and safely through their environments with mobility devices, they must be able to think and reason. In particular, powered mobility requires that a child can follow instructions, understand indirect cause and effect, and comprehend directions involving location (directionality). Therefore, a certain level of cognition (e.g., between 18 months and 2 years) is needed before use of a mobility device can be considered. Studies have shown that when children are provided with powered mobility and become independent in mobility, they make gains in cognition and demonstrate increased motivation to explore and interact with the environment.

Family Variables. A family's cultural values influence its acceptance of a mobility device. In families who greatly value independence, the idea of a self-propelled or powered wheelchair is enthusiastically accepted. Families that value interdependence of family members may consider a wheelchair unnecessary and a disruption to their family's interaction.

In general, family members may be concerned about the appearance of the child when in a wheelchair. The wheelchair conveys that the child has a disability, thus carrying with it a stigma. For this reason, parents may select to use a stroller for a number of years, to deemphasize the child's motor disability and nonambulatory status.

Important to the success of the child in using a wheelchair is accessibility of all of his or her environments. Parents are naturally unprepared for the child's use of a wheelchair; therefore, the home may lack accessibility. All of the child's environments need to be assessed for accessibility to ensure success in using wheeled mobility. Transporting the wheelchair needs to be considered because it is a large and often heavy piece of equipment.

Selecting a Wheelchair and Wheelchair Components

The type of mobility device that best matches the child's skills and needs is a team and family decision. The critical variables were defined previously and include the child's motor skills; the child's visual perception; the child's cognition; the family's values, resources, and concerns; and the child's environments. These variables are discussed as they relate to the available selection of mobility devices.

Transport Chairs

Child considerations. The first mobility device of the young child is usually a stroller because it is lightweight and practical for community travel. Strollers with firm seats and backs that can be adjusted to different angles provide greater postural support and are appropriate for young children with trunk instability. Large, sturdy strollers offer a convenient means for transportation. If the child has poor trunk and head control, a seat insert can fit into the stroller to provide additional external support. Commercial seat inserts have secure strapping systems, footrests, and lateral supports if needed.

When the child reaches the age and size when a stroller is no longer appropriate or no longer offers adequate support, another mobility device is considered. If the child is unable to self-propel, a transport chair is recommended (see Figure 6.9). Transport chairs can be customized to fit the needs of the child by selecting optional features that assist in maintaining postural stability and alignment. The options available include head and trunk supports, wedged or contoured seats, various strapping systems, and lap trays. Complete modular systems with replaceable and adjustable components can be modified to assist the child. These features allow for correct trunk and pelvic alignment and for postural stability (Bergen, 1990). The entire seat tilts from upright to various reclining angles, offering the child a variety of functional positions. The upright position is selected for most fine motor activities. The semireclined position may be appropriate for feeding and can be used intermittently throughout the day to provide the child with rest in a relaxed position. All parts of the chair can be adjusted to improve the fit and to increase the child's function.

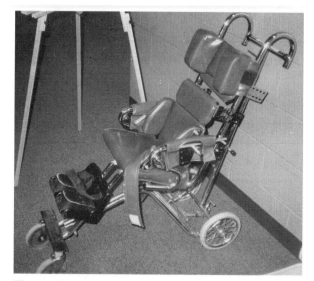

Figure 6.9 A travel chair can tilt at its base.

Family and environmental considerations. Parents may prefer strollers because a child in a stroller appears "normal" and does not carry the stigma of a child in a wheelchair. A stroller is also less expensive and more lightweight than a transport wheelchair. If the stroller provides security and good positioning, it can be a temporary option for the family before considering the purchase of a wheelchair.

A stroller collapses easily and can be transported in a car, making it ideal for shopping, public events, or appointments away from home. The stiff structure of the stroller base does not allow for a smooth and comfortable ride over rough terrain, however. Rough terrain may also cause damage to its structure and wheelbase. The stroller is most appropriate for use outdoors on smooth surfaces. Because strollers do not support trays and are usually fixed in a semireclined position, they cannot be converted into functional chairs for use in the classroom or home.

Although transport chairs are much more expensive than strollers, they are more durable and more versatile and can grow with the child. These chairs and their special features allow for good fit and positioning of the child's posture. They also offer the child security and stability during feeding and fine motor activities, freeing the parents from the need to provide postural support.

Although these chairs are now lighter than the first models, they remain fairly heavy, which may present a problem for a parent who has physical limitations. Yet because the chair fits the child well and provides optimal postural support, the older child can stay in it for extended periods. This fact may be helpful during social and meal times, especially if the tilting feature is used to help the child shift his or her weight on the buttocks. Travel chairs can be placed in most cars' front seats by collapsing the wheelbase; however, they do not always fit into small, compact cars. They are also difficult to lift into sport utility vehicles and vans. The family should evaluate the fit of the chair into its automobile before purchase.

Transport chairs are versatile in that they serve as functional chairs within the home and classroom. They are usually sturdy and provide smooth riding over rough terrain. However, because of the slanting base of four small wheels, the chair requires more space in the classroom and is more difficult to maneuver than the small wheelchairs. The tilting feature offers the child an optimal view of the room on the basis of his or her visual field, and because the travel chair's frame does not easily fit at a table, it is routinely ordered with a tray. Large trays with bordering rims make ideal surfaces for play but are sometimes awkward in small spaces.

Self-Propelled Wheelchairs

Child-related considerations. The variety of manual wheelchairs available has dramatically increased in recent years. A manual wheelchair is considered for children who have the arm strength, control, and endurance for self-propulsion and who have the cognitive and visual skills to direct a chair within their environment. Most manual wheelchairs are lightweight and are easily handled and transported. Small chairs that are low to the ground match the needs of the young child to be at the height of his or her peers. These small wheelchairs may not have the maneuverability of larger chairs, but they are most appropriate for the classroom environments of young children (see Figure 6.10).

Regular-sized wheelchairs offer a choice of seat and back sizes and shapes, and they should be ordered to fit the child, with projected growth considered. Manual sport or ultralight wheelchairs are about half the weight of a standard chair (Cook & Hussey, 1995). The amount of support the chair provides can be adjusted by adding or eliminating lateral supports, trays, and strapping. Footrests, a firm back and seat, and armrests are standard items and are available with different features and functions. Armrests can be adjusted to change the height of the lap tray for various activities. For example, the tray may be raised during self-feeding to support the hand-to-mouth movement. Most manufacturers also offer a variety of back and seat designs and dimensions. Seating may also be customized by companies specializing in designing and fabricating contour

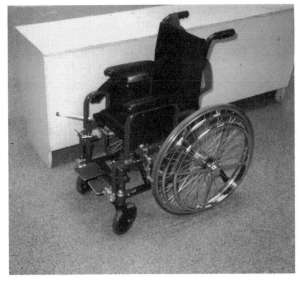

Figure 6.10 A wheelchair with a left-arm drive. The long extension on the brake enables the child to reach with his or her left hand to the opposite side to lock the wheels.

seating and wheelchair equipment. Ultralight chairs do not have as many seating options.

Family and environment considerations. Self-propelled wheelchairs, as with transport chairs and strollers, come in various weights, but they are typically lightweight and are easily collapsed and lifted into a car. Cost is a consideration, particularly when evaluating the purchase of optional features. Appearance of the chair is important, and the current chairs (such as the sports wheelchairs) are available in a range of colors and styles. The space available in the home, the child-care center, and the school may be factors in wheelchair choice should any of these environments lack wheelchair accessibility.

Powered Chairs. In general, children who do not have the upper-extremity strength or control necessary to propel a chair but have the cognitive and perceptual skills to plan and direct chair movement from one location to another are candidates for powered mobility. Advancements in technology allow children with severe physical and cognitive disabilities to use this option.

Powered mobility can also be appropriate for children who can walk or propel a chair short distances but who have limited strength and endurance and cannot independently manage long distances. Powered mobility may be a choice for the older child who, on entrance to high school or college, has long distances to cover daily, sometimes over rough terrain. Below are several options for the child who would benefit from powered mobility.

Scooters. Motorized scooters are typically used as additional systems for long distances by children who have adequate upper-body control to sit with minimal trunk support. Although the scooter is usually considered a vehicle for community travel, it is available in a front-wheel drive, lightweight model that has enhanced maneuverability for indoor use (Wright-Ott & Egilson, 1996).

Standard powered chairs. The child can control or drive a powered chair with a variety of input devices. The most typical control for a powered chair is the proportional joystick. The child moves the joystick in the direction he or she wants the chair to go. The chair's speed is proportional to the amount of joystick deflection. Digital control, using a microswitch, provides the child with less control over direction and starting or stopping the chair than the proportional joystick, but speed is usually programmed into the switch system. Although switch systems offer less control, they also require less control on the part of the child. These systems include a press pad, arm slot, and individual switches (Cook & Hussey, 1995).

Switches enable the child to control the chair through sip and puff or by the head, knee, arm, foot, or other body parts using different mounting of switches. The child with fair control, but poor strength and endurance, can easily operate and direct a chair using microswitch control. When the child has poor control and forceful movement, the switch can correct for the degree of force by responding with a programmed speed and a limited choice of directions. Accurate knowledge of vision and cognition abilities can guide the practitioner in the selection of an appropriate control interface for the chair and in training the child to use the powered mobility.

Family and environmental considerations. Although powered chairs may offer the child the first and only opportunity for independent mobility, a number of variables must be considered by the family before investing resources. If the powered chair is an additional mobility device for the child who already has a manual chair, the cost of an additional chair may not be covered by insurance. Because powered chairs are heavy, transporting them requires a van and a lift even when the battery pack can be detached and lifted separately. Moreover, the home environment must be made accessible, with wide spaces to accommodate the chair's limited maneuverability. Overall, the expenses of powered mobility may be unmanageable for the family and must be considered.

Recent literature has advocated use of powered mobility for the young child (i. e., 18–24 months of age) who is immobile (Butler, 1986; Swinth, 1997; Trefler & Taylor, 1988). Although it may be developmentally appropriate to obtain powered mobility for a child before 24 months of age, the family may not be ready yet to accept the need for mobility assistance. At this early age, the family may be reluctant to accept this physical symbol of the child's disability. In addition, given the expense of the chair, the growth and development of the child should be considered when ordering the size and features. The powered chair needs ongoing maintenance and may require relatively frequent repair. The family must be willing to undertake this ongoing responsibility.

Positioning and Fitting the Child to the Chair

Functional use of self-propelled or powered mobility travel chairs requires correct positioning and seating. Occupational therapy practitioners and other team members evaluate the child's neuromotor, sensory, and orthopedic status to make recommendations regarding seating (Wright-Ott & Egilson, 1996). The goals when recommending and selecting seating are to promote normal muscle tone while inhibiting abnormal or primitive reflexes, to prevent the development or progression of orthopedic deformities, to increase functional skills, to accommodate impaired sensation, and to provide comfort. An extensive range of commercial seating systems is available (Cook & Hussey, 1995).

Taylor (1987) described three components of evaluation for seating and positioning. They are

- functional assessment of the child that includes his or her daily activities and educational goals;
- evaluation of specific positions by observing the child in different positions or on a seating simulator; and
- selecting a seating system with appropriate material, size, angle, and shape.

Trunk support and pelvic alignment are critical to positioning in the chair. To maintain the pelvis in neutral alignment with the hips flexed at 90°, strapping at a 45° angle is recommended. Additional straps for the trunk can provide support and stability when the child lacks internal control. Straps that cross the chest in a V, H, or X design can assist with alignment, with upright posture, and with maintenance of posture when fatigue becomes a factor. Straps that originate on the chair back below the level of the shoulders and fit over the top of the shoulders effectively maintain postural alignment.

The lower extremities should be well supported, with neutral rotation at the hips and 90° flexion at the hips, knees, and ankles. This position promotes neutral pelvic alignment and prevents posterior pelvic tilt and lower-extremity extension. Contoured seats prevent the child from scooting forward in the chair (i.e., in the child with strong extensor tone).

Additional features may be added to the chair when shoulder retraction and head control are issues. Shoulder protraction wings encourage midline positioning of the upper extremities. Head supports can assist the child in maintaining his or her head at midline. When head control is poor and frequently pulls into flexion, head straps or a cervical collar can be considered; however, these devices must be selected and used with care because the head often slips into an undesirable position, reinforcing, rather than helping, poor neck alignment. Stabilization of the head may not be as important as neck alignment for swallowing and as head tilt for adequately seeing the environment. Head straps may feel restrictive and uncomfortable. A better choice may be to tilt the seating unit backward, thus allowing gravity to assist in maintaining head alignment against the chair's back.

Functional Use of the Mobility Device in the Child's Daily Activities

Occupational therapy practitioners often focus on improving function while the child is seated in the chair (Deitz, Jaffe, Wolf, Massagli, & Anson, 1991). A primary method is to give the child a tray surface to support hand use. Wheelchair trays are standard features with transport chairs and some powered chairs. Self-propelled chairs may come with desk arms to accommodate sitting at a table.

Wheelchair trays can provide a surface for eating, for working on school or vocational tasks, or for play. The tray may also provide a surface for a communication device or computer. Augmentative communication devices must remain with the child; therefore, mounting them on the wheelchair tray is ideal. The tray has the additional benefits of helping the child maintain an upright posture by supporting the midtrunk and of maintaining the upper extremities in a functional position (Bergen & Colangelo, 1985). Following are other functional issues to be assessed with the child in his or her chair.

- Can the child reach with adequate range to manage the environment (e.g., turn faucets on and off; write on the blackboard; and reach shelves, the floor, and a light switch)?
- Can the child turn the chair and maneuver it through rooms and hallways?
- Can the child propel or drive up to a table or desk and position himself or herself comfortably for tabletop activities?
- Can the child propel or drive the chair over grass, rough terrain, and other outdoor surfaces in his or her environment (Wolf, Massagli, Jaffe, & Deitz, 1991)?
- Can the child transfer in and out of the chair independently?

The family and occupational therapy practitioner can identify the functional limitations of the environment that require accommodation. Together, they help the child overcome the functional limitations. In some cases, the environment can be adapted; for example, table heights can be adjusted, and home or school modifications can be made. The child may become independent in transferring into the chair with adapted environmental supports and modified techniques. (Features on the chair itself must accommodate the child's ability to step out of and into the chair and to stand and pivot next to the seat.) Other interventions may include improving sitting balance and arm strength, and increasing arm range and arm and hand control.

Summary

Children with developmental disabilities often require assistance with self-care and daily living skills. The child's ability to achieve independence and mastery in self-care is important to self-esteem. Autonomy in self-care also enhances the child's interaction with family members. Occupational therapy practitioners are particularly skilled and resourceful in enhancing the child's daily living skills by analyzing the performance components inherent in self-care tasks and by maintaining a perspective of the child's occupation as it relates to his or her culture, family, and home. Occupational therapy practitioners work closely with family members and other disciplines to ensure that a consistent, comprehensive approach is implemented that places the family's priorities first, that enables the child, and that enlists appropriate community resources. Occupational therapy practitioners recognize that the self-care issues of the child with developmental disabilities are often long term and sometimes even lifelong. Methods appropriate for the young child are adapted and expanded for older children.

Many of the variables in the child's home and school environment that can affect development of self-care independence have been described in this chapter. A holistic approach that considers the child, the family, and the living environment enables the occupational therapy practitioner to offer a therapeutic approach that is based on a comprehensive understanding of the child. This understanding creates opportunities for increased mastery of the important tasks of self-care. ◆

Study Questions

1. What are the primary personal (intrinsic) variable and contextual variables that influence the young child's development of feeding skills?

2. When a child has severe motor impairment, what are the priorities for intervention? List five strategies that should be considered in intervention to improve feeding skills.

3. How do behavioral problems often result from feeding dysfunction? How can a practitioner evaluate the basis of negative behaviors at mealtime; what variables should be considered?

4. Describe good positioning for a young child to begin self-feeding.

5. Give three reasons why a child's transport wheelchair should be considered for feeding the child.

6. List three types of adapted equipment that might be used when a child with a motor disability first learns to dress. For each, explain why the equipment would be used and what type of child would benefit from its use.

7. What two recommendations for bathing should a therapist give to the parents of a child who demonstrates severe hypersensitivity to the bath?

8. What recommendations should the occupational therapy practitioner make for selecting an appropriate augmentative communication device for the child with poor motor control and infant-level communication skills?

9. What is the role of the occupational therapy practitioner in helping to integrate use of an augmentative communication device into the daily life of a young child at preschool?

10. What variables need to be considered when recommending powered mobility to the family of a young child? Discuss the advantages and disadvantages of initiating use of powered mobility by 2 years of age in the child with multiple disabilities.

References

Barnard, K. E., & Kelly, J. F. (1990). Assessment of parent–child interaction. In S. Meisels & J. Shonkoff (Eds.), *Handbook of early childhood intervention* (pp. 278–302). Boston: Cambridge University Press.

Bergen, A. F. (1990). *Positioning for function: Wheelchairs and other assistive devices.* Valhalla, NY: Valhalla Rehabilitation Publications.

Bergen, A. F., & Colangelo, C. (1985). *Positioning the client with CNS deficits: The wheelchair and other adapted equipment* (2nd ed.). Valhalla, NY: Valhalla Rehabilitation Publications.

Boehme, R. (1988). *Improving upper body control.* Tucson, AZ: Therapy Skill Builders.

Brandenburg, S., & Vanderheiden, G. (1987). *Communication, control, and computer access for disabled and elderly individuals. Resource Book 2: Switches and environmental controls.* San Diego, CA: College-Hill Press.

Butler, C. (1986). Effects of powered mobility on self-initiated behaviors of very young children with locomotor disability. *Developmental Medicine and Child Neurology, 28,* 325–332.

Case-Smith, J., & Humphry, R. (1996). Feeding and oral motor skills. In J. Case-Smith, A. Allen, & P. Pratt (Eds.), *Occupational therapy in children* (3rd ed., pp. 430–460). St. Louis, MO: Mosby.

Chan, S. (1992). Families with Asian roots. In E. Lynch & M. J. Hanson (Eds.), *Developing cross-cultural competence: A guide for working with young children and their families.* Baltimore: Brookes.

Chiulli, C., Corradi-Scalise, D., & Donatelli-Schultheiss, L. (1988). Powered mobility vehicles as aids in independent locomotion for young children. *Physical Therapy, 68,* 997–999.

Cook, A., & Hussey, S. (1995). *Assistive technologies: Principles and practice.* St. Louis, MO: Mosby.

Danella, E., & Vogtle, L. (1992). Neurodevelopmental treatment for the young child with cerebral palsy. In J. Case-Smith & C. Pehoski (Eds.), *Developmental of hand skills in the child.* Rockville, MD: American Occupational Therapy Association.

Deitz, J., Jaffe, K. M., Wolf, L. S., Massagli, T. L., & Anson, D. (1991). Pediatric power wheelchairs: Evaluation of function in the home and school environments. *Assistive Technology, 3,* 24–31.

Einarsson-Backes, L. M., Deitz, J., Price, R., Glass, R., & Hayes, T. (1994). Effect of oral support on feeding efficiency in preterm infants. *American Journal of Occupational Therapy, 46*, 490–498.

Gisel, E. G., Applegate-Ferrante, T., Benson, J., & Bosma, J. F. (1995). Effect of oral sensorimotor treatment on measures of growth, eating efficiency and aspiration in the dysphagic child with cerebral palsy. *Developmental Medicine and Child Neurology, 37*, 528–543.

Glass, R. P., & Wolf, L. S. (1997). Feeding and oral-motor skills. In J. Case-Smith (Ed.), *Pediatric occupational therapy and early intervention* (pp. 127–166). Andover, MA: Andover Medical Publishers.

Humphry, R. (1991). Impact of feeding problems on the parent-infant relationship. *Infants and Young Children, 3*(3), 30–38.

Humphry, R., & Case-Smith, J. (1996). Working with families. In J. Case-Smith, A. Allen, & P. Pratt (Eds.), *Occupational therapy for children* (3rd ed., pp 67–98). St. Louis, MO: Mosby.

Humphry, R., & Rourk, M. H. (1991). When an infant has a feeding problem. *Occupational Therapy Journal of Research, 11*(2), 106–120.

Kellegrew, D. H. (1998). Creating opportunities for occupation: An intervention to promote the self-care independence of young children with special needs. *American Journal of Occupational Therapy, 52*, 457–465.

Klein, M. D. (1988). *Pre-dressing skills.* Tucson, AZ: Therapy Skill Builders.

Klein, M. D., & Delaney, T. A. (1994). *Feeding and nutrition for the child with special needs.* Tucson, AZ: Therapy Skill Builders, Psychological Corporation.

McNaughton, D., & Light, J. (1989). Teaching facilitators to support the communication skills of an adult with severe cognitive disabilities: A case study. *Augmentative and Alternative Communication, 5*, 35–41

Morris, S. E., & Klein, M. D. (1987). *Pre-feeding skills.* Tucson, AZ: Therapy Skill Builders.

Musselwhite, C., & St. Louis, K. (1988). *Communication programming for persons with severe handicaps: Vocal and augmentative strategies.* Boston: College-Hill Press.

Scherzer, A., & Tscharnuter, I. (1991). *Early diagnosis and therapy in cerebral palsy.* New York: Marcel Dekker.

Shepherd, J., Coley, I., & Proctor, S. (1996). Self-care and adaptations for independent living. In J. Case-Smith, A. Allen, & P. Pratt (Eds.), *Occupational therapy for children* (pp. 461–503). St. Louis, MO: Mosby.

Smith, R. O. (1991). Technological approaches to performance enhancement. In C. Christiansen & C. Baum (Eds.), *Occupational therapy: Overcoming human performance deficits* (pp. 747–788). Thorofare, NJ: Slack.

Swinth, Y. (1997). Technology for young children with disabilities. In J. Case-Smith (Ed.), *Pediatric occupational therapy and early intervention* (pp. 277–300). Andover, MA: Andover Medical Publishers.

Taylor, S. J. (1987). Evaluating the client with physical disabilities for wheelchair seating. *American Journal of Occupational Therapy, 41*, 711–716.

Trefler, E., & Taylor, S. J. (1988). Power mobility for severely physically disabled children: Evaluation and provision practices. In K. M. Jaffe (Ed.), *Childhood power mobility: Developmental, technical and clinical perspectives* (pp. 117–126). Washington, DC: RESNA.

Wolf, L. S., Massagli, T. L., Jaffe, K. M., & Deitz, J. (1991). Functional assessment of the Joncare Hi-Lo Master power wheelchair for children. *Physical and Occupational Therapy in Pediatrics, 11*(3), 57–72.

Wright-Ott, C., & Egilson, S. (1996). Mobility. In J. Case-Smith, A. Allen, & P. Pratt (Eds.), *Occupational therapy for children* (pp. 562–580). St. Louis, MO: Mosby.

7

Independent Living Strategies for Adults With Developmental Disabilities

Karen Twilligear Babola

Karen Twilligear Babola, MOT, OTR, is Assistant Professor, Department of Occupational Therapy, School of Allied Health Sciences, University of Texas Medical Branch at Galveston, Texas.

Key Terms

ecological inventory

self-advocacy

self-efficacy

situational observation

topographical orientation

Objectives

On completing this chapter, the reader will be able to

1. Explain the benefits of using a client-centered treatment approach.

2. Identify issues that affect the transition to adult roles.

3. Discuss methods for assessing clients with developmental disabilities.

4. Describe approaches for increasing independence in self-maintenance tasks.

5. Identify techniques for developing home management skills.

"When human being flows into human doing, persons become world makers and life makers" (Peloquin, 1997, p. 168).

Developmental disabilities include a broad range of illnesses or disorders that affect a person's ability to perform meaningful occupations. These include cerebral palsy, mental retardation, autism, learning disabilities, and genetic disorders. Although a developmental disability must be diagnosed before the person is 18 years of age, the sensorimotor, cognitive, and psychosocial impairments resulting from these disorders often continue to affect the person throughout adult life. The type and severity of impairment vary from person to person and may affect the person's functional level. One person with mental retardation may participate independently in a variety of satisfying occupations, whereas another may require maximum assistance to engage in simple tasks.

Although a person's functional abilities may be limited by his or her specific impairments, another limiting factor may be a lack of opportunity to develop needed skills. Persons with developmental disabilities often begin receiving occupational therapy and other supportive services early in life. These interventions usually focus on basic self-care and school-related skills. However, as the person enters adolescence, a variety of other skills are needed to prepare for the assumption of adult roles. Supportive services may need to continue throughout adulthood, either continuously or intermittently, to enhance the person's success in establishing and maintaining a meaningful adult occupation.

This chapter focuses on ways to assist persons who are capable of living semi-independently or independently to acquire the skills needed to function as adults in mainstream society. The importance of using a client-centered approach during treatment is examined first. Next, several issues that may influence the successful transition to adult roles during adolescence and early adulthood are presented. General guidelines for evaluation of the client are then discussed. Finally, methods for helping clients develop self-maintenance and home management skills are reviewed.

Client-Centered Approach

Several models for client-centered practice have emerged within the past 20 years (Baum & Christiansen, 1997; Canadian Association of Occupational Therapists, 1997; Dunn, Brown, & McGuigan, 1994; Kielhofner, 1995; Kielhofner & Burke, 1980; Law et al., 1996; Schkade & Schultz, 1992), and it is beyond the scope of this chapter to review these in detail. In general, a client-centered approach is one that emphasizes that "clients and families have ultimate responsibility for decisions about their daily occupations and the occupational therapy services they receive" (Law & Mills, 1998, p. 10). The practitioner functions as a facilitator, respecting the person's choices and providing the support he or she requires to work toward personal goals within the usual environment. It is the client rather than the practitioner who prioritizes issues on which to focus and defines the desired outcomes of any services provided (Law & Mills, 1998).

There are several benefits to using a client-centered approach when working with adults with developmental disabilities. First, this approach facilitates the most efficient use of the practitioner's and client's time and resources. Because the treatment planning process is collaborative, energy is directed only toward goals or activities that are meaningful to the client. As Hammell (1998) said, "Clients may share a diagnosis with other clients, but intervention must be applicable to the unique environment, life stage, and goals of the person and must consider the meaning that the disability holds for him or her" (p. 124). This recommendation is particularly important within the current health care environment where resources may be limited.

Second, use of a client-centered approach fosters the development of a sense of self-efficacy within the client. Clients are more likely to engage in activities in which they believe they can be successful, continue with these activities in spite of challenges, and generalize new skills from one situation to another (Gage & Polatajko, 1994). Bandura and Wood (1989) found that a person's perception of control in a situation contributed to a stronger feeling of self-efficacy. In client-centered therapy, the client controls the process and is supported in the successful completion of identified actions, which should improve the client's sense of self-efficacy and provide motivation for tackling future challenges.

Finally, a client-centered approach helps clients develop the ability to manage chronic disabilities throughout their lifetime. The client's capacity to identify solutions to problems and to learn problem-solving skills is emphasized. Baum (1998) encouraged practitioners to

> view clients in the context of their lives and help them acquire the skills to handle not only the immediate issues that are influencing their

health, but to learn strategies that will promote, protect, and improve their health over the long-term. (p. 30)

Campbell (1997) emphasized the need to prevent the occurrence of secondary problems, such as repetitive motion and cardiovascular disorders, by helping clients with chronic disabilities take personal responsibility for their health. The use of a client-centered approach helps clients with chronic disabilities develop these critical strategies.

One issue that may arise when using a client-centered approach with adults with developmental disabilities is what to do if the client is not able to identify needs. This can be a problem if a client has cognitive impairments that affect insight or judgment. Attempts should first be made to help the client talk about needs through more structured or guided questions. If the client is not able to identify needs with assistance, then input from family members and others who are greatly involved in the client's daily life should be used to establish treatment priorities.

Transition to Adult Roles

Although expectations may differ somewhat from culture to culture, the transition from childhood to adulthood involves several key issues. These include "the evolution from dependence to independence, from residing at home to living in the community, from attending school to becoming employed, and from being part of one family to establishing a new nuclear family" (Hayes, Bain, & Batshaw, 1997, p. 757). Persons typically learn the skills needed for adult roles gradually, through opportunities and responsibilities available in family, school, and early work experiences. Through assigned chores at home, a teen learns to wash clothes, clean house, and cook simple meals. Basic reading, writing, and math skills mastered at school are used to balance a checkbook and fill out a job application. Time management and interpersonal skills are practiced during early work experiences.

Children with developmental disabilities may not experience the situations and activities that prepare them for assuming adult roles. The focus of services at school often continues to be on basic self-care and academic tasks if these have not been mastered. Family members may underestimate the child's abilities and, therefore, not expect the performance of chores at home. Anderson, Clark, and Spain (1982) found that only 21% of children with disabilities are given chores to do at home, whereas 69% of children who are developing typically are

given such responsibilities. Early work experiences outside the home may also be limited for teens with disabilities. Wysocki and Neulicht (1998) reported that the unemployment rate in the United States among teens with disabilities ranged from 44% to 64% from the late 1980s to the mid 1990s, as compared with 5% to 9% for persons without disabilities. Children with disabilities need to be exposed to as many of the usual experiences and activities of childhood as possible to help them develop a level of independence that is consistent with their abilities. Parents should be encouraged to include them in household activities such as setting the table for meals, washing dishes, washing clothes, or cleaning their rooms. Practice of home maintenance tasks can also be incorporated into classroom activities, such as planning and preparing food for a holiday party, cleaning up the classroom, or planning and carrying out a fund-raising activity.

By the time a child is 14 to 16 years old, it is important to begin prioritizing the ways in which limited time, resources, and energy will be spent to maximize the teen's ability to transition to adult roles. This should be a collaborative process involving the teen, family members, school personnel, and health care providers. As these future plans develop, it is helpful to use a tool such as the Canadian Occupational Performance Measure (COPM) to focus treatment efforts. The COPM (Law et al., 1994), which is described in greater detail in chapter 3, allows the teen and the family members to identify and prioritize specific individualized goals in the areas of self-care, productivity, and leisure. Specific questions regarding self-care to be explored at this point include the following:

- What is the expected level of independence the client will eventually attain in self-maintenance tasks?
- Where will the person be living after graduation from high school?

To make informed decisions about the future, the teen and family members must understand the nature of the teen's disability. Although it is likely that the family members have received information about the child's disability at some point, family members may have difficulty integrating this information early on. General information about a specific condition may not always be helpful because there is such variability in the way developmental disabilities affect a person. Instead, the therapist needs to teach the teen and family members about current abilities and how these abilities may change over time so that the client becomes the "expert" on managing his or her disability throughout life (Campbell, 1997).

As occupational therapy practitioners assist the teen and family members to identify future goals, it is especially important to be familiar with any legislation that influences the opportunities and rights of clients with developmental disabilities. Legally mandated and privately funded initiatives and programs that support independent living options, paid employment, and other aspects of community integration can be integral to the person's successful transition to adulthood. As teens prepare to graduate from school and assume more adult roles, it is important to help them be aware of and use all available resources that will support independent functioning in the community. Although the practitioner or a family member may initially serve as an advocate for the teen with developmental disabilities, the goal should be for the person to develop the ability to do this independently, if possible. Educating the person regarding legal rights, practicing needed skills through role-playing, assisting the person to write letters or complete necessary paperwork, and providing support during initial attempts will help the person develop the capacity to become an advocate for his or her own circumstances.

Evaluation

When treatment issues are prioritized by the client through a structured interview process, such as the COPM, the occupational therapy practitioner needs to gather additional information about the factors that limit the client's abilities in the identified areas of concern. Few standardized tests exist for use with clients with complex disabilities. Therefore, the benefit of using standardized, developmentally referenced instruments with this group is questionable (Falvey, 1986; Transition Ad Hoc Committee, 1986). Functional, environmentally referenced assessments, such as situational observations or environmental inventories, are recommended. These assessments provide specific information about discrepancies between the person's abilities and environmental demands (Spencer & Sample, 1993).

Environmentally referenced assessments involve watching a client perform a specific task in the usual environment in which the task occurs, such as shopping for groceries at the store. The focus of a situational observation is on the client's performance: For example, is there adequate range of motion to reach items on the shelf or sufficient strength to push the grocery cart? An ecological inventory not only considers the client's abilities but also takes into

account factors in the environment that may affect the client's capacity to complete desired tasks: For example, is lighting in the grocery store adequate or the noise level too distracting? Through such observations, the therapist identifies problems that can then be addressed through the practice of needed skills, training in compensatory techniques, or modification of the environment.

Spencer and Sample (1993) developed a Performance Inventory that can be used as an interview or observation guide with teens or young adults during the assessment process. The inventory looks at a client's performance in five domains:

- Domestic or home
- General community
- Vocational
- Recreational and leisure
- School

Items in the domestic or home and general community domains are particularly relevant to a client's ability to perform self-care and home maintenance tasks (see Appendix to this chapter). The Performance Inventory is completed by interviewing the client, family members, or both and then observing the client complete specific tasks in the usual environment in which they occur.

As with other clients, the evaluation process is an ongoing one among persons with developmental disabilities. As different interventions are tried, the client's performance and satisfaction are monitored so that adjustments can be made as needed. Whenever possible, services should be provided in the client's usual environment rather than a clinical setting. Because the desired outcome is to help the client achieve identified functional goals, working in the usual environment allows problems specific to that particular situation to be resolved more effectively.

Self-Maintenance Tasks

According to the American Occupational Therapy Association's (AOTA) Uniform Terminology for Occupational Therapy—Third Edition (1994), self-maintenance tasks include grooming, oral hygiene, bathing, toilet hygiene, personal device care, dressing, feeding and eating, medication routine, health maintenance, socialization, functional communication, functional mobility, community mobility, emergency response, and sexual expression. Techniques for addressing many of these tasks are contained elsewhere in this text and can be generalized to persons with developmental disabilities. The following section will focus on issues in self-maintenance that are particular to each group of persons as they assume adult roles.

Basic Self-Care

Not all clients with developmental disabilities will become completely independent in basic self-care, or it may take so much time and energy to complete these tasks independently that opportunities to participate in other meaningful occupations are limited. In either case, the focus should shift to teaching the client how to direct others to complete these tasks. Campbell (1997) suggested that teens could practice directing an attendant or requesting help from others through role-play. She also emphasized that teens should schedule their own medical appointments and take the lead in interactions with all health care providers early on. Further information about developing the skills needed to manage personal care attendants is contained elsewhere in this book.

Some persons with developmental disabilities may never complete self-care tasks independently; others may complete these tasks physically yet not follow socially acceptable standards for cleanliness or appearance because of cognitive impairments. While acknowledging the influence of cultural and familial values on a person's decisions in this area, the therapist should emphasize the health benefits of regular bathing and grooming. For some persons, the appropriateness of makeup and clothing may also need to be addressed. They may wear winter garments during summer or party-type clothes to the work setting. The use of magazine pictures or video clips as visual aids can be helpful in discussing situationally appropriate dress while exploring the range of acceptable individual expression. Group discussions are particularly helpful because of the opportunity for peer feedback. Some clients may benefit from a system of cue cards or coding of clothing items to assist them in matching clothing and selecting items appropriate for different occasions. A behavior modification program to reinforce cleanliness and acceptable appearance may also be needed if problems in these areas limit the client's opportunities in work or social situations.

Health Maintenance

Health maintenance, according to the Uniform Terminology for Occupational Therapy—Third Edition (1994), includes activities that help a client develop a healthy lifestyle and prevent illness. Adults with developmental disabilities face the same challenges as those without disabilities as they try to eat a healthy diet, exercise regularly, avoid harmful substances, and manage stress in their lives. However, several studies have indicated that this population has a higher rate of secondary conditions that limit their quality of life, such as cumulative trauma disorder (CTD), arthritis, and bursitis (Murphy, Molnar, & Lankasky, 1995; Turk, 1994); respiratory and cardiovascular problems (Dorval, 1994); and depression (Lollar, 1994). The use of compensatory techniques or adaptive equipment often involves the use of different muscle groups, stressful postures, or extra energy expenditure that may contribute to the development of secondary problems. Clients with existing disabilities may also have more difficulty recovering from minor injuries or illnesses, leading to periods of increased disability(Campbell, 1997).

Health maintenance behaviors are learned, and training should start during childhood. The child should begin to manage his or her disability by learning to take medications under supervision. Training should also be provided to take care of the adaptive equipment used. The child should also be taught to tell others when feeling ill. By adolescence, the client should be able to meet alone with health care professionals or at least talk directly to them rather than have a parent talk for them (Hayes, Bain, & Batshaw, 1997). Adolescents should also be taught how to teach others, such as care providers, about their specific condition and needs.

Children and adolescents with disabilities should be included in health education classes and activities with their peers, whenever possible, to begin learning about good nutrition and healthy behaviors. Adolescent and adult clients should be encouraged to develop and maintain a personal fitness program, including the use of energy conservation and work simplification techniques during daily activities. These programs will reinforce overall good health. In addition, persons should be given specific information about secondary problems for which they are at higher risk, considering their particular physical impairments and lifestyle. For example, a person who uses a wheelchair for mobility needs information about how to avoid or minimize the development of bursitis or CTD in the shoulder. A person with cardiovascular problems may benefit from training in stress management techniques. These types of information can be discussed on an individual or group basis, provided in handouts or other written formats, or practiced during individual or group sessions. It may also be helpful to refer clients to community organizations that provide educational materials and have support groups for dealing with particular problems on a long-term basis.

Socialization

By the time they become adults, most clients with developmental disabilities have developed a means for functional communication with others. Appropriate socialization skills are likely to have been taught throughout childhood and adolescence. But as clients move from the structure of nuclear families and school programs into the community at large, they may need support to develop satisfying social relationships. As Schwier (1994) reminded us,

> Perhaps one of the most important things for families and advocates to remember is that initial connections for any of us aren't based on extraordinary links. People meet, connect, continue, or fade away in everyone's life; the trick is to provide a dynamic range of possibilities. (p. 23)

The trick, then, is to help clients explore ways of making connections with others at work and in the community. Two ways in which adults make such social connections are through common interests and service to others. If clients do not have well-defined interests, a leisure interest survey, such as the NPI Interest Checklist (Rogers, 1988), can be used to help them identify possible activities. Whether clients want to develop a new interest or find opportunities to participate in already valued activities, such things as taking classes at a community college, civic center, or private facility or joining a special interest club or group give them opportunities to socialize with other adults with similar interests. Clients may also want to take advantage of extracurricular activities offered at work, such as bowling leagues or golf tournaments.

Helping clients find opportunities to be of service to others can also be very important. As Schwier (1994) said,

> Traditionally, people with disabilities have been the recipients, beneficiaries, the "done-for" rather the "do-for" someone else. Imagine life spent without ever giving; without ever being expected to be more than a recipient of someone else's "good deed" or paid service. We have ignored the basic human need to give something to another human being. (p. 25)

Community service agencies, hospitals, public schools, and nursing homes all offer chances for regular volunteer work. Projects sponsored by churches, special interest groups, employers, or the community-at-large present other opportunities for service.

Initially, clients may need help in locating and connecting with desired groups or organizations for both leisure and service activities. In some cases, physical or attitudinal barriers may limit their participation. If so, assisting them to educate others regarding their abilities and to advocate for the removal of discriminatory policies may be necessary. Specific tasks or environments may also have to be modified to enable them to successfully participate in new activities.

Community Mobility

Community mobility can be accomplished through a variety of methods, including driving a car, riding a bicycle, walking, riding the bus, or using other public transportation systems such as a taxi or van service. The ability to use any of these methods depends on the client first having developed functional mobility. Training in the use of one or more community mobility methods should begin in adolescence or early adulthood. The focus of intervention will depend on the client's abilities and preferences, the reason for traveling, and the availability of public transportation services in the area.

Before clients can travel independently in the community, their ability to find their way (topographical orientation) should be evaluated. Clients should be observed completing a variety of tasks, ranging from moving from one area to another within a familiar public building to using a map to find a route to an unfamiliar destination. Visual–spatial or memory impairments may interfere with a client's ability to do this easily. Clients may develop the needed skills if they practice traveling specific routes within the usual environment, using landmarks or signs to help mark the way. If they have difficulty remembering routes, clients may need instruction sheets or maps. These can be kept in a personal planner for easy reference.

No matter what means of travel clients decide to use, they should be familiar with basic traffic rules, such as when and where to cross the street safely and how to ask others for directions or help if needed. These skills can be taught through worksheets, discussion, role-playing, and practice of skills in simulated and real situations. Clients who ride bikes should be encouraged to wear a helmet at all times and reflective clothing at night. If available, many clients will use some form of public transportation. To access a taxi or van service, the client must be able to call and arrange for the service and to give directions to where they want to go. Cue cards containing needed information can help a client complete these tasks independently.

McInerney and McInerney (1992) described a program for training adult residents of a community-based facility to use the bus independently for recreational outings. They developed a rating scale based on a task analysis (see Figure 7.1) in which 14 performance and social skills were identified as necessary for independent and safe bus travel. Training was provided in groups of four to five clients and took place in three phases, progressing from simulated practice on a van to supervised bus riding leading to unsupervised bus riding. It took an

average of 6.58 weeks for clients to master the targeted skills. Sessions of 60 to 90 minutes were provided three or five times per week for this training. Within the year after completion of the program, clients who had completed the training made an average of 9.38 independent bus trips for leisure purposes, indicating that they maintained the skills over time.

The ultimate level of independence in community mobility for most clients is being able to drive a car. Driver training is undertaken only after extensive evaluation of a client's sensorimotor, cognitive, and psychosocial abilities. Visual and perceptual skills, reaction time, self-control, and general

Competency Domain	Skill Steps	Rating Scale			
		NEVER (0 pts.)	YES/ SELDOM (1 pt.)	YES/ sometimes (2 pts.)	Always (3 pts.)
Bus Riding (first bus)	1. Knows/carries correct fare				
	2. Locates/walks to bus stop				
	3. Gets on appropriate bus				
	4. Placces fare in box				
	5. Asks for transfer if needed				
	6. Pushes buzzer at appropriate time				
	7. Gets off at appropriate stop				
Bus Riding (second bus)	8. Locates/walks to transfer point				
	9. Gets on appropriate bus				
	10. Gives transfer to driver				
	11. Pushes buzzer at appropriate time				
	12. Gets off at appropriate stop				
Social Skills (both buses)	13. Displays appropriate social behaviors				
	14. Is able to demonstrate recovery skills				

Figure 7.1 Task analysis of independent and safe bus travel skills. From "A Mobility Skills Training Program for Adults With Developmental Disabilities," by C. A. McInerney and M. McInerney, 1992, *American Journal of Occupational Therapy, 46,* pp. 233–239. Copyright 1992 by the American Occupational Therapy Association, Inc. Reprinted with permission.

driving knowledge should be evaluated through clinical screening and driving simulator tests before progressing to behind-the-wheel training (Okkema, 1994). Clients may use adaptations, such as hand controls, to compensate for physical impairments, but there is really no effective way to compensate for major perceptual or cognitive impairments when driving. Behind-the-wheel training should take place in a variety of situations, progressing from driving in an empty parking lot to navigating in heavy traffic. Practitioners must be familiar with local procedures and requirements for driver's training to help a client through this process successfully.

Emergency Response

Emergency response includes the ability to recognize and respond in a positive way to hazardous situations. Both the awareness of what makes a situation an emergency and the skills needed to deal with specific problems are best developed through practice in simulated situations that mirror the client's usual environments as much as possible. The very nature of an "emergency" means that its location or time of occurrence cannot be predicted. Therefore, practice of needed skills should occur in the client's usual environments to enable him or her to develop the flexibility of response required in different situations. Discussing what is happening, using pictures of possible hazards, or video clips of emergency situations may also help increase a client's ability to respond appropriately.

Specific emergency response skills that should be taught include basic first aid techniques, cardiopulmonary resuscitation (CPR), extinguishing small fires, and strategies for handling being lost. Clients also need to know how to contact emergency services in their area when a situation is beyond their ability to handle. Emergency phone numbers and basic procedures, or information such as an address and telephone number that a responding agency will likely need, can be posted on cue cards near telephones in the home or residential facility. Clients may also need to keep a similar cue card with them, in a wallet or personal planner, when out in the community. A personal cue card might also contain basic identifying information about the client, a description of any serious medical conditions or special needs, and personal emergency contact information.

Sexual Expression

Sexual expression is a self-maintenance activity that is often neglected when working with clients with developmental disabilities. There is a societal reluctance to admit that persons with disabilities experience the same desires and needs for sexual expression as those without disabilities. As Schwier (1994), author and parent of a child with a disability, reminded us,

> Although attitudes have changed dramatically since Jim was born in 1974, "intellectual disability" is not often listed among the top ten most desirable characteristics in a mate. Worse, society seems determined to conspire against people with intellectual disabilities and their chance for a loving sexual relationship with another person. Commonplace is the attitude that a relationship for someone with a disability, particularly one in which sexuality is physically expressed, is disgusting, repulsive, and somehow perverse. . . . For so long, we've been denying dignity and companionship, making life needlessly lonely for so many people already facing difficult challenges in their daily life. (p. 5)

Parents may also attempt to protect their children from possible victimization by denying their emerging sexuality during puberty and limiting their knowledge about sex. Sexuality education, however, is considered one of the most effective ways to protect children from sexual abuse and the consequences of unprotected sexual activity (Hayes, Bain, & Batshaw, 1997). Such education also helps persons explore their own values and develop responsible decision-making skills regarding sexual expression.

The Council on Child and Adolescent Health of the American Academy of Pediatrics (1996) suggested that sexuality education should include the following:

- developing an appreciation of one's own body;
- interacting with both genders in respectful and appropriate ways;
- learning appropriate ways to express affection and love;
- encouraging the development of interpersonal relationships;
- learning to be assertive in protecting the privacy of one's own body; and
- learning about conception, contraception, and protection from sexually transmitted diseases.

The use of multimedia materials, such as *Sex Education for Persons With Disabilities That Hinder Learning: A Teacher's Guide* (Kempton & Caparulo, 1989) or *Circles: A Multi-Media Package To Aid in the Development of Appropriate Social/Sexual Behavior in the Developmentally Disabled Individual* (Champagne &

Walker-Hirsch, 1987), may be helpful in teaching basic information about sexuality. Role-playing and the discussion of situations observed in movies or television shows are also useful strategies in helping persons develop the awareness and social skills needed in more intimate relationships.

When clients decide to become sexually active, they may need help in overcoming individual problems or environmental barriers. A person with physical impairments may need specific information about alternative positioning or adaptive techniques to use during sexual activity. Physical assistance from attendants may also be needed for initial positioning during sexual activity. Models, diagrams, pictures, and open discussion are all helpful in clarifying any problems that exist and proposing usable solutions (Frank, 1991).

Self-advocacy skills can be especially important for those living in supervised situations. For instance, a person living in a residential facility may need to negotiate with a roommate or with staff members for private time in the bedroom. Frank (1991) described the case of a couple with disabilities who had to get help from house staff members in a group home to wire two single beds together so that they could have adequate space for safe intercourse. Assisting the client to identify needs, any environmental barriers that exist, and possible solutions to the problems will help with successful self-advocacy.

Environmental barriers also exist in the form of policies and laws that limit the sexual freedom of persons with disabilities. Some communities still have laws that restrict marriage between persons with cognitive impairments or other disabilities. Residential facilities may even prohibit sexual contact between consenting adult residents. Governmental disability benefits are often less for married couples than they are for two single adults. Practitioners may need to educate clients regarding their rights and help them address discriminatory policies and practices. Schwier (1994) encouraged us to work together with our clients to ensure a more compassionate future for all.

Anyone can exist, anyone can go through the motions of life. But to share that life with another human being, to be cared for and loved, to be appreciated and valued is quite another thing. People no longer are content to be catalogued and shelved as "disabled." They want, and deserve, to be part of the whole. As Dennis Robertson, a self-advocate at a Washington conference, said, "I think people take one look at me and say in their minds: He won't ever have sex, so why talk about it and get his hopes up? This makes me angry ... because they could be wrong." (pp. 26–27)

Home Management Skills

Home management includes all the tasks necessary to get and keep up personal and household items—clothing care, cleaning, meal preparation and cleanup, shopping, money management, household maintenance, and safety procedures (AOTA, 1994). The client's expected living situation is an important factor to consider when prioritizing goals in this area. Clients in the community may have options ranging from personal care homes to independent living. In any of these living situations, clients may be interested in participating in home management tasks to some degree. Because the clients' abilities and the environmental demands vary so much, the best way to increase independence in home maintenance tasks is through the practice of needed skills in the actual environment in which the tasks usually occur. Modifications to compensate for physical or cognitive impairments can then be made as needed.

Clothing Care

The main tasks involved in maintaining clothing are cleaning and storage. For proper cleaning, clothes should be sorted according to whether they are to be hand washed, machine washed, or dry cleaned. Items to be hand or machine washed must then be sorted into white or light-colored versus dark-colored items. Next, correct cleaning supplies and equipment are located. Clothes are then washed, dried, and put away. Some items may need to be ironed before being put away.

Each step in this process may be adapted if needed. For clients with visual, perceptual, or cognitive impairments, instructional sheets or cue cards in either word or picture form may be used to correctly sequence the entire task or to help complete specific steps, such as sorting light from dark clothes or setting machine dials. Clothing labels can be marked so that the proper cleaning method can be easily identified, as well as whether items to be washed should be sorted with light or dark clothes. Supplies such as detergent, bleach, and fabric softener can be clearly labeled, with simplified instructions for correct use highlighted. Correct settings for different types of loads can be marked with bold-colored markers or stickers directly on the washing machine and dryer dials. Drawers, shelves, and closets can be clearly labeled using words or pictures to indicate where different items are to be stored.

For clients with decreased upper-extremity strength, poor endurance, or unsteady gait, a wheeled cart may be needed for transporting items to and from the laundry area. Clients who use a wheelchair for mobility may need to carry small loads or have someone carry larger loads for them. If front-loading machines are not available, clients who use wheelchairs may also need assistance getting wet clothes out of the bottom of the washer. Clients may be able to use a reacher to accomplish this task independently. Areas for storing cleaning supplies and clothing may have to be modified so that they are within easy reach of clients using wheelchairs or with limited upper-extremity range of motion.

Learning to properly hang up garments within closets is also an important part of maintaining clothing. Folding clothes, such as underwear, shirts, and socks, for storage in an appropriate drawer is also necessary for easily locating items of clothing when they are needed. Developing these clothing storage skills is also an important element in keeping a clutter-free living environment.

Cleaning

Cleaning includes such tasks as picking up and putting away items, dusting, sweeping, mopping, vacuuming, scrubbing, making beds, and removing trash (AOTA, 1994). Each of these tasks can be analyzed and broken down into steps and then modified as needed if the client is having difficulty. For clients with visual, perceptual, or cognitive impairments, cue cards, checklists, or labels on supplies and equipment can increase the ability to complete tasks independently. It can also be helpful to schedule the different tasks on a weekly or monthly calendar for clients with memory or time management problems.

Cleaning tasks can also be modified to compensate for physical problems. Reachers, adapted handles on brooms or mops, and hand mitts or extended handles for dusting or scrubbing can compensate for decreased range of motion or strength. A wheeled cart can be used to carry items to be put away or cleaning supplies from room to room and to collect trash. Clients with poor endurance can benefit from using energy conservation and work simplification techniques.

Meal Preparation and Cleanup

Cooking and serving a meal can be a chore or a creative venture depending on a person's interests and lifestyle. In many cultures, it is also an important activity for meaningful socialization among family members and friends. Holiday celebrations, intimate dinners, or delivering cookies to a friend who is sick are all meaningful social activities that involve food. Because of the possible psychosocial benefits of being able to participate in these activities, meal preparation can be a major focus for intervention.

Persons without disabilities commonly use many of the strategies that help clients with disabilities participate independently in cooking tasks. A computer program guides a person through the process of planning meals, even to the point of making up the required shopping list. Choppers, electric mixers, jar openers, and ergonomically designed utensils make tasks easier. Precut vegetables, prepared mixes, and frozen dinners save time and effort. Disposable plates and utensils cut down on the cleanup required.

Some clients may require additional modifications of meal preparation tasks. Meal planning can be structured by using a checklist or cue card. Recipes can be simplified, with the print enlarged and pictures used to show the required steps. Labeling of kitchen cabinets and drawers makes it easier to locate equipment and supplies. Cue cards can be posted showing how to use the stove, oven, microwave, dishwasher, and other appliances. Timers with enlarged numbers are also helpful for clients with visual problems.

Work simplification principles can be used to arrange supplies and equipment in the most efficient way. Specialized equipment exists for clients with the use of only one hand, decreased strength, or decreased range of motion—cutting boards and mixing bowls with nonskid or suction feet, rocker knives, two-handled pots, bowl or pan holders, wheeled trivets, scrubbing brushes with suction bases, and more. A wheeled cart can be used to carry items from the kitchen to the table. Other energy conservation techniques are also useful for clients with decreased endurance.

Shopping

More than the other home management tasks discussed thus far, shopping requires interacting in the community. Adequate socialization and community mobility skills are prerequisites as clients go to various locations for shopping. Planning what to buy can be simplified by using a list or checklist of needed items. Checklists or lists organized by grouping together similar types of items, such as canned goods or dairy products, are helpful, as is a layout of the store. Many stores have maps showing what is in each aisle; these maps can be very useful when making up a shopping list. Reachers can also help clients who use wheelchairs or have limited range of motion to get desired items while shopping. Motorized carts and personal assistance are available in most stores if needed.

If they are using cash to pay for items, clients may want to organize their money in advance so that it is easier to access. A coin holder keeps change sorted according to value, and paper money can be arranged by denomination. If bank checks are to be used, many stores now have the capability of filling these out electronically so a signature is all that is required. Signature stamps can be used to sign checks or credit card receipts if writing is difficult.

Money Management

Money management includes budgeting, paying bills, and using the banking system (AOTA, 1994). Clients can use templates for filling out checks and deposit slips for their bank account. Many bank statements include a checklist or form that can be used to balance the account each month. Calculators are useful for checking the accuracy of the math involved in this process. Budgets can be set up in advance and dates for paying monthly bills marked on a calendar. Computer programs are available that will help a person set up a budget, pay bills on time, and balance accounts. Checks can be printed in hard copy or payments can be made directly by electronic transfer. These technological advances reduce the effort and paperwork previously required for money management tasks.

Household Maintenance

Like cleaning, many different tasks are grouped together under the category of household maintenance. All activities that keep the home, yard, and transportation vehicles in safe and efficient working condition are included in this category. As clients identify different maintenance tasks they are interested in doing, any problems that arise can be addressed. As with other home maintenance tasks, cue cards or a checklist can be used to sequence or recall the steps for a particular task. Adapted equipment and compensatory techniques are helpful for clients with physical impairments, and the environment can be modified using work simplification principles.

Safety Procedures

Home safety is an important issue regardless of the client's living situation. Clients with visual impair-

ments need adequate nonglare lighting in all areas. Reflective tape, enlarged letters and numbers, and high contrast colors may also be beneficial. Environmental cues, such as warning signs or stickers, can alert clients with cognitive impairments to possible hazards. Furniture should be arranged with plenty of space allowed for movement by clients who use wheelchairs, crutches, canes, or walkers. Clutter, throw rugs, electrical cords, and small pets can all present hazards for clients with unsteady or assisted gait. Home and personal emergency call systems reduce the risk of serious consequences from personal injury or victimization for all clients.

Conclusion

Persons with developmental disabilities may have a variety of impairments that affect their ability to engage in meaningful occupations. As they work toward assuming adult roles in the community, they may need continuous or intermittent support to successfully participate in desired activities. Collaborative efforts between a client and therapy professionals to analyze problems and generate useful solutions, as outlined in this chapter, can make a major difference in the quality of a client's life. ◆

Study Questions

1. What are three benefits of using a client-centered approach with adults with developmental disabilities? How can this approach be adapted for use with clients who have difficulty identifying needs?

2. What are three ways the therapist can help an adolescent and family members begin the transition to adult roles? Which two questions can help direct intervention during this period?

3. What type of assessment is recommended for clients with complex disabilities—standardized, developmental, or environmentally referenced instruments? Why is this type of assessment recommended?

4. Compare and contrast situational observation and ecological inventory.

5. Describe two methods for addressing issues in each of the following self-maintenance areas: basic self-care, health maintenance, socialization, community mobility, emergency response, and sexual expression.

6. Describe three methods for adapting home maintenance tasks for clients with cognitive impairments.

7. What are two ways to adapt tasks for clients with physical impairments for each of the following home maintenance areas: clothing care, cleaning, meal preparation, shopping, money management, household maintenance, and safety procedures?

References

American Academy of Pediatrics, Council on Child and Adolescent Health. (1996). Sexuality education of children and adolescents with developmental disabilities. *Pediatrics, 97,* 275–278.

American Occupational Therapy Association. (1994). Uniform terminology for occupational therapy—Third edition. *American Journal of Occupational Therapy, 48,* 1047–1054.

Anderson, E. M., Clark, L., & Spain, B. (1982). *Disability in adolescence.* New York: Methuen & Company.

Bandura, A., & Wood, R. (1989). Effect of perceived control-lability and performance standards on self-regulation of complex decision making. *Journal of Personality and Social Psychology, 56,* 805–814.

Baum, C. (1998). Client centered practice in a changing health care system. In M. Law (Ed.), *Client-centered occupational therapy* (pp. 29–45). Thorofare, NJ: Slack.

Baum, C. M., & Christiansen, C. (1997). The occupational therapy context: Philosophy-principles-practice. In C. Christiansen & C. Baum (Eds.), *Occupational therapy: Overcoming human performance deficits* (pp. 4–43). Thorofare, NJ: Slack.

Campbell, S. K. (1997). Therapy programs for children that last a lifetime. *Physical and Occupational Therapy in Pediatrics, 17,* 1–15.

Canadian Association of Occupational Therapists. (1997). *Enabling occupation: An occupational therapy perspective.* Ottawa, ON: Canadian Association of Occupational Therapists Publications ACE.

Champagne, M., & Walker-Hirsch, L. (1987). *Circles: A multi-media package to aid in the development of appropriate social/sexual behavior in the developmentally disabled individual.* Santa Barbara, CA: James Stanfield Publishing.

Dorval, J. (1994). Achieving and maintaining body system integrity and function: Clinical issues. In D. J. Lollar (Ed.), *Preventing secondary conditions associated with spina bifida or cerebral palsy* (pp. 65–77). Washington, DC: Spina Bifida Association of America.

Dunn, W., Brown, C., & McGuigan, A. (1994). Ecology of human performance: A framework for considering the effect of context. *American Journal of Occupational Therapy, 48,* 595–607.

Falvey, M. (1986). *Community-based curriculum: Instructional strategies for students with severe handicaps.* Baltimore: Paul Brookes.

Frank, D. I. (1991). Sexual counseling with a developmentally disabled couple: A case study. *Perspectives in Psychiatric Care, 27,* 30–34.

Gage, M., & Polatajko, H. (1994). Enhancing occupational performance through an understanding of self-efficacy. *American Journal of Occupational Therapy, 48,* 452–461.

Hammell, K. W. (1998). Client-centred occupational therapy: Collaborative planning, accountable intervention. In M. Law (Ed.), *Client-centered occupational therapy* (pp. 123–143). Thorofare, NJ: Slack.

Hayes, A., Bain, L. J., & Batshaw, M. L. (1997). Adulthood: What the future holds. In M. L. Batshaw (Ed.), *Children with disabilities* (4th ed., pp. 757–772). Baltimore: Paul Brookes.

Kempton, W., & Caparulo, F. (1989). *Sex education for persons with disabilities that hinder learning: A teacher's guide.* Santa Barbara, CA: James Stanfield Publishing.

Kielhofner, G. (1995). *A model of human occupation: Theory and application* (2nd ed.). Baltimore: Williams & Wilkins.

Kielhofner, G., & Burke, J. (1980). A model of human occupation, part one: Conceptual framework and content. *American Journal of Occupational Therapy, 34,* 572–581.

Law, M., Baptiste, S., Carswell, A., McColl, M. A., Polatajko, H., & Pollock, N. (1994). *Canadian occupational performance measure* (2nd ed.). Toronto, ON: Canadian Association of Occupational Therapists.

Law, M., Cooper, B. A., Strong, S., Stewart, D., Rigby, P., & Letts, L. (1996). The Person–Environment–Occupation Model: A transactive approach to occupational performance. *Canadian Journal of Occupational Therapy, 63,* 9–23.

Law, M., & Mills, J. (1998). Client-centered occupational therapy. In M. Law (Ed.), *Client-centered occupational therapy* (pp. 1–18). Thorofare, NJ: Slack.

Lollar, D. J. (1994). Encouraging personal and interpersonal independence. In D. J. Lollar (Ed.), *Preventing secondary conditions associated with spina bifida or cerebral palsy* (pp. 17–25). Washington, DC: Spina Bifida Association of America.

McInerney, C. A., & McInerney, M. (1992). A mobility skills training program for adults with developmental disabilities. *American Journal of Occupational Therapy, 46,* 233–239.

Murphy, K. P., Molnar, G., & Lankasky, K. (1995). Medical and functional status of adults with cerebral palsy. *Developmental Medicine and Child Neurology, 37,* 1075–1084.

Okkema, K. (1994). Self-care strategies following stroke. In C. Christiansen (Ed.), *Ways of living: Self-care strategies for special needs* (pp. 227–254). Rockville, MD: American Occupational Therapy Association.

Peloquin, S. M. (1997). The spiritual depth of occupation: Making worlds and making lives. *American Journal of Occupational Therapy, 51,* 167–168.

Rogers, J. C. (1988). The NPI interest checklist. In B. Hemphill (Ed.), *Mental health assessments in occupational therapy* (pp. 93–114). Thorofare, NJ: Slack.

Schkade, J. K., & Schultz, S. (1992). Occupational adaptation: Toward a holistic approach to contemporary practice. Part 1. *American Journal of Occupational Therapy, 46,* 829–837.

Schwier, K. M. (1994). *Couples with intellectual disabilities talk about living and loving.* Bethesda, MD: Woodbine House.

Spencer, K. C., & Sample, P. L. (1993). Transition planning services. In C. B. Royeen (Ed.), *AOTA self study series: Classroom applications for school-based practice* (Lesson 10). Rockville, MD: American Occupational Therapy Association.

Transition Ad Hoc Committee. (1986). *Transition: A team approach. A process handbook.* Bismark, ND: Department of Public Instruction, Department of Human Services, and State Board for Vocational Education.

Turk, M. A. (1994). Attaining and retaining mobility: Clinical issues. In D. J. Lollar (Ed.), *Preventing secondary conditions associated with spina bifida or cerebral palsy* (pp. 42–53). Washington, DC: Spina Bifida Association of America.

Wysocki, D. J., & Neulicht, A. N. (1998). Adults with developmental disabilities and work. In M. Ross & S. Bachner (Eds.), *Adults with developmental disabilities: Current approaches in occupational therapy* (pp. 45–87). Bethesda, MD: American Occupational Therapy Association.

Appendix

PERFORMANCE INVENTORY
Performance Domain: <u>Domestic/Home</u>

School: _____   Student: _____

Age: _____   Date: _____

Directions: Address the following areas through interviews with the student, family members, or others as appropriate, or through student observation.

Goal Area	Activity	Current Level of Functioning
Eating and food preparation	1. Meal planning	
Interview with parents and school cafeteria staff	2. Preparing meals and snacks • gathers ingredients and equipment • opens containers (i.e., soda cans, milk cartons, cereal box) • follows recipes • uses microwave • uses stove top • uses oven • users other appliances	
Observation of student's home kitchen layout	3. Eating a meals/snack • oral motor skills (i.e., swallowing, chewing) • uses utensils • uses manners	
	4. Preparing eating area • sets table • gets condiments	
	5. Cleaning up after meal • puts away leftovers • wipes off work surface	

Domestic/Home Domain (*continued*)

Goal Area	Activity	Current Level of Functioning

	• washes dishes
	  – handwashing
	  – using dishwasher	

	6. Accessibility to kitchen • uses adaptive equipment	

Grooming and dressing	1. Grooming
	  • brushes teeth
	  • uses mouthwash
	  • brushes/combs hair
	  • styles hair
	  • skin care
	  • maintains appearance	

Interview with parents/
caregivers and student
	2. Dressing/undressing
	  • undresses self
	  • chooses appropriate clothes
	  • dresses self
	  • dresses appropriate for season/weather conditions	

Priorities:		

Hygiene and toileting
 	
Interview with parents/
caregivers and student
	1. Uses private and public toilets
	  • wipes self
	  • flushes toilet
	  • washes hands
	2. Washing hands and face
	3. Bathing/showering
	4. Shampooing/rinsing hair
	5. Shaving
	  • men
	6. Using deodorant	

Priorities:		

Household maintenance	1. Keeping room neat
	  • makes bed
	  • changes bed linens
	  • straightens room	

Interview with parents/
caregivers
	2. Handling household chores
	  • does laundry
	  • vacuums/dusts
	  • cleans bathroom
	  • sweeps	

	3. Maintaining outdoors
	  • rakes leaves
	  • mows lawn
	  • weeds
	  • waters lawn
	  • cleans up after animals	

Domestic/Home Domain (*continued*)

Goal Area	Activity	Current Level of Functioning
Priorities:		
Social skills	1. Telephone use • telephone etiquette • takes message • dials telephone • can use telephone for emergency • can use assistive devices if necessary • can use telephone directory	
Interview with parents/ caregivers	2. Caring for others • pet care • sibling care • babysitting • care of elderly	
	3. Reciprocal relationships • gift giving • remembers birthdays • sends thank you cards	
Priorities:		
Sexuality/health/safety Hygiene and toileting	1. Awareness of public versus private sexual activities • closes door for bathing, toileting, dressing, etc. • chooses appropriate place to masturbate	
Interview with parents/ caregivers	2. Appropriate show of affection	
	3. Awareness of bodily and sexual functions	
	4. Knowledge and use of birth control methods	
	5. Knowledge of sexually transmitted diseases	
	6. Knowledge of general health concerns • disease transmission (i.e., covers mouth when sneezing, coughing, controls drooling, blows nose, etc.) • health concerns specific to disability (i.e., skin care, range of motion, positioning of weight) • takes medication (i.e., knows medication schedule, ability to swallow, related behavioral concerns) • cares for minor injury	
	7. Awareness of home hazards and emergency procedures • poisons • fire • accidents	
Priorities:		

PERFORMANCE INVENTORY
Performance Domain: General Community

School: _____

Student: _____

Age: _____ Date: _____

Directions: Address the following areas through interviews with the student, family members, or others as appropriate, or through student observation.

Goal Area	Activity	Current Level of Functioning
Travel	1. "Walking" (wheeling) to and from destination • safety when crossing streets • arrives at destination	
	2. Riding bicycle • knows safety rules • able to find way • locks bicycle	
	3. Riding school bus/city bus • demonstrates appropriate behavior when on bus • communicates with bus driver • can find appropriate bus • can read bus map • can make a transfer • knows how to pay an appropriate amount • shows bus pass	
	4. Driving own vehicle • knows laws • demonstrates safe and defensive technique • can physically handle task • uses appropriate adaptive equipment • uses seat belts	
	5. Orienting skills • identifies signs • carries identification • asks for help • responsible for possessions • uses caution with strangers • reads maps	
Priorities:		
General shopping	1. Handling money/budgeting • makes shopping lists • recognizes budget constraints • handles money exchanges	
	2. Locating/getting items • pushes cart • uses store directory • asks for help • follows list • makes choices • does cost comparisons	
	3. Clothes/personal items • plans for trip • selects appropriate store	

General Community Domain (*continued*)

Goal Area	Activity	Current Level of Functioning
	• selects items within budget • makes wise choices • handles money exchanges	
Priorities:		
Restaurant	1. "Reads" menu (or alternative) 2. Communicates to wait person 3. Uses manners 4. Locates restrooms 5. Tallies bill (including tip) 6. Handles money exchanges	
Priorities:		
Using services	1. Uses pay telephone 2. Uses relay system (if hearing impaired) 3. Uses beauty parlor 4. Makes appointments 5. Uses banking services 6. Uses/communicates with dentist, doctor, etc. 7. Uses laundromat/dry cleaner	
Priorities:		

Note. From "Transition Planning Services" by K. C. Spencer and P. L. Sample, 1993, in C. B. Royeen (Ed.), *AOTA Self Study Series: Classroom Applications for School-Based Practice* (Lesson 10). Copyright 1993 by the American Occupational Therapy Association, Inc. Reprinted with permission.

8

Self-Care Strategies for Persons With Rheumatic Diseases

Jeanne L. Melvin

Jeanne L. Melvin, MEd, OTR, FAOTA, is Program Manager, Fibromyalgia and Chronic Pain Management Programs, Cedars-Sinai Medical Center, Los Angeles, California.

Key Terms

ankylosing spondylitis

enthesopathy

fibromyalgia syndrome

juvenile rheumatoid arthritis

osteoarthritis

polyarticular

psoriatic arthritis

osteolysis

osteophytes

resorption

rheumatoid arthritis

systemic lupus erythematosus

systemic sclerosis

Objectives

On completing this chapter, the reader will be able to

1. Define new trends in rheumatologic rehabilitation.

2. Explain the difference between self-management and self-care.

3. Explain the physical limitations associated with seven rheumatic diseases.

4. Explain how medications can alter function.

5. Define the specific factors related to arthritis that affect self-care.

6. Define the revised American College of Rheumatology functional classification.

7. Provide a listing of assistive devices for limitations in a specific joint or for limitations in a functional activity.

8. Provide information on community resources for patients.

This chapter emphasizes the unique aspects of evaluating and treating self-care limitations in persons with rheumatic diseases. *Rheumatic disease* is a classification that includes diseases that have muscle or joint pain as a primary symptom. The term *arthritis* means joint inflammation; it is not a specific disease but a symptom of more than 100 different diseases. Fibromyalgia syndrome (FMS) is considered a rheumatic disease because of the predominance of muscle and tendon pain, but it does not involve arthritis, inflammation, or degeneration and, therefore, is in a class by itself among the rheumatic diseases.

Over the past 10 years, three major trends or factors have influenced rehabilitation for patients with rheumatoid arthritis (RA) and other inflammatory rheumatic diseases. First, RA is no longer considered just a disabling disease but one that can shorten life. One study showed that persons with RA die an average of 10 years earlier than the general population (Pincus & Callahan, 1989). Predictors of shorter life expectancy include more involved joints and poorer functional status, greater age, lower socioeconomic status, and cardiovascular disease. Patients with the poorest overall function fare more poorly than those with good function (Pincus et al., 1984). Thus, improving or maintaining function not only improves the quality of life but also helps prevent premature death in patients with RA.

Second, outcomes studies have shown that medications offer a 20% to 50% improvement in arthritis symptoms for most patients and that self-management training can reduce symptoms an additional 15% to 30% (Hirano, Laurent, & Lorig, 1994). In clinical situations these outcomes can be even greater, with self-help education based on individual assessment and goal setting. This means that implementation of self-management measures are very effective in controlling symptoms and improving the quality of life. In some cases, self-management has been shown to be as effective as medications.

Third, research on fitness exercise for controlling symptoms, reducing fatigue, and improving the functional capacity of persons with rheumatic diseases has shown dramatic results (Minor, 1998) and is now a major component in self-management training. Additionally, a new approach to fatigue management training for persons with rheumatic diseases has evolved; it combines fitness training with patient education, on-time management, planning, pacing, prioritizing, and efficient use of energy (Belza, 1996; Cordery & Rocchi, 1998). Energy conservation is now only a small part of fatigue management training for persons with rheumatic diseases, increasing in importance as a person's function becomes more limited.

The basis for therapy for RA is changing to a self-management model within a systems-oriented treatment context. In the 1970s and 1980s, patient education focused on teaching patients about the disease, medications, joint protection, exercises, and pain-relieving physical agents. The goal was to have patients comply with instructions. In the 1990s, patient education evolved into teaching self-management within a wellness context. *Self-management*, defined by Lorig (1993) as "learning and practicing the skills necessary to carry on an active and emotionally satisfying life in the face of chronic illness," involves helping patients acquire a complex set of skills and attitudes. These skills and attitudes are designed to help maintain or improve health, slow disease progression, minimize dysfunction, and promote optimal participation in normal activities by teaching patients how to effectively use activity, exercise, fatigue management, nutrition, sleep, and rest. These techniques are taught to help patients control symptoms and to improve their overall health. Approaches for teaching self-management have been reviewed and organized into a practical model by Boutaugh and Brady (1998). Self-care training is a part of improving function within the self-management model. The more disabled a person becomes, the more important self-care training is and the greater effect it can have on that person's psychological health and immune system.

The most common rheumatic diseases that limit a person's ability for self-care are osteoarthritis (OA), FMS, RA, psoriatic arthritis (PA), ankylosing spondylitis (AS), systemic lupus erythematosus (SLE), systemic sclerosis (SSc), and juvenile rheumatoid arthritis (JRA). Each of these diseases is discussed in this chapter with special emphasis on hand involvement, functional limitations, and assistive technology solutions. RA is a particularly important disease to understand, because it provides a model for treating chronic inflammation of all the extremity joints. In other words, knowing how to treat inflammation of the wrist in an adult with RA provides the practitioner with knowledge useful to understanding inflammatory arthritis of the wrist in any other disease.

In occupational therapy settings, patients with rheumatic diseases may present with limitations, such as limited shoulder motion or bilateral knee arthritis, in one or a few joints. In these cases, clinical decision making starts with the joint problem. When patients have disease involving many joints (polyarticular) and severe functional limitations, intervention begins with a focus on functional tasks, such as improving dressing ability.

In the following sections, the major rheumatic diseases will be reviewed from the standpoint of their typical symptoms and progression. Emphasis will be placed on the functional consequences of these conditions and the types of intervention that may be used to reduce symptoms, inhibit the progression of permanent disability, and enhance the patient's ability to function. Joint impairment and functional activity are used to categorize common assistive devices for the different types of conditions described.

Osteoarthritis (Degenerative Joint Disease)

OA is the most common rheumatic disease, affecting both men and women equally during their middle age and beyond (45 years of age and older), with its prevalence increasing with age (Bland, Melvin, & Hasson, 2000). The progression of OA involves a two-stage process. First, the articular cartilage wears down or deteriorates; and, second, bone builds up around the margin of the joint, creating a lumpy, enlarged appearance. This two-stage process is frequently painless, with stiffness and limited range of motion (ROM) as the primary problems, or there may be inflammation and associated pain and swelling. Joints typically affected by OA include the hands, spine, knees, hips, and the metatarsophalangeal joint of the large toe, shoulders, and elbows. Traumatic arthritis is OA that results from injury to a joint. This condition is common in athletics and can occur in any joint.

Hand Involvement

In the past, OA was described as typically affecting the interphalangeal joints and thumb carpometacarpal joint. These are the joints that tend to be the most symptomatic. However, osteophytes (bony outgrowths) or osteophytosis can also occur at the metacarpophalangeal (MCP) joints (where they can interfere with gliding, triggering problems in the wrist) and in the intercarpal joints where they cause limited motion and pain with wrist motion over the volar side of the thumb MCP joint (Buckland-Wright, MacFarland, & Lynch, 1991; Moratz, Muncie, & Miranda-Walsh, 1986; Swanson

& DeGroot-Swanson, 1985). Several studies on hand involvement have shown that women often have more symptoms, more distal finger involvement, and more generalized OA than men (Carmen, 1989; Moratz et al., 1986).

In the hand, limitations in ROM are caused by the buildup of bone around the joint, which may result in the inability to grip fully to hold onto objects or to fully extend the fingers. Specific ROM exercises are not necessary or helpful when the limitation is caused by excess bone tissue, because persons already use their full available ROM during daily activities (Melvin, 1989). The main therapeutic intervention for hand conditions includes splints to stabilize joints, treatment for inflammation or prevention of tendon triggering (Colditz & Melvin, 2000), joint protection techniques (JPT) (Cordery & Rocchi, 1998), and assistive devices or adaptive methods.

Other Joint Limitations and Treatment in OA

Limitations in hand, elbow, shoulder, and neck function due to pain and stiffness can have a major effect on the performance of self-care skills. Table 8.1 provides a list of common joint limitations experienced with OA and the intervention approaches often recommended by occupational therapy practitioners and other health care providers.

Fibromyalgia Syndrome

FMS is a chronic and painful disorder characterized by widespread discomfort and tenderness to palpation at anatomically defined "tender points." The term *fibromyalgia* refers to pain that seems to emanate from muscles and fibrous soft tissues. *Syndrome* refers to the somewhat variable spectrum of associated symptoms (Russell & Melvin, 2000). It is believed to be the result of a disturbance of the neuroendocrine, biorhythmic, and nociceptive systems. A functional definition that may be used with patients is, FMS is a hypersensitivity syndrome throughout the entire body associated with a sleep disorder. Characteristic associated symptoms may include pain, fatigue, anxiety, depression, diminished cognition and memory, headaches and altered function of the nasopharyngeal tract, stomach, bowel, skin, nerves, muscles, tendons, heart, and eyes. It is noninflammatory and nondegenerative. There is no arthritis associated with it, and pain around the joints is usually the result of noninflam-

Table 8.1 Osteoarthritis: Common Limitations and Interventions

Limitation	Intervention
Severe stiffness in morning	Thermoelastic gloves at night; active ROM exercises in warm water; gentle stretching exercises before bed
Inability for full grip secondary to decreased finger ROM	Enlarged or nonslip handles on equipment and devices
Inability to hold objects secondary to pain	Joint protection techniques; enlarged handles; adaptive methods; patient education on optimal treatment for inflammation
Inability to open hand flat to neutral	Assistive devices for specific activities
Inability to apply pinch because of CMC or pantrapezial pain	MCP–CMC orthosis to restrict CMC motion during activities; pantrapezial arthritis also requires wrist immobilization
Inability to hold objects because of thumb metacarpal adduction contracture (the most common thumb deformity)	Reduced handles to accommodate diminished web space
Inability to apply pinch because of thumb IP, MCP, or CMC instability	Thumb orthosis to stabilize IP joint alone, MCP joint alone, or MCP–CMC or CMC–MCP–IP joints combined
Shoulder pain: decreased upper extremity dressing and bathing	Adaptive methods and assistive devices (see Table 8.6)
Back pain: decreased toilet, tub, and low seat transfer, and more difficult lower extremity dressing and bathing	Assistive devices to don pants, shoes, and socks, to tie shoes, and to remove shoes; transfer bars, bathing aids, adapted seats (see Tables 8.10 and 8.12)
Decreased hip flexion: more difficult lower extremity dressing and toilet or low seat transfer	Assistive devices to don pants, shoes, and socks and to tie shoes (see Table 8.9)
Decreased hip abduction: decreased perineal care	Adaptive bathing and toileting devices
Decreased knee flexion or pain: more difficult lower extremity dressing and low seat transfer	Assistive devices to don pants, shoes, and socks and to tie shoes plus walker adaptations if necessary
Cervical pain and decreased ROM (Note: nerve root compression with decreased hand strength)	Joint protection techniques Assistive devices Soft collar for positioning (not immobilization)
First MTP joint pain or stiffness: limits ambulation endurance	Foot orthoses and lightweight shoes with cushioned soles
Decreased ambulation and coordination, risk of falling	Home safety evaluation and education and adaptation

Note. CMC = carpometacarpal; IP = interphalangeal; MCP = metacarpophalangeal; MTP = metatarsophalangeal; ROM = range of motion.

matory enthesopathy; that is, pain amplified from tenderness at sites where tendons attach to bones.

Patients with primary FMS and no other regional injuries generally have normal ROM, but because the muscles are sore and stiff, patients report that they often have to move slower and with more caution during activities of daily living (ADL). They often have their greatest pain in the neck and shoulder region. Thus, activities requiring heavy lifting or sustained positioning at shoulder height are difficult or avoided. Some patients have diffuse pain in their hands, preventing them from using a forceful grip. Patients with FMS severe enough to be referred for rehabilitation often have limited endurance for sitting, standing, and walking. In one study, persons with FMS exhibited limitations of physical function nearly comparable to that of RA, even though they were limited by different factors (Cathey, Wolfe, & Kleinheksel, 1988).

Functional ability may also be limited by impaired cognition, such as decreased short-term memory; decreased reading retention; and decreased ability to focus, organize, and plan. Persons with FMS may also have difficulty with motor planning and exhibit clumsiness. These difficulties result from a neurotransmitter imbalance that affects the nervous system rather than an organic lesion. When cognitive problems are evident, all home programs should be provided to the patient in writing.

The current recommended treatment for FMS is self-management training. This includes therapeutic exercise (stretching), cardiovascular fitness, good nutrition, sleep retraining, coping skills training, and stress management. Cognitive problems and fatigue tend to resolve as the patient becomes able to correct his or her sleep disorder behaviorally without medication. All patients may benefit from a fatigue management program as described above and training in proper body mechanics (Melvin, 1996, 1998). Assistive devices are usually limited to cervical and spine pillows, car seats, and positioning devices that encourage good alignment during activities

Rheumatoid Arthritis

RA is a systemic disease with inflammation of the synovium, which lines the inside of joint capsules, tendon sheaths, and bursa, as a primary symptom. RA primarily affects women between the ages of 20 and 50 years, but may also affect men as well as adolescents more than 16 years of age. Exacerbations and remissions characterize the course of RA. It primarily affects the extremity joints and the neck (the back and trunk joints are generally not affected). For many persons with RA, joint disease is the sole problem. However, a small number of persons have involvement of internal organs, such as the lungs, blood vessels (vasculitis), heart, and eyes. Organ involvement is referred to as *extraarticular manifestation*. Because it is a systemic disease, RA affects every cell in the body, even if obvious pathology can be identified only in the joints. When these patients have a flare up of their arthritis, they feel as though they have the flu. Symptoms include joint pain and swelling, fatigue, malaise or flu-like feelings, muscle weakness, and pain (Sanford, Silverman, & Wolfe, 2000).

Hand Involvement

Most persons with RA have bilateral hand involvement. The disease may involve only a few joints such as the wrists or the MCP joints, or it may affect all of the joints and tendon sheaths. The disease may be mild or severe and progress slowly or rapidly, with or without remissions. Acute involvement includes warm, swollen, painful joints and swelling in the flexor and extensor tendon sheaths (this tenosynovitis may be painless or painful). As the synovitis persists, the synovium in the joints and tendon sheaths grows and thickens (called *pannus*), thus damaging and distending the joint capsules and their supporting ligaments. The inflammation erodes the cartilage in the joints. In RA, joints become lax or unstable, which tends to be more of a problem than joint stiffness. The damage to joint structures is caused by biochemical changes as well as by wear and tear from forces resulting from movement.

During active inflammation, therapy focuses on reducing inflammation and swelling with splinting, cold modalities, JPT, assistive devices, and adaptive methods to reduce stress to the joints and to prevent contractures. During periods of remission, some soft tissue contractures can be corrected with exercise and splints.

Patients with end-stage RA of their hands frequently have severe fixed deformities but no pain or inflammation. Treatment in these cases focuses primarily on adaptive devices and compensatory methods, as well as splints, to stabilize the thumb interphalangeal or MCP joints (Melvin, 1989). In selected cases, splints that improve the alignment of the MCP joints may be helpful, but they are recommended only if they improve function. Many splints to reduce ulnar drift actually limit function. Before a splint is given to a patient, it is critical to evaluate function with and without the splint to determine its effectiveness.

Table 8.2 lists common limitations associated with involvement to joints of the hand during RA and the types of intervention commonly associated with these limitations. Measures to reduce swelling and pain are frequently coupled with the use of assistive devices and splints to increase function, provide joint protection, and stabilize joints. Table 8.3 lists other types of upper-extremity involvement and their functional consequences that can interfere with the performance of self-care tasks.

Table 8.2 Rheumatoid Arthritis: Hand Limitations for Self-Care and Interventions

Limitations	Interventions
Swollen, painful joints: limited ROM, inhibited strength, decreased function in all activities	Cold modalities to decrease swelling and inflammation; JPT; adaptive devices; splints
Joint contractures diminish grip	Adaptive handles, devices, and methods (some soft tissue contractures can be reduced with serial splinting)
Joint instability in thumb or finger: decreased function and prehension strength	Individual joint orthosis to stabilize joint
Severe (reducible) MCP ulnar drift decreases function	MCP ulnar drift positioning splint (static or dynamic)
Active ROM is limited because of flexor tenosynovitis	Cold modalities to decrease swelling (if not effective; an injection is the next treatment of choice)
Limited wrist flexion or wrist splints: limited ability to manage proximal dressing, fasteners, toileting, and hygiene	Adaptive methods or equipment; flexible wrist splint

Note. JPT = joint protection techniques; MCP = metacarpophalangeal; ROM = range of motion.

Table 8.3 Other Joint Involvement in Rheumatoid Arthritis: Limitations to Self-Care and Activities of Daily Living

Joint Involvement	Limitation
Radioulnar synovitis, proximal or distal	Decreased supination or pronation
Elbow synovitis	Decreased extension limits ability for transfer push off, LE dressing, and desk activities; decreased flexion limits ability for feeding and face and upper-body care
Elbow nodules	Pain that limits bed mobility, chair transfer at a table
Shoulder synovitis	Decreased shoulder ROM (less than 90°) limits ability for reach and dressing; pain results in decreased ability for lifting, carrying, pushing, and grip
Neck pain or limited ROM	Reduced visual field for safety and interpersonal communication, requiring persons to turn their whole body to see around the room
Hip and knee pain and limitations producing the same functional problems as OA (see Table 8.1)	OA limitations are often secondary to stiffness, pain, and decreased ROM, whereas RA limitations are secondary to swelling, inflammation of soft tissue, laxity, or contracture

Note. LE = lower extremity; OA = osteoarthritis; RA = rheumatoid arthritis; ROM = range of motion.

Intervention for Joints Not in the Hand

A combination of therapeutic strategies is required to decrease joint stress and inflammation. These strategies include joint protection techniques that address both energy conservation and appropriate body mechanics for accomplishing necessary tasks. Other strategies include the use of thermal modalities, adaptive methods, and assistive devices. Proper body mechanics can serve the person with arthritis in two ways: (a) by reducing the stress on the joints during activities and (b) by reducing the work load on the muscles, thus increasing efficiency and conserving energy. It is helpful to incorporate the principles of body mechanics relevant to a person with RA as a part of instruction in joint protection. Most literature on body mechanics is directed toward the patient with back pain, who typically has healthy hands, arms, and knees. Thus, instruction in body mechanics must be modified for persons with RA.

Maintaining normal body weight can play an important role in reducing stress to the hips, knees, ankles, and toes. For example, in gait stride, force exerted per square inch over the joint surface in the hip is four times the body weight. Consequently, for every pound of weight loss, there is a 4-pound reduction of force, per square inch, on the hip joint.

Padded elbow sleeves can reduce pressure on nodules, thus reducing pain during desk work and bed mobility. Often, the elimination of pressure can help reduce the size of the nodules. Soft neck collars can also be used to improve postural alignment during activities. Persons with restricted neck rotation can use swivel chairs with adequate stability. Proper positioning during sleep, work, and leisure activities is critical in the treatment of cervical arthritis (Melvin, 1989).

Psoriatic Arthritis

PA is a systemic disease in which psoriasis is associated with inflammatory arthritis. Psoriasis is a chronic dermatitis consisting of discrete pink or dull red lesions surrounded by a characteristic silvery scaling. Five distinct subgroups are based on clinical patterns (Moll & Wright, 1973).

1. Asymmetric, oligoarticular arthritis affects a single or a few joints of the fingers or toes accounts for 70% of all PA.

2. Symmetrical polyarthritis is similar to the pattern seen in RA, and rapid joint stiffness and contractures can occur.

3. AS is similar to idiopathic ankylosing spondylitis and is associated with severe peripheral joint disease.

4. The predominant involvement of the distal interphalangeal (DIP) joints of the hands is associated with psoriatic nail involvement and asymmetric peripheral joint arthritis.

5. Arthritis mutilans (osteolysis or dissolution of the bone ends in involved joints) creates floppy joints and may be associated with spinal arthritis.

Subgroups 2, 3, and 5 have the greatest functional impairment and are the subgroups most likely to be referred to occupational therapy.

Occupational therapy for PA is essentially the same as for RA for peripheral involvement and AS for spinal involvement. Intervention focuses on accommodating limitations in joint movement and methods for improving self-care and ADL. However, treatment of the arthritis and skin requires the following specific considera-tions (Melvin, 1998; Rahman, Gladman, Gall, & Melvin, 2000).

• The diffuse digital "sausage" swelling or dactylitis of PA reflects inflammation of the tendon sheath and swelling of surrounding tissue and is extremely difficult to treat. It is resistant to mechanical methods for edema reduction, such as Coban™ wrapping, stretch gloves, and compression sleeves. Cold modalities can help reduce joint swelling, but they are generally ineffective for treating the sausage swelling. Even drug therapy may not help manage this problem.

• Patients with severe, acute PA are prone to developing rapid contractures and have a tendency for bony ankylosis. These patients need to have their ROM carefully monitored. Proper bed positioning, especially for the neck, wrists, knees, and ankles, is critical. Hand and ankle orthoses may be the only effective means of preventing dysfunctional contractures.

• Psoriatic skin lesions may restrict options for splinting. Plastic orthoses should not be applied directly to involved skin. A cotton (not nylon) stockinet can be used to protect the skin. All splints and liners should be washed daily. Moleskin and soft foam liners should not be used.

• Patients often have to cope with disfigurement as well as pain and joint limitations.

Several new medications are available for psoriasis. Patients should be referred to the National

Psoriasis Foundation and the Arthritis Foundation for the latest treatments.

Ankylosing Spondylitis

AS is a chronic systemic disease in which the primary sites of inflammation are the ligamentous, capsular, and tendinous insertions into the bone (the entheses). AS primarily involves the sacroiliac, spinal apophyseal, and axial joints. Other symptoms may include asymmetric or peripheral arthritis or ocular, cardiac, or pulmonary involvement (Arnett, Gall, & Slonaker, 2000). Hand involvement in AS tends to be mild and episodic, usually involving one or a few joints in an asymmetrical pattern. Shoulder involvement is more common than elbow or hand synovitis. Treatment for peripheral joint limitations in these areas is the same as for RA.

Spinal involvement in AS creates a stiff or "poker" spine. The goal of rehabilitation is to educate the patient early regarding posture so the spine becomes stiff or ankylosed in a straight, upright posture. Positioning during leisure activities, work, and bed rest is critical to this goal. Persons who have not had adequate posture education use multiple pillows to support their head and knees. This can result in spinal kyphosis, with patients exhibiting a bent-over, rigid posture with their face toward the ground, rendering them unable to see ahead of them. In some cases, fixed ankylosis can occur in a few days (Arnett, Gall, & Slonaker, 2000).

Spinal rigidity and pain can restrict patients' ability for bed mobility, lower extremity dressing and bathing, transferring, driving, and vocational skills. Safety precautions against falling require special attention. Persons with fused backs can lose their balance and fall during activities requiring bending, which can result in a broken neck and quadriplegia.

Systemic Lupus Erythematosus

SLE is a systemic inflammatory disease characterized by small vessel vasculitis with a diverse clinical picture. It occurs most often in women. Manifestations of the disease depend on the organ systems involved and may include any or all of the following: fever; erythematous rash; polyarthritis; pneumonitis; polyserositis (especially pleurisy and pericarditis); myositis; anemia; thrombocytopenia; and renal, neurological, psychological, and cardiac abnormalities (Walker, Sotosky, & Melvin, 2000). Stroke, psychosis, depression, and memory difficulties can occur as central nervous system manifestations of the disease (Liang, Roger, & Larson, 1984).

Hand involvement in SLE may look just like RA, but the deformities are usually caused by soft tissue damage rather than bone erosions. The arthritis has the same pattern of involvement as in RA; only a small percentage of SLE patients develop severe arthritis limitations (Nalebuff & Melvin, 2000).

This disease is often treated with moderate to high doses of corticosteroids. Patients on this medication are often slightly euphoric, making retention of verbal instructions difficult. All instructions for patients exhibiting this euphoria need to be provided in writing and reviewed in a follow-up session if possible (Walker et al., 2000).

Systemic Sclerosis

Scleroderma is an umbrella term for a group of disorders that include sclerosis of the skin as a predominant feature. SSc is the generalized or systemic form. Morphea or linear scleroderma are the localized forms. Patients often prefer the term scleroderma because it is easier to say and to understand. Therefore, scleroderma is often used as the common term for SSc.

SSc is a generalized disorder of the small blood vessels and connective tissues characterized by fibrotic, ischemic, and degenerative changes in the skin and internal organs. The skin and underlying tissues become tight, hard, and restricted. There are two main subtypes:

1. *Limited cutaneous systemic sclerosis* is the most common. Involvement of the skin is limited to the distal extremities and the face (the trunk is spared). The skin changes may be stable or slowly progressive, and Raynaud's phenomenon is present long before skin thickening occurs. These patients may maintain hand ROM for years or develop only moderate proximal interphalangeal (PIP) joint flexion contractures. Involvement of internal organs occurs 10 to 20 years later (Melvin, LeRoy, & Elrod, 2000).

2. *Diffuse cutaneous systemic sclerosis* often demonstrates with rapid progression of skin thickening, beginning as edema in the hands and feet and progressing to include the trunk. Raynaud's phenomenon occurs within 1 year of the onset of skin changes. Polyarthritis is common (Medsger, 1988). These patients are at a higher risk for developing early, and often severe, involvement of internal organs, including kidney failure, heart disease,

interstitial lung disease, and gastrointestinal involvement (Melvin et al., 2000).

Diffuse cutaneous systemic sclerosis has the most severe hand and joint limitations. The characteristic hand deformity includes restriction of the wrist to midrange, loss of thumb palmar abduction, loss of MCP flexion, and severe flexion contractures of the PIP joints resulting in a claw deformity pattern. In the early stages, it is crucial to maintain thumb abduction and MCP flexion, as well as to prevent wrist flexion contractures. Some patients have severe resorption or dissolution of the ends of their distal phalanges, thus shortening their digits, and a few develop gangrene from artery fibrosis or occlusion. These patients can develop joint restrictions in any body region affected. Self-care evaluation is a key part of occupational therapy for these patients. In addition to hand and face ROM therapy, these patients need deep breathing to maintain rib cage excursion and instruction in maximizing gravity assist for esophageal motility and instruction in managing Raynaud's phenomenon. (Melvin, 1994; Melvin et al., 2000).

Juvenile Rheumatoid Arthritis

JRA is considered a different disease from adult RA. It is delineated into three major types and seven subtypes, defined by the symptoms present during the first 6 months following onset. The major types are systemic onset, polyarticular onset, and pauciarticular onset. These types have been further divided according to the type of course the disease follows. All forms of JRA are systemic in nature and have an element of fatigue, fever, and malaise associated with the active disease (Mier, Wright, & Bolding, 2000).

The most severe involvement of polyarticular disease occurs in children with young-age onset. The type of hand involvement in these children is totally different from that of adult RA. These children tend to have flexion contractures of the wrists and digit joints, with ulnar deviation at the wrist and secondary radial drift at the digits. It is not uncommon for lateral pinch to be their main prehension pattern. Children with late-age onset may develop hand problems similar to those of adults with RA (Melvin, 1989).

Self-care training is a critical part of treatment of JRA. For older children, the ADL and self-care evaluation must extend into the school (Szer & Wright, 2000). An extensive review of occupational therapy evaluation and treatment of JRA has been presented by Bolding and Sanders (2000).

Self-Care Evaluation and Intervention for Persons With Arthritis

For most disabilities, the ADL or self-care evaluation is designed to determine a person's ability or inability to perform a task. This is also true for arthritis, but with joint disease, *how* a person performs an activity is almost as crucial as their ability to complete it, for this information provides the data necessary for JPT (Melvin, 1989). Observing patients perform daily activities provides an opportunity to determine whether their method causes unnecessary fatigue or jeopardizes their safety (Schweidler, 1984).

The self-care evaluation should answer the following questions regarding functional ability (questions 1–4), energy conservation (5 and 6), and safety (7 and 8):

1. Is the patient performing any daily tasks that are causing pain to, or placing potentially deforming stress on, the involved joints?
2. Are there adaptive methods or equipment that could minimize or eliminate the pain or joint stress caused by these activities?
3. Does physical limitation interfere with the patient's performance of daily tasks?
4. Are there adaptive methods or equipment that could increase the patient's ability to be self-reliant in these tasks?
5. Is the patient's method of performing activities causing fatigue?
6. Can the activity be done in a more energy-efficient manner?
7. Is the patient performing the activity safely?
8. Could assistive devices or instruction improve safety?

The need for physical treatment is determined by the musculoskeletal evaluation. The purpose of self-care treatment is (a) to reduce pain and inflammation by reducing stress on the joints; (b) to increase functional independence; and (c) to eliminate or reduce forces that could cause deformity or unnecessary fatigue, as well as to reduce safety risk factors.

In a study of the self-care needs of persons with RA, the most frequently reported self-care needs were the maintenance of a balance between activity and rest (83%), the promotion of normalcy (66%), and prevention of hazards (58%). Concerns were the same for both women and men (Ailinger & Dear, 1997).

Special Factors To Consider During the Self-Care Evaluation

Medications. Have you ever had trouble opening a childproof bottle? Imagine if you had to take medicine at 6:00 a.m., when you are tired, stiff all over, and your hands are so sore that you can hardly use them. This is the situation for most persons with hand involvement or severe active disease. Many patients wake up early to take their medications, then go back to sleep for an hour so that they are less stiff when they get up. Others schedule functional activities or exercise in accord with their optimal medication benefit, which may be a half hour or an hour after taking medications.

It is important to remember that fast-acting medications (e.g., nonsteroidal anti-inflammatory drugs, aspirin, or other analgesics) can alter a patient's performance on objective assessments such as dressing time, grip strength, and ROM in as little as 30 minutes. Therefore, it is important to note the use of anti-inflammatory and analgesic medications before the self-care evaluation. This is also the ideal time to find out whether the patient is taking the medications as prescribed and whether he or she can manipulate the bottles and pills without problems. Patients with limited hand function should ask the pharmacist to dispense pills in easy-to-open bottles (Melvin, 1989).

Effective drug management of inflammation is central to the management of the illness and the person's overall functional ability. These medications may influence psychological as well as physical functioning. If patients are having trouble with side effects or drug compliance, they should be encouraged to discuss the difficulty with their physician or pharmacist.

Morning stiffness. Morning stiffness refers to the prolonged generalized difficulty in joint movement that occurs in association with inflammatory polyarthritides upon awakening. The stiffness tends to be generalized and may last from 10 minutes to several hours. It is indicative of systemic involvement. Morning stiffness contrasts with the stiffness of OA, which is localized and occurs only in involved joints after inactivity and tends to disappear within 30 minutes of active motion.

Morning stiffness is an objective indicator of the degree of disease activity present in patients with RA. Patients with uncontrolled or untreated RA may have up to 3 to 5 hours of generalized stiffness in the morning. As the disease becomes less active or controlled by medications, the duration of morning

stiffness decreases to perhaps 15 to 30 minutes' duration. Patients are considered well controlled if they have less than 30 minutes of morning stiffness. Morning stiffness is a distinct feeling of excessive stiffness that wears off at a certain point. Patients often describe the situation thus: "My morning stiffness wears off about 10:00 a.m.; then I have my regular stiffness the rest of the day." Morning stiffness is calculated from the time the patient wakes up until the stiffness wears off, and it is recorded in hours (Melvin, 1989, p. 258).

How morning stiffness affects functional ability varies from person to person. Many patients feel stiff but are able to get around and to perform self-care functions, whereas others are totally dependent during periods of morning stiffness. Some patients may need assistive devices specifically during this period.

The following questions can assist in determining the patient's duration of morning stiffness (Melvin, 1977, 1989).

- Are your joints usually stiff in the morning when you awaken?
- What time do you usually awaken?
- What time do you usually get out of bed?
- What time does this morning stiffness wear off, leaving you with the regular stiffness you have during the day? (This question may sound awkward, but patients frequently respond "never" if you ask them what time their stiffness wears off, because they have some degree of stiffness all day.)

Fatigue and endurance. Becoming easily fatigued is one of the complications of all systemic diseases. It can limit a person's ability to carry out bathing, meal preparation, child care, shopping, work, and socializing. For the purpose of planning treatment, it is helpful to determine the patient's energy pattern by asking the following questions (Melvin, 1977, 1989).

- What is the pattern or times of peak and low energy?
- At what time of day does fatigue occur?
- What is the duration of the fatigue?
- How do you handle the fatigue?
- What do you do to improve endurance or reduce fatigue?
- What factors, beside illness, contribute to your fatigue or endurance? For example, do you have to take medications, experience sleep difficulties, or have depression or a poor physical condition that might explain the fatigue or contribute to it?

Disease variability. We all have good days and bad days, but when persons with arthritis say this, they are usually referring to their level of pain and function. It is critical when evaluating a person with arthritis to find out what they are like on their good and bad days, and how many of each are in a typical week. Some persons may need assistive devices only on the bad days or when their disease is periodically flaring up, which may be 1 or 2 days a week or 3 or 4 days a month.

American College of Rheumatology Functional Status Classification (Revised 1991 Criteria)

A general classification system for RA (Hochberg et al., 1992) was designed for identifying functional levels for research. This classification system is limited insofar as it is general and can reflect only gross changes in the patient's progression or regression. However, it is often helpful in providing a quick overall picture of the patient's status.

- *Class I:* Completely able to perform usual activities of daily living (self-care, vocational, and avocational).
- *Class II:* Able to perform usual self-care and vocational activities, but limited in avocational activities.
- *Class III:* Able to perform usual self-care activities, but limited in vocational and avocational activities.
- *Class IV:* Limited ability to perform usual self-care, vocational, and avocational activities.

Joint Protection Techniques

There are two reasons for recommending an assistive device to persons with rheumatic disease: (a) to help them become more self-reliant or capable and (b) to help them implement joint protection principles. Because one of the overriding goals in therapy for arthritis is to reduce stress and inflammation in the joints, it is of paramount importance that all self-care instruction incorporate joint protection principles. The concept of JPT was developed by Joy Cordery (1965), an occupational therapy practitioner. Major principles include having respect for pain; maintaining muscle strength and ROM; using each joint in its most stable, anatomically and functionally correct, plane; avoiding positions of deformity and forces in their direction; using the strongest joint available for the job; using correct patterns of movement; avoiding staying in one position for long periods of time; avoiding starting an activity that cannot

be stopped immediately; balancing rest and activity; and reducing force. Assistive devices and work simplification techniques facilitate implementation of these principles. The case descriptions in the next section illustrate examples of incorporating these principles throughout the care plan.

Equipment Recommendations— Factors To Consider

The determination of the patient's equipment needs is part of the ADL evaluation. For persons who are employed, the ADL evaluation should extend to the workplace. When selecting or designing equipment for a person with arthritis, it is important to keep the considerations listed below in mind (Melvin, 1989).

- The patient's equipment needs in the morning may differ from those in the afternoon; they may also differ during periods of exacerbation and remission.

> Mrs. S. is a 53-year-old married woman who has had RA in all of her peripheral joints for 7 years. She has had several remissions, but the inflammation has been steadily active for the last 2 years and particularly bad the past couple of months. Her morning stiffness is severe and lasts 2 hours. Her joints are also very stiff at night, making it difficult for her to use the toilet during the night and early morning. However, after she has showered, taken her medications, and exercised, she is much more limber and has no problem rising from a low seat.
>
> To help her specifically during the night and early morning, the occupational therapist recommended she raise her bed up 3 inches on specially made wood blocks with a well for the bed leg. She also ordered arm bars that attach to the back of the toilet seat and a lightweight, plastic-molded raised toilet seat (the easiest to clean). The patient puts it on the toilet before she goes to bed and stores it in a closet during the day when she no longer needs it, reducing the inconvenience to other family members. She is also able to take the toilet seat with her on overnight trips. Next year, she plans to remodel her home and install a high toilet, like the ones used in accessible bathrooms. This would be the ideal solution, for it looks the most normal and eliminates an extra cleaning chore.
>
> Her response to the equipment is this: "I hate having to use special devices, but it makes it easier to get out of bed to go to the bathroom, knowing I'm not going to have the excruciating pain in my knees and hands trying to get up from a low seat. Raising the bed was also helpful and makes me feel less disabled. I avoided getting a raised toilet seat for years, because I thought they

were ugly, with clamps that were permanently attached, requiring everyone to use it."

• Activities and equipment involving a strong grasp are contraindicated for patients with active MCP joint involvement.

Nancy W. is 40 years old and has had RA for 5 years. She has low-level inflammation in her hands, wrists, shoulders, and knees. Recently, while in a general hospital for MCP joint surgery, the occupational therapy practitioner gave her a long-handled back brush and squeeze-grip long reachers to facilitate her ability in ADL. However, both of these devices hurt her hands. (These devices function as a long lever, increasing the forces on the hand.) When she complained to her rheumatologist, he referred her to an outpatient arthritis treatment program.

The occupational therapy practitioner, experienced in arthritis treatment, issued her a long, terry cloth back scrubber with loop handles that are held with the palms of the hands. Nancy has fragile hands, with active inflammation and beginning joint deformity; consequently all dynamic grip reachers would cause undesirable force to the hand.

The therapist did an extensive ADL evaluation, carefully analyzing all reach activities. More than 50% of the activities for which Nancy wanted to use the reacher could be eliminated by reorganizing her cupboards and putting items she did not use in the basement. Many others could be eliminated by use of a lightweight step stool (one that is easy to lift and open) in the kitchen. After the therapist instructed Nancy in joint protection principles and the importance of using her palms bilaterally to lift heavy objects and avoiding a strong grip, Nancy began to actively find ways to eliminate grip and stressful reach from her activities. The therapist carefully reviewed how lever forces work and how Nancy could use them to her advantage (for example, using an extended handle on a stiff faucet).

• The equipment may affect other joints of the body.

Susan T. is a 30-year-old secretary who has had RA for 1 year. Physicians are still experimenting with different drugs, trying to bring her inflammation under control, but so far nothing has worked. She has recently started on gold therapy, which will take 3 to 4 months before it is effective. Her wrists and MCP and finger joints are swollen, as are her toes and left knee. The physical therapist recommended a cane to take the weight-bearing forces off the knee and improve her ability to get around. The occupational therapy practitioner was concerned about the stress the cane would cause to her right

hand—both the grip and the wrist radial deviation required by the cane are powerful forces that can cause MCP ulnar drift. Using a rigid wrist splint with the cane just made the forces on the MCP joints worse. The occupational therapy practitioner recommended to the physical therapist that a lightweight forearm crutch with a padded grip be used instead. This crutch would allow the wrist to be in the desired ulnar deviation or neutral and thus would reduce much of the force on the hand. The physical therapist agreed, but the patient flatly refused the forearm crutch because it made her look handicapped. She was reluctant but willing to use the cane.

When Susan returned to the occupational therapy practitioner with a cane, the therapist listened to all of her concerns about looking disabled and her fears about her boyfriend rejecting her. The therapist acknowledged that these are valid and natural concerns. Then the therapist explained in depth, using pictures, how radial deviation of the wrist and grip can cause the MCP ulnar drift deformity that the patient feared. She also explained that deformities occur during periods of swelling, and that the goal of therapy was to protect the joints during periods of inflammation. They agreed that the objective was for her to have strong functional joints when the medications brought the disease under control or when it went into remission.

The therapist reinforced the notion that the forearm crutch was a short-term measure, to be used only until the medicines became effective. The patient acknowledged that it would be helpful to be able to tell others that the crutch was only temporary, and that she was more worried about getting hand deformities than what other persons might think of the crutch. She walked across the room with the forearm crutch and sheepishly admitted that it was less painful to her hands than was the cane.

In the next therapy session, the therapist instructed Susan in JPTs for her MCP joints. This instruction included doing tasks with both hands, using the palms, and adapting handles to keep the MCP joints in extension.

• Some patients with wrist or hand involvement are unable to grip standard transfer assist equipment.

Marsha M. is a 55-year-old bookkeeper with severe OA in her hands; she is limited in both flexion and extension. Because she cannot make a full grip, when she tries to grasp something narrow, she feels weak because she cannot hold on tight. Her PIP and DIP joints are frequently inflamed and painful, making it difficult to hold onto things. She was referred to occupational therapy for a general ADL evaluation. One of Marsha's chief concerns was being able to get in and out of the tub safely. She reported that taking a daily hot tub bath was her "lifesaver" and the best thing she could do for her arthritis. However, she had not been able to take a bath for a month: the last time she had tried, she almost could not get out, which was particularly frightening to her because she lives alone. The occupational therapy practitioner had her demonstrate her transfer technique in the clinic model bathroom, and together they determined the type and placement of grab bars and the helpfulness of two different kinds of low tub seats. They settled on a chrome grab bar that fits over the tub rail. This device would allow the patient to pull herself up by hooking her forearm around it instead of gripping it. The patient reiterated how helpful it was to be able to practice with the therapist at the clinic, so that she could prove to herself that she could do it and that she was doing it correctly or the best way possible.

• Convenience appliances are not always convenient for patients with arthritis. This principle does not need a case example—everyone has some personal experience with appliances that are difficult to use. The most common examples are electric can openers. Both puncturing the can top and pressing the lever can be difficult for normal hands. Electric knives and toothbrushes can be heavy and often have buttons too small or difficult for some patients to use. It is imperative that practitioners be familiar with the strength and dexterity required to operate an appliance before ordering or recommending it to patients.

• A change in ambulation aids requires instruction in ADL.

Leslie T. is a 27-year-old fashion designer who developed severe hip pain. The orthopedist diagnosed the problem as avascular (aseptic) necrosis of the femoral head and advised her to avoid bearing weight on the hip for 4 to 6 months. He inquired whether she knew how to use crutches, to which she answered yes. He gave her a brief demonstration. He then gave her a prescription for both crutches and a walker. Two days later she called the orthopedist in tears and panic, stating her situation quite graphically, "When I'm using the walker or crutches I feel like a triple amputee, I can't do anything with my hands. Isn't there anything else I can do?" He referred Leslie to the physical therapy department for functional training, but when the physical therapist heard the reason for referral, they decided on a course of occupational therapy.

The occupational therapy practitioner did an ADL evaluation, reviewed transfer techniques, and issued Leslie the following helpful devices: crutch bag, walker basket, pocket apron, and shower seat. She recommended that Leslie purchase a high stool for the kitchen and reviewed possibilities for having groceries delivered and simplifying meals. She also instructed her in energy conservation techniques to counteract the fatigue of using ambulation aids.

Persons who are on crutches or walkers for extended periods find the experience frustrating as well as exhausting (mentally and physically). Nevertheless, reliance on these ambulation devices is a common situation; total hip replacement surgeries, for example, require no or partial weight-bearing for 3 months.

• Lower extremity dressing aids sometimes do more harm than good.

Dan R. is a 40-year-old computer executive who has had AS since age 22. He received extensive rehabilitative services early in the course of his illness. On his last visit to his physician, he reported having increasing difficulty putting on his socks and shoes. He was referred to occupational therapy specifically for assistive devices for this area of dressing. The occupational therapy practitioner had the patient demonstrate donning and doffing his socks and shoes. He was able to do the tasks with difficulty. The activity did not cause him pain, but he was limited by stiffness in his back and hips. She also ascertained that he had stopped doing his stretching exercises about a year ago. She showed Dan the devices available but would not recommend them for him, because this dressing activity was forcing him to use his available sitting hand-to-floor ROM on a daily basis. Assistive devices at this time would eliminate this daily stretch and encourage a loss of flexibility. She recommended that he obtain a referral to physical therapy for reevaluation of his home stretching program. She suggested that he be diligent in a daily stretching routine for 2 weeks to see whether his hand-to-floor range would improve and make dressing and bathing easier. She asked him to call her in 2 weeks with a progress report so she could determine whether further therapy is needed.

Note: If the dressing activity was causing hip or back pain and aggravating inflamed joints, then the appropriate treatment would be teaching an adaptive method that does not cause pain or require assistive devices.

Common Functional Limitations and Possible Solutions

Assistive devices can make a major difference in the ability of persons with arthritis to participate in daily tasks. Practitioners play a very important role in evaluating these persons for appropriate devices, including offering the opportunity to try various products. Practitioners also assess the environment and the role of other persons and use this information in making recommendations. Training is important with many assistive devices, and follow-up is essential (Mann, 1998).

A relationship between assistive device training and patient compliance or usage has been demonstrated. In Great Britain, assistive device training programs resulted in higher use rates, improved satisfaction, and safer bathing practices (Chamberlain, Thornley, Stowe, & Wright, 1981; Stowe, Thornley, Chamberlain, & Wright, 1982).

In addition to catalogs for ADL equipment, there is *Abledata*, a database of more than 20,000 assistive devices available from approximately 2,500 manufacturers (*Abledata* is available on the Internet at www.abledata.com). It provides detailed information and, for many devices, pictures are included. It may be useful to use several search directories to find an item on the Internet.

Aids for hand impairment. The hand joints are particularly vulnerable to stress because they are small and highly mobile with complex biomechanical forces acting on them. The muscles are used to move the joints, rather than to stabilize and support them. Moreover, the accumulated force of using the hands over the course of a day is considerable, even if they are used gently.

The activities that tend to cause the greatest pain and damage are those that require a tight grip or pinch force. All of the aids recommended in Table 8.4 are designed to reduce the force required of the hands in activities.

Aids for elbow impairment. Loss of elbow flexion can severely interfere with one's ability to eat, wash, or touch one's face. Loss of extension can interfere with one's ability to touch the feet and perform lower-extremity dressing, as well as push off from chairs. Pressure or repetitive trauma may aggravate rheumatoid nodules. Severe bilateral limitations are extremely disabling and constitute an indication for surgery. (See Table 8.5.)

Aids for shoulder impairment. A considerable amount of shoulder ROM (approximately 50%) can be lost before causing a major restriction of functional activities. Persons with 90° of shoulder flexion or less generally need some aids to assist with reach or dressing. Painful shoulders can reduce the ability of the upper extremity in all strength tasks such as lifting, carrying, or pushing. (See Table 8.6.)

Aids for neck impairment. In the early stages of inflammation, the facet joints of the spinal cord can be aggravated by repetitive motion or posture in extremes of range, such as forward flexion while reading. In cases of severe involvement (e.g., JRA or AS), neck immobility restricts the visual range. This development is particularly critical in activities in which safety is a concern, such as driving or child care. An immobile neck also makes it difficult to participate in conversation in a group setting, where conversation may originate from different directions. If ankylosis is inevitable, aids should be considered to help maintain optimal alignment. (See Table 8.7.)

Aids for knee impairment. Knee pain inhibits muscle strength of the knee extensors, reducing the ability to rise from a sitting position, to stand, and to ambulate. Loss of extension greater than 30° can severely limit ambulation. A minimum of 100° of knee flexion is needed to sit in a chair or climb steps comfortably.

To prevent joint contractures and to reduce joint stiffness, patients with knee involvement should be advised to change the position of their legs when sitting, so that the knees are often stretched out. Use of a footstool to support the legs may be recommended. It is important to alternate frequently between sitting and standing. Table 8.8 lists several devices that can be used to avoid excessive strain on the knees during self-care activities.

Aids for hip impairment. A minimal hip flexion contracture can encourage knee flexion contractures and other such problems or cause compensatory spinal changes, such as lordosis. These conditions in turn reduce efficiency in gait and movement. An impaired hip may limit or restrict participation in sports but may not prevent functional activities. A moderate contracture increases the problems noted above and would make it difficult for the person to lie supine.

Loss of hip flexion (an extension contracture) creates greater functional limitations. Ninety degrees of hip flexion is necessary to sit comfortably in a regular chair. If a person has less than 90° of flexion, his or her back will press into the chair, which can cause back pain. Severe loss of flexion, for example, to 45°, makes it impossible to sit normally in a chair. Shallow seats or sitting on the edge of a seat may provide an answer in some situations. For any person with this type of problem who is not a candidate for surgery, obtaining comfortable seating is a critical part of therapy. If proper seating would make a difference in the person's

Table 8.4 Aids for Hand Impairment

Device	Comments
Adapted, built-up, or narrowed handles	Adhesive foam, foam tubing, or custom handles made out of orthotic material are the most common methods. On forearm crutches, the plastic handle can be removed and the narrow stem lightly padded.
Nonslip or plastic sheets (e.g., Dycem mats)	These are used to reduce force required to stabilize items (e.g., when used under a dinner plate); a person only has to cut food, not cut and press down.
Faucet turners	When possible, it is worth investing in lever fixtures for taps or faucets.
House or car key adaptations	Commercial key holders that increase leverage are available. If only one or two keys are a problem, each can be adapted by sealing the end between two pieces of orthotic material. Caution: custom adaptations may not fit the recessed area for ignition keys.
Lamp switch extenders and switches in extension cords	
Soaped runner on kitchen drawers for easier gliding	Silicon spray (e.g., WD-40®) can ease operation of sliding doors, locks, and hinges.
Lightweight kitchen utensils	
Electric can opener	Before ordering, therapists should be familiar with the strength required to operation openers.
Jar opener	Wall-hung or under-counter openers that allow bilateralpalmar holding of the jar are the best choice for people with active hand inflammation.
Bowl holders	There are now round bowls with a rubber stabilizing ring that allows the bowl to be positioned at any angle.
Saucepan stabilizers	If a full tea kettle is kept on the stove, the saucepan can be stabilized against it while stirring.
Spring-loaded clipping scissors	
Suction bottle/glass brushes	These fit into the bottom of the sink and are very helpful if there is no dishwasher.
Electric scissors	These take practice to learn to use easily.
Cutting boards with stainless steel nails	These are used to stabilize vegetables for cutting.
Strap loops for forearm for oven doors, drawers, sliding doors	Straps allows the person to slip forearm through loop to open door. In the kitchen, they can be made out of attractive, sturdy ribbon or colored webbing.
Shoulder straps and pads for handbags, suitcases, shopping bags	Commercial shoulder pads are available at luggage stores.
Blanket cradles or ribbon handles sewn on blankets	These are used to make blanket manipulation easier.

(continued)

Table 8.4 (*continued*)

Device	Comments
Electric blankets	These are used to minimize bulk and aid in reducing morning stiffness.
Sheet tucker (small wooden paddle)	
Universal cuff	These are used to hold brushes, silverware, and pencils.
Book racks, newspaper holders	These are used to keep books and newspapers at an upright angle without manually holding them. Plastic ones are available for cookbooks.
Pen or pencil holding devices	Many styles are available. My favorite for reducing hand strain is to stick the pen or pencil through the center of a small (2-in. diameter), firm (not hard), foam ball (usually neon red).
Electric shaver holders	
Cup holders, lightweight mugs, mugs with open handles	The open handle can accommodate deformity.
Button hooks	Depending on the hand problem, these may need to be built up or narrowed; padded or firm.
Soap on a rope (for shower or tub)	These prevent soap from falling.
Car door openers	Styles are available to open all types of doors.
Aerosol can holder	Grip pressure can be used to press spray knob.
Plastic open handles for milk cartons and large soda bottles	
Pop top and screw cap openers	
Plastic bag and box top openers	
Luggage carrier	These can be used to cart other things around the house.

Note. From *Rheumatic Disease in the Adult and Child: Occupational Therapy and Rehabilitation* (3rd ed., pp. 441–442), by J. L. Melvin, 1989, Philadelphia: F. A. Davis. Copyright 1989 by F. A. Davis. Adapted with permission.

employment or attendance in school, rehabilitation agencies may be able to assist with funding for equipment. Equipment for this problem includes specially adapted chairs and toilet seats that allow the patient to sit upright with the hips in less than 90° of flexion.

Table 8.9 lists devices that are applicable to restrictions that limit hand-to-foot or floor range. These devices are useful for those with back or elbow restrictions as well as limited hip flexion.

Aids for limitations in dressing. During dressing, limited range in proximal upper-and lower-extremity joints may make it difficult to get clothing over the feet or over the head. Poor grasp strength and loss of fine prehension skills create problems in manipulating fasteners. Upper-extremity weakness interferes with putting on coats or jackets.

It is useful to advise patients that clothing selection is important as part of a management strategy. Clothes should be easy to put on. For example, turtlenecks should be avoided, along with trousers with tight-fitting elastic at the waist or sleeves. Fasteners (buttons and zippers) can be a particular problem, so care should be taken to purchase garments with closures or fasteners in front. For exist-

Table 8.5 Aids for Elbow Impairment

Devices	Comments
Elbow protectors with foam pad (Heelbos®) or gel pad (Roylan®)	These can be worn to bed to reduce pressure on nodules or sensitive skin and to facilitate bed mobility or during the day to increase comfort. The foam pads are lighter and may cause less strain on fragile shoulders than gel pads.
Extended handle tableware for feeding, extended straws	These aids compensate for loss of elbow flexion and inability to bring hand to mouth.
Lower extremity dressing aids	These compensate for loss of elbow extension.
Chairs that are easy to rise from for patients with limited ability to push off	The inability to straighten the elbow limits ability to push off during transfer. Higher chairs require less push off with the arms.

Note. From *Rheumatic Disease in the Adult and Child: Occupational Therapy and Rehabilitation* (3rd ed., p. 442), by J. L. Melvin, 1989, Philadelphia: F. A. Davis. Copyright 1989 by F. A. Davis. Adapted with permission.

Table 8.6 Aids for Shoulder Impairment

Device	Comments
Extended handles with enlarged grip on hairbrushes, combs, toothbrushes, tableware, back brushes	Caution: Extended handles increase the forces on the hand and wrist—use lightweight devices
Long, cloth, back scrubbers	Preferred over other back brushes; often available at notions counters
Extended drinking straws	To compensate for severe loss of shoulder flexion
Coat holder	Available from European companies; bracket with clips holds coat while donning, releases with foot pedal
Lightweight down winter coat	Heavy coats are difficult to take on and off, and the weight hangs on the shoulders
Reacher	Caution: Increases forces on the hand and wrist—use lightweight devices
Dressing stick (cup hook on one end, adapted coat hook on other end)	Also helpful for reaching, pulling, or pushing items other than clothing
Front-opening clothes	Pullover clothes require considerable shoulder flexion
Sponges and dustpans with extended handles for floor care	Kneeling to do activities in front of the body requires more shoulder flexion than using extended-handle devices
One-handed hair rollers	Self-fastening covering holds hair in place without clips, so hair can be rolled without using the affected shoulder

Note. From *Rheumatic Disease in the Adult and Child: Occupational Therapy and Rehabilitation* (3rd ed., p. 443), by J. L. Melvin, 1989, Philadelphia: F. A. Davis. Copyright 1989 by F. A. Davis. Adapted with permission.

Table 8.7 Aids for Neck Impairment

Device	Comments
Chairs that swivel	Neck stiffness or immobility requires turning the entire body to see to the sides. Swivel chairs allow the patient visual range without getting up. Executive office chairs can have wheels removed and be used in the living room.
Wide-angled rearview mirror	Available at most auto parts stores.
Expandable/mounted mirror	Allows adjustment to create correct angle for viewing.
Typing draft holder	Holds pages at eye level next to the monitor; eliminates need for repetitive turning or extension.
Adjustable book holder	For students, I recommend using a simple wire holder on top of a stack of books to bring the book to eye level (works well in the library).
Cervical contour pillows	Available from medical distributors; the Jackson Cervipillo® is a good one to start with.
Telephone receiver headset	For people who work on the telephone, a lightweight headset receiver is a worthwhile investment; contact your local telephone company for resources.
Step stool and reacher for upper cabinets	Step stool reduces need to hyperextend neck.

Note. From *Rheumatic Disease in the Adult and Child: Occupational Therapy and Rehabilitation* (3rd ed., p. 443), by J. L. Melvin, 1989, Philadelphia: F. A. Davis. Copyright 1989 by F. A. Davis. Reprinted with permission.

Table 8.8 Aids for Knee Impairment

Device	Comments
Elevated chairs in the living room, kitchen, at work (and in the clinic)	Sofas and office waiting room chairs can be adapted by setting them on top of a 3-in. carpeted platform.
High kitchen stool	It is important that these be lightweight as well as sturdy so they can be moved easily.
Raised toilet seat	If possible, have an elevated toilet installed; if it has to be removed frequently, the weight and ease of attachment should be considered.
Arm bars for toilet	These help reduce stress on the knees by transferring some lifting work to the arms.
Shower bench	Benches that block shower curtain closure allow water to get on the floor; patient's ability to clean up the water must also be a consideration; a hand-held showerhead may be helpful.
Tub grab bars	These reduce the weight-bearing load and provide stability during transfers.
Walking aids	Canes should have wide rubber tips that are replaced when worn; there are several adaptations for making cane use safe on icy streets.
"Half step" or short steps	Steps can be adapted so they are half the height of regular steps.

(continued)

Table 8.8 (*continued*)

Device	Comments
Mobile cart for transporting	Make sure the cart is sturdy if it will be used a lot.dishes and other items
Shopping carts	These eliminate weight bearing required by carrying; carts should be pushed all the way to the car.

Note. From Rheumatic Disease in the Adult and Child: Occupational Therapy and Rehabilitation (3rd ed., p. 444), by J. L. Melvin, 1989, Philadelphia: F. A. Davis. Copyright 1989 by F. A. Davis. Adapted with permission.

ing clothes, hook-and-loop fasteners can be used to replace buttons (with the buttons attached permanently to the buttonhole) (Dallas & White, 1982). Alternatively, a buttonhook can be useful for managing buttons. Large rings or leather loops are useful aids on zipper tabs.

Dressing sticks are useful for pulling on pants. Stocking devices are valuable for putting on socks or stockings. For women, a useful strategy for putting on panty hose is to dust thighs with powder before pulling the panty hose into place. Rolling panty hose from top to bottom before putting them on facilitates dressing. The garments can be unrolled once the legs have been inserted.

Shoes should be purchased with care. Desirable characteristics include adjustable closures to accommodate swelling; low heels (less than 1 inch); cushioned soles; wide toe area; and soft, stretchable upper materials. Many of the currently manufactured athletic shoes are satisfactory. Adaptations for shoes are also available, including cushioned inserts, pads, and elastic shoelaces. Table 8.10 provides a summary of clothing devices.

Aids for limitations in grooming. Decreased shoulder movement impedes hair care, makeup application, shaving, and dental hygiene. The loss of hand dexterity also interferes with these tasks, as well as with nail grooming. Temporomandibular joint disease may complicate dental care. See Table 8.11 for suggested assistive devices.

Aids for limitations in bathing. Limitations in ambulation and transfer skills may make getting in and out of the tub or shower fatiguing, unsafe, or impossible. Loss of upper-extremity strength and range interferes with management of faucets, washcloths, soap,

Table 8.9 Aids for Hip Impairment

Device	Comments
Reachers	A wide selection is available.
Sock donners	Also available for pantyhose.
Elastic shoestrings	Elastic strings allow shoes to be put on with greater ease, tying is eliminated, and the need for extreme hip flexion is avoided.
Boot jack	This device catches the head of the shoe and helps to pull it off.
Dressing sticks, pants dressing poles, extended shoehorns	These devices help compensate for loss of hip flexion, although dressing without aids may be the daily activity necessary for maintaining hip flexion; use aids only if essential.
Double-faced tape on the end of a stick	Helps in picking up small items such as pills or broken glass.

Note. From Rheumatic Disease in the Adult and Child: Occupational Therapy and Rehabilitation (3rd ed., p. 444), by J. L. Melvin, 1989, Philadelphia: F. A. Davis. Copyright 1989 by F. A. Davis. Adapted with permission.

Table 8.10 Aids for Facilitating Dressing Tasks

Device	Comments
Dressing stick, pants dressing poles	These reach-extending devices compensate for loss of hand-to-toe ROM or loss of shoulder flexion and elbow extension.
Reaching devices	Reachers increase the lever force on the hands and need to be used with caution by persons who have active hand or wrist inflammation. Lightweight passive reachers are the least stressful.
Shoe and sock aids	Reach-extending devices compensate for a lack of hand-to-toe ROM. The boot jack can reduce stress on the hands or compensate for loss of hip or back ROM.
Stocking donner	
Long-handled shoe horn	
Boot jack	
Adaptive closures: elastic shoelaces, button hook, zipper pull, zipper loop or ring, zipper tab	A wide variety of commercial and homemade closures are available. Shoes can be adapted with hook-and-loop fasteners, zippers, or clip-style closures.
Adapted clothing	Patterns or specially made garments to facilitate dressing may be purchased. Difficult closures may be replaced with simpler fasteners or Velcro® strips. Clothing with elasticized waists, front closures, or wraparound skirts may be selected.

Note. From *Rheumatic Disease in the Adult and Child: Occupational Therapy and Rehabilitation* (3rd ed., p. 445), by J. L. Melvin, 1989, Philadelphia: F. A. Davis. Copyright 1989 by F. A. Davis. Adapted with permission. ROM = range of motion.

shampoo, and so on. Limited range in proximal upper- and lower-extremity joints creates problems in reaching body parts, and fatigue could prevent a patient from completing a bath independently. Cleaning up water spilled on the floor during bathing is a safety concern for many patients, and this problem may deter patients from taking a shower. (See Table 8.12.)

Aids for limitations in toileting. Limitations in knee and hip flexion and extension and in transfer skills make it difficult to get on and off a toilet. Decreased range in proximal upper-and lower-extremity joints or loss of hand skills may interfere with managing perineal hygiene and cause problems in dressing and undressing for toileting. Table 8.13 lists devices that may be helpful in these activities.

Aids for limitations in housekeeping. Aids and adaptations may be necessary because of limitations in

mobility, proximal upper-and lower-extremity ROM and strength, or hand deformity. It is critical to consider aids that will promote joint protection and energy conservation (see Table 8.14).

Aids for limitations in meal preparation. A person with arthritis may need special aids to compensate for impaired mobility, limited range in reaching and bending, or lack of strength and endurance. Because many kitchen tasks are resistive or repetitive, it is especially important to consider joint protection and energy conservation principles. (See Table 8.15.)

Aids for limitations in eating. Limited proximal upper-extremity range may impair the person's ability to get food to the mouth. Lack of supination or fine prehension may impair the ability to manipulate utensils. Weakness may make it difficult to cut food or lift a glass or cup. See Table 8.16 for a list of devices and approaches for making mealtime easier.

Table 8.11 Aids and Devices for Facilitating Grooming

Device	Comments
Enlarged or extended handles on toothbrushes, combs, razors	Lightweight materials to build up handles include cylindrical foam, adhesive foam, small wooden doweling, and aluminum tubing. Plastic coating or applications of low-temperature plastic splinting material will foster a better grip.
Dental hygiene aids, Electric toothbrushes, Water jet appliances, Floss and toothpick holders, Toothpaste tube key	Careful selection of these devices is advised because some are heavy, have an awkward grip, or require too much grip.
Nail care devices, Electronic nail files, Padded contour nail file holders, Long handled toenail scissors	These compensate for weakness and loss of fine pinch. Clippers may be mounted on a wooden block or extensions may be placed on the handles.
Adaptations for cosmetic containers	An attachment for aerosol spray cans acts as a lever to press the spray button. Cosmetics may be selected for accessible containers (e.g., push-up lipsticks, deodorants with larger tops).

Note. From *Rheumatic Disease in the Adult and Child: Occupational Therapy and Rehabilitation* (3rd ed., p. 445), by J. L. Melvin, 1989, Philadelphia: F. A. Davis. Copyright 1989 by F. A. Davis. Adapted with permission.

Table 8.12 Aids To Facilitate Bathing Activities

Device	Comments
Safety mats, grab bars	These aid transfer and increase safety; vertical poles or bars attach to tub to assist weak grasp by using forearm as a substitute.
Tub shower seats	These aid transfer and increase safety; available in a wide variety of styles and heights.
Lever faucet handles, tap-turning devices	These allow use of lever force to turn handles, thus reducing stress on hand joints.
Bathing supplies: shower caddies, tub trays, soap dispensers	These aid limited strength and increase range; wide variety is available.
Washing and drying: long-handled sponge, wash mitts, adapted washcloths, terry cloth robes	These aid limited range in proximal joints. Long-handled sponges are impractical if wrists or hands are involved. Mitts aid limited grasp. Terry cloth robe saves energy required for drying after bath.

Note. From *Rheumatic Disease in the Adult and Child: Occupational Therapy and Rehabilitation* (3rd ed., p. 446), by J. L. Melvin, 1989, Philadelphia: F. A. Davis. Copyright 1989 by F. A. Davis. Adapted with permission.

Table 8.13 Aids to Facilitate the Performance of Toileting Activities

Device	Comments
Elevated toilet seats	Wide variety of temporary and permanent adaptations possible
Commodes, grab bars	Aid transfer and increase safety
Dressing: adapted clothing, dressing aids	See Table 8.10
Toilet paper holder	Device holds paper and extends reach for cleaning after elimination. Several different styles; needs to be lightweight

Note. From *Rheumatic Disease in the Adult and Child: Occupational Therapy and Rehabilitation* (3rd ed., p. 446), by J. L. Melvin, 1989, Philadelphia: F. A. Davis. Copyright 1989 by F. A. Davis. Adapted with permission.

Summary

It is not enough for persons with arthritis or pain to be able to do self-care or other valued activities—they need to be able to perform them safely in a way that will not cause pain or damage their joints. To achieve this goal, occupational therapy practitioners need to understand the biomechanics of joint pathology and the way in which functional activities, splints, assistive devices and methods, and JPTs affect the joint. This is especially important when assisting the patient in managing self-care needs, because these tasks and activities constitute daily regimens that are repeated over and over for weeks and years. The occupational therapy practitioner must also be aware that such factors as medications, fatigue, and duration and severity of morning stiffness can influence the ADL evaluation and must be considered when prescribing self-care interventions. ◆

Table 8.14 Devices and Approaches for Facilitating Housekeeping Tasks

Device	Comments
Kitchen or utility carts	These help conserve energy, reduce joint stress, and compensate for limited strength. Wheeled carts eliminate lifting and carrying because many items can be carried in one trip.
Lightweight sweepers, self-propelled vacuum cleaners, electric brooms, lightweight vacuums	These conserve energy and reduce joint stress. Lightweight sweepers may be used to reduce frequency of heavier vacuuming.
Shortened handles on broom and dustpan for wheelchair use	Brooms need to be small and lightweight (ordinary brooms can be viewed as heavy weights on the end of long levers, which increase stress to the wrist joints).
Laundry aids: platforms to raise washer and dryer height, lowered clothes racks and lines, adjustable-height ironing board, lightweight travel iron or plastic regular iron	These help compensate for strength and range limitations. Automatic washers and dryers should be selected for accessibility and easy-to-operate controls, and clothes selected for easy care, little ironing.

Note. From *Rheumatic Disease in the Adult and Child: Occupational Therapy and Rehabilitation* (3rd ed., p. 446), by J. L. Melvin, 1989, Philadelphia: F. A. Davis. Copyright 1989 by F. A. Davis. Adapted with permission.

Table 8.15 Approaches and Devices for Facilitating Meal Preparation Tasks

Device	Comments
Lightweight utensils, cookware, and dishes	Less strength and energy are required, which reduces joint stress. Ceramic plates may range in weight from 11 oz to 29 oz each.
Devices to open containers: jar openers, can openers, boxtop openers, bag openers	These compensate for weak grasp or loss of fine prehension. Electric appliances must be selected so that controls are easy to operate. Those that allow two hands to hold a jar are best.
Aids for cutting and chopping	These compensate for weak grasp and loss of fine hand skills; they also reduce joint stress. Knives and scissors should be maintained with sharp cutting edges to reduce the force required in cutting. The Swedish knife has a vertical handle helpful for people with limited wrist motion. Spring-style scissors are less stressful to joints. Cutting boards may be adapted with rustproof nails to hold food.
Labor-saving appliances	These generally lessen joint stress, because less strength and energy are required. Examples include microwave ovens, electric skillets, blenders, and food processors. Appliances should be selected so that controls are easy to operate and parts that must be lifted are lightweight.
Small suction brush	Using these inside the sink makes cleaning tableware easier.
Adaptations for storage: pegboard, vertical storage, pull-out shelves	These conserve energy. They may compensate for loss of range and strength. Work areas should be arranged so that tools and equipment are stored where they are first used. Adaptations may be permanent and built-in or temporary, commercially available items.

Note. From *Rheumatic Disease in the Adult and Child: Occupational Therapy and Rehabilitation* (3rd ed., p. 447), by J. L. Melvin, 1989, Philadelphia: F. A. Davis. Copyright 1989 by F. A. Davis. Adapted with permission.

Table 8.16 Devices and Approaches for Making Mealtime Easier

Device	Comments
Adapted utensils: enlarged or extended handles, utensil cuffs, swivel forks and spoons	Attractive utensils with enlarged handles are commercially available. Handles or cuffs of standard utensils may be enlarged with foam or plastic to eliminate tight grasp of utensil. Swivel handles compensate for loss of supination.
Aids for drinking: long straws, lightweight and spill-proof cups, thermal mugs, trays, table height adjustments	Thermal mugs with wide handles allow both hands to be used with MCP joints in less stressful positions. Severely disabled or hospitalized patients may need meals served at a more accessible table height.

Note. From *Rheumatic Disease in the Adult and Child: Occupational Therapy and Rehabilitation* (3rd ed., p. 447), by J. L. Melvin, 1989, Philadelphia: F. A. Davis. Copyright 1989 by F. A. Davis. Adapted with permission. MCP = metacarpophalangeal.

Study Questions

1. How are hand deformities different between a young child with JRA and an adult with RA?

2. What medication makes it difficult for persons with SLE to learn instructions?

3. What are the three components for fatigue management for persons with rheumatoid diseases?

4. For all persons with disabilities, the purpose of the ADL evaluation is to determine the levels of ability and disability. What additional process needs to be determined when evaluating persons with arthritis?

5. What are the three major trends or factors that have influenced rehabilitation of persons with arthritis over the past 10 years?

References

Ailinger, R. L., & Dear, M. R. (1997). An examination of the self-care needs of clients with rheumatoid arthritis. *Rehabilitation Nursing 22*(3), 135–140.

Arnett, F., Gall, V., & Slonaker, D. (2000). Ankylosing spondylitis. In J. Melvin & K. M. Ferrell (Eds.), *Rheumatologic rehabilitation series: Vol. 2. Adult rheumatic diseases.* Bethesda, MD: American Occupational Therapy Association.

Belza, B. L. (1996). Fatigue. In S. T. Wegener, B. L. Belza, & E. P. Gall (Eds.), *Clinical care in the rheumatic diseases.* Atlanta, GA: American College of Rheumatology.

Bland, J., Melvin, J. L., & Hasson, S. (2000). Osteoarthritis. In J. Melvin & K. M. Ferrell (Eds.), *Rheumatologic rehabilitation series: Vol. 2. Adult rheumatic diseases.* Bethesda, MD: American Occupational Therapy Association.

Bolding, D., & Sanders, M. A. (2000). Occupational therapy for children and adolescents with juvenile rheumatoid arthritis. In J. L. Melvin & F. V. Wright (Eds.), *Rheumatologic rehabilitation series: Vol. 3. Pediatric rheumatic diseases.* Bethesda, MD: American Occupational Therapy Association.

Boutaugh, M. L., & Brady, T. J. (1998). Patient education for self-management. In J. L. Melvin & G. Jensen (Eds.), *Rheumatologic rehabilitation series: Vol. 1. Assessment and management.* Bethesda, MD: American Occupational Therapy Association.

Buckland-Wright, J. C., MacFarland, D. G., & Lynch, J. A. (1991). Osteophytes in the osteoarthritic hand: Their incidence size, distribution and progression. *Annals of Rheumatic Disease, 50*(9), 627–630.

Carmen, W. J. (1989). Factors associated with pain and osteoarthritis in the Tecumesh community health study. *Seminars in Arthritis and Rheumatism, 18* (4), 10–13.

Cathey, M. A., Wolfe, F., & Kleinheksel, S. M. (1988). Functional ability and work status in patients with fibromyalgia. *Arthritis Care and Research, 1,* 85–98.

Chamberlain, M. A., Thornley, G., Stowe, J., & Wright, V. (1981). Evaluation of aids and equipment for the bath: II. A possible solution to the problem. *Rheumatologic Rehabilitation, 20*(1), 38–43.

Colditz, J., & Melvin, J. L. (2000). Splinting for arthritis of the hand. In J. L. Melvin & E. A. Nalebuff (Eds.), *Rheumatologic rehabilitation series: Vol. IV. The hand: Evaluation, therapy, and surgery.* Bethesda, MD: American Occupational Therapy Association.

Cordery, J., & Rocchi, M. (1998). Joint protection and fatigue management. In J. L. Melvin & G. Jensen (Eds.), *Rheumatologic rehabilitation series: Vol. 1. Assessment and management.* Bethesda, MD: American Occupational Therapy Association.

Cordery, J. C. (1965). Joint protection: A responsibility of the occupational therapy practitioner. *American Journal of Occupational Therapy, 19,* 285–294.

Dallas, M. J., & White, L. W. (1982). Clothing fasteners for women with arthritis. *American Journal of Occupational Therapy, 36,* 515–518.

Hirano, P. C., Laurent, D. D., & Lorig, K. (1994). Arthritis patient education studies, 1987–1991: A review of the literature. *Patient Education and Counseling, 24*(1), 9–54.

Hochberg, M. C., Chang, R. W., Dwosh, I., Lindsey, S., Pincus, T., & Wolfe, F. (1992). The American College of Rheumatology 1991 revised criteria for the classification of global functional status in rheumatoid arthritis. *Arthritis & Rheumatism, 35*(5), 498–502.

Liang, M., Roger, M., & Larson, M. (1984). The psychosocial impact of systemic lupus erythematosus and rheumatoid arthritis. *Arthritis and Rheumatism, 27,* 13–21.

Lorig, K. (1993). Self-management of chronic illness: A model for the future. *Generations, 17*(3), 11–14.

Mann, W. C. (1998). Assistive technology for persons with arthritis. In J. L. Melvin & G. Jensen (Eds.), *Rheumatologic rehabilitation series: Vol. 1. Assessment and management.* Bethesda, MD: American Occupational Therapy Association.

Medsger, T. A. (1988). Systemic sclerosis and localized scleroderma. In R. Schumacher, Jr. (Ed.), *Primer on the rheumatic diseases.* Atlanta, GA: Arthritis Foundation.

Melvin, J. L. (1977). *Rheumatic disease: Occupational therapy and rehabilitation.* Philadelphia: F. A. Davis.

Melvin, J. L. (1989). *Rheumatic disease in the adult and child: Occupational therapy and rehabilitation* (3rd ed.). Philadelphia: F. A. Davis.

Melvin, J. L. (1994). *Scleroderma: Caring for your hands and face*. Bethesda, MD: American Occupational Therapy Association.

Melvin, J. L. (1996). *Fibromyalgia syndrome—Getting healthy*. Bethesda, MD: American Occupational Therapy Association.

Melvin, J. L. (1998). Self-management for fibromyalgia. *OT Practice, 3*(11), 39–43.

Melvin, J. L., LeRoy, C., & Elrod, C. (2000). Systemic sclerosis (scleroderma). In J. L. Melvin & K. M. Haralson-Ferrell (Eds.), *Rheumatologic rehabilitation series: Vol. 2. Adult rheumatic diseases*. Bethesda, MD: American Occupational Therapy Association.

Mier, R., Wright, F. V., & Bolding, D. (2000). Juvenile rheumatoid arthritis. In J. L. Melvin & F. V. Wright (Eds.), *Rheumatologic rehabilitation series: Vol. 3. Pediatric rheumatic diseases*. Bethesda, MD: American Occupational Therapy Association.

Minor, M. (1998). Exercise for health and physical fitness. In J. L. Melvin & G. Jensen (Eds.), *Rheumatologic rehabilitation series: Vol. 1. Assessment and management*. Bethesda, MD: American Occupational Therapy Association.

Moll, J. M. H., & Wright, V. (1973). Psoriatic arthritis. *Seminars in Arthritis and Rheumatism, 3*, 55–57.

Moratz, V., Muncie, H. L., Jr., & Miranda-Walsh, H. (1986). Occupational management in the multidisciplinary assessment and management of osteoarthritis. *Clinical Therapeutics, 9*(Suppl. B), 24–29.

Nalebuff, E. A., & Melvin, J. L. (2000). Orthotic treatment for arthritis of the hand. In J. L. Melvin & E. A. Melvin (Eds.), *Rheumatologic rehabilitation series: Vol. 4. The hand: Evaluation, therapy and surgery*. Bethesda, MD: American Occupational Therapy Association.

Pincus, T., & Callahan, L. F. (1989). Reassessment of twelve traditional paradigms concerning the diagnosis, prevalence, morbidity and mortality of rheumatoid arthritis. *Scandinavian Journal of Rheumatology, 18*(Suppl. 79), 67–96.

Pincus, T., Callahan, L. F., Sale, W. G., Brooks, A. L., Payne, L. E., & Vaughn, W. K. (1984). Severe functional declines, work disability, and increased mortality in seventy-five rheumatoid arthritis patients studied over nine years. *Arthritis and Rheumatism, 27*, 864–872.

Rahman, P., Gladman, D. D., Gall, V., & Melvin, J. L. (2000). Psoriatic arthritis. In J. L. Melvin & K. M. Ferrell (Eds.), *Rheumatologic rehabilitation series: Vol. 2. Adult rheumatic diseases*. Bethesda, MD: American Occupational Therapy Association.

Russell, I. J., & Melvin, J. L. (2000). Fibromyalgia. In J. L. Melvin & K. M. Ferrell (Eds.), *Rheumatologic rehabilitation series: Vol. 2. Adult rheumatic diseases*. Bethesda, MD: American Occupational Therapy Association.

Sanford, M., Silverman, S., & Wolfe, T. (2000). Rheumatoid arthritis. In J. L. Melvin & K. M. Haralson-Ferrell (Eds.), *Rheumatologic rehabilitation series: Vol. 2. Adult rheumatic diseases*. Bethesda, MD: American Occupational Therapy Association.

Schweidler, H. (1984). Assistive devices, aids to daily living. In G. K. Riggs & E. P. Gall (Eds.), *Rheumatic diseases rehabilitation and management*. Boston: Butterworth.

Stowe, J., Thornley, G., Chamberlain, M. A., & Wright, V. (1982). Evaluation of aids and equipment for the bath and toilet: Survey II. *British Journal of Occupational Therapy, 45*, 92–95.

Swanson, A. B., & DeGroot-Swanson, G. (1985). Osteoarthritis in the hand. *Clinics of Rheumatic Disease, 11* (2), 393–420.

Szer, I., & Wright, F. V. (2000). School integration for children and adolescents with juvenile arthritis. In J. L. Melvin & F. V. Wright (Eds.), *Rheumatologic rehabilitation series: Vol. 3. Pediatric rheumatic diseases*. Bethesda, MD: American Occupational Therapy Association.

Walker, S. E., Sotosky, J. R., & Melvin, J. L. (2000). Orthotic treatment for arthritis of the hand. In J. L. Melvin & E. A. Melvin (Eds.), *Rheumatologic rehabilitation series: Vol. 4. The hand: Evaluation, therapy and surgery*. Bethesda, MD: American Occupational Therapy Association.

9

Self-Care Strategies After Spinal Cord Injury

Suzanne Eberle

Susan L. Garber

Theresa L. Gregorio-Torres

Nancy W. Pumphrey

Pamela Lathem

Suzanne Eberle, OTR, is Assistant Director, Occupational Therapy, Kessler Institute of Rehabilitation, West Orange, New Jersey.

Susan L. Garber, MA, OTR, FAOTA, is Associate Professor, Department of Physical Medicine and Rehabilitation, Baylor College of Medicine, Houston, Texas, and is Rehabilitation Research Specialist, Veterans Administration Medical Center, Houston, Texas.

Theresa L. Gregorio-Torres, MA, OTR, is Unit Coordinator, SCI/Amputee/ Comprehensive Rehabilitation Unit, Department of Occupational Therapy, The Institute for Rehabilitation and Research (TIRR), Houston, Texas.

Nancy W. Pumphrey, OTR, is Occupational Therapist, University of Texas M. D. Anderson Cancer Center, Houston, Texas.

Pamela Lathem, OTR, is Senior Occupational Therapist, University of Texas M. D. Anderson Cancer Center, Houston, Texas.

Key Terms

autonomic dysreflexia

ball-bearing forearm orthosis (BBFO)

Frankel scale

mobile arm support (MAS)

paraplegia

tetraplegia

universal cuff

Wanchik device

Objectives

On completing this chapter, the reader will be able to

1. Understand how a spinal cord injury affects every aspect of a person's daily life.

2. Distinguish between paraplegia and tetraplegia.

3. Identify functional limitations and interventions necessary to accomplish self-care tasks for various levels of spinal cord injury.

4. Appreciate that self-care tasks for persons with high-level tetraplegia can be tedious and demanding.

5. Appreciate that the client and his or her family members should participate in selecting among the self-care options available for improving independence.

Spinal cord injury represents one of the most devastating and challenging types of disabling trauma seen by occupational therapy personnel. Young adults, nearly 80% male, incur most injuries, which are caused by motor vehicle crashes, falls, violence, and sports injuries (Go, DiVivo, & Richards, 1995).

The role of occupational therapy in the treatment of persons with spinal cord injury has evolved over several decades into a multifaceted and complex array of intervention categories. Therapy personnel assume responsibility for training in activities of daily living (ADL), designing and fabricating assistive devices, strengthening the upper extremities, exploring avocational and vocational interests and skills, and providing mechanisms to promote maximum independence (Garber, 1985).

The effective rehabilitation of patients with spinal cord injuries depends on these traditions and employs new evaluation and treatment efforts in such areas as environmental control systems, pressure-ulcer prevention programs, and technology and adaptive skills training (Garber, 1985). New challenges include reducing the length of hospital stays and developing community-based programs for persons with severe disabilities in concert with new developments in vocational rehabilitation and independent living (Tate, Heinrich, Paasuke, & Anderson, 1998).

Objective documentation of function and progress after spinal cord injury is most often accomplished using the Functional Independence Measure (FIM™), but the FIM needs to be supplemented by other objective scales that provide the sensitivity and detail necessary to document progress (Watson, Kanny, White, & Anson, 1995).

The functional levels of the spinal cord for the upper and lower extremities are described in Tables 9.1 and 9.2. Although the functional levels of spinal cord injury form the basis of this chapter, the neurological completeness of an injury warrants a brief description. The American Spinal Injury Association has adopted the Frankel grading system to describe the neurological extent of injury, which is shown in Table 9.2 (American Spinal Injury Association, 1996).

Because higher-level injuries in the cervical spine result in greater loss of function, challenges for practitioners and their clients are greater for these types of injuries. Table 9.3 provides an overview of the expected functional outcomes in ADL for different levels of injury. It is important to note that because not all lesions are complete, the actual abilities and levels of independence achieved by patients with injuries at different levels will vary. Motivation, preinjury lifestyle and circumstances, other injuries, and age will all influence the success of rehabilitation efforts.

High-Level Tetraplegia: Levels C-1–C-4

High-level tetraplegia refers to the paralysis that results from an injury to the spinal cord at any segmental level between the C-1 and C-4 vertebrae. For the purpose of this chapter, *high-level tetraplegia* describes those persons with any or all of the following conditions: (a) neurological level of C-4 or above, complete motor and sensory deficits bilaterally; (b) total or partial dependence on respiratory or other breathing aids; (c) long-term medical and personal care needs; and (d) limited expected functional recovery (Garber, Lathem, & Gregorio, 1988).

Although persons with high-level spinal cord injuries are usually dependent in self-care, learning to be verbally independent so they may instruct others in their care allows for some control in their life. There are three major objectives in the rehabilitation of persons with C-1–C-4 tetraplegia: (a) education regarding their care, (b) exposure to functional activities, (c) and adaptation through the use of high technology. Persons with injuries at the C-1 or C-2 level are ventilator dependent. Primary muscle innervation will be sternocleidomastoid (neck flexion and head rotation). At the C-4 level, the key muscles innervated are the diaphragm and the upper trapezius. The person may need a ventilator at first, but he or she is usually weaned from the ventilator. Movement includes full neck rotation, neck extension and flexion, and some scapular elevation. Little or no scapular depression exists (Trombly, 1995).

For a high-level (C-1–C-3) spinal cord–injured person, a mouthstick serves as a substitute for the hand. Traditional mouthstick training enables the person with this level of injury to achieve some independence and control in his or her life.

K. T. was an active high school senior when he dove into a shallow pool and hit his head on the bottom, resulting in a C-3 spinal cord injury. He received comprehensive rehabilitation, including strengthening of preserved neck musculature and mouthstick training. He learned to turn pages of a book, type, and write. Once discharged from the hospital, he decided to pursue

Table 9.1 Functional Levels of the Cervical Spinal Cord

Roots	Muscles	Function
C-2, C-3	Sternocleidomastoid	Neck flexion and head rotation
C-3, C-4	Trapezius	
	Superior	Neck extension and scapular elevation
	Middle	Scapular adduction
	Inferior	Scapular adduction and depression
C-3, C-4, C-5	Diaphragm	Respiration
C-4, C-5	Rhomboids	Scapular medial adduction, retraction, and elevation
C-5, C-6	Deltoid	
	Anterior	Shoulder flexion to 90°
	Middle	Shoulder abduction to 90°
	Posterior	Shoulder extension and horizontal abduction
	Supraspinatus	Shoulder abduction
	Infraspinatus	Shoulder lateral rotation
	Teres minor	
	Subscapularis	Shoulder medial rotation
	Teres major	
	Biceps brachii	Elbow flexion and forearm supination
	Brachialis	Elbow flexion
	Brachioradialis	
	Extensor carpi radialis longus	Wrist flexion and abduction
C-5, C-6, C-7	Serratus anterior	Shoulder forward thrust; scapular rotation for shoulder abduction
C-5-T-1	Pectoralis major	Shoulder adduction, flexion, and medial rotation
	Pectoralis minor	Shoulder forward and downward
C-6, C-7	Supinator	Forearm supination
	Pronator teres	Forearm pronation
C-6, C-7, C-8	Latissimus dorsi	Shoulder medial rotation
	Triceps brachii	Elbow extension
	Extensor digiti communis	MCP extension
	Extensor digiti minimus	Little finger extension
C-7, C-8	Extensor indicis proprius	Index finger MCP extension
	Extensor carpi ulnaris	Wrist extension
	Extensor pollicis longus	Thumb IP extension
	Extensor pollicis brevis	Thumb MCP extension
	Abductor pollicis longus	Thumb abduction
C-7, C-8, T-1	Flexor digitorum superficialis	IP flexion
	Flexor digitorum profundus	DIP flexion

(continued)

Table 9.1 (*continued*)

Roots	Muscles	Function
C-8, T-1	Flexor carpi ulnaris	Wrist flexion and adduction
	Interossei	MCP flexion
	Dorsales	Finger abduction
	Palmares	Finger adduction
	Flexor pollicis longus	Thumb IP flexion
	Flexor pollicis brevis	Thumb MCP flexion
	Abductor pollicis	Thumb abduction
	Adductor pollicis brevis	Thumb adduction
	Opponens pollicis	Thumb opposition
	Lumbricales	MCP flexion

Note. DIP = distal interphalangeal; IP = interphalangeal; MCP = metacarpophalangeal. From *Specialized Occupational Therapy for Persons With High Level Quadriplegia* by S. L. Garber, P. Lathem, and T. L. Gregorio, 1988, Houston: TIRR. Copyright © 1988 by TIRR. Reprinted by permission. There may be some variation among references regarding actual nerve roots and innervated muscles (Burke & Murray, 1975; Chusid, 1985; *Dorland's Medical Dictionary*, 1962; Hoppenfeld, 1977; Sharrard, 1964).

Table 9.2 The Frankel Grading System: Neurological Extent of Spinal Cord Injury

Grade Level	Description
Frankel A	Complete No sensation or motor function
Frankel B	Incomplete Preserved sensation only Preservation of any demonstrable sensation, excluding subject phantom sensations Voluntary motor function is absent
Frankel C	Incomplete Preserved motor (nonfunctional); sensation may or may not be preserved
Frankel D	Incomplete Preserved motor (functional)
Frankel E	Complete recovery Complete return of all motor and sensory function; abnormal reflexes may persist

From *Spinal Cord Injury: The Facts and Figures* (p. 27) by S. L. Stover and P. R. Fine, 1986, Birmingham: University of Alabama Press. Copyright © 1986 by University of Alabama Press. Reprinted by permission.

a college degree in computer science. He was independently mobile with a chin-controlled power wheelchair and, therefore, was able to travel across the college campus without difficulty. However, he sometimes did find himself in buildings with elevators, and he had no way of depressing the elevator buttons. Frequently, passers-by would depress the buttons for him; but if no one was nearby, he had to wait, which often made him late for class. Finally, he decided to call the occupational therapist who had worked with him originally and to set up an outpatient appointment.

After consultation and evaluation, the therapist devised a small, triangular-base-shaped mouthstick holder with suction cups on the bottom that was positioned on K. T.'s lapboard. It was strategically placed close to his body so that he could flex his head forward and bite the mouthstick to pick it up independently. He was instructed to drive his chin-controlled wheelchair close to the elevator buttons, positioning it so the side where the mouthstick holder was mounted was closest and parallel to the buttons. Then he could lift the mouthstick and call the elevator. Once inside the elevator, he repeated the process to select the floor he desired. Fortunately, the elevator buttons are accessible to him most of the time. However, he has found that he is unable to depress the buttons in all elevators, and, at those times, he politely asks for assistance. This relatively inexpensive mouthstick holder and a little creativity went a long way toward enhancing this young man's ability to pursue his education. ■

Table 9.3 Typical Functional Outcomes for Persons With Complete Spinal Cord Injuries

Location of Injury	Mobility	Orthotic Devices	Community Transport	Communication	Feeding	Grooming	Bathing	Dressing	Toilet Needs
C-3–C-4	Can use pneumatic or chin-control power W/C with power recliner	UE externally powered orthosis, dorsal cock-up splint, BBFO	Needs assistance of others in accessible van with lift, cannot drive	Can use phone and typewriter with adapted equipment	Usually needs feeding assistance, may use BBFO with universal cuff and adapted utensils; drinks with long straw after setup	Must rely on personal care assistance	Must rely on personal care assistance	Must rely on personal care assistance	Must rely on personal care assistance
C-5	Can use powered W/C indoors and outdoors; short distances in manual W/C with adapted hand rims indoors	UE externally powered orthosis, dorsal cock-up splint, BBFOs	Can drive with specially adapted van	Can use phone and typewriter with adapted equipment	Can self-feed with specially adapted equipment for feeding after setup	Can be independent with adapted equipment	Must rely on personal care assistance	Requires assistance with UE dressing; dependent for LE dressing	Needs assistance from others and equipment
C-6	Can travel short distances with manual W/C with adaptations; assistance needed outdoors; independent in hand-driven W/C	Wrist-driven orthosis, universal cuff, writing devices, built-up handles	Independent driving in specially adapted van	Can use phone, can also type and write with adapted equipment; can turn pages without assistance	Can be independent with adapted equipment, can drink from glass	Can be independent with adapted equipment	Independent in UE and LE bathing with adapted equipment	Independent with UE dressing; assistance needed for LE dressing	Independent for bowel routine; needs assistance with bladder routine

(continued)

Table 9.3 (*continued*)

Location of Injury	Mobility	Othotic Devices	Community Transport	Communi-cation	Feeding	Grooming	Bathing	Dressing	Toilet Needs
C-7	Can use manual W/C indoors and outdoors except on stairs	None	Independent driving a car with hand controls or specially adapted van; can independently place W/C in car	Independent with adapted equipment for phone, typing, and writing; independent in turning pages	Independent	Independent	Independent with equipment	Independent	Independent
C-8–T-1	Can use manual W/C indoors with curbs, escalators	None	As above	Independent	Independent	Independent	Independent	Independent	Independent
T-2–T-10	Independent	KAFO with forearm crutches or walker	As above	Independent	Independent	Independent	Independent	Independent	Independent
T-11–L-2	Independent	KAFO or AFO with forearm crutches	As above	Independent	Independent	Independent	Independent	Independent	Independent
L-3–S-3	Independent	KAFO or AFO with forearm crutches or canes	As above	Independent	Independent	Independent	Independent	Independent	Independent

Note. AFO = ankle–foot orthosis; BBFO = ball-bearing forearm orthosis; KAFO = knee–ankle–foot orthosis; LE = lower extremity; UE = upper extremity; W/C = wheelchair.

S. K. had sustained a spinal cord injury at the C-3 level. Before his injury, he had been an avid collector of small fish, which he kept in his aquarium at home. He had always enjoyed taking care of the aquarium; however, because he also enjoyed simply watching the fish, he was determined to find a way to care for them, even if it only involved feeding. He devised a plan to stabilize a small cup that held the fish food on a platform above the aquarium. He mounted a mouthstick holder at the level where he could drive is wheelchair up to it, access the mouthstick (which he had had adapted with a small spoon), and scoop the food up and into the aquarium. This task was not only fun for him, but it greatly increased his sense of accomplishment, self-esteem, and independence.

Eating, Medication, and Meal Preparation

Eating. Head position and sitting angle may affect the person's ability to chew and successfully swallow food or medications, especially if there is any involvement of the brain stem. It is important for the person to be verbally independent in directing another person about proper positioning at mealtime so that the food can be swallowed safely and the meal thus made more enjoyable.

Depending on the strength of the deltoid and biceps muscles, a person with a lesion at C-4 may find a ball-bearing forearm orthosis (BBFO) or mobile arm support (MAS) useful for self-feeding or self-propulsion in a powered wheelchair or both (see Figure 9.1). A MAS with a wrist support and an adapted utensil is one device that can help the person with a muscle grade of fair to poor in the anterior and posterior deltoid and biceps reach his or her maximum potential for self-care activities. An automated, automatic feeder is another option for self-feeding (see Figure 9.2).

Medication. Persons with C-1–C-4 tetraplegia should be knowledgeable about all their medications. They should be able to identify them visually and know the dosage, purpose, and side effects of the medication and be prepared to inform others about their medication history in case of an emergency. The person taking the medications should commit the information about dosage, purpose, and side effects to memory and should be tested on the accuracy of the details. In addition, workbooks that list the specific medications the person is taking can be provided to the family members—it is not enough for this information to be given just to the caregiver.

Meal preparation. The person with C-1–C-4 tetraplegia uses oral instructions to fulfill roles common in family life, such as instructing a child in preparing a simple meal or using household appliances. During rehabilitation, a goal of occupational therapy may be for the patient to be independent in instructing the therapist on how to make a sandwich and how to use the microwave. It will then be the practitioner's responsibility to give direct feedback to the patient on the effectiveness of the instructions. It is important to remember that voice volume and word choice are just as important as accuracy of direction in determining others' willingness to listen and assist.

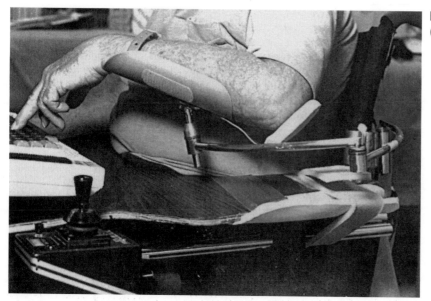

Figure 9.1 Mobile arm support (MAS).

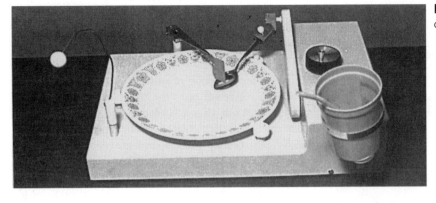

Figure 9.2 Electronic feeding device.

Hygiene and Grooming

Dental care. Brushing teeth, rinsing the mouth, and using mouthwash can be done independently by using commercially available dental devices (see Figure 9.3). This specially mounted device can be set at the height from the floor that will allow a person with C-1–C-4 tetraplegia to drive the wheelchair to it and use its components to complete dental hygiene tasks. Flossing of teeth must be performed by a caregiver. Dental hygiene is extremely important, because a person with a C-1–C-4 injury may use a mouthstick to accomplish certain tasks, and the structure and health of teeth can affect a person's ability and comfort in using the mouthstick (see Figure 9.4). The person should be encouraged to have annual or more frequent dental evaluations to ensure healthy oral hygiene. A caregiver must clean dentures because of the high level of dexterity necessary for this task.

For tasks such as washing, shaving the face, combing hair, or applying makeup, stable head support is important for safety and comfort. These tasks, as well as feminine hygiene and bowel and bladder care, must be performed by a caregiver. As with any task, the person with tetraplegia has preferences about how personal hygiene and grooming tasks are to be performed. It is important for the person to be accurate with directions so that the tasks are completed satisfactorily.

Bathing. Although the person with C-1–C-4 tetraplegia will be totally dependent in the task of bathing, a caregiver can accomplish that task efficiently and effectively in several different ways. Many times, because a person's bathroom is not accessible or appropriate equipment is not available, bathing is done in bed. Some types of plastic covering are made to be placed under the person while he or she is being bathed to protect the bedding from

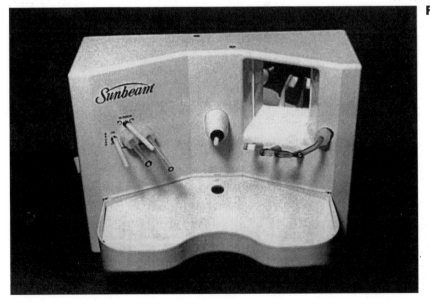

Figure 9.3 Dental hygiene device.

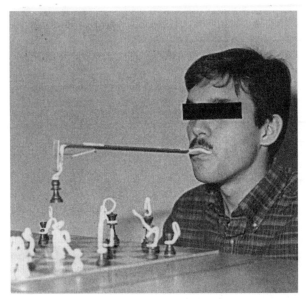

Figure 9.4 Mouthstick activity performed by a person with high-level quadriplegia.

getting wet. Alternatively, a commercially available inflatable bathtub can be used on top of the bed to hold water; the inflatable bathtub is portable, which allows bathing while traveling. A basin of water and other necessary items (i.e., soap, washcloth and towels, shampoo, razor) should be brought to the bedside before the bath begins to reduce the time the person is exposed to the water and room air. An inflatable shampoo basin can be used to wash the person's hair while he or she is in bed.

If the bathroom is accessible, a tall-back shower lift with head and neck support may be used to support the body while the person sits in a shower chair, to assure safe transfer and body support in perhaps slippery conditions. For those persons using a ventilator, protection to prevent water from entering the trachea must be assured.

Bowel and bladder care. The person with C-1–C-4 tetraplegia requires assistance in all bowel and bladder management and feminine hygiene, except for emptying a legbag. This task can be accomplished with an electric legbag emptying device, which receives its power from the electric wheelchair battery. A breath control or lever switch mounted in an accessible place activates it. The emptying device is connected to the clamp that surrounds the legbag tubing. When not activated, the tube is held closed by pressure and does not allow urine to pass. When the electric switch is activated, the pressure is released from the tube, allowing the urine to leave the legbag. This device limits a person to emptying the legbag into a floor drain, basin, cat litter box, or

outdoors. For those persons active in the community, this can be a very liberating device, because they do not have to ask others to perform this personal task for them.

Another method of urine collection is to mount a sealed container onto the wheelchair. The legbag tubing extends to reach around the wheelchair and into the container. The container must be emptied daily by another person and cleaned regularly to avoid development of an odor. A sitting position during a bowel program can assist in bowel evacuation. A commode chair with a high back and head positioner is needed to give proper body support during this procedure.

It is important for the person with C-1–C-4 injury to be able to verbally, independently instruct others on how to manage *autonomic dysreflexia*, which is an increase in blood pressure caused by bladder or bowel distension, suppository insertion, skin irritation, clothing or legbag straps that are too tight, or pressure ulcers. This condition can lead to a cerebrovascular accident or death if not relieved.

Ovulation and fertility are usually not altered in the female with spinal cord injury once spinal shock resolves. Caregivers, who must manage the menstrual and birth control needs of women with C-1–C-4 tetraplegia, should fully respect choices of those women regarding these intimate and personal activities.

Mobility

Transfers. Transfers of persons with C-1–C-4 tetraplegia can be accomplished in three ways: (a) with a mechanical lift transfer, (b) with a three-person lift, or (c) with a dependent slideboard transfer. The practitioner should decide which method is the safest and most effective, taking into account the patient's size and the ability of the caregiver. It is important for the patient to be able to direct each step of the transfer with complete and accurate instructions.

Wheelchair mobility. A person with C-1–C-4 tetraplegia can use a powered wheelchair for independent mobility. With this level of spinal cord injury, a person would be able to use a sip-and-puff, chin-controlled head array as a fiber optic switch for the driving mechanism (see Figure 9.5). A manual wheelchair is recommended as backup for the powered wheelchair.

A person with a C-4 spinal cord injury can achieve power mobility in three ways. One is by using a small remote joystick mounted on a midline

A power reclining system on a powered wheelchair will allow the person to perform independent weight shifting to reduce the risk of pressure ulcers. If spasticity is a problem, a power tilt system is an alternative that allows for weight shifting 45° to 60° depending on the system (Lathem, Gregorio, & Garber, 1985).

Transportation. The person with C-1–C-4 tetraplegia requires assistance with all community transportation. Information regarding adapted vans with power wheelchair lifts and tie-down systems must be discussed with the person and caregiver. The wheelchair itself must have adequate positioning devices to support the person's body and to maintain stability while the van is in motion. These devices may include head supports, chest straps, seatbelts, and lateral supports.

The clearance through the van door is a critical measurement, because the wheelchair back with head support tends to be higher than a conventional van doorway opening. The safest position for securing the wheelchair to the floor is facing forward. Visual restriction by the headliner of the van is sometimes a problem. Those persons who are unable to afford a modified van for personal transportation should be educated in the use of public transportation systems. Going on a community outing with supervision is the best preparation for a person with high-level tetraplegia to learn how to access public transportation.

Dressing and Undressing

A person with C-1–C-4 tetraplegia will depend on others for dressing (and undressing) tasks. However, the person can retain control over the task by making daily clothing selections. When clothing is purchased, consideration should be given to reducing the effort needed to dress and undress. Some suggestions are loose-fitting clothing, stretchable fabrics, touch-fastener closures, slip-on shoes, minimal zippers and buttons, and elastic sleeves and waistbands (Farmer, 1986).

Because persons with injuries at these levels have impaired sensation, fabrics that do not irritate the skin should be selected. Clothing made of breathable materials, such as cotton, is best for air exchange between the atmosphere and the skin. Pants with double-welted seams and studs or rivets should be avoided, because these can cause excessive pressure. Rear pockets of pants may be removed to reduce the risk of pressure from seams. In addition, it is important to make sure that jew-

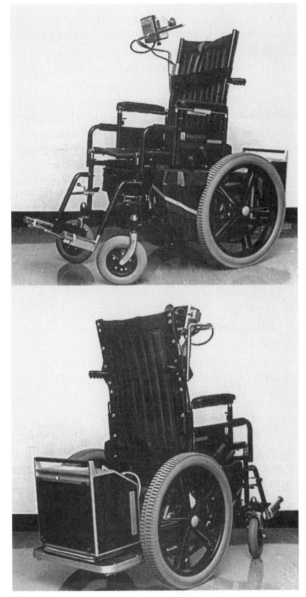

Figure 9.5 Powered mobility with chin control for the person with high-level quadriplegia (front and back view).

swing-away bar under the person's chair. The person is then able to control a proportional drive joystick through jaw movements. Another option is to use a sip-and-puff (breath control) switch. This device works by sealing the lips around a strawlike tube and then blowing soft or hard or sucking air back into the tube to make the chair move in the desired direction. The third option is to use a MAS to operate a standard joystick. Positioning of the joystick is important for safe and reliable hand placement and control. It is helpful to have on/off and high/low push button or toggle switches relocated on top of the joystick box for easy access when needed.

elry is not too tight, lest it restrict circulation and need to be cut off.

Upper extremity. Upper-extremity dressing is done by the caregiver by putting clothing on the patient overhead, side to side, or around the back. The person with a C-1–C-2 injury needs assistance to extend the neck; the person with C-2–C-4 injury is able to assist in flexing the neck forward. Bras with front touch fasteners or hooks are easier to put on using the around-the-back method; bras with back closures can be fastened first and then slipped over the head. Clip-on ties or ties fastened midway are the easiest for a caregiver to put on a person with a C-1–C-4 injury.

The same techniques are performed in reverse to undress the upper extremities. If sitting in a wheelchair, the patient must be well-supported to maximize trunk balance.

Lower extremity. Lower-extremity dressing presents additional concerns. Brief-style underpants can cause pressure over the ischial tuberosities, resulting in skin breakdown. Moreover, if the person is rolled from side to side for the garment to be pulled up over the hips, the skin could be damaged through shearing and friction. Loosely fitting socks are much easier to pull over the foot than tight, elasticized socks. Slip-on or self-fastening closure shoes are also recommended.

The task of dressing and undressing the person with a C-1–C-4 injury provides a convenient opportunity for the caregiver to perform a complete skin inspection. Pressure sores or other lesions should be carefully noted and treated promptly.

Communication

Persons with C-1–C-2 tetraplegia have limited head and neck control. Consequently, they are more successful in completing tasks such as turning pages, typing, and activating a tape recorder and telephone if they use electronic equipment. Persons with C-3–C-4 tetraplegia may use either electronic devices or a mouthstick to accomplish these tasks. Mouthsticks often are used to enable the person with a spinal cord injury at this level to participate in leisure and avocational activities, such as board games (see Figure 9.4). Other equipment used to improve communication skills includes elevating tables, modified workstations, mouthstick holders, environmental control units, computers, electric typewriter keyguards, bookholders, electric page turners, voice amplifiers, speaker phones, phone flippers, and gooseneck supports, some of which are pictured in Figure 9.6.

Environmental control systems and computer input devices now operate reliably with voice commands. Access to phone systems may require a combination of mouthstick skills, voice activation, and setup by another person.

Tetraplegia: Levels C-5–C-8

Persons with C-5 tetraplegia have functional biceps and are therefore able to feed themselves and perform simple grooming tasks with the aid of adapted equipment. At level C-6 wrist function occurs, which means that the person with the spinal cord injury requires only minimal to moderate assistance in grooming, bathing, and meal preparation. Many

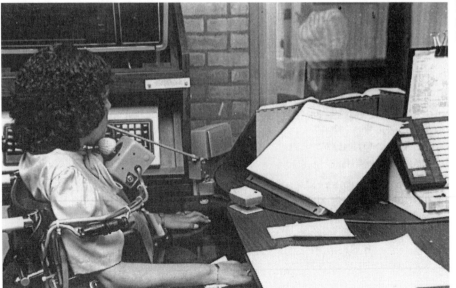

Figure 9.6 Workstation modified for the person with high-level quadriplegia.

persons with injuries at the C-7 and C-8 levels can live without assistance or alone with home modification (Stover & Fine, 1986).

Eating, Medication, and Meal Preparation

Eating. A variety of adaptive devices enable persons with spinal cord injuries at levels C-5–C-8 to feed themselves. The universal cuff (an elastic or self-fastening strap attached to a leather pocket) is easily donned and simply used with a regular utensil inserted into the palmar pocket (see Figure 9.7).

The person with a spinal cord injury at levels C-5–C-6 is able to pick up a modified cup or glass using a wrist-stabilizing device. A cup or glass can be given a modified handle so that the hand can passively lift it to the mouth, although some prefer using a long straw so they do not have to lift the cup or glass from the table. A straw holder is usually used to keep the straw pointed toward the face for ease of reach. If a ratchet-type orthosis or an electric prehension orthosis is already being used, the orthosis itself can be positioned around the cup or glass for lifting. Once the container is in position, the person with the injury is usually independent with drinking. A nonbreakable, lightweight cup or glass is safer than heavier containers and gives less stress to arm musculature.

Eating with utensils can be accomplished with a variety of adaptations, such as a hand orthosis with a utensil pocket, a long opponens orthosis, or a wrist-stabilizing splint to which a spoon or fork can be attached. If arm movements are weak, a BBFO or monosuspension feeder can help the person be independent in eating.

Swivel utensils may be used if inadequate forearm rotation makes it difficult to keep food on the utensil. Plateguards may also be useful, because food

can be scooped against them. Initially, persons with spinal cord injuries at this level may not be able to self-feed an entire meal because of decreased upper-extremity strength and endurance. A ratchet-type or electric prehension orthosis can be used to hold utensils in the conventional way, however, which allows independent feeding.

Cutting food takes much practice, and the person with tetraplegia at levels C-5–C-6 usually requires minimum to moderate assistance and adapted equipment. A rocker knife can be used if the person has good internal rotation in the shoulder. A knife with a serrated edge can be used if a sawing motion is required for cutting. Some persons with lesions at the C-5 level choose to have the food cut up by others; their choice should be respected.

Persons with lesions at levels C-7–C-8 need only minimal assistive devices to eat. They may intertwine the utensil in their fingers for stability. However, to cut food, they may use both hands or some adaptation, such as a cuff, to secure the knife. These persons may drink independently from a cup or glass using a tenodesis grasp or using both hands.

Medication. Medications can be placed in an easy-to-open container or an open cup. A person with C-5 tetraplegia may use an electric prehension orthosis to independently pick up and place the medication in his or her mouth. If the medication is placed in a small shallow cup, a person whose wrists are stabilized will be able to raise the cup between two hands and bring them together to the mouth. Safety issues must be considered with this method, such as the consequences of dropped medications or of open containers, which could be handled by small children in the home.

The person taking medications should try different types of containers and request that the pharmacist provide the simplest type to open, which have either flip-top or screw-top lids. The most difficult styles to open are the push and turn, childproof type.

Meal preparation. Meal preparation can be a very difficult and time-consuming task for persons with C-5 tetraplegia, and persons with lesions at the C-6 level may require moderate assistance. Use of an electric prehension orthosis or ratchet-type orthosis makes meal preparation tasks easier than does a passive wrist-stabilizing orthosis.

A major challenge is the safe lifting of pans into and out of the oven. A microwave or toaster oven may eliminate the problem and generally proves adequate if meals are prepared for just one or two persons. Stovetop cooking can be accomplished

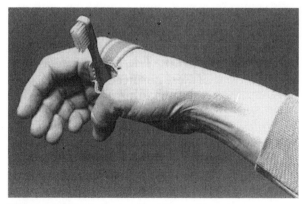

Figure 9.7 Universal cuff with toothbrush.

with over-the-stove mirrors, long-handled utensils, large-handled pots, shallow fry pans, and long oven mitts to prevent burns. A suction stabilizer that holds the pans steady contributes to safety when preparing hot food. Using adapted utensils or a palm-to-palm method to grasp utensils, a person with an injury at the C-5–C-8 level can accomplish many mealtime tasks.

The easiest way to transport food from one place to another is to slide the item along the counter or to use a laptray. Commercially available one-handed can openers with adjustable stands to support the can are difficult for a person with C-5 tetraplegia to use, but with practice the device may be mastered. A blender or mixer can conserve the person's energy; controls should be levers or push buttons.

Cutting can be done with an adapted knife and a cutting board with a stainless or aluminum nail through it to stabilize the food. Suction cups on the bottom provide stability on the countertop. This device allows both hands to be used in a palm-to-palm method, or one hand can stabilize while the other cuts. A table or low counter is helpful because objects are close and elbows are supported. Persons with C-5–C-8 injuries lack triceps and trunk balance and are therefore most successful when working close to the body. Jars can be opened by holding them between both hands and pushing the tops against serrated edges while turning. The jar lids should be kept loosely engaged for ease of opening.

Ovens can be difficult to handle, because of the weight or spring action of the door. Lifting pans into and out of the oven can be very unsafe; usually using a toaster oven or a broiler on a low tabletop is a safer way to bake. Lever action is used to open the door and depress buttons. Microwave ovens are also safer than conventional ovens, if they are placed on a table at an accessible height. A button or lever often controls the door. Loops can be added to the door handle to aid in opening.

The refrigerator door can be made easier to open by adding loops to the door handle. Frequently used items should be placed on the shelves of the refrigerator that are at eye level or lower. Food storage containers should be lightweight plastic, in case they are dropped or slip from the person's grasp.

Several items are useful for dishwashing.

- An accessible sink makes cleanup easier.
- A scrubber with soap in the handle is a useful step saver.
- Brushes with large open handles that the hand can fit through provide a good grasp.

- A rubber pad on the bottom of the sink will decrease the likelihood of breakage.
- An adapted scrub brush and a liquid soap dispenser, a bottlebrush, a wash mitt, and levers on sink controls can help during dish washing.

The dishes can be dried either in the sink or in a sink rack. A dishwasher can be used if the weight of the door is not a problem; a loop can be added to assist in opening the door.

Prepared foods and microwave dishes may be relatively expensive, but they save time and energy and reduce frustration. Conventional meal preparation presents challenges that may include getting the food out of the pantry, refrigerator, or freezer; reaching the pots and pans; opening plastic or metal containers or packages of frozen items; operating manual and small electric kitchen appliances; setting the table; and using large kitchen appliances.

The kitchen area should have room for easy wheelchair maneuvering to open drawers and doors. The cabinets should be easy to open, with glides and handles to assist those with limited strength and hand function. Items need to be placed within reach at wheelchair level, and one may choose to remove cabinet doors altogether. A reacher can be used to get to those items that are above the head. The preferred refrigerator design is a side-by-side style, because both the freezer and the refrigerator compartments are accessible.

Small manual kitchen appliances need to be on a work surface at desk height so that they can be operated with little or no adaptation, but they require more energy than electric ones to operate, and often they are not as effective. Several electric appliances are available for performing common meal preparation tasks: electric can openers, electric peelers, food processors, and mixers are a few examples. Small electric appliances, such as electric can openers, may require a supporting base and lever switches or special push buttons for efficient and safe operation.

The person with an injury at this level needs to be careful around sharp surfaces and extreme temperatures because of sensory deficits. Switches or knobs on the range or oven should be at eye level and within reach to eliminate the need to reach over hot burners.

It takes creativity to adapt the kitchen environment to meet the needs of a person with C-5–C-8 tetraplegia. Careful planning can help save time and promote efficiency in meal preparation.

Hygiene and Grooming: Levels C-5–C-6

Dental care. The first prerequisite for effective tooth-brushing is to develop a functional hand-to-mouth pattern. The person with C-5 tetraplegia can use several different types of orthoses or assistive devices to get hand to mouth, and a person who is unable to lift his or her arm against gravity can use a MAS for this task. A person using a MAS must be set up with the toothbrush in a utensil holder and toothpaste on the brush. The person then brushes one side of the mouth, turns the toothbrush around, and brushes the other side. The toothbrush can be turned within the utensil holder by holding the brush between the teeth and rotating the head or by grasping the brush between the teeth, removing it from the holder, then reinserting it into the holder. A cup of water with a straw, previously set up by another person, can be used to rinse the mouth.

If a person has adequate muscle strength to move his or her arm against gravity, other orthotic devices, such as a universal cuff, a long opponens splint, or an electric or reciprocal orthosis, can substitute for lack of wrist extension to stabilize the hand (see Figure 9.7). Other assistive devices, such as a Wanchik writer, dorsal wrist cock-up splint, or elastic wrist brace, may also be used for this activity. These devices are usually less expensive than the other ones mentioned above. A toothpaste tube with a flip-top cap is preferred by most persons because it can be easily opened by bringing it to the mouth with both hands and using the teeth to open it. A pump tube can be mounted on a fabricated stand to stabilize it when toothpaste is dispensed.

Combing hair. Brushing and styling the hair require maximum assistance if one lacks the use of the triceps. A person with C-5 tetraplegia who uses a MAS is unable to perform this task without assistance. Using a curling iron also requires a lot of assistance. To minimize the time and amount of assistance needed for hair grooming, the person with a C-5 injury may wish to get a permanent or a low-maintenance hairstyle. A person with this level of injury who can move his or her arm against gravity needs to use an orthosis to stabilize the wrist. A comb with an extended handle stabilized in the previously mentioned orthoses or assistive devices is best, and long-handled brushes are also useful. A phone holder or universal cuff can also be used in conjunction with these devices.

Shaving. Shaving the face can be performed with either an electric or safety razor, depending on personal preference. Many persons use electric razors

to avoid the cuts and nicks experienced with blades. Inability to keep the razor from falling is a major problem, but one that can be overcome with a two-handed technique. The therapist should be sensitive to this fact and work to achieve safety and independence in the selected shaving method. A person using a MAS needs assistance setting up the razor and shaving cream. In some cases, assistance is needed to shave difficult-to-reach contours of the face and neck.

Using a reciprocal orthosis, an electric prehension orthosis, or a specially adapted cuff enables the person with C-5 tetraplegia to hold an electric razor (see Figure 9.8). The razor's weight is a major consideration; the limb must be able to support the razor. Safety razors can be adapted with a variety of low-temperature plastics for ease of handling. If the person can move his or her arm against gravity, a utensil holder can be used to stabilize the razor. Commercially available razor holders can be purchased, but they must be used in conjunction with a wrist-stabilizing brace. Commercially available shaving cream dispensers with a long lever handle can assist with this aspect of the activity.

Most women with C-5 tetraplegia require assistance in shaving their underarms and legs because the trunk needs to be stabilized during forward leaning and upright balance has to be maintained while using both upper extremities for the task.

Washing face and hands. To be independent with face and hand washing, the person with C-5–C-6 injury must be able to maneuver the wheelchair up

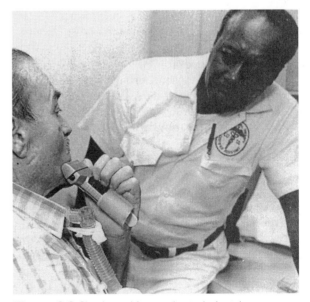

Figure 9.8 Shaving with an adapted electric razor (C-5–C-6 quadriplegia).

to a sink. The water faucets must have a lever so the person can operate easily, and a wash mitt with a D-ring strap must be placed on the person's hand. Some persons may want to use a stabilizing wrist device under the mitt. Soap can be secured to the sink by a suction pad. If a MAS is employed, the person uses a combination of head, neck, and upper-extremity movements to reach all areas. Excess water is squeezed out of the wash mitt by pushing it against the side of the sink.

Makeup application. The female with an injury at level C-6 can use a reciprocal orthosis to grasp make-up brushes, pencils, or wands. Sanding or slightly filing the clasps on blush and eye shadow compacts makes them easier to open. Small tubes, such as those containing mascara, can be held in the mouth and opened, allowing greater independence.

Bathing. A person with C-5 tetraplegia requires maximum assistance from another person for safety during bathing. If an accessible shower is available, a shower commode chair is used for bathing.

A D-ring wash mitt may be used to perform a small part of the bathing task independently, namely, washing of the face, neck, anterior chest, and upper legs. Long-handled brushes help in getting hard-to-reach places such as the feet and between the toes. A handheld showerhead may be useful, but the occupational therapist may need to add an adapted handle to it. Skin protection, postural support, and adapted handles make bathing a more independent, more private activity. Bed baths are an alternative for those persons whose homes are not modified or for when equipment is not available.

Washing and drying hair. Washing the hair is most easily performed while showering or bathing. Because the ability to stabilize the trunk while leaning forward over a sink is necessary, most persons with injury at this level choose to have someone else wash their hair. A commercially available shampoo basin can be used when bathing in bed is required; this basin holds the water, and a tube attached to the basin drains the excess water into a bucket.

Because it can be difficult to hold a hair dryer against gravity, mounting a blow dryer on a gooseneck stand and moving the head toward the direction of the blowing air is the easiest way to dry the hair.

Hygiene and Grooming: Levels C-7–C-8

Persons with C-7–C-8 injury can perform upper-body grooming and hygiene at the sink independently with few or no adaptive devices. Sink accessibility is important: the person with the injury must be able to reach and use the faucets. Lever controls are easiest for the person to use, although some persons may be able to use some twisting controls. Towels should be placed close to the sink and at a low level for greater independence.

Dental care. Persons with injured spinal cords may position the toothbrush between their fingers to secure it or use a built-up handle to strengthen their grip. Some may choose to use an electric toothbrush. Getting the toothpaste onto the brush may require using the countertop to get enough pressure to push the paste out, or the paste may be put in the person's mouth before the brush. A small, prethreaded dental flossing tool is also helpful.

Washing face and hands, combing hair, shaving, and applying makeup. Persons with C-7–C-8 tetraplegia can independently use a washcloth and soap for upper-body hygiene. Hair can be groomed with a regular brush and comb, but, if the hair is very thick, an adapted handle may be necessary. Men with injuries at this level may decide to use an electric razor to shave; a strap may be needed, however, to secure the razor. A lightweight safety razor can be used instead, but it may not be as secure in the hand as an electric razor and may require frequent repositioning. Women with injuries at this level can usually apply most makeup independently, except for application of eye makeup. Applicators for eyeliner, eye shadow, and mascara may need to be built up, and containers may need to be adapted for easier opening.

Bathing and hair washing. Persons with this level of injury need assistance with bathing for safety and to assure that every area is cleansed well. They may either use a roll-in shower with a shower chair or transfer into the tub to a bath bench with a back. They may use a handheld showerhead and long-handled bath brushes to reach areas not accessible without bending. They probably will not be able to reach their buttocks well because of poor balance, and they will need assistance also with washing their feet. They should be able to shampoo their hair if they are well-supported on the bath bench or in the shower chair. Rinsing the soap out is best accomplished with a handheld showerhead. Towels should be placed where they will stay dry but still be within reach. Transfers can be tricky when one is wet, so drying off well is very important for safety.

Bowel and bladder management. Persons with a spinal cord injury at level C-5 require assistance in bowel and bladder care, because they lack hand function and cannot position themselves independently. The person receiving assistance in bowel and bladder care, however, should be able to verbally direct the caregiver in this task.

A person with C-5 tetraplegia may be able to empty his or her legbag with the use of either a manual pneumatic legbag clamp or an electric legbag emptier. The emptying clamp is released by a switch that the person can easily reach. The legbag may be emptied into a floor basin or cat litter box or onto grass. The automatic legbag emptier must be mounted on the wheelchair. Gravity assists in draining urine from the tubing.

Proper food intake regulates waste elimination. Foods with a proper balance of fiber, nutrients, and liquids aid bladder and bowel regulation.

For the person with C-6–C-7 tetraplegia, self-catheterization may be made easier with bilateral reciprocal orthoses. However, the need to manage clothes and to transfer may make it difficult to manage this activity every 4 hours. Persons who must rely on themselves are usually more motivated to develop the fine-motor coordination essential to managing bowel and bladder care. Practicing fine-motor skills—by sewing, lacing, and writing, for example—promote the problem-solving abilities necessary to successfully complete a clean, safe, self-catheterization.

Persons with spinal cord injuries at levels C-7–C-8 need assistance managing a regular bowel program because of difficulty with body positioning. However, they should be knowledgeable in the task and be able to verbally direct the caregiver. Two examples of devices for bowel management are illustrated in Figure 9.9. The person with injuries at this level may be able to manage an intermittent catheterization program if he or she is independent with proper body positioning in the wheelchair or in bed. He or she should be able to empty the legbag with minimal adaptations. A woman with this level of injury should be able to position a sanitary napkin appropriately when dressing, but she may have difficulty inserting a tampon.

Self-care is a tedious and demanding regimen for a person with a spinal cord injury, involving tasks that are often difficult and frustrating to master. Support, humor, praise, and practice are the practitioners' tools to encourage the patient to reach his or her maximum potential for independent living.

Mobility

Transfers. For the person with C-5–C-6 tetraplegia, transferring or moving the body from one surface to another calls for a tremendous amount of effort. Many persons with injuries at this level choose to rely on others to perform the entire task for them because of the energy expenditure necessary for completion. In most cases, moderate assistance from another is needed for transferring to and from level surfaces. In transfers between positions of different heights, maximal to total assistance is required, however. A transfer board provides a smooth surface to slide across, which decreases resistance during the task. Persons with a level C-7–C-8 injury can use a sliding board to transfer to and from the wheelchair, although eventually, they may be able to transfer without using the board. Removable armrests and footrests make transferring safe for both the person with the injury and the assistant.

Manual wheelchair. A person with C-5 tetraplegia can be independent in wheelchair mobility over both level and uneven surfaces with a manual wheelchair. The wheelchair must be measured accurately to accommodate the body for proper support and function (see Figure 9.10). The wheelchair's back must be high enough to support the trunk, so arm function

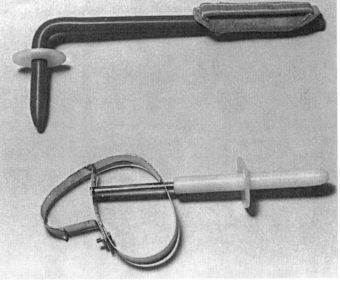

Figure 9.9 Bowel management devices.

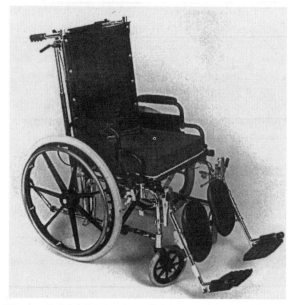

Figure 9.10 High-back reclining manual wheelchair for persons with quadriplegia.

can be maximized, and vertical or oblique rim projections are recommended for pushing the wheelchair forward and in reverse. The scapular stabilizing musculature must be strengthened to avoid overstretching the supporting shoulder structures. A wrist-stabilizing splint is used to enhance hand placement between the rim projections.

A grade aid (or hill climber), a secondary braking device, is recommended for propelling the wheelchair up an incline or ramp. The grade aid, which is mounted under the wheelchair brakes, is engaged by pushing the lever handle downward. The device lies on the surface of the tire, allowing the tire to be pushed forward. When the push stroke is completed, the grade aid clutches the tire, preventing it from rolling in reverse, and thereby maintains the ground gained. After the incline or ramp has been climbed, the lever is disengaged by pushing the lever upward.

Also useful are brake extensions, which make it easier to operate the lever that controls the wheelchair brakes. Antitip bars are a safety option to consider for lightweight wheelchairs, because they prevent the wheelchair from tipping backwards on an uneven surface.

For some persons with spinal cord injury, propelling the weight of a manual wheelchair takes too much effort, and endurance is compromised. Sometimes the slowness of the propulsion limits functional mobility in the community. Rough terrain, long distances, or shoulder pain can challenge

the person's abilities and may necessitate a powered wheelchair. Use of a powered wheelchair may conserve energy and allow the person greater mobility, as well as expand the opportunities for school or work. A manual wheelchair is usually purchased as a backup to the powered wheelchair.

The person with an injury at level C-7–C-8 can be independent using a manual wheelchair. Friction-coated hand rims may be used to assist in propulsion. This person will still have difficulty pushing up steep inclines or over rough terrain, but as endurance builds up, that person may become able to participate in wheelchair sports.

Motorized wheelchair. A motorized wheelchair with a hand control is usually the choice of mobility for spinal cord-injured persons at the C-5–C-6 level. The ease of powered mobility allows for the conservation of energy and the time efficiency needed for community accessibility. A person who uses a MAS needs extensive practice initially to master driving a hand-controlled powered wheelchair; it is important to position the MAS in the way that provides the greatest mechanical advantage.

The hand control may need to be adapted with an extended joystick for moving the wheelchair effectively and safely. The wrist may be supported with an orthosis or assistive device. A powered recliner or tilt may be necessary for weight shifting if the person is unable to lean from side to side or push up independently to relieve pressure.

Persons with injuries at the C-7–C-8 level will be independent with a joystick-operated, powered wheelchair. Powered mobility conserves energy and allows other functional tasks, such as dressing and vocational activities, to be carried out.

> S. M. is a 21-year-old male who sustained a C-4–C-5 level spinal cord injury in a motor vehicle accident. He underwent spinal stabilization and was placed in a halo brace postoperatively. He was transferred to The Institute for Rehabilitation and Research for comprehensive rehabilitation. During the first 4 weeks of hospitalization, S. M.'s occupational therapy program focused on progressive wheelchair sitting (to enable him to achieve the 90° sitting angle), strengthening and range of motion to the upper extremities, and the initiation of independent living skills training. At week 5, he was fitted with a BBFO to facilitate such activities as feeding, turning pages, and typing. He particularly practiced the skill of typing because this encouraged fine placement control. S. M. gradually improved his ability to move the BBFO in the directions he desired. After 2 weeks of prac-

tice, it was time to mount the BBFO onto a powered wheelchair so he could develop skill in accessing and moving the joystick control. Initially, he found this to be a difficult task because the momentum of the wheelchair interfered with the movement control of his arm in the BBFO. With continued practice, encouragement, and motivation, he improved both his skills and his self-esteem. His occupational therapist reports that she will never forget the excitement or the look on his face when, for the first time, he independently drove the wheelchair in a straight direction for approximately 10 feet. This independence in mobility boosted S. M.'s spirits and gave him the needed motivation to work even harder to achieve the goals he had set for himself.

Although S. M. quickly learned to drive the wheelchair forward and to the right, driving in reverse and turning left were more difficult. An orthotist was consulted and, together with the occupational therapist and the patient, devised a spring assist to add to the proximal arm of the BBFO. This spring served as an active resist to retract the shoulder to the point that these difficult directions (reverse and left) of the drive path were also accomplished with relative ease. Except for the placement of his arm in the BBFO trough, S. M. became totally independent in driving the wheelchair in approximately 4 weeks.

Community transportation. New technology in adapted driving—modified vans with low-or zero-effort steering and electric lifts, for example—enables some persons with injuries at the C-7–C-8 level to be independently mobile (see Figure 9.11).

Some assistance is necessary for transfers, as the person usually drives while seated in a motorized wheelchair that is stabilized on the floor with a four-point electric tie-down system. Evaluation and supervised driver's training are critical to ensure safety. Those who cannot achieve this level of independence must rely on another person to drive. The person with C-5 tetraplegia can either be transferred into the passenger seat of a van or have the wheelchair tied to the floor for transport safety. Whenever the van is in motion, the wheelchair seat belt, as well as the van safety restraint, should be fastened.

If the person does not own a van, he or she must be transferred into a car with assistance. The wheelchair itself is loaded by the caregiver into the back flooring or into the trunk of the car. Loading a motorized wheelchair is very difficult and time-consuming because of the necessary dismantling and handling of the batteries. Therefore, a manual wheelchair is usually used, which may mean less function for the person at his or her destination.

In some cities, van or bus service with modified lifts is available. If trunk balance is a problem, the use of a chest strap assures upright sitting to counter the force of the bus or van's motion. Wheelchair lifts on buses, paratransit, and agreements with cab companies for transporting persons in wheelchairs are more widely available than they used to be before passage of the Americans With Disabilities Act.

Persons with a C-7–C-8 injury should be able to drive personal vehicles adapted with appropriate controls. Most should be able to transfer independently into a passenger car, but they will need assistance with wheelchair loading, cartop loaders, or

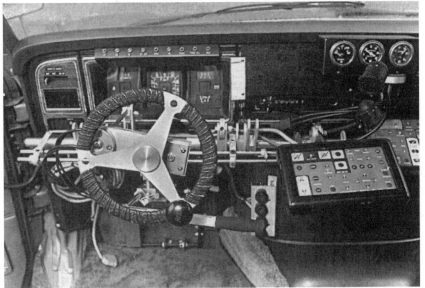

Figure 9.11 Driving controls in a adapted van.

special lifts. Some of these persons may choose to drive a modified van while seated in their wheelchairs. This option conserves the person's energy, but it is more expensive than using adapted controls.

Dressing and Undressing

Upper extremities. The person with a C-5 spinal cord injury, who has decreased upper-extremity range of motion and lack of trunk stability, may require moderate assistance with upper-body dressing for pullover clothes.

To don a front-fastening shirt or jacket, the spinal cord-injured person can use the around-the-back method; moderate assistance will be required. A buttonhook–zipper pull device can be used to be independent with closures. Bras that either close in the front or use self-fastening closures can be donned by putting the thumb through sewn-in loops added to the garment. As for ties, many men will choose either to use a clip-on style or to have the caregiver fasten a conventional tie.

Lower extremity. Because the person with injury at the C-5 level lacks bed mobility skills, assistance is required in lower-extremity dressing. Slacks and skirts that are slightly loose fitting in the hips and relatively long in length are easier to put on and better fit a person sitting in a wheelchair with flexed knees. Modified clothing is commercially available through catalogs, and modified sewing patterns are available to assure a more functional fit for a person with a physical disability.

A person with a C-6–C-8 spinal cord injury may be independent with upper-and lower-body dressing through use of the rolling side-to-side method in bed, but this technique consumes a lot of energy. Donning and doffing footwear generally require assistance but may be accomplished independently with the use of specially adapted shoes.

Communication

Communication, whether written or oral, is critical for any person. Many adaptations can help the person with a spinal cord injury carry out this important activity.

Writing. Initially, devices to assist in writing—a MAS in conjunction with an electric prehension, reciprocal, or long opponens orthosis, for example—may be indicated. Most persons gradually reduce their use of the MAS, but they continue to need a wrist-stabilizing orthosis with an adaptation to hold a pen or pencil.

The first attempts at writing may be very difficult; it may be a good idea to start by drawing lines or circles. To ask the person to form letters or numbers early on can lead to disappointment or frustration, because arm movements have not yet been refined. Assistive devices, such as a Wanchik writer (see Figure 9.12), a flexor hinge orthosis (see Figure 9.13), or a dorsal wrist cock-up splint with cuff, can help hold the wrist in a neutral position, as well as position the writing utensil. A Dycem nonslip pad is useful for holding the paper in place while writing. When arm control improves, letters and numbers may be attempted. Practice is the key to improving this skill.

Typing may be the preferred method for written communications, but it too can be frustrating if too much skill is called for before arm control has developed. The most efficient typing is achieved using either an electric typewriter or a computer. The wrists must be stabilized, and a typing implement attached, so that the typewriter keys can be depressed. In most cases, another person must remove the typed text from the typewriter or computer printer.

The fine control of the arm necessary to select the keys to depress makes typing a good exercise

Figure 9.12 Wanchik device for daily living activities.

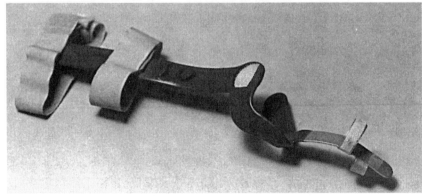

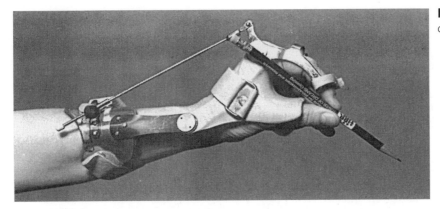

Figure 9.13 Flexor hinge/reciprocal orthosis.

for those using a MAS. Usually the person is asked to type each row of keys individually from right to left, left to right, and then up and down before actually typing words. Once control of arm placement is achieved, words can be typed.

Telephone use. Telephone accessibility is very important for persons with spinal cord injury, and there are several ways to achieve it. Some choose to use a gooseneck stand to hold the telephone receiver at ear height while using a phone flipper (an extended lever) to depress the hang-up switch on the phone base. This lever is lifted to obtain a dial tone or to receive a call when the phone rings. Most persons using MAS use this method because of their inability to hold the receiver to the ear.

Persons who have adequate arm strength and are able to hold the receiver to the ear may use a phone holder for independence with handling. Telephones that have the functions of automatic dialing, memory, or redial often increase efficiency. A speaker phone also decreases necessary hand function, although its use interferes with privacy. A telephone with the dialing buttons on the receiver is usually not recommended because its manipulation requires increased hand function.

For persons with a spinal cord injury at levels C-6–C-8, using the phone can be made easier with an adapted handset, universal cuff, or reciprocal orthosis used to press the buttons. In a vocational setting, earphones or a headset can streamline the requirements of simultaneous note writing and phone use. Most persons with this level of spinal cord injury do not require wrist support and can don and doff a simple device independently. The same device selected to dial a phone can be used to type or use the computer. The wrist-driven orthosis gives dynamic grasp, which is useful for loading paper and computer disks and for picking up and moving objects.

Paraplegia: Levels T-1–T-6

The muscles of the trunk and thorax have their roots from T-1 to L-4. They include the intercostals (T-1–T-10), serratus posterior superior (T-1–T-4), rectus abdominis and external oblique abdominis (T-5–T-12), transverse abdominis (T-7–L-1), internal oblique abdominis (T-8–L-1), serratus posterior inferior (T-9–T-12), and quadratus lumborum (T-12–L-4). In general, they are responsible for elevation and depression of the ribs during respiration, contraction of the abdomen, and anterolateral flexion of the trunk.

Persons with a spinal cord injury at the T-1–T-6 level have full use of their upper extremities and should be able to live independently in a wheelchair-accessible environment. Although breathing improves at this level, trunk balance is still compromised, and appropriate safety precautions should therefore be implemented. The wheelchair is the primary mode for mobility, although ambulation may be encouraged for exercise purposes (Hoppenfeld, 1977).

Eating and Meal Preparation

Persons with a T-1–T-6 spinal cord injury are independent with eating and preparing meals at the wheelchair level; poor trunk control, however, may necessitate their use of adaptive devices or modifications. Some modifications may include lowered countertops or work surfaces. A mirror positioned over a standard range is helpful for seeing inside of pans and avoiding hot areas that are not visible from the wheelchair level. It is important to consider the accessibility of the oven and the refrigerator from the wheelchair. Usually a side approach is best for securing items from each, as well as for maintaining balance. Dishes, glasses, and cooking pans are most accessible if located at a level no higher than the shoulders (see Figure 9.14).

Sink Hygiene and Grooming

Persons with a T-1–T-6 level of injury are independent with upper-level grooming and hygiene at the sink, if the bathroom is wheelchair accessible.

Bathing. The person with this level of injury needs some adaptations to accomplish bathing. Use of a shower commode chair in a roll-in shower probably provides the best level of independent functioning for bathing. A bathtub bench could be used to transfer into the tub independently, although assistance may be needed for transfers when the person is wet. A handheld showerhead allows for greatest independence in showering. There may be some difficulty reaching the buttocks and lower back for cleansing, but long-handled sponges or brushes should allow access, so long as the person can maintain his or her balance. Hair washing is best done when the person is supported in the shower or tub.

Bowel and bladder. Men are able to apply an external catheter and, if using an intermittent catheterization program, can do it independently. Women with a T-1–T-6 injury can catheterize but need

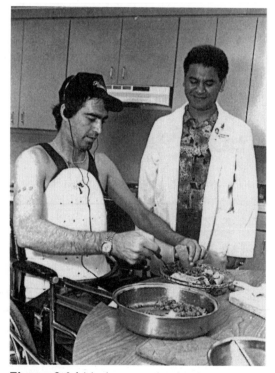

Figure 9.14 Meal preparation by the person with paraplegia: Level T-6.

assistance with special positioning of their legs and may need adaptive equipment. Bowel program management is accomplished independently by use of suppositories. Again, positioning may be the one area requiring assistance. Women can place sanitary napkins independently, but they may need a mirror and an adaptive device to help position their legs when inserting a tampon.

Mobility

Persons with this level of paraplegia have the arm strength to transfer independently; however, several factors—body weight and height, transfer surfaces, wheelchair position, and general endurance level—can complicate transfer independence. Extremes in weight and height, in combination with the poor trunk control, may complicate independent transfer enough for some persons to require assistance with this task. Transfers into and out of the car frequently require assistance. Low-level spasticity and good muscle tone can help in some instances; without those conditions, safe transfer can be compromised.

Mobility is usually achieved independently in a manual wheelchair. The wheelchair should be lightweight, and the height of its back should be below the scapula for optimal propulsion. Armrests and footrests should be removable to allow for maximal independence (see Figure 9.15). Some persons with T-1 through T-4 injuries may choose to use a powered wheelchair to conserve energy and time.

Persons with this level of injury are able to drive a vehicle using hand controls, a steering knob, and an emergency brake extension (see Figure 9.16). The person's transfer skill and overall endurance will determine the decision about the type of vehicle. Transferring independently into a car is possible, but loading the wheelchair requires additional energy. Some may choose to use a wheelchair-loading device or to drive a van. If the person decides to drive a van, he or she should transfer from the wheelchair to the captain's chair to drive safely.

Dressing

Persons with a T-1–T-6 injury can dress without assistance. Dressing loops and larger-sized clothing enhance independence in lower-extremity dressing. These persons do not require assistance in upper-extremity dressing, but they may have to support themselves on the bed or wheelchair to maintain their balance. Shoes and socks can be put on independently if there is good range of motion in the hip and little interference from spasms.

those with injury below level T-8. The paraplegic person with a spinal cord injury at levels L-4–S-2 can ambulate with short leg braces and forearm crutches.

Functionally, these persons are independent in all self-care tasks, although they may use some adapted equipment for energy conservation, efficiency, and maximum control. One of the major concerns is preventing secondary complications for the person of the spinal cord injury. These include urinary tract infections and pressure ulcers (Pearman, 1985; Turner, 1985). Although management of these potentially serious problems is usually addressed during the initial rehabilitation, once the person returns to the community, family, employment, or school, secondary complications are often ignored until the situation reaches crisis level. Persons who return to outpatient clinics at facilities where they originally were rehabilitated are reeducated or updated at follow-up visits on advances in medical technology.

Equipment: From Tradition to High Technology

The appropriate prescription of upper-extremity assistive devices is a major focus during the rehabilitation of persons with spinal cord injury. Until recently, little was reported in the literature about the use of these devices once the patient returned to family, community, and employment. In 1990, Garber and Gregorio reported the results of their study of the use of, and satisfaction with, devices prescribed during initial rehabilitation to persons with tetraplegia secondary to spinal cord injury. The first part of the study focused on the categorization of devices and described the frequency with which they had been prescribed to a population of 56 persons with spinal cord injury and resultant tetraplegia. The device categories included feeding (71%), splints and slings (79%), dressing (29%), hygiene and grooming (23%), communication (41%), and miscellaneous (23%) (Garber & Gregorio, 1990). They found that 54% of the devices prescribed were still in use 1 year after discharge from the rehabilitation hospital, representing a significant decline in use. Furthermore, by the end of the second year after discharge, only 35% of all prescribed devices were still in use.

Feeding devices and splints and slings were the categories prescribed most often for the largest number of subjects. These categories, which include the more expensive devices, most frequently continued to be used (Garber & Gregorio, 1990). In contrast,

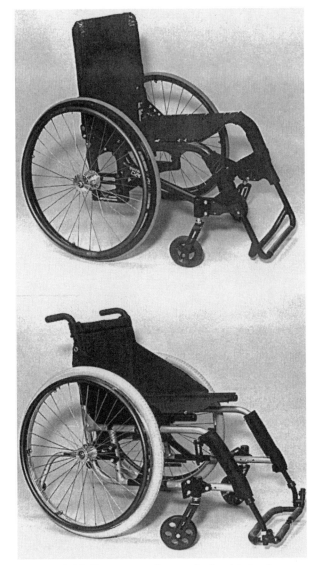

Figure 9.15 Two types of manual wheelchairs for persons with paraplegia.

Communication

Persons with this level of injury are independent in all communication skills, such as typing, writing, and using the telephone. By using either a standard keyboard or a mouse, these persons can easily operate computers.

Paraplegia: Levels T-7–S-5

For the person with paraplegia affecting levels T-7–S-5, upper-extremity and thoracic function are intact, which improves trunk stability, wheelchair sitting balance, and transfers. Functional ambulation with long leg braces and crutches is possible for

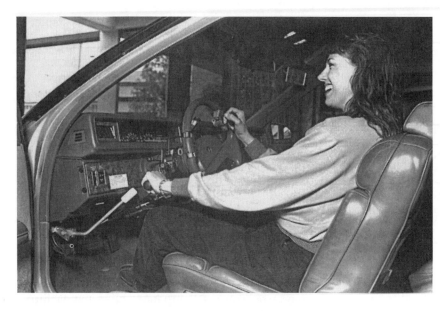

Figure 9.16 Adapted vehicle with hand controls.

dressing and hygiene devices were prescribed for the fewest number of subjects and, in combination with the miscellaneous device category, showed the greatest decline in use. The investigators concluded that practitioners must identify ways to prescribe only the most necessary equipment, even though the most frequently discarded items were low in cost. One approach would be to provide devices to patients during their rehabilitation hospitalization, but help them learn to function without them before discharge.

Advances in technology influence every aspect of daily life and thus the overall quality of life for persons with spinal cord injury. From the automatic teller machines in banks to voice-activated telephone systems, technology often provides unique and dynamic solutions to otherwise insoluble problems. For the person with a spinal cord injury, technology expands opportunities for independence and productivity.

In the early 1970s, the U.S. government demonstrated its commitment to improving the vocational and self-care goals of persons with severe physical impairments through the establishment of rehabilitation engineering centers. These centers combined the efforts of medicine, engineering, and related sciences to identify practical solutions to problems that limited the integration of persons with physical impairments into productive community life (Traub & LeClair, 1975).

In 1988, with the passage of the Technology-Related Assistance for Individuals With Disabilities Act (Pub. L. 100–407), the U.S. government further demonstrated its support for the development and use of technological systems and devices that would enhance the outcome of rehabilitation of persons with severe physical disabilities. Assistive technology, then, has become the byword of the 1990s for consumers and health care providers alike. *Assistive technology* is defined as "any item, piece of equipment or product system, off-the-shelf, modified, or customized that is used to increase, maintain or improve function" (Pub. L. 100–407). It consists of both high and low technology that includes, but is not limited to, environmental control units, computer access systems, augmentative communication devices, and mobility and seating systems.

Occupational therapy practitioners have a prominent role in the assistive technology clinics that operate in many rehabilitation facilities or are established in the private sector. Practitioners evaluate each person with spinal cord injury and other neuromuscular and musculoskeletal dysfunction for the potential to use technology to enhance and expand the skills needed to be more independent in self-care, return to school, or become involved in other aspects of daily life. The occupational therapy practitioner, as part of the assistive technology team, makes recommendations and trains these persons to use technology to achieve their maximum potential (Mann & Lane, 1991).

Occupational therapy practitioners have played a leading role in evaluating and recommending environmental control units (ECUs) for persons with significant disability. These electronic devices enable a person to access and manipulate objects in the environment known as target devices, such as lamps, televisions, thermostats, blinds, and stereo systems.

ECUs are now commonly used by able-bodied persons to automate and facilitate routine household tasks. A simple example of a prevalent ECU is the remote control device for the television or stereo. More specialized units, which can be voice activated, are also available. These devices are particularly useful for persons with impaired motor function, especially those with high-level spinal cord injury (Swenson et al., 1998).

Surveys have shown that, although these units are often used in hospitals and rehabilitation facilities, they have not been widely recommended for use in home settings. This is primarily because of their high cost and limitations in reimbursement (Holme, Kanny, Guthrie, & Johnson, 1997).

A number of robotic devices have been developed and evaluated at rehabilitation centers in the United States, Canada, and England (Glass & Hall, 1987). Their primary purpose is to help persons with very limited upper-extremity function perform daily living and vocational activities. This technology has the potential to reduce dependency on full-time attendant care and provide the person with severe physical impairment with a mechanism of control.

Most robotic systems are voice activated and microprocessor based. They are usually mounted either on a workstation or on the wheelchair. Practitioners and patients reported positive experiences with robotic systems, and several systems are being modified to make them more functional.

Acceptance and use of robotic systems will depend on several factors. Because a robotic system can be very costly, cost-benefit analyses must be done. The system's reliability and durability must be determined to assess how many hours the physically disabled person could depend on the system and not on attendant care. Another factor is its acceptance by the health care professional, who must learn the system and transmit the crucial information to the consumer. Advances in robotic technology can provide opportunities for new levels of self-care, independence, and employment. More important, robotic technology can return a measure of personal autonomy that until recently was only imagined.

Summary

Few fields in rehabilitation are changing more rapidly than occupational therapy. The effect of high technology has not yet been fully realized, but it must be anticipated. It is apparent that systems and devices that maximize functional potential will continue to be a major concern in the rehabilitation of persons with spinal cord injuries. With the explosive expansion of electronic technology, microprocessor-controlled preprogrammed "smart" devices are forthcoming in the areas of wheelchair mobility, environmental control, adapted driving, and vocational training (Swenson, Barnett, Pond, & Schoenberg, 1998). The area of technological innovation presents new challenges to occupational therapy practitioners, who must continue to balance the promise of technology with the practicalities of everyday life and the preferences and lifestyles of the persons they serve. ◆

Study Questions

1. Define the grades of the Frankel scale for completeness of spinal cord injury. At what grade is sensory but not motor function preserved below the neurologic level of the lesion (including sacral segments S4–S5)?

2. Below what level of injury can a person expect to be independent in upper-extremity dressing?

3. What are the ways in which occupational therapy personnel can help manage or prevent pressure sores?

4. Define dysreflexia and cite examples of its causes.

5. What two types of orthoses might be worn by a person with C-5 tetraplegia? Identify the daily living functions associated with each.

6. What three ways can a person with C-4 tetraplegia operate a powered wheelchair?

References

American Spinal Injury Association. (1996). *International standards for neurological and functional classification of spinal cord injury.* Chicago: American Spinal Injury Association.

Farmer, A. R. (1986). Dressing. In J. P. Hill (Ed.), *Spinal cord injury—A guide to functional outcomes in occupational therapy* (pp. 125–143). Rockville, MD: Aspen.

Garber, S. L. (1985). New perspectives for the occupational therapist in the treatment of spinal cord-injury individuals. *American Journal of Occupational Therapy, 39,* 703–704.

Garber, S. L., & Gregorio, T. L. (1990). Upper extremity assistive devices: Assessment of use by spinal cord-injured patients with quadriplegia. *American Journal of Occupational Therapy, 44,* 126–131.

Garber, S. L., Lathem, P., & Gregorio, T. L. (1988). *Specialized occupational therapy for persons with high level quadriplegia* (Monograph). Waco, TX: Baylor University College of Medicine and The Institute for Rehabilitation and Research (TIRR).

Glass, K., & Hall, K. (1987). Occupational therapy practitioners' views about the use of robotic aids for people with disabilities. *American Journal of Occupational Therapy, 41,* 745–747.

Go, B. K., DeVivo, M. J., & Richards, J. S. (1995). The epidemiology of spinal cord injury. In S. L. Stover, J. A. DeLisa, & G. G. Whiteneck (Eds.), *Spinal cord injury* (pp. 21–55). Gaithersburg, MD: Aspen.

Holme, S. A., Kanny, E. M., Guthrie, M. R., & Johnson, K. L. (1997). The use of environmental control units by occupational therapy practitioners in spinal cord injury and disease services. *American Journal of Occupational Therapy, 51,* 42–48.

Hoppenfeld, S. (1977). *Orthopaedic neurology—A diagnostic guide to neurological levels.* Philadelphia: Lippincott.

Lathem, P., Gregorio, T. L., & Garber, S. L. (1985). High-level quadriplegia: An occupational therapy challenge. *American Journal of Occupational Therapy, 39,* 705–714.

Mann, W. C., & Lane, J. P. (1991). *Assistive technology for persons with disabilities: The role of occupational therapy.* Rockville, MD: American Occupational Therapy Association.

Pearman, J. W. (1985). Prevention and management of infection—The urinary tract. In G. M. Bedbrook (Ed.), *Lifetime care of the paraplegic patient* (pp. 54–65). Edinburgh, Scotland: Churchill Livingstone.

Stover, S. L., & Fine, P. R. (1986). *Spinal cord injury: The facts and figures.* Birmingham, AL: University of Alabama at Birmingham.

Swenson, J. R., Barnett, L. L., Pond, B., & Schoenberg, A. A. (1998). Assistive technology for rehabilitation and reduction of disability. In J. A. DeLisa & B. M. Gans (Eds.), *Rehabilitation medicine: Principles and practice* (3rd ed., pp. 745–762). Philadelphia: Lippincott-Raven.

Tate, D. G., Heinrich, R. K., Paasuke, L., & Anderson, D. (1998). Vocational rehabilitation, independent living, and consumerism. In J. A. DeLisa & B. M. Gans (Eds.), *Rehabilitation medicine: Principles and practice* (3rd ed., pp. 1151–1162). Philadelphia: Lippincott-Raven.

Traub, J. E., & LeClair, R. R. (1975). The rehabilitation engineering program. *American Rehabilitation, 1*(2), 3–7.

Trombly, C. A. (1995). Spinal cord injury. In C. A. Trombly (Ed.), *Occupational therapy for physical dysfunction* (4th ed., pp. 795–814). Baltimore: Williams & Wilkins.

Turner, A. N. (1985). Prevention of tertiary complications and management—Decubiti. In G. M. Bedbrook (Ed.), *Lifetime care of the paraplegic patient* (pp. 54–65). Edinburgh, Scotland: Churchill Livingstone.

Watson, A. H., Kanny, E. M., White, D. M., & Anson, D. K. (1995). Use of standardized activities of daily living rating scales in spinal cord injury and disease services. *American Journal of Occupational Therapy, 49,* 229–234.

10

Self-Care Strategies After Stroke

Judith A. Jenkins

Judith A. Jenkins, MA, OTR, is Occupational Therapy Team Leader, Rehabilitation Unit, University of Texas Medical Branch at Galveston, Texas.

Key Terms

aphasia

ataxia

dysarthria

hemiplegia

hemianopia

hemorrhage

unilateral neglect

Objectives

On completing this chapter, the reader will be able to

1. Understand the risk factors that contribute to stroke, the location of involvement, and the resulting deficits.

2. Understand the prognosis for recovery from stroke.

3. Understand what important precautions to take when treating patients with stroke.

4. Illustrate and explain the Functional Independence Measure (FIM™) self-care assessment tool.

5. Define and compare the difference between remediation and compensatory treatment approaches.

6. Explain the discharge planning process.

The challenge for occupational therapy in treating the patient recovering from a stroke is to recognize that a stroke has the potential to affect every aspect of a person's life. Hemiparesis occurs in approximately 75% of patients. Persisting neurological impairments lead to partial or total dependence in activities of daily living (ADL) in 25% to 50% of stroke survivors (Wojner, 1996). It is important to assist the patient and his or her caregiver in establishing achievable goals, given the many motor, cognitive, and perceptual deficits that may occur. Because most stroke survivors are cared for in the home, the focus of assessing the home environment and training the caregiver before discontinuing treatment becomes a vital focus during the rehabilitation phase.

Medical and Functional Problems Associated With Stroke

Approximately 550,000 people suffer a stoke each year in the United States, and about 3 million Americans are currently living with varying degrees of disability resulting from strokes (American Heart Association, 1992). Stroke is the third leading cause of death in the United States and the leading cause of disability in adults.

High blood pressure, high cholesterol levels leading to arteriosclerosis, cigarette smoking, obesity, cocaine use, coronary heart disease, and diabetes are some risk factors associated with onset of stroke. The frequency of stroke increases with advancing age, doubling with every decade after age 55 (Bonita, 1992). Strokes occur more frequently in men than women and among African Americans more frequently than whites.

Stroke Subtypes

A stroke is a sort of "brain attack" caused by a disruption in blood supply to the brain from a blockage or bleeding in the brain. Thromboembolic strokes and hemorrhagic strokes are the two major types of stroke. A thromboembolic stroke results when a plaque fragment or blood clot lodges in an artery and restricts blood flow to the brain. A blood clot that forms within an artery that supplies the brain is called a *thrombus*. An *embolus* is a plaque fragment or blood clot that travels to the brain from the heart or an artery supplying the brain. Thrombi and emboli together account for approximately 60% of all cases of stroke (Brandstater, 1998).

The second major type of stroke, the hemorrhagic stroke, occurs when a blood vessel is ruptured by a head injury or an aneurysm. An *aneurysm* is a weak and bulging portion of an arterial wall. Long-term high blood pressure can weaken blood vessels in the brain and cause them to bulge and eventually burst. When the blood vessel ruptures, blood is spilled into the brain, causing damage to brain cells.

Another type of stroke occurs when there is an occlusion in small vessels near the end of the arterial course. This is called a *lacunar stroke*. Such strokes affect a relatively small segment of the brain. Twenty percent of all cerebral infarctions can be characterized as lacunar strokes (Brandstater, 1998).

A *transient ischemic attack* (TIA) occurs when there is a temporary block of blood flow to an artery inside the brain or leading to the brain. The symptoms of a TIA are generally temporary, lasting just a few seconds or up to 12 to 24 hours; most of them last 2 to 15 minutes (Lamsback & Navrozov, 1993).

Location of Strokes and Associated Syndromes

Knowledge of common symptoms associated with various lesion sites can help the practitioner anticipate possible functional deficits. Individual variations in the extent and location of the lesion will result in a unique presentation of symptoms. The therapist's evaluation can be adapted to detect the most common symptoms associated with the location of brain injury. Table 10.1 summarizes the clinical picture presented by lesions at various sites.

Prognosis

Several studies have concluded that most stroke recovery occurs in the first 30 days, and improvement may continue as long as 6 to 12 months after stroke (Kelly-Hayes et al., 1989; Skilbeck, Wade, Langton-Hewer, & Wood, 1983). The longer the delay in onset of recovery, the poorer the prognosis.

If recovery does not begin in 1 to 2 weeks, the potential for the return of motor skills and language becomes unfavorable. Deficits such as constructional apraxia, uninhibited anger, and neglect tend to diminish and may disappear in a few weeks. Hemianopia that has not resolved in a few weeks will usually be permanent, although reading and color discrimination may continue to improve. In lateral medullary infarction, difficulty in swallowing may be protracted, lasting 4 to 8 weeks or longer; relatively normal func-

Table 10.1 Summary of Lesion Sites and Associated Impairments

Site of Lesion	Clinical Picture
Middle cerebral artery	Contralateral hemiplegia, more upper-extremity involvement, hemisensory loss, and hemianopia Dominant hemisphere: expressive aphasia, receptive aphasia, or both; apraxia; and astereognosis Nondominant hemisphere: visual spatial deficits, impaired body awareness, and visual construction deficits
Internal carotid artery	Hemiplegia, unilateral sensory loss, and aphasia
Anterior cerebral artery	Diminished behavioral control, arousal, and attention; contralateral hemiplegia with the lower extremity more involved than the upper extremity; urinary incontinence, and gait apraxia
Posterior cerebral artery	Contralateral hemiplegia, hemianesthesia, and homonymous hemianopia Dominant hemisphere: aphasia Nondominant hemisphere: visual spatial deficits
Bilateral hemisphere	Bilateral hemianopia, cortical blindness with denial of visual disturbance, and amnesia
Brain stem	Lateral medullary or Wallenberg syndrome may include loss of pain and temperature sensation on the ipsilateral face and contralateral body, dysarthria, dysphagia, ipsilateral limb ataxia, vertigo, and nystagmus; other dysfunctions associated with brain-stem involvement include contralateral hemiplegia, contralateral ataxia, and a contralateral increase in the pain and temperature threshold
Vertebrobasilar artery	Cranial nerve palsy; unilateral or bilateral motor, sensory, or cerebellar signs; nystagmus; or coma
Lacunar infarct	In contrast to the multitude of symptoms that may result from large vessel occlusion, one or two striking features are evident. These features have been used to classify four lacunar syndromes. A pure motor stroke results in hemiplegia, a pure sensory stroke leads to paresthesia, and ataxic hemiparesis leads to hemiparesis and ipsilateral ataxia. The fourth syndrome, dysarthria and clumsy hand syndrome, are self-descriptive in that they result in difficulty with speech and fine-motor incoordination of the involved upper extremity.

tion is restored in most cases. Aphasia, dysarthria, cerebellar ataxia, and walking may improve for 1 year or longer, although it is frequently reported that whatever motor and language deficits remain after 5 to 6 months will be permanent (Lamsback & Navrozov, 1993). The patient with a lacunar infarct and pure motor hemiparesis has a good chance for full recovery, which may start within 1 to 2 days, with almost complete restoration in a week (Lamsback & Navrozov, 1993).

Predictors of Successful Outcome

Studies that attempted to determine the factors associated with favorable functional outcome after stroke (Granger, Hamilton, & Gresham, 1988; Granger, Hamilton, Gresham, & Kramer, 1989) found that 80% of stroke survivors will be able to attain inde-

pendence in mobility, whereas 67% will attain independence in ADL. Mauthe, Haaf, Hayn, and Krall (1996) showed that more than 70% of the variance in discharge destinations after stroke rehabilitation is determined by the ability to function independently in the performance of self-care tasks necessary for bathing, toileting, social interaction, dressing, and eating. Independence in bowel and bladder control, eating, and grooming have a cumulative influence on predicting the ability of a survivor to live independently in the community after discharge.

Davidoff, Keren, Ring, and Solzi (1991) found that patients receiving inpatient rehabilitation services were able to maintain the gains in functional independence 1 year after discharge, and that outpatient therapy services permitted further gains, particularly in patients with unilateral neglect, impaired joint position sense, urinary incontinence, or complete upper-or lower-extremity hemiplegia.

Bernspang, Viitanen, and Eriksson (1989) found that even several years after a stroke, deficits in vision and visual perception were more significant than motor impairment in determining the extent to which survivors could manage self-care requirements. The authors speculated that it may be easier for persons to compensate for motor impairment than for perceptual limitations.

Precautions

Cardiac. The therapist must be aware of specific precautions and secondary diagnoses—hypertension, coronary artery disease, and congestive heart failure, for example—that are frequently associated with stroke (Roth, 1988). A careful review of the patient's medical chart should be conducted before therapy begins. Physicians may provide parameters for heart rate, oxygen saturation, and blood pressure for patients whose condition may be unstable. These patients must be monitored before, during, and after activity to determine whether the activity is too strenuous. Isometric, resistive, and overhead activities increase cardiac stress and should be carefully monitored or avoided, depending on the patient's cardiac status. In addition, community activities in extremely cold or hot weather should be postponed.

Dysphagia. Dysphagia, or difficulty in swallowing, often accompanies stroke and may affect as many as one third of stroke patients (Roth, 1988). The speech pathologist may conduct a videofluoroscopic or modified barium swallow exam. In some facilities this is done by the occupational therapist, or the occupational therapist may assist with proper positioning of a patient during the exam. This is the best tool for detecting deficits in oral control and swallowing. Food and liquid of various consistencies are mixed with barium, which makes the swallowed substance visible on the video monitor. This mixture is given to the patient in small quantities. The movement of the food is observed in the mouth, through the pharynx, and into the esophagus. Any abnormality that suggests risk of aspiration (getting food in the trachea) can readily be detected, and specific recommendations about the types of food that are safe can be made.

In patients with swallowing dysfunction, specific guidelines may include avoid drinking with a straw, take one or two sips of liquid before eating solid foods, tilt the head while swallowing, and limit environmental distractions while eating. During feeding training, the occupational therapist should be aware of possible restrictions, such as no oral intake, as well as specifications for texture or consistency of food and beverages. The dietitian will also be consulted to ensure that protein and caloric needs are met and dehydration is prevented.

Gastrostomy tube. If the patient has severe dysphagia, he or she may have a gastrostomy tube. The tube must be monitored so that it is not disturbed during activity. When gastrostomy feedings are given, the patient must be maintained in an upright position (at least 45°) generally for 1 hour after meals (see Figure 10.1). That position prevents backflow of the feeding, which can lead to aspiration pneumonia. Practitioners should also be aware of the tube's location to avoid pressure on it from clothing or a gait belt.

Fall risk. Stroke survivors are more likely to fall than any other population (Vlahov, Myers, & Al-Ibrahim, 1990). Studies report that from 41% to as much as 83.3% of patients who fell had a diagnosis of stroke (DeVincenzo & Watkins, 1987; Grant & Hamilton, 1987; Mion et al., 1989; Vlahov et al., 1990). Patients with impaired balance or vision, lower-extremity weakness, impulsivity, confusion, gait disturbances, or perceptual deficits such as depth perception and unilateral neglect are at an increased risk for falls. They may require constant or intermittent supervision. Safety belts should be used in wheelchairs and on the toilet if sitting balance or judgment is impaired. A gait belt is recommended when transferring, standing, or walking with a patient. Brakes on the wheelchair, bed, or other unstable items should be locked before attempting a transfer.

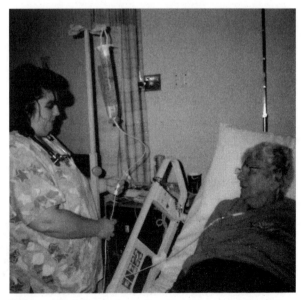

Figure 10.1 Illustration of gastrostomy tube feeding.

Shoulder pain. Elderly patients frequently have some degree of joint damage caused by preexisting conditions such as osteoarthritis. Proper alignment of all joints must be maintained during self-care and passive range of motion to avoid impingement and injury to soft tissues. The affected shoulder is particularly vulnerable to injury after stroke. The patient and caregiver should be taught to position the affected arm correctly during all tasks. All caregivers must be careful to avoid pulling on the affected arm and should mobilize the scapula before attempting overhead movement of a spastic arm. The therapist should be alert for signs of shoulder-hand syndrome, or *reflex sympathetic dystrophy*, including:

- swelling of the hand;

- trophic changes, including altered skin color, nail appearance, sweating, or hair growth; and

- pain at rest or upon motion, especially during metacarpophalangeal and shoulder flexion, abduction, or external rotation (Eto, Yoshikawa, Ueda, & Hirai, 1980).

The Self-Care Skills Assessment

Before initiating the ADL or self-care skills assessment, the practitioner should complete an evaluation of the patient's physical, cognitive, and perceptual abilities. General mobility skills, such as ability to transfer and ambulate, should also be evaluated. A comprehensive evaluation will assist in planning a safe and successful ADL treatment program. For example, a patient who has poor sitting balance may need to perform bathing and dressing activities in a supine position from the bed, not sitting on the side of the bed unsupported.

Phillips and Wolters (1996) noted that during the self-care evaluation the following abilities should be observed:

- Ability to sustain antigravity posture
- Ability to maintain head and trunk control
- Ability to maintain midline orientation during dynamic activity
- Functional use and quality of movement of the involved upper extremity
- Ability to perform bilateral movement
- Ability to use objects appropriately
- Endurance for self-care tasks
- Level of cognitive functioning in the areas of initiation, attention, organizational skills, and sequencing abilities

- Ability to visually attend to self-care tasks
- Presence of perceptual difficulties interfering with task performance

In addition to noting the above items, it is important to obtain information from the patient and family members regarding the patient's normal daily routine. Having an understanding of the physical design of the patient's discharge destination will assist the therapist in planning training sessions that will best simulate the home environment. Finally, the most important result of the occupational therapy evaluation is the collaboration with the patient and the caregiver to establish realistic, attainable goals.

This chapter will focus on using the Functional Independence Measure (FIM™) to assess levels of independence in ADL. The Barthel Index and the FIM have been tested extensively in rehabilitation for reliability, validity, and sensitivity, and they are the most commonly used measures (Gresham et al., 1995).

The FIM is a measure of disability (measured in terms of burden of care) for patients, regardless of impairments or limitations (*Guide for the Uniform Data Set*, 1993). It assesses self-care, sphincter control, transfers, locomotion, communication, and social cognition on a 7-level scale (see Table 10.2).

FIM items are to be assessed within 72 hours after admission. If it is not safe to assess a particular area within the 72-hour window of time, or the assistance of two persons is required to perform the activity, then the recorded level is 1—total assistance (*Guide for the Uniform Data Set*, 1993). The score should reflect the person's actual performance, not a simulation of the task.

Assessment

The following case histories will provide information on the type of stroke, resulting impairments suffered, and occupational therapy intervention. Results of an occupational therapy evaluation and a measure of the subject's disability based on the FIM scale are included.

Case Study I

Joyce is a woman 58 years of age who suffered a multiple ischemic stroke with multiple vascular distribution. The primary distributions were left anterior cerebral and right occipital stroke. The strokes resulted in weakness of the right side, ataxia, impaired sensation to the right side, major

Table 10.2 Description of the Levels of Function and Their Scores

Score	Level of Function
7	Complete Independence: All of the tasks described as making up the activity are typically performed safely, without modification, assistive devices, or aids, and within reasonable time.
6	Modified Independence: Activity requires an assistive device or more than reasonable time, or there are safety (risk) considerations.
5	Supervision or Setup: The subject requires no more help than standby, cueing, or coaxing, without physical contact; or, helper sets up needed items or applies orthoses.
4	Minimal Assistance: The subject requires no more help than touching, and subject expends 75% or more of the effort.
3	Moderate Assistance: Subject requires more help than touching, or expends half or more (up to 75%) of the effort.
2	Maximal Assistance: Subject expends less than 50% of the effort, but at least 25%.
1	Total Assistance: Subject expends less than 25% of the effort.

Note. From *Guide for the Uniform Data Set for Medical Rehabilitation (Adult FIM™)* (Version 4.0), 1993, Buffalo, NY: State University of New York at Buffalo. Reprinted with permission.

vision impairment, and blindness in the left field of vision in both eyes (*hemianopia*).

Before her hospitalization, Joyce was employed as a nurse and lived alone in a single-story home. She was independent in all ADL and instrumental activities of daily living (IADL). The occupational therapy evaluation revealed that active range of motion was within normal limits in bilateral upper extremities. Her sitting balance was graded as good, but standing balance was graded as poor. She was considered at high risk for falls because of her impulsivity and impaired balance and vision. Joyce required minimal assistance for most self-care tasks. Table 10.3 shows her FIM scores at evaluation and discharge. Her rehabilitation stay was 3½ weeks.

Plan of Care

The occupational therapist used the FIM as a guideline in establishing the short- and longer-term goals listed below. The FIM levels to which the goals correspond are shown in parentheses.

Within 2 weeks, the patient will:

- perform grooming activities with setup (5);
- perform upper-extremity and lower-extremity dressing with setup (5);
- perform tub transfers with minimal assistance (4), using a tub transfer bench and grab bars;
- perform toilet transfers with supervision (5); and
- feed herself with setup assistance (5).

Within 3 to 4 weeks the patient will feed herself with modified independence (6) and perform tub transfers with supervision (5), using the tub transfer bench and grab bars. The caregiver will be independent in appropriate setup of the patient for participation in ADL.

Treatment Strategies

Occupational therapy intervention consisted of scheduled ADL training sessions in Joyce's room. The occupational therapist coordinated with the nursing staff members to ensure a consistent arrangement of her meal trays to improve her ability to locate food items. It was recommended that she be placed in a private room, because she was severely distracted by environmental stimuli such as conversations between other persons, the television, the ringing telephone, and minor changes in the physical arrangement of her room. The structure of Joyce's rehabilitation program allowed her to improve her level of independence in feeding, grooming, and toileting from minimal assistance to modified independence.

In the occupational therapy treatment room, the therapist focused on activities to improve visual scanning, right upper-extremity coordination, and motor control. Joyce was encouraged to follow the movement of her hand with her eyes to compensate for impaired proprioception. Bimanual use of the upper extremities was facilitated through activities such as

Table 10.3 FIM Scores for Patient in Case Study 1

Activity	Score at Admission	Score at Discharge
Eating	4	6
Grooming	4	6
Bathing	4	6
Dressing, upper extremity	4	5
Dressing, lower extremity	4	5
Bladder control	4	7
Bowel control	4	6
Bed, chair transers	4	5
Toilet transfers	4	5
Tub, shower transfers	3	5

folding clothes and towels, rolling out thera-putty with a rolling pin, and using a bimanual sander box placed on an incline board (see Figure 10.2). Joyce was then asked to reach for small blocks with her right hand, pick them up one at a time, place them in front of the sander box, and push the box up the incline board until the block fell over the top. The blocks were placed to her right side (the involved side), both within and outside her field of vision. This activity addressed her impaired motor planning and coordination through reaching with her involved extremity; picking up the small blocks involved fine-motor function. Pushing the sander upwards improved upper-extremity strength in her shoulder flexors. Placement of some of the blocks outside her visual field required her to use head-turning strategies to compensate for the hemianopia.

During lower-extremity dressing, Joyce had difficulty putting on her right sock and shoe. She was unable to maintain the position of crossing her right leg over her left, and she lost her balance when she reached down. In addition to routine practice and training in donning and doffing her socks and shoes, Joyce was asked by the occupational therapist to sit on the edge of the treatment mat and reach for items located just below her knees and, eventually, on the floor. This activity helped improve her sitting balance, and by discharge she was able to don and doff both shoes and socks with setup.

Because Joyce would be unsupervised for some periods of the day after her discharge from the hospital, the occupational therapist worked with Joyce and her caregiver on strategies for storing food items, so that she could retrieve a cold snack from the refrigerator. Joyce practiced making a sandwich and arranging snacks in a familiar container that she could located easily. The caregiver participated in several training sessions with the therapist before Joyce's discharge from the hospital to ensure follow-through with learned compensatory strategies. ∎

Case Study 2

Benjamin is man 55 years of age who suffered a right middle cerebral artery distribution stroke with associated left-side weakness, slurred speech, and decreased alertness. His hospital course was complicated by a left atrial myxoma excision with cardiopulmonary bypass. He also presented with decreased vision in the left eye, a left homonymous hemianopia, and left-side neglect. His sensation was impaired on the left side.

During his acute care hospitalization, a modified barium swallow revealed paralysis of the left side of his tongue and vocal cords. A gastrostomy tube was placed to avoid the possibility of aspiration. It is important to note that while in acute care, he had fallen twice while attempting to walk to the bathroom unassisted.

Before his hospitalization, Benjamin was self-employed as a handyman. He lived with his daughter in a single-story home. He was independent in all ADL and IADL. His plans

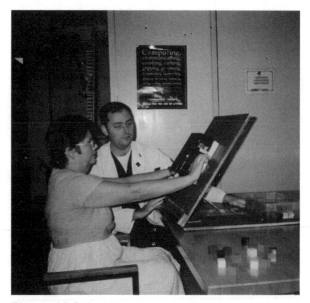

Figure 10.2 Activity using an incline board.

on discharge were to move into an apartment for senior citizens. The occupational therapy evaluation revealed that active range of motion in his right upper extremity was within normal limits and strength was normal. Active range of motion in the left upper extremity was within functional limits, although movement patterns were athetoid. Edema was present in the left forearm, wrist, and hand. He had complaints of pain at the shoulder at the end of passive range. Benjamin was oriented to person only and was able to follow one-step directions. He was impulsive and easily distracted by environmental stimuli. His sitting balance was fair and standing balance was poor. He was graded as needing total assistance with feeding, because he was not being fed orally and depended on the nursing staff members for his gastrostomy tube feedings. Benjamin required moderate assistance with most of his basic self-care tasks (see Table 10.4). His rehabilitation stay was 3½ weeks and continued with therapy through outpatient services.

Plan of Care

As in the other case study, the occupational therapy practitioner used the admission FIM scores as a guide to establish the following goals. Within 2 weeks, the patient will:

• perform grooming activities with setup (5);

• perform upper-extremity dressing with minimal assistance (4);

• perform lower-extremity dressing with minimal assistance (4);

• bathe with minimal assistance (4); and

• perform shower transfer with minimal assistance (4), using a tub transfer bench, grab bar and handheld shower.

Within 4 weeks, the patient will:

• perform upper-extremity dressing with setup (5);

• perform lower-extremity dressing with setup (5); and

• bathe with supervision and setup (5).

Intervention Strategies

Occupational therapy intervention consisted of daily ADL training sessions in the patient's room. Treatment activities focused on improving motor control in the left upper extremity, improving trunk control, devising compensatory strategies for left hemianopia and left-side neglect, and improving safety during transfers. Because of Benjamin's left-side neglect and impaired sensation, he did not use his left hand spontaneously. He also became very frustrated during ADL training. Because of poor motor control in his left hand, he avoided using it altogether. Benjamin was initially taught one-handed dressing techniques (see Figure 10.3). He improved his level of independence and was then more receptive to occupational therapy intervention. Functional use of the left upper extremity was encouraged by teaching him to use his left upper extremity as a gross assist to stabilize fabric when zipping his

Table 10.4 FIM Scores for Patient in Case Study 2

Activity	Score at Admission	Score at Discharge
Eating	1	1
Grooming	4	5
Bathing	3	5
Dressing, upper extremity	3	5
Dressing, lower extremity	3	4
Bladder control	2	5
Bowel control	3	4
Bed, chair transfers	3	5
Toilet transfers	3	5
Tub, shower transfers	1	5

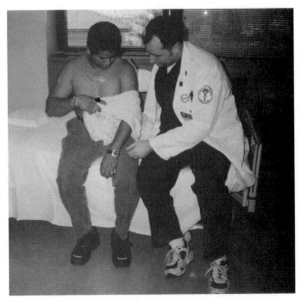

Figure 10.3 One-handed dressing.

pants, bathing his right upper extremity, and pulling up his pants. He eventually progressed to using his left upper extremity as a fair assist and performed activities such as donning and doffing socks, putting his belt through the loops, and propelling his wheelchair.

Treatment activities to improve trunk control were similar to those used in case study 1. Grooming activities were done while standing in front of the mirror to assist with improving dynamic standing balance. Benjamin was able to return home with his daughter, who would provide intermittent supervision. Occupational therapy services were recommended for continuation through home health services. Home health therapy would give him the opportunity to focus on improving independence and safety in basic ADL. The goal would be to eliminate the need for supervision and allow him to live independently in a senior apartment, which was his primary goal. ∎

Setting of Goals

Setting treatment goals involves estimating the amount of time it will take for the patient to achieve a specific level of independence. The following factors may determine the length of stay and assist in establishing realistic and attainable goals with the patient and his or her family members.

• Funding sources
• Personal financial resources
• Prior level of functioning
• Age
• Lifestyle and role responsibilities
• Family member support
• Presence of cognitive and perceptual deficits
• Degree of physical dysfunction
• Discharge disposition

A goal that is well written should suggest a functional outcome and describe the result that treatment intervention is expected to achieve (Daniel & Strickland, 1992). The American Occupational Therapy Association's *Guidelines for Documentation* (Kron et al., 1988) suggest that short- and long-term goals should be measurable and related to the occupational therapy problem list. Goals may be measured by the level of assistance required to perform an activity, as in the case assessments; the FIM or any other ADL scale can be used as guidelines. Methods of measurement may also involve speed, accuracy, or frequency of the skill required. A goal must also include a time frame for goal attainment.

It is most important for the occupational therapist to consider functional measures in motor recovery when writing goals. For example, when writing a goal to improve grip strength, the therapist should focus on skills, such as ability to hold and drink from a glass, not on a number of pounds in grip strength as measured by a dynamometer. Consider what specific activity will be affected by improvement of range of motion, coordination, endurance, balance, or strength. Other examples of useful goals would be to improve the active range of motion so that the patient is able to retrieve items from a cabinet or groom hair, to improve fine-motor control to enable the patient to button a shirt with a front closure or hook a bra, and to improve dynamic standing balance to enable the patient to adjust his or her clothing after toileting. Establishing functional, measurable goals helps reflect the uniqueness of occupational therapy.

Treatment Approaches

Once the evaluation is complete and functional goals have been established, treatment begins. A variety of treatment approaches can be used and combined to maximize both the level and the quality of independence. It is important to note that component skill-training activities should be related to improving the patient's ability to perform self-care tasks (A. Woodson, personal communication, August 20, 1998). Motor learning theory, as described by Carr and Shepherd (1987), uses a sequential clinical reasoning process. A functional performance problem is identified; the limiting motor components are analyzed; the impaired components are practiced in isolation through visual, verbal, and manual guidance; and, finally, the motion is practiced in the context of the functional task, with the intent of integrating the components.

Remediation Techniques

Gresham et al. (1995) recommended that patients who have functional deficits and some voluntary movements of the involved arm or leg be encouraged to use the limb in functional tasks. Exercise and functional training should be directed at improving strength, motor control, and functional performance and relearning sensorimotor relationships.

Motor facilitation and retraining techniques help improve upper-extremity function and trunk control, which are necessary for optimal performance of self-care skills. Motor retraining is directed at correcting impaired motor activity of the affected extremity, at preventing overuse of the unaffected side, and at preventing the development of abnormal movement patterns on the affected side. They can be used in the clinic to build the prerequisite skills needed for ADL. Specific techniques can enhance functional mobility for rolling, sitting, standing, or kneeling. Working on various surfaces, such as a table mat, bench, chair without arms, bed, ball, or rocker board, can provide graded challenges to balance. Reaching activities and eye-hand coordination games can introduce speed and control. Skilled use of remediation techniques can be the most efficient way to promote positive changes that ultimately enhance ADL performance.

Compensation Techniques and Contextual Training

In the compensatory model, the emphasis is on achieving independence in ADL to improve function rather than on enhancing motor recovery or minimizing impairments (Gresham et al., 1995). Gresham and the other panel members also recommended that patients with persistent functional deficits be taught compensatory techniques for performing ADL, using the affected extremity when possible and, when not, the unaffected limb. The traditional method involved using only the unaffected extremity, as in one-handed dressing techniques.

Contextual training involves practicing a task in a specific environment until it becomes learned or habitual. This repetition of specific task sequences has been found to be effective in improving independence in the brain-injured population (Soderback, 1988). Practice is most effective when it is specific to the context in which the task is used and when it is performed in a consistent sequence (Bukowski, Bonavolonta, Keehn, & Morgan, 1996). In addition to offering the benefit of practicing familiar functional activity, contextual training requires the patient to integrate various motor, cognitive, and perceptual skills. The activity should initially begin with a low level of challenge and gradually increase in complexity as the patient masters each step. For example, in the treatment of Benjamin in case study 2, the occupational therapist first allowed him to perform dressing activities with one hand and progressed to incorporating the use of his involved extremity. Another example would be progressing from placing a patient's clothing articles within the area of reach or field of vision (setup) to having the patient search a cluttered drawer or a closet for specific articles.

IADL, such as home care, child care, community living skills, and work, provide cognitive, perceptual,

and motor challenges. These activities are best performed in the actual environment in which they will take place after therapy. Because the therapist often cannot conduct therapy outside the hospital, he or she should attempt to simulate the discharge situation to identify problem areas and improve performance. With guidance, patients are frequently able to apply principles learned in simulated settings to their own situation.

Discharge Planning

When a reasonable number of goals have been met or changes in functional ability no longer occur, it may be time for discharge from the rehabilitation unit. Gresham et al. (1995) recommended that absence of progress on two consecutive evaluations should lead to reconsideration of the intensive rehabilitation setting. It is frequently said that discharge planning should begin from the day of admission to the unit. The occupational therapist, in conjunction with the rehabilitation team, the patient, and his or her caregiver must determine whether the patient will be safe in the discharge environment.

Therapeutic day pass. A therapeutic day pass, which permits the patient to visit the home environment for a period of 4 to 6 hours with a caregiver, can be a useful for identifying problems that may require specific environmental adaptations or further functional training. Reliable friends or family members may report on the patient's performance during a home pass. The pass should include information on what kinds of activities the patient undertook and any problems he or she may have encountered with, for example, household ambulation, wheelchair mobility, kitchen and bathroom mobility, and general accessibility in and around the home. The patient's companion should note any problems that would prevent the patient from using any of the recommended equipment. (See Table 10.5 for a list of techniques and assistive devices commonly recommended after stroke.)

Home safety assessment. Another valuable tool for discharge planning is the home safety assessment. This assessment generally involves the occupational therapist, the physical therapist, the patient, and, if necessary, the caregiver visiting the home. The main purpose of the home safety assessment is to ensure the patient's safety in the home environment and to determine whether the patient has had sufficient training to safely negotiate the environment. The therapist should assess whether the patient was able to generalize to the home setting

Table 10.5 Techniques and Assistive Devices Used After Stroke

Activity	Problem	Technique	Assistive Device
Feeding	Weak or absent grip; weak supinators; difficulty loading utensil; difficulty bringing hand to mouth; unilateral neglect	Facilitating gross grasp and strengthen grip; cueing to locate all items on the tray	Universal cuff, built-up or extended utensils or handles; swivel spoon; lip plates; scoop dish; plate guard
Grooming	Weak or absent grasp; hemiplegia		Built-up handles or universal cuff; suction cup denture or nail brushes; wash mitt with liquid soap
Bathing	Hemiplegia; unable to reach lower body; impaired sitting or standing balance		Same as for grooming, plus long-handled sponge; tub bench or shower chair; handheld shower; grab bars
Toileting	Impaired ability to transfer safely; weak pinch and grasp; hemiplegia	Raise or lower the height of surface to accommodate the patient	Commode chair over toilet; toilet safety frame with elevated toilet seat; grab bars
Dressing, upper extremity	Hemiplegia unilateral neglect dressing apraxia	One-handed dressing contextual training visual scanning cues	Button aid, zipper pull, Velcro® closures
Dressing, lower extremity	Poor sitting or standing balance; hemiplegia; weak grasp or pinch	Practice dressing while supine in bed; have patient roll from side-to-side or bridge to pull up underwear or slacks; simplify clothing	Reacher; dressing stick; elastic shoe laces; long-handled shoe horn; hook-and-loop closures; button aide

some of the basic skills learned in the rehabilitation setting—stair climbing, tub and toilet transfers, kitchen mobility, and household ambulation, for example. The advantage of the home safety assessment is that it allows the therapist to see the physical structure of the home and determine whether there is adequate space to use recommended equipment, such as a tub transfer bench. During the home safety visit, the therapist can make recommendations specific to the patient's environment.

Caregiver training. A caregiver should be trained when the patient is unable to carry out his or her home exercise plan independently. Approximately 70% to 90% of stroke victims are cared for in the home (Ozer, Materson, & Caplan, 1994). It may be very difficult for one person to be responsible for all aspects of the patient's care at home, especially if he or she is also caring for other family members. Hasselkus (1991) reported that caregivers often experience ethical dilemmas when faced with conflicts between taking good care of the patient and meeting other family and personal responsibilities. Evans, Bishop, and Haselkorn (1991) found that patients at risk for less-than-optimal home care had caregivers who were more likely to be depressed, had below-average knowledge of stroke care principles, and had a greater incidence of family dysfunction.

The therapist should collaborate with the caregiver to develop a home program that meets the patient's needs and is realistic for the caregiver to perform. Before discharge, the home program should be demonstrated and plenty of opportunity given for practice. Showing picture diagrams or photographs of each activity may be helpful.

Continuity of care. The final concern in discharge planning is continuity of care. Arrangements should be made if therapy is to continue through home health services or through an outpatient or skilled nursing facility. It is important at this time to establish a plan for follow-up care, which may be done by the patient's primary care physician or the rehabilitation physician.

Summary

Current trends in health care continue toward shorter hospital stays. One third of all patients with stroke are being moved from an acute care setting to rehabilitation units within 14 days of onset, and length of stay has been declining since 1989 (Joe, 1995). The challenge for the occupational therapy practitioner is to provide the treatment approach that will best enable the patient to achieve maximal benefits and functional gains within the shortened time frames. Another challenge for the occupational therapy profession is to be diligent in conducting outcome studies showing a correlation between remediation and compensatory training with improvements in ADL. ◆

Study Questions

1. What aspects of basic self-care tasks may be affected when a person suffers a middle cerebral artery stroke?

2. What factors are considered when determining the prognosis for recovery?

3. Discuss the precautions associated with swallowing difficulties and their effect on feeding training.

4. What abilities should be observed during the self-care evaluation?

5. Discuss the factors that may determine the length of the inpatient rehabilitation stay.

6. Describe the difference between remediation techniques and compensation techniques.

References

American Heart Association. (1992). *1992 stroke facts.* Dallas, TX: Author.

Bernspang, B., Viitanen, M., & Eriksson, S. (1989). Impairments of perceptual and motor functions: Their influence on self-care ability 4–6 years after a stroke. *Occupational Therapy Journal of Research, 9,* 38–52.

Bonita, R. (1992). Epidemiology of stroke. *Lancet, 339,* 342–344.

Brandstater, M. (1998). Stroke rehabilitation. In J. DeLisa & B. Gains (Eds.), *Rehabilitation medicine: Principles and practice* (pp. 1165–1189). Philadelphia: Lippincott-Raven.

Bukowski, L., Bonavolonta, M., Keehn, M. T., & Morgan, K. A. (1996). Interdisciplinary roles in stroke care. *Nursing Clinics of North America, 21,* 359–374.

Carr, J. H., & Shepherd, R. B. (1987). *A motor relearning programme for stroke* (2nd ed.). Rockville, MD: Aspen.

Daniel, M. S., & Strickland, R. L. (1992). Writing goals for documentation. In *Occupational Therapy Protocol Management in Adult Physical Dysfunction* (pp. 389–407). Gaithersburg, MD: Aspen.

Davidoff, G. N., Keren, O., Ring, H., & Solzi, P. (1991). Acute stroke patients: Long term effects of rehabilitation and maintenance of gains. *Archives of Physical Medicine and Rehabilitation, 72,* 869–873.

DeVincenzo, D. K., & Watkins, S. (1987). Accidental falls in a rehabilitation setting. *Rehabilitation Nursing, 12,* 248–252.

Eto, F., Yoshikawa, M., Ueda, S., & Hirai, S. (1980). Post hemiplegic shoulder-hand syndrome, with special reference to related cerebral localization. *Journal of the American Geriatrics Society, 28*(1), 13–17.

Evans, R. L., Bishop, D. S., & Haselkorn, J. K. (1991). Factors predicting satisfactory home care after stroke. *Archives of Physical Medicine and Rehabilitation, 72,* 144–147.

Granger, C. V., Hamilton, B. B., & Gresham, G. E. (1988). The stroke rehabilitation outcome study: Part I. General description. *Archives of Physical Medicine and Rehabilitation, 69,* 506–509.

Granger, C. V., Hamilton, B. B., Gresham, G. E., & Kramer, A. A. (1989). The stroke rehabilitation outcome study: Part II. Relative merits of the Total Barthel Index Score and a four item subscore in predicting patient outcomes. *Archives of Physical Medicine and Rehabilitation, 70,* 100–103.

Grant, J., & Hamilton, S. (1987). Falls in a rehabilitation center: A retrospective and comparative analysis. *Rehabilitation Nursing, 12,* 74–76.

Gresham, G. E., Duncan, P. W., Stason, W. B., Adams, H, P., Jr., Adelman, A. M., Alexander, D. N., Bishop, D. S., Diller, L., Donaldson, N. E., Granger, C. V., Holland, A. L., Kelly-Hayes, M., McDowell, F. H., Myers, L. R., Phipps, M. A., Roth, E. J., Siebens, H. C., Tarvin, G. A., & Trombly, C. A. (1995, May). *Post-stroke rehabilitation clinical practice guideline, No. 16* (AHCPR Publication No. 95-0622). Rockville, MD: U.S. Department of Health and Human Services,

Public Health Service, Agency for Health Care Policy and Research.

Guide for the Uniform Data Set for Medical Rehabilitation (Adult FIM) (Version 4.0). (1993). Buffalo, NY: State University of New York at Buffalo.

Hasselkus, B. (1991). Ethical dilemmas in family caregiving for the elderly: Implications for occupational therapy. *American Journal of Occupational Therapy, 45,* 206–212.

Joe, B. E. (1995, October 19). Accelerating stroke rehab. *OT Week,* pp. 14–15.

Kelly-Hayes, M., Wolf, P. A., Kase, C. S., Gresham, G. E., Kannel, W. B., & D'Agostino, R. B. (1989). Time course of functional recovery after stroke: The Framingham Study. *Journal of Neurologic Rehabilitation, 3,* 65–70.

Kron, L., McGourty, L., Foto, M., Kronsnoble, S., Lossing C., Rask, S., & DeRenne, S. C. (1988). Guidelines for occupational therapy documentation. In E. Hopkins & H. Smith (Eds.), *Willard and Spackman's occupational therapy* (7th ed., pp. 811–813). Philadelphia: Lippincott.

Lamsback, W. J., & Navrozov, M. (1993). Cerebral vascular diseases. In R. D. Adams & M. Victor (Eds.), *Principles of neurology* (5th ed., pp. 669–748). New York: McGraw-Hill.

Mauthe, R., Haaf, D., Hayn, P., & Krall, J. (1996). Predicting discharge destination of stroke patients using a mathematical model based on six items from the Functional Independence Measure. *Archives of Physical Medicine and Rehabilitation, 77,* 10–30.

Mion, L. C., Gregor, S., Buettner, M., Chwurchak, D., Lee, O., & Paras, W. (1989). Falls in the rehabilitation setting: Incidence and characteristics. *Rehabilitation Nursing, 14,* 17–21.

Ozer, M. N., Materson, R. S., & Caplan, L. R. (1994). *Management of persons with stroke.* St. Louis, MO: C. V. Mosby.

Phillips, M. E., & Wolters, S. (1996). Assessment in practice: Common tools and methods. In C. B. Royeen (Ed.), *Stroke: Strategies, treatment, rehabilitation, outcomes, knowledge, and evaluation* (pp. 1–47). Bethesda, MD: American Occupational Therapy Association.

Roth, E. J. (1988). The elderly stroke patient: Principles and practices of rehabilitation management. *Topics in Geriatric Rehabilitation, 3,* 27–61.

Skilbeck, C., Wade, D., Langton-Hewer, R., & Wood, V. (1983). Recovery after stroke. *Journal of Neurology Neurosurgery Psychiatry, 46,* 5–8.

Soderback, I. (1988). The effectiveness of training intellectual functions in adults with acquired brain damage. *Scandinavian Journal of Rehabilitation Medicine, 20,* 47–56.

Vlahov, D., Myers, A. H., & Al-Ibrahim, M. S. (1990). Epidemiology of falls among patients in a rehabilitation hospital. *Archives of Physical Medicine and Rehabilitation, 71,* 8–12.

Wojner, A. W. (1996). Optimizing ischemic stroke outcomes: An interdisciplinary approach to poststroke rehabilitation in acute care. *Critical Care Nursing Quarterly, 19*(2), 47–61.

11

Self-Care Strategies for Persons With Movement Disorders

Margaret McCuaig
Janet L. Poole

Margaret McCuaig, MA, OT(C), is Coordinator of Rehabilitation Services for a multilevel care facility in Victoria, British Columbia, Canada.

Janet L. Poole, PhD, OTR/L, FAOTA, is Assistant Professor, Occupational Therapy Program, Department of Orthopaedics, University of New Mexico, Albuquerque, New Mexico.

Key Terms

adaptive strategies

augmentative communication

dysphagia

independent living movement

routines

transparent equipment

Objectives

On completing this chapter, the reader will be able to

1. Identify the difference between occupational therapy aimed at remediation of impairment and occupational therapy aimed at independent living.

2. Describe factors to consider when recommending adaptive strategies.

3. Describe adaptive strategies using equipment and techniques for meal management, mobility, and communication for persons with movement disorders.

4. Describe adaptive strategies using routines and social support for communication, homemaking, and meal management for persons with movement disorders.

5. Identify ways in which routines and social supports can be facilitated.

This chapter presents anecdotal accounts of how adults with movement disorders view and manage their self-care. Principles for problem solving from the perspectives of the client and the occupational therapy practitioner are drawn from case examples. Emphasis is given to the person's perspective and experience of self, within the context of his or her social and physical environments, as they relate to the management of self-care requirements. Also described is the practitioner's role in helping the person with movement disorders develop adaptive strategies. A framework is used that considers techniques, equipment, routines, and social supports as categories of adaptive strategies that help persons with movement disorders compensate for the lack or excess of movement with which they must contend.

Persons With Movement Disorders

Persons with movement disorders face the challenge of living with too much or too little movement, associated with some degree of paralysis or weakness. For persons with these disorders, actions are frequently difficult to start, stop, or control. Many conditions carry with them a progressive component, often rapid, and some create a disturbance in cognitive functioning. Memory, concentration, and an ability to organize and sequence events may be affected. Sensory abilities, including *proprioception*, or knowledge of the body's posture, movement, and position in space, may be impaired. Problems with functional abilities are often intensified by stress as well as the aging process, even if the medical condition itself is stable (Lohr & Wisniewski, 1987). Many persons with movement disorders experience pain and have constant fatigue and low energy; poor balance; and difficulties with most areas of self-care, including communication, mobility, eating, dressing, toileting, bathing, and grooming.

The scope of this chapter includes persons with movement disorders, including amyotrophic lateral sclerosis, cerebral palsy, dystonia, Huntington's chorea, multiple sclerosis, muscular dystrophy, Parkinson's disease, tardive dyskinesia, and Tourette's syndrome. This list provides examples of conditions of both hyperkinetic and hypokinetic movement disorders, but it is not exhaustive (Jain & Kirshblum, 1993). A list of supplementary readings presented at the conclusion of the chapter provides sources for detailed descriptions of the medical conditions under discussion. Table 11.1 provides common definitions of frequently used terms, and Table 11.2 describes features and problems of selected movement disorders.

Framework for Identifying Problems in Self-Care

A person's environment can support or inhibit independence. Social supports, cultural beliefs and values, environmental designs and furnishings, and the availability of structures and tools are all important factors in a person's ability to perform tasks of daily living. For this reason, when addressing problems of self-care, it is important to assess and to intervene within the context of the person's social, cultural, and physical environments (Christiansen, 1991).

Problems related to self-care are often addressed through adaptive strategies within the domains of techniques and equipment, routines, and social supports. In this chapter, case studies describe specific occupations of self-care within these adaptive domains. The emphasis of this approach differs from the traditional presentation of problems according to disability and of solutions in terms of physical performance.

Traditionally, medical rehabilitation focused on the assessment and elimination of the impairment (Christiansen, 1991). Consistent with the themes expressed elsewhere in this book, this chapter focuses on the process of adaptation of a person to his or her physical and social environments. The objective is to show that self-care needs can be met despite the presence of movement disorders and without emphasizing remediation of physical dysfunction. The importance of a person's social and physical contexts is highlighted as a critical consideration in the assessment of self-care problems and in intervention (Corbin & Strauss, 1988).

Occupational Therapy and Adults With Movement Disorders

The occupational therapist's role in working with adults with movement disorders is to be knowledgeable about the context of a person's life and committed to supporting the perspective of the consumer, using nontraditional approaches reflecting principles of the independent living movement. This framework requires occupational therapy practitioners to support a person's acquisition of skills and capabilities for self-direction and to acknowledge the

Table 11.1 Movement Disorder Terms and Examples of Associated Conditions

Term	Description	Example
Ataxia	Movement, usually of the extremities, that is reduced in speed and distorted in terms of timing and direction	Multiple sclerosis; Charcot–Marie–Tooth
Athetosis	Slow sinuous movement with fluctuations in tone and most commonly found in the distal extremities; more rhythmic and slower than choreiform movements; exacerbated by anxiety and attempted voluntary movements	Cerebral palsy; tardive dyskinesia
Bradykinesia	Slowness of movement resulting in a person "freezing"; often misinterpreted as depression and withdrawal; presents as a loss of spontaneity	Parkinson's disease
Chorea	Usually describes a random pattern of rapid, irregular, unpredictable, and involuntary contractions of a group of muscles; resulting clinical picture may be one of a "dancing" or "clownish" gait with the distal extremities more involved than the proximal ones; movements attenuated during sleep, exacerbated with stress and attempts at action	Huntington's chorea; tardive dyskinesia
Dystonia	Although often found as a clinical descriptor, is in fact used to describe a neurological syndrome in which there is an abnormality of tone; affects muscle groups in the trunk, neck, face, and proximal limbs; presents with slow, sustained, involuntary twisting movement patterns that may be generalized, segmental, or focal; confused with athetosis when slow, and chorea when rapid	
Hyperkinesia and hypokinesia	An excess and a paucity of movement, respectively; difficulty with initiation and enactment of a normal speed of movement	All movement disorders, with exception of amyotrophic lateral sclerosis
Spasticity	Extreme or excessive muscle tone; presents as resistance to passive movement; a constant cocontraction of muscle groups inhibiting relaxation pulls the body into abnormal patterns, rendering it vulnerable to deformities; exacerbated by effort	Cerebral palsy; multiple sclerosis
Rigidity	Resistance of proximal and axial muscles to passive movement; frequently experienced as stiffness and associated with pain	Parkinson's disease
Tremor	Simple, involuntary, rhythmic movement, frequently starting in the hands; difficult to differentiate from generalized shivering or shaking; frequently found at rest, but disappears in sleep; most pronounced under stress	Parkinson's disease; multiple sclerosis

person's ability to be a manager who can communicate effectively, identify and use resources, make choices and decisions, set priorities, and make sound judgments (Hammel, 1996).

Teaching strategies that minimize fatigue, conserve energy, enhance safety, and foster adequate stability (particularly postural) are essential for managing self-care for persons with movement disorders

(Gauthier, Dalziel, & Gauthier, 1987). Auditory and visual cues may be necessary to facilitate initiation and speed of movement in persons with movement disorders. In particular, occupational therapy practitioners should consider equipping clients with an array of adaptive strategies from which they can choose for managing their self-care. A person who fatigues easily through the course of the day may

Table 11.2 Summary Data of Major Motor Control Disorders: Manifestations and Presenting Problems

Condition	Features	Movement Problems
Amyotrophic lateral sclerosis	Motor neuron disease of rapid onset; more prevalent in men over 30; affects central and peripheral motor neurons	Progressive muscle weakness and atrophy distally, then proximally; fatigue
Cerebral palsy	Motor disorder resulting from a nonprogressive lesion in the developing brain, resulting in abnormal and fluctuating in abnormal and fluctuating muscle tone and reflexes	Ataxia; athetosis; flaccidity; spasticity; or mixed pattern of movement affecting the limbs, trunk, head, and neck
Charcot–Marie–Tooth	Inherited, progressive, sensorimotor disorder of nervous system; included mild loss of sensation	Progressive muscle weakness starting in extremities, resulting in loss of balance and tripping
Duchenne muscular dystrophy	Hereditary and progressive disease of the muscles; onset in males ages 2 to 6 years of age; marked wasting of proximal muscle groups; moves distally	Rapidly progressive muscle weakness, initially affecting pelvic and pectoral groups; fatigue
Huntington's chorea	Hereditary, progressive disorder of the basal ganglia; characterized by abnormal, involuntary choreiform movements; amplified by progressive cognitive impairment	Abrupt, involuntary choreiform movements; exacerbated by stress and effort
Multiple sclerosis	Lesions in the central nervous system; demyelination results in a series of exacerbations and remissions; progressive weakness; sensory disturbances; cognitive damage	Progressive muscle weakness and spasticity; tremors, ataxia, and fatigue
Parkinson's disease	Degeneration of the basal ganglia; progressive; found most frequently in men and women more than 50 years of age; results in muscle rigidity, postural changes, dementia, loss of autonomic reflexes	Slowness in motor planning; difficulty initiating movement; tremors at rest and with intention; shuffling gait; slurred speech; symptoms exacerbated by fatigue and stress
Tourette's syndrome	Involuntary movement disorder; onset 2 to 5 years of age, primarily males; includes sensory disturbances, impulsivity, compulsive and ritualistic behaviors, with possible attention deficits	Recurrent involuntary, repetitive, rapid movements; hyperactivity; symptoms increase with stress

need to have at least three strategies for getting to the toilet: one using bars on the wall, one using a sliding transfer board, and one requiring the presence of another person for physical support. The choice of strategy will depend on the person's energy level, resources available, urgency, and timing.

Choice of Adaptive Strategy

This chapter is organized according to adaptive strategies in the domains of (a) techniques and equipment and (b) routines and social supports. Strategies consist of actions a person uses to accomplish certain tasks, which in turn organize life.

Within these domains of adaptive strategies, examples of self-care activities such as eating, communicating, mobility, and homemaking are described, and strategies for occupational therapy intervention are discussed.

A person's choice of a specific adaptive strategy is not based on function alone (McCuaig & Frank, 1991). Deciding how to accomplish a task is highly dependent on values that determine the importance and order of potential actions. The decision to choose one piece of equipment, technique, or routine rather than another is also based on the context, possibilities, and requirements of the situation.

All too often, the clinical focus in occupational therapy intervention has been to increase function without consideration of the context in which it is performed. Living with a movement disorder involves more than learning several techniques in a clinical setting or choosing a particular piece of equipment. Physical and social supports and limitations, as well as individual constraints and beliefs, strongly influence behavior and adaptation. A person's choice of action or adaptive strategy will be shaped by temporal factors, personal values, and beliefs about the activity, self, and environment (Fleming, 1991).

Meghan, a woman with cerebral palsy, has personal criteria for choosing her adaptive strategies in self-care activities. Her criteria include being viewed as mentally competent, physically able, and socially acceptable (McCuaig & Frank, 1991). To carry out her activities, she chooses from a variety and combination of strategies that include techniques and equipment, routines, and social resources. As might be expected, Meghan's choice of strategy is frequently based not on functional efficiency but on self-presentation, or how she wishes to appear to others. The techniques, pieces of equipment, routines, or persons supporting her appearance as a competent and socially and physically able person are preferred as adaptive strategies.

Meghan's athetosis, physical deformities, and inability to speak affect her ability to function. Therefore, if she makes tea for her sister, whom she believes views her as incompetent and dependent, she completes every step herself, from boiling the water to pouring the cream in the cups and serving the food. When she is with those who she feels acknowledge her as a competent person, her desire to present a social self and to communicate are more important than her physical abilities. Under these circumstances, she will ask her guest to fix and serve the tea. This leaves her free to use her hands for pointing to her communication system to "chat" with her visitors. However, Meghan directs the activity, indicating which dishes to use and noting where the items are located and where tea will be served. Thus, Meghan has a repertoire of strategies for "making tea" and chooses one based on the context of the event. Who is present and how she is perceived are more important considerations than simply getting the tea from the kettle into the cups.

Adaptive Strategies Using Equipment and Techniques

Adaptive strategies to address self-care management for persons with movement disorders often include methods or techniques involving either specialized or commonplace equipment. See Table 11.3 for factors to consider when making recommendations.

Equipment. Highly specialized equipment used by persons with movement disorders might include powered wheelchairs for those unable to walk (which are discussed later in the chapter) and environmental control systems. Stereo sound systems, telephones, apartment intercoms, lights, fans, and televisions can be accessed with environmental control units using a wide variety of switching devices. Persons lacking the dexterity, coordination, or strength to turn knobs or push buttons directly have easy access to many functions within their living environments through the use of environmental controls (Bain, 1996; Cook & Hussey, 1995).

By contrast, equipment may be "transparent" and not readily identifiable as an adaptive device. Included in this category are conventional items that are widely available commercially yet considered adaptive because of specific characteristics and applications. There are several important advantages to such equipment, including cost, availability, and service and maintenance warranties, which frequently accompany major items. Useful equipment can be found in shopping malls and local hardware stores or through consumer catalogues. Often, commercially available items have easily replaceable parts, minimizing the downtime for malfunctioning equipment. To ensure that such adaptations will not jeopardize the item's warranty, manufacturers should be contacted before making modifications (Gordon & Kozole, 1984).

Examples of transparent adaptive equipment include a typewriter with widely spaced keys for

Table 11.3 Factors To Consider When Recommending Adaptive Strategies

---

What is important to the individual about the task?

Is the strategy viewed as compatible with the particular social context?

Does the strategy enhance the person's sense of personal control?

Does the strategy minimize effort?

Does the strategy interfere with social opportunities or diminish the presentation of self?

Is the recommended strategy temporally realistic, given the context?

Does the strategy provide for safety?

---

someone who lacks the coordination and dexterity to type; felt-tipped pens for a person too weak to exert pressure to write; and front-opening, lightweight clothing to make dressing easier for someone with a movement disorder. Wall-mounted grab bars, which are becoming common in many apartment dwellings, provide stability for someone transferring to and from the toilet. Many persons with movement disorders use commercially available nonskid mats and adhesive strips for bathtubs and showers.

Assessment, prescription, and adaptation of equipment are familiar activities for occupational therapy practitioners. Batavia and Hammer (1990) noted the general absence of consumer-based criteria for the evaluation of equipment. Criteria formulated by consumers could benefit designers, manufacturers, funding agencies, occupational therapy practitioners, and, ultimately, the consumers themselves in the process of choosing appropriate equipment. Batavia and Hammer cited research showing that, in addition to identifying the need for the equipment, important criteria from the consumers' perspectives included effectiveness, affordability, operability, and dependability. It is also interesting to note that the ranking of criteria changed according to the function of the equipment. Acceptability (the esthetics, or psychological "fit") was a high priority for something as personal as a powered wheelchair, but of little consequence in an environmental control unit to operate the stereo.

Among criteria for equipment to be used specifically by persons with a movement disorder is the ability to withstand unusual physical force or stress, which includes falling and inadvertent, uncoordinated hitting. Equipment often needs to be both lightweight to compensate for weakness and durable to withstand being dropped or struck through excess movement. If a person has involuntary movement, safety factors such as stability, absence of sharp edges, and flexibility must be considered. Equipment may need extra padding, bolts may need to be covered, and raw edges may need to be smoothed or sanded. If the person has difficulty initiating and sustaining movement, then sensitivity to touch and the use of lightweight material are important features of equipment. If the person's condition is deteriorating, the equipment must be easy to adapt at little expense to meet changing requirements.

Techniques. Techniques refer to the methods a person has developed or been taught to accomplish a task; techniques often include equipment. Adults frequently use methods that have evolved over the years, often by trial and error, through family member intervention, persistence, and experimentation. Often techniques that appear to be awkward, uncoordinated, and precarious are in fact finely honed and efficacious elements of a highly integrated system.

The occupational therapist's role in teaching adaptive techniques to persons with movement disorders is to observe closely and evaluate the person within his or her traditional environment, giving attention to the larger and potentially fragile system of movement. Techniques designed for persons with movement disorders require observation of timing and an understanding of a person's adaptive use of his or her physical abilities and limitations. Body postures that decrease excessive movements and provide trunk support and proximal stability need to be taught and developed. For those with decreased movement, as in seen in Parkinson's disease, finding the body part that provides consistent, voluntarily controlled movement and does not fatigue easily is important. Rhythmic counting may assist someone who has difficulty initiating movements.

Meal management. Occupational therapy practitioners have paid considerable attention to the development of equipment and specialized techniques for meal management. Very sophisticated feeding apparatus, such as the Winsford and Beesons feeder (Cook & Hussey, 1995), move food from the plate to the mouth by means of a spoon set in motion with an electronic switch, which is useful for adults with cerebral palsy. In other instances, highly individualized devices are fabricated, such as a feeding harness developed for a man with amyotrophic lateral sclerosis, as reported by Takai (1986). Stability for persons with movement disorders is often enhanced by the use of nonskid mats, plate guards, weighted utensils, and utensil holders, such as the universal cuff (Foti, Pedretti, & Lillie, 1996). Commonplace equipment, such as straws and heavy mugs, may be used by persons with poor coordination.

Dysphagia, or difficulty swallowing, frequently occurs in persons with movement disorders, particularly those with amyotrophic lateral sclerosis, cerebral palsy, multiple sclerosis, or Parkinson's disease. This condition is potentially life threatening because of the possibility of aspiration and inadequate nutrition. Weakness of the tongue and palate leads to food retention in the mouth and throat and difficulty maneuvering food in the mouth, such that food may slip into the airway. Poor lip closure may result in drooling. Often, correct assessment and diagnosis, coupled with simple intervention, helps to normalize oral food intake. Occupational therapy intervention for persons with dysphagia has been well documented (Asher, 1986; Nelson, 1996).

We return to the example of Meghan, a woman with athetoid cerebral palsy, for nontraditional examples of how techniques and equipment can be part of an adaptive strategy for meal management. Meghan, who has deformities in her trunk and limbs and an inability to communicate verbally, uses her body as a tool to compensate for the changes in tone that make her movements difficult to predict and control (McCuaig & Frank, 1991). She holds a fork woven unconventionally in and out of the fingers of her right hand. She spears the food with her fork and, balancing on her forearm and elbow, brings the food to her mouth. Her chin rests on her chest with her neck rotated so that her left ear is almost touching her shoulder. This seemingly contorted body position provides the balance she lacks when sitting erect and decreases the effects of the excess movements in her arms when her elbow is not stabilized. A colorful, plastic-coated mat stabilizes her dishes, countering the excess movement in her hands. Meghan is not set apart as different from her mealtime partners by her use of "adapted" equipment. She uses ordinary utensils in extraordinary ways.

Equipment and techniques address only the functional aspect of moving food from the plate to the mouth. Of equal or greater importance for Meghan is the social context of meal management and eating. Although Meghan often invites others for tea or lunch, she rarely eats at these functions. The physical stress of eating, the ensuing fatigue, and the fact that when she is eating she cannot use her hands to access her communication systems, has led to her decision not to eat with others. She explains her decision with this comment: "The reason I very often don't eat with people is I feel I can eat after they go, but I won't be able to talk [after they are gone]." Like most of us, Meghan uses the occasion of tea or a meal for social purposes. Occupational therapy practitioners who emphasize the functional and nutritional aspects of mealtime management have sometimes overlooked this social aspect.

Thus, important considerations for therapy personnel in recommending equipment and techniques may be the extent to which they permit social interaction and whether independence in meal management is important to the person. Is eating viewed as a social occasion? Is eating "independently" with equipment more important than the length of time or the physical effort it takes to finish a meal? Is appearance important, and, if so, are the utensils attractive and pleasant to hold to the tongue and lips? Does the plate guard blend with the plate? Does the color of the nonskid mat clash with that of the table? Do the techniques, such as sliding rather than lifting, minimize effort? Does the independent use of the equipment detract from the potential social opportunities available when a person is fed by another (Einset, Deitz, Billingsley, & Harris, 1989)? What are the time considerations and the fatigue factors? Would several small meals a day be more manageable than the traditional three main meals? These are some of the questions that may be important to determine appropriate adaptive strategies for mealtimes. Further suggestions for adaptive strategies for meal management are described below in the section on adaptive strategies using routines and social supports.

Mobility. Another factor identified as central for adults with movement disorders is independent mobility, both within and outside the person's dwelling (DeJong, 1979; Neuman, Schatzlein, & Sparks, 1987). The physical control a person has over the environment and the ease and freedom with which he or she can move within it influence feelings of independence, dignity, and competence. Physical control also helps to conserve energy.

Equipment recommended for mobility must be considered from perspectives other than function. Stronger than the desire to be mobile may be the need to maintain the view of an able self, which may not include using a wheelchair.

Persons with movement disorders may have substantial changes in ability and endurance over time, even during the course of a day. Accordingly, they may require highly flexible mobility systems. For example, a person with multiple sclerosis may wish to use a manual wheelchair for exercise in the morning and a powered chair for transportation as the day and as his or her fatigue progress.

Particular concerns for occupational therapy practitioners in addressing powered mobility for persons with movement disorders are physical and cognitive control, flexibility, and safety. Positioning for maximum stability is critical and may require special seating, with trunk and head supports. Proximal joints and limbs must be stabilized and extraneous movements controlled to enhance distal control. In general, persons with severe movement disorders involving abnormal or fluctuating muscle tone require customized seating systems. Typically, these include carefully fabricated seating surfaces. Cook and Hussey (1995) and Pederson (1996) provided a useful overview of the issues of seating and positioning for clients with varying levels of need.

Once the most reliable, consistent, voluntarily controlled body movement and location have been determined, the powered wheelchair's control mechanism (usually a joystick) can be adapted to compensate for almost any degree of excess or lack of movement. Wheelchair control mechanisms can be mounted easily in various places on the chair—on the right, the left, centrally, under the chin, or at the back or side of the head. *Latching*, or "cruise control," is an option for those who fatigue easily. *Tremor dampening* is a mechanical means for adjusting the sensitivity of switches so unintentional movement does not activate them. With this feature, switches can be adjusted to work appropriately with almost any degree of excess movement. The speed at which the braking system engages can also be adjusted for someone with a sensitive startle reflex.

For persons with cognitive impairment, occupational therapy practitioners may provide safe environments for practice, extended time to experiment with moving in the powered wheelchair, obstacle courses, and simulation exercises. Practitioners may need to emphasize demonstration and going over verbal instruction.

Particular safety points for powered mobility systems include replacing square-headed bolts with round ones, padding sharp edges, removing heel loops if necessary, and using safety belts and antitipping devices.

Meghan uses a conventional powered wheelchair with a joystick, with the footrests removed. This chair, along with ramped sidewalks, paved roads, and an accessible apartment, gives her the independence she requires to get about in her home environment, go to her appointments, do her shopping, and visit friends who are within commuting distance. She can approach and leave clerks, friends, store displays, and buildings with the same timing, speed, and grace as the general public. She can move across busy streets during the prescribed "walk" interval.

Meghan's ability to extend her body image to include the wheelchair appears to be an important adaptation in her mastery of techniques and the use of equipment. A straight cloth sack made by a friend hangs over the wheelchair handles, allowing Meghan to carry items in the same manner in which a person might use a backpack or a tote bag over a shoulder. Meghan hangs her purse on the right side of the chair. She has personalized the chair with a sticker saying, "Writers have the last word." When looking at Meghan, one has the sense not of a person sitting in a wheelchair, but of a unit, a goodness of fit.

Communication. People engage in different modes of communication. *Conversation*, commonly a brief, temporal, and often spontaneous verbal exchange, is usually thought of as the most common. These verbal exchanges include changes in intonation and timing and are accompanied by facial expressions, gestures, and body language. Conversation takes place in face-to-face situations, over the telephone, or simultaneously with an activity. *Messaging*, another mode of communication, is the delayed presentation of previously prepared information. Common tools for messaging include pens or pencils, typewriters, facsimile machines, telephone answering devices, and computers. When a person is unable to use the conventional modes and tools of communication for conversation or sending messages, the dynamics and quality of the interaction are affected.

Augmentative communication includes any personal or technical system that enhances a person's present communication abilities. These devices may produce speech, a visual display, or a written message. Body parts, such as a hand, the head, or eyes, are used to access the devices directly or indirectly.

Communication aids may take many forms. A man unable to move from the neck down uses a pointer held in his teeth to dial his telephone. He has learned to use his mouth to manipulate the pointer as a substitute for his hand, and he uses the pointer as his finger to dial the numbers (Zola, 1982).

Meghan has a wide variety of universal or commonplace communication devices, including felt-tipped pens, an electric typewriter with widely spaced keys, a computer, and a telephone. She also uses specialized equipment, including an 8 in. by 11 in. letter board indicating the letters of the alphabet to which she points to spell her message (see Figure 11.1); a Canon Communicator™, which is a small, portable, battery-operated device with keys that she presses to produce a ticker tape-printed message; and a Vocaid, a device that produces synthesized sounds in the form of letters and is

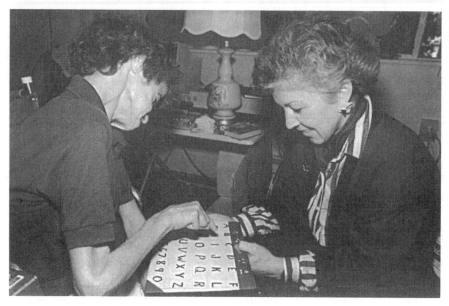

Figure 11.1 Meghan communicating through her letter board.

attached to her telephone, enabling her to spell messages to her caller. Meghan also uses her voice, facial expressions, and gestures to convey a message. She has a repertoire of equipment and techniques from which to choose, based on the context of the communication that is taking place.

Meghan's decision regarding which piece of equipment to use is based not only on wanting to present an able self but also on her perceptions of the demands of the situation and on her expectations of the exchange. If Meghan is having a conversation with a friend, she likes to sit close to that person with the letter board on her lap, point to the letters as she spells out her message, and have her friend repeat the letters and say the resulting words. Although this method is slow (approximately 12 words per minute), it allows Meghan to make frequent eye contact and to stay engaged with her partner. She can use her other hand to gesture, and she can use her face and body to express feelings. The "voice" is personal and not synthesized.

When Meghan is in a place such as the drug store, a situation that engenders fewer personal communication expectations, she uses her electronic Canon Communicator. This device resembles a small pocket calculator, looks attractive, produces a written message that is easy to see, and is understood by all who can read. Meghan has tried to use her letter board in public, but says, "People just think I'm retarded pointing to this dumb piece of paper, and ignore me." She finds that persons are interested in her Canon Communicator, and that it can be an icebreaker for persons who are not

familiar with her methods. With a store clerk, Meghan needs only to deliver a message that will not be ignored and that will get her the items she requires. Meghan's desire to present a sophisticated and capable image is supported by her use of this device in public.

In assessment and intervention for communication needs, occupational therapy practitioners work closely with speech and language pathologists to determine the ease of access to the equipment and the requirements of the social and physical environment. For persons with movement disorders, specific recommendations for communication needs include enlarged pencils, writing aids that hold a pen or pencil, and felt-tipped pens. For persons who can use typewriters, computers, or electronic communicators, key guards that prevent more than one key from being pressed at the same time can help those with poor coordination. Enlarged keyboards for computers are useful for persons who lack the fine-motor skills to access a standard-size keyboard. Mini keyboards are available for persons who lack range and muscle strength in their upper extremities.

Often a person has sufficient control of the head and neck to permit the use of mouthsticks or head wands for operating augmentative communication devices. Mouthsticks made of lightweight doweling or arrow shafts with rubber tubing on the end may be useful for persons with adequate neck and jaw control and movement. Smith (1989) noted that inadequate attention has been given to the potential problems of improperly fitted mouthsticks.

In addition to oral problems, consequences of improperly fitting mouthpiece components include fatigue, gagging, and temporomandibular joint dysfunction. Practitioners are urged to consider the standards developed by Blaine and Nelson (1973) when prescribing mouthsticks. Head pointers offer another option for using augmentative communication devices, and these can be custom made or obtained commercially.

Other important considerations when determining appropriate equipment and techniques for communication are rate of transmission, portability of the system, reliability, flexibility, spontaneity, and the system's potential for expressing the fullness of the message. An augmentative system should require as little expenditure of energy as possible, for both the sender and the receiver of the message. It must enhance one's personal abilities and, wherever possible, encourage physical gestures and expressions of sound. The equipment must also meet the requirements of the physical and social environments.

Adaptive Strategies Using Routines and Social Supports

Behaviors, repeated over time and organized into patterns and habits, form routines. Routines and the use of social supports can be considered adaptive strategies for persons with movement disorders, because they compensate for the inability to perform certain activities, the extended length of time and energy required to accomplish a task, and the limited coordination and strength available to the person with a movement disorder. Frequently, a person's strategy for accomplishing a task employs a unique combination of equipment, techniques, routines, and social supports. These social supports may take the form of family members and friends, casual acquaintances, formal and informal organizations, or health care workers within and without institutions.

The use of adaptive strategies employing routines and social supports often depends on specific factors. The person needs to know that a certain activity or interaction is going to take place and what the requirements of the situation will be. The person must also have time to plan, have a well-developed ability to organize personal and environmental resources, have the perception of how long an activity will take, understand what the specific steps will involve, and know how much energy will be needed. Routines generally have a sense of predictability and familiarity, in that they have usually been used successfully in the past under similar, if not identical, conditions. Social supports need to be initiated, nurtured, and developed.

Communication. Emma, a woman who has amyotrophic lateral sclerosis and lives in a long-term-care facility, uses a variety of techniques and pieces of equipment for communication to adapt to her inability to speak and to her lack of movement in her limbs. She has a letter and word board to which she can point with hand movements that are slow and difficult. She also has a computerized message system, which she operates with a microswitch in her palm; and a system of eye blinking, which she uses in conjunction with the communication partner's verbal spelling. In addition, Emma has established routines for communication that are considered adaptive because of their premeditated, compensatory nature.

Emma, like Meghan, determines which strategy to use after considering outcome, context, and values. She decides in advance the purpose of the communication, the intended recipient of the message, what she expects from the exchange, and what is important for her to achieve. Emma decides ahead of time whether it is more important to save the other person time by having information ready, or whether the conversation process and the elements of the interaction are of greater significance than the message itself. One of Emma's routines for communicating is to provide her communication partner with the bulk of information in the format of a printout from her computer. This routine requires Emma's knowledge of the visit before it occurs, adequate time to compose her thoughts and messages at the computer, and the ability of her communication partner to read. She is very aware of the importance of her social support system and consciously works at sustaining these networks. It requires much more of Emma's time, but considerably less of her partner's, if she puts her thoughts on paper before the interaction. It also provides the partner with something to read and on which to focus. Emma can work at her own pace at her computer when she has the energy, and she can take rest periods, which in conversation would be awkward and possibly stressful for the partner.

Many persons with movement disorders that include loss of speech struggle with the assumption of one disability based on the presence of another (Wright, 1983). The inability to speak is frequently equated with the inability to think. The strategy Emma has developed for communicating with per-

217

sons through a prepared note helps to dispel any misconceptions the partner might have of her cognitive abilities. The notes contain witticisms, inquiries about the partner's well-being, social comments about the news or weather, descriptions of her sons' activities, and her feelings about events on the ward. Emma presents herself as a socially competent woman, full of ideas and feelings, and actively engaged in life.

Homemaking. The following incident demonstrates the use of routines and social supports as an adaptive strategy for homemaking activities. Lee is a woman who has Parkinson's disease with resulting intention tremor in her upper extremities, head, and neck; a slow and shuffling gait; rigidity in her trunk; and slurred speech. She shares a home with her elderly husband. Having friends in for tea once a week is an important social event for Lee. When her guests arrive, the cups and saucers are out on a cart, along with the cream, sugar, napkins, and a cake. During the tea, Lee plays the host, directing the event. She manages everything, deciding when to hold the tea, what to serve, and who will pour. She has a keen sense of timing, is extremely gracious and social in her requests, is well-organized, and gives clear directions.

For Lee to execute the activities of this very ordinary but important occasion, she must invest considerable planning time and effort. She needs to travel in her scooter to the local mall to buy the cake and other grocery items, and she must transport them safely home. She has to have her cups clean and arranged on the tray ahead of time. Her problems with strength, balance, dexterity, and coordination make an apparently easy task one that requires a great deal of orchestration.

Meal management. For many persons with movement disorders, eating can be an exhausting and undignified experience, whether managing food independently or being fed. The physical and emotional strain of getting the food on the utensil, bringing it safely to the lips, keeping it in the mouth, chewing adequately, swallowing smoothly, and maintaining a comfortable posture can be great. Weighted handles, nonskid mats, plate guards, and even automatic feeding devices are often not adequate to support a person's nutritional, social, and personal needs related to eating. As with other self-care activities, function alone is not sufficient for a satisfying experience at mealtime. While being fed brings its own set of problems, it is often the strategy of choice for persons unable to manage a meal in a

reasonable amount of time and with a minimum of effort.

Catherine, a young woman with cerebral palsy living in an extended-care facility, prefers to be fed rather than to feed herself. She has spent countless hours practicing, trying different pieces of equipment and physical positions. The combination of her severe athetoid movements, poor head control, and general weakness makes eating independently an unpleasant chore. She now prefers to spend her energy writing at her computer, visiting with friends, and going to school. To make her mealtime pleasant, she has asked to be fed in her room, and she invites one other person who also needs to be fed to join her and the aide who is feeding her. When she orders her meal she includes an extra tea and biscuit for the aide. This is a treat for the aide and adds to the feeling of the meal being more of a shared and social experience. Catherine also has the television turned on to her favorite soap opera at noon and to the news in the evening. This too is a treat for the aide and gives both Catherine and the aide something on which to focus and discuss. The conversation, the meal, and the company promote a relaxed atmosphere and help to minimize the potential boredom, and therefore the stress, of the aide.

When occupational therapy practitioners plan mealtime interventions, they should always think about how to create an environment that promotes eating as an enjoyable social event rather than simply a nutritional exercise. At its best, eating is an intimate affair; at its worst, it is traumatic. Wherever possible, the physical environment should promote relaxation and comfort. Attention should be given to room temperature, noise level, and visual stimulation, particularly if the person has a sensitive startle reaction. A quiet room may suit one person, whereas another person might prefer company. Persons who need to be fed can be taught how to engage the interest and attention of the person feeding them. They can be encouraged to take control of choices, determining what food to eat and when and how quickly items are presented and in what order. They can also help to identify what elements of the mealtime event are stressful and collaborate with the practitioners in addressing them.

Facilitating the Development of Routines and Social Supports

Research in multiple sclerosis (Brooks & Matson, 1982) has suggested that social psychological variables are the most important explanatory models of adjustment to the disease. In particular, integrating the realities of the disease into the lifestyle, and depending on strong social support networks, have each been identified as important variables for persons with this progressive, episodic, and debilitating neuromotor condition. Thus, research has shown that the development of adaptive routines and social supports is an effective therapeutic strategy.

Practitioners can help persons with all types of movement disorders to develop strategies that use routines and social supports by facilitating a person's repeated action beyond basic problem solving until a routine is established and acceptable to the persons and those in his or her environment. During this process, practitioners should help develop routines that minimize stress and conserve energy. Routines require planning and organization to allow persons to do the most important activities when they have the most energy, maximizing both safety and enjoyment.

Therapy sessions can be planned to support a person's shift from focusing on the physical to the cognitive domain. A person who is no longer able to execute an activity physically may need to learn to organize and plan to direct care. Overvaluing the concept of independence may lead to goals that seek to achieve levels of function that are too costly in terms of expended energy. Assistance with personal care may be preferable to independence in activities of daily living if the physical and mental costs of attaining independence interfere with social interaction or life satisfaction (Gillette, 1991). Social supports must be sought out, developed, nurtured, and maintained. Attention must be given to ways in which the distress, enormous effort, and tedium of living with and supporting someone with a physical disability can be managed so that important social supports can be maintained as integral components of a person's adaptive strategies.

Summary

Strategies that minimize fatigue, enhance safety, and reduce stress are important. Attention to organization, pacing, timing, and energy conservation are also important for managing self-care by persons with movement disorders. A philosophy of independent living that emphasizes the importance of a person's acquisition of skills and capabilities for self-direction in managing physical and social resources has been embraced. However, this philosophy also acknowledges that a person can exhibit an independent spirit while accepting assis-

tance from others, and that all adaptive strategies must be considered in terms of their contribution to overall well-being and life satisfaction. In working with persons with movement disorders, the role of the therapist is to identify, in conjunction with the client, an array of adaptive strategies that can be used comfortably within the context of the client's daily life. ◆

Study Questions

1. What are adaptive strategies?

2. List two examples of adaptive strategies for communication, mobility, home management, and eating.

3. Why should persons with movement disorders be equipped with an array of adaptive strategies?

4. What are important factors to consider when recommending equipment for persons with movement disorders?

5. How can routines and social supports be facilitated?

References

Asher, I. E. (1986). Dysphagia in the adult population: The role of occupational therapy. *Occupational Therapy in Health Care, 3,* 5–21.

Bain, B. (1996). Environmental controls and robotics. In J. Hammel (Ed.), *Technology and occupational therapy: A link to function.* Bethesda, MD: American Occupational Therapy Association.

Batavia, A. I., & Hammer, G. S. (1990). Toward the development of consumer-based criteria for the evaluation of assistive devices. *Journal of Rehabilitation Research, 27,* 425–436.

Blaine, H. L., & Nelson, E. P. (1973). A mouthstick for quadriplegic patients. *Journal of Prosthetic Dentistry, 29,* 317–322.

Brooks, N., & Matson, R. R. (1982). Social psychological adjustment to multiple sclerosis. A longitudinal study. *Social Science and Medicine, 16,* 2129–2135.

Christiansen, C. (1991) Occupational performance assessment. In C. Christiansen & C. Baum (Eds.), *Occupational therapy: Overcoming human performance deficits* (pp. 376–424). Thorofare, NJ: Slack.

Cook, A. M., & Hussey, S. M. (1995). Technologies that aid manipulation and control of the environment. In A. M. Cook & S. M. Hussey (Eds.), *Assistive technologies: Principles and practice* (pp. 575–629). St. Louis, MO: Mosby-Yearbook.

Corbin, J. M., & Strauss, A. (1988). *Unending work and care: Managing chronic illness at home.* San Francisco: Jossey-Bass.

DeJong, G. (1979). Defining and implementing the independent living concept. In N. M. Crewe & I. K. Zola (Eds.), *Independent living for physically disabled people* (pp. 4–27). San Francisco: Jossey-Bass.

Einset, K., Deitz, J., Billingsley, F., & Harris, S. R. (1989). The electric feeder: An efficacy study. *Occupational Therapy Journal of Research, 9,* 38–52.

Fleming, M. (1991). The therapist with the three-track mind. *American Journal of Occupational Therapy, 45,* 1007–1014.

Foti, D., Pedretti, L. W., & Lillie, S. (1996). Activities of daily living. In L. W. Pedretti (Ed.), *Occupational therapy: Practice skills for physical dysfunction* (4th ed., pp. 463–506). St. Louis, MO: Mosby.

Gauthier, L., Dalziel, S., & Gauthier, S. (1987). The benefits of group occupational therapy for patients with Parkinson's disease. *American Journal of Occupational Therapy, 41,* 360–365.

Gillette, N. (1991). The challenge of research in occupational therapy. *American Journal of Occupational Therapy, 45,* 660–662.

Gordon, R. E., & Kozole, K. P. (1984). Occupational therapy and rehabilitation engineering: Team approach to helping persons with severe physical disability to upgrade functional independence. *Occupational Therapy and Health Care, 1*(4), 117–129.

Hammel, J. (Ed.). (1996). *Technology and occupational therapy: A link to function.* Bethesda, MD: American Occupational Therapy Association.

Jain, S. S., & Kirshblum, S. C. (1993). Movement disorders, including tremors. In J. DeLisa & B. Gans (Eds.), *Rehabilitation medicine: Principles and practice* (2nd ed., pp. 700–715). Philadelphia: Lippincott.

Lohr, J. B., & Wisniewski, A. A. (1987). *Movement disorders: A neuropsychiatric approach.* New York: Guilford.

McCuaig, M., & Frank, G. (1991). The able self: Adaptive patterns and choices in independent living for a person with cerebral palsy. *American Journal of Occupational Therapy, 45,* 224–243.

Nelson, K. L. (1996). Dysphagia: Evaluation and treatment. In L. W. Pedretti (Ed.), *Occupational therapy: Practice skills for physical dysfunction* (4th ed., pp.165–191). St. Louis, MO: Mosby.

Neuman, S. S., Schatzlein, J. E., & Sparks, R. (1987). Technology. In N. M. Crewe & I. K. Zola (Eds.), *Independent living for physically disabled people* (pp. 245–270). San Francisco: Jossey-Bass.

Pederson, J. P. (1996). Seating and wheeled mobility for OTs. In J. Hammel (Ed.), *Technology and occupational therapy: A link to function.* Bethesda, MD: American Occupational Therapy Association.

Smith, R. (1989). Mouthstick design for the client with spinal cord injury. *American Journal of Occupational Therapy, 43,* 251–255.

Takai, V. L. (1986). Case report: The development of a feeding harness for an ALS patient. *American Journal of Occupational Therapy, 40,* 359–361.

Wright, B. (1983). *Physical disability: A psychosocial approach* (2nd ed.). New York: Harper & Row.

Zola, I. K. (1982). *Missing pieces: A chronicle of living with a disability.* Philadelphia: Temple University Press.

Suggested Readings

Carroll, D. L., Dudley, J., & Dorman, M. D. (1993). *Living well with MS: A guide for patient, caregiver, and family.* New York: Harper Perennial.

Duvoisin, R. C. (1996). *Parkinson's disease: A guide for patients and family* (4th ed.). Philadelphia: Lippincott.

Goetz, C. G. (1997). Tardive dyskinesia. In R. L. Watts & W. C. Koller (Eds.), *Movement disorders: Neurological principles and practice* (pp. 519–526). New York: McGraw-Hill.

Lynch, S. G., & Rose, J. W. (1996). *Disease-a-month: Multiple sclerosis.* Chicago: Year Book Medical.

McGill, F. (1980). *Go not gently: Letters from a patient with amyotrophic lateral sclerosis.* New York: Arno.

Montgomery, M. A. (1984). Resources of adaptation for daily living: A classification with therapeutic implications for occupational therapy. *Occupational Therapy in Health Care, 1*(4), 9–24.

Rose, F. C. (Ed.). (1990). *Amyotrophic lateral sclerosis.* New York: Demos.

Trombly, C. A. (1995). *Occupational therapy for physical dysfunction* (4th ed.). Baltimore: Williams & Wilkins.

12

Managing Self-Care in Adults With Upper-Extremity Amputations

Diane J. Atkins

Diane J. Atkins, OTR, is Coordinator, Amputee Program, The Institute for Rehabilitation and Research, Houston, Texas, and Assistant Professor, Department of Physical Medicine and Rehabilitation, Baylor College of Medicine, Houston, Texas.

Key Terms

amputee center of excellence

biscapular abduction

body-powered prostheses

desensitization

disarticulation

electric prostheses

functional use training

humeral flexion

hybrid prosthesis

preprosthetic program

terminal device

Objectives

On completing this chapter, the reader will be able to

1. Identify the important elements to be considered in a preprosthetic program.

2. Understand important prosthetic training principles as they relate to body-powered and electric prostheses.

3. Identify the major differences between the hook and the myoelectric hand.

4. Discuss what accounts for the successful rehabilitation of a person with an amputation.

5. Understand appropriate functional outcomes as they relate to persons with unilateral and bilateral amputations.

We are often enriched by the personal aura and spirit of persons who manage life with disabilities, each in his individual special way. (*Marquardt, 1989*)

Upper-extremity amputation presents a complex loss for the patient. The hand functions in prehensile activities as a sensory organ and as a means of communication. Any loss will interfere with the patient's productivity and feeling of completeness, as well as alter his or her interactions with the environment (Bennett & Alexander, 1989).

Each person with an upper-extremity amputation is unique, and no two amputations are identical. Because each of us is so dependent on arms and hands, the person with an upper-extremity amputation—particularly one who has lost both arms—is initially devastated and unprepared to perform even a simple task. Therefore, rehabilitation of that person can be one of the most challenging and rewarding clinical opportunities a practitioner can experience. Additionally, the occupational therapy practitioner becomes the key player in assisting the person with an upper-extremity amputation to become confident and self-reliant.

Independence in all functional activities is the goal of almost every person with an upper-extremity amputation, and this goal is entirely possible. The exception to the outcome of total independence, however, is seen in bilateral, very short, above-the-elbow amputations and in bilateral amputations at the shoulder. Although some persons with upper-extremity amputations may choose not to wear a prosthesis, the goal of occupational therapy is to enable that person to feel complete in his or her self-image and to be as independent and self-reliant as possible. Every person with an upper-extremity amputation should be given the opportunity to use a prosthesis, and it is ultimately his or her choice as to whether that prosthesis will become a part of daily life.

In this chapter, the preprosthetic and prosthetic training process will be reviewed, and several case studies presented. These case studies demonstrate the vital, essential link the occupational therapy practitioner provides in the total rehabilitation experience of the person with an upper-extremity amputation.

The Preprosthetic Therapy Program

The preprosthetic therapy phase begins when the sutures are removed and the wound has healed, generally about 2 to 3 weeks after surgery. Occupational therapy personnel are the primary professionals who will manage and monitor this program. The nursing staff members should be thoroughly familiar with these goals as well, and often the occupational therapy practitioner can assist with their instruction.

The goals of the preprosthetic therapy program are to:

- promote residual limb shrinkage and shaping,
- promote residual limb desensitization,
- maintain normal joint range of motion,
- increase muscle strength,
- provide instruction in the proper hygiene of the limb,
- maximize self-reliance in the performance of tasks required for daily living,
- explore the patient's goals regarding the future,
- inform the patient about prosthetic options, and
- determine the electrical potential provided by various muscles (this procedure, known as *myoelectric site testing*, is necessary if myoelectric prosthetic components are prescribed) (Atkins, 1989a).

The Prosthetic Training Program

Before initiating a program of upper-extremity prosthetic training, one must realistically orient the patient as to what the prosthesis can and cannot do. If the patient has an unrealistic expectation about the usefulness of the prosthesis as a replacement arm, he or she may be dissatisfied with the ultimate functioning of the prosthesis and may reject it altogether. Alternatively, if the expectations of the patient are realistic at the beginning of training, ultimate acceptance will be based on the ability of the prosthesis to improve the person's performance. It is imperative, then, that the practitioner be honest and positive about the function of the prosthesis. If the person with an amputation "believes in" and understands the functional potential of the prosthesis, successful rehabilitation is more likely (Atkins, 1989b).

It is recommended that a person with a recent amputation be taken to a quiet room without distractions, where the practitioner can begin to familiarize him or her with the new prosthesis. The training progression includes learning prosthetic terminology, donning and doffing the prosthesis, and orienting the person to the body movements required to operate the prosthesis. Simple grasp-and-release activities follow the orientation. As the treatment program progresses and the patient becomes more comfortable with a new body image, the practitioner should involve him or her in the clinic treatment area. The practitioner may introduce the patient to and try to encourage socialization with others. If possible, it is useful to schedule another person with a similar level of limb loss during the same treatment time (Atkins, 1994).

To reduce anxiety and frustration, early learning experiences for patients should be selected with success in mind. It is important to practice activities of daily living that are useful and purposeful. Thus, cutting food, using scissors, dressing, opening jars and bottles, washing dishes, using household tools (such as a hammer), and driving are all functionally important activities that can be practiced during treatment. Atkins (1989b) stressed the importance of careful positioning before attempting functional tasks, because most difficulties result from improper positioning. To facilitate proper positioning, the patient should be instructed to orient the components of the prosthesis in space to a position resembling that of a normal limb engaged in the same task.

A few techniques should be mentioned here. The prosthesis always functions as the nonpreferred extremity did, as the stabilizer of objects. When cutting meat, the fork is placed between the hook fingers and behind the prosthetic thumb. The knife is held in the unaffected extremity. Principles of dressing are the same as for a person after a stroke: The prosthesis is dressed first and undressed last.

Success can be defined as the patients' daily wearing of their prostheses and their incorporation of their new arm in most bilateral activities. It is important that persons with amputations view this new tool as an important extension of the body. A revised body image should incorporate this new look and presentation. The level of a unilateral amputation largely influences whether the prosthesis is both used and accepted. Successful outcomes in rehabilitation for the unilateral and bilateral amputee can be attributed to the following factors:

- Early posttraumatic intervention
- Experienced team approach
- Patient-directed prosthetic training
- Patient education
- Patient monitoring and follow-up (Atkins, 1989b)

Functional Outcomes at Various Levels of Amputation

Persons with unilateral upper-extremity amputations will often be able to accomplish most of their activities of daily living with one arm. With this in mind, it is extremely important to fit the unilateral upper extremity with a prosthesis within 3 months of losing the arm. If fitted within 3 months, the persons with an amputation will generally still be thinking about accomplishing tasks in a two-handed way and will automatically use the prosthesis appropriately. Those amputees who have been without a prosthesis for longer than 3 months will generally choose to accomplish a task unilaterally rather than try to think how the task used to be performed with two hands. It, therefore, becomes more difficult to train a person with a prosthesis, because he or she has become dependent on the sound arm to accomplish most tasks.

Unilateral Below-Elbow Amputation

Following the loss of a hand, a wrist disarticulation or a long below-elbow amputation is desirable, because supination and pronation are preserved. It is important that the prosthesis fits comfortably and that the components function well before beginning functional training. The practitioner should communicate openly and frequently with the prosthetist not only initially but also when the patient is fit for the prosthesis or when concerns about its operation arise.

Body-Powered or Electric Prosthetic Prescription

The question of which upper-extremity prosthetic device is appropriate—an all body-powered, all-electric, or a hybrid (combination of body-powered and electric)—is a challenging one. Some of the advantages of the hook-type, body-powered prosthesis include lighter weight, better durability, increased sensory feedback, less expense, and greater ease in seeing the manipulated object. Advantages of the electric arm include better appearance, moderate or no harnessing, less body movement to operate, greater ability to reach overhead and to grasp larger objects, and better grip strength.

The most effective method for determining the appropriate prosthetic prescription is accomplished with the amputee rehabilitation team. This team includes a physiatrist, prosthetist, occupational and physical practitioners, nurse, and social worker. The patient, of course, is also a critical team player. His or her needs and desires need to be heard and addressed in the final prescription.

Finances may restrict the purchase of an all-electric prosthetic arm, which can cost from $15,000 to $80,000. A less expensive, hybrid prosthesis may be a better choice, although the body-powered prosthesis is the arm of choice for many persons with upper-extremity amputations who have had the opportunity to try both types. Referring the person with a complex or bilateral upper-extremity amputation to a specialized "center of excellence" may be a desirable option—personnel there have many years of extensive experience with hundreds of upper-extremity amputees.

Achieving Successful Amputee Rehabilitation

An unusually high rejection rate of upper-extremity prostheses can often be attributed to the following reasons (Burrough & Brook, 1985):

- Development of one-handedness, which removes the functional need for the prosthesis
- Lack of sufficient training or skill in using the prosthesis
- Poor comfort of the prosthesis or a poorly made prosthesis
- Unnatural look or profile of the prosthesis
- Reactions that the wearer gets from others

The motions that are required to operate a body-powered, below-elbow prosthesis are humeral flexion and biscapular abduction. These motions separately, or accomplished together, open the terminal device of a hook or hand. If a person with a below-elbow amputation is performing activities at midline, such as buttoning a button, fastening a buckle, or cutting meat, scapular abduction alone will enable the person to open the hook or hand in the area immediately in front of him or her.

Functional use training is the most challenging and prolonged stage of the prosthetic training process. The success or failure of the patient's acceptance and use of the prosthesis depends on (a) the motivation of the patient, (b) the comprehensiveness and quality of the tasks and activities practiced, and (c) the experience and enthusiasm of the occupational therapy practitioner (this is critical). The functional training experience is most effective if the same practitioner remains with the patient throughout the entire process (Atkins, 1989b).

The decision to use a myoelectrically controlled below-elbow prosthesis must be evaluated by the entire team, and particularly by the person who will be using it. So far, there is no definitive standard by which to determine the ideal candidate for myoelectric use.

The myoelectric arm did not achieve widespread commercial availability until the 1960s. The concept of myoelectric control is very simple: One uses an electric signal from a muscle to control the flow of energy from a battery to a motor. In a myoelectric prosthesis, the control signal comes from a muscle remnant (the wrist flexor and wrist extensor in a below-elbow amputation) that still has normal innervation and thus is subject to voluntary control. The motor actuates a prosthetic hand, wrist, or elbow.

The person with a unilateral below-elbow amputation should be expected to achieve complete independence. The sound arm and hand will accomplish the major part of any bilateral task, with the prosthesis providing a gross functional assist. Certain activities, such as buttoning, tying shoes, and cutting meat, may initially require special adaptive equipment. Eventually, however, many persons with unilateral wrist disarticulation and below-elbow amputations reject adaptive devices and learn their own techniques for accomplishing virtually all of their activities (Atkins, 1994). The following case study provides an example of the management of this type of patient.

Case Study I

L. G. is a woman 20 years of age from Houston, Texas. She lost her left hand below the elbow in 1990, in an automobile accident. Within 3 months of the amputation, L. G. was involved in a preprosthetic program, which included wrapping the residual limb in elasticized bandages to shape it properly, practicing desensitization techniques, and performing range of motion and muscle-strengthening exercises.

L. G. was initially fitted and trained with a body-powered prosthesis, because that was the only prosthesis the state would pay for through her insurance. L. G. was never satisfied with the appearance of a hook-type, body-powered prosthesis, and, although she wore and used the prosthesis, she hoped to acquire a myoelectric prosthesis. Approximately 2 months after receiving her body-powered prosthesis, L. G. received funding from a philanthropic charity in Houston, which allowed her to purchase a myoelectric arm.

Her myoelectric arm training included an orientation to many two-handed activities, such as opening jars (see Figure 12.1). L. G. was instructed to use her myoelectric hand as the functional assist (holding the jar) and her sound hand to do the major part of the activity. Today L. G. is totally independent in all activities of daily living. She works full time and has a young daughter. She uses both body-powered and electric prostheses and sometimes chooses to use no prosthesis at all.

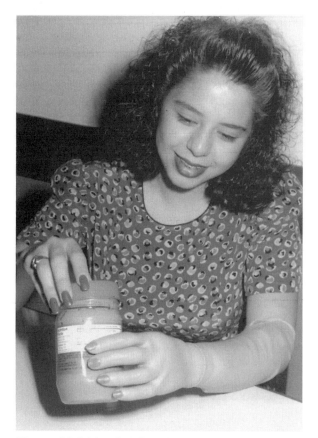

Figure 12.1 Myoelectric training includes two-handed activities such as opening a jar.

Unilateral Above-Elbow Amputation

In the case of an amputation above the elbow, the decision regarding which components to use takes additional time, planning, and discussion with the amputee team and patient. The human elbow joint is an extremely valuable joint, and its loss seriously affects the ease with which one learns to use an above-elbow prosthesis. At best, the above-elbow prosthesis provides a good functional assist in most bilateral activities. Developing the ability to use an above-elbow prosthesis takes time, commitment, and strong motivation on the part of the patient.

Body-powered elbows or electric elbows may be included in the prosthetic prescription. If myoelectric operation of the elbow unit is selected, control with remnant biceps and triceps muscle contractions is usually possible. Financial sponsorship is an important factor in the determination of the components of an above-elbow prosthesis. A totally electric prosthesis can cost as much as $80,000, whereas a totally body-powered prosthesis is approximately $10,000.

Various combinations of body-powered and electric elbows, used in conjunction with myoelectric hands and body-powered hooks, can be used in a hybrid prosthesis. Some hybrid prostheses offer an interchangeable hook and myoelectric hand in the same prosthesis. A device of this type is an excellent alternative for persons who value function and appearance (see Figure 12.2).

The principles of training a person with an above-elbow amputation are identical to those for training someone with a below-elbow amputation. In addition to using scapular abduction and humeral flexion to open the terminal device, the body-powered elbow locks and unlocks through a combination of shoulder abduction depression and extension. This process is often described as an "out, down, and back" motion. Learning to lock and unlock the elbow can be one of the most frustrating aspects of learning to use an above-elbow prosthesis. It is extremely important that patients be proficient at locking and unlocking the elbow before attempting two-handed functional tasks.

When bilateral activities are initially attempted, the person with an amputation should be given simple and positive learning experiences. More ad-

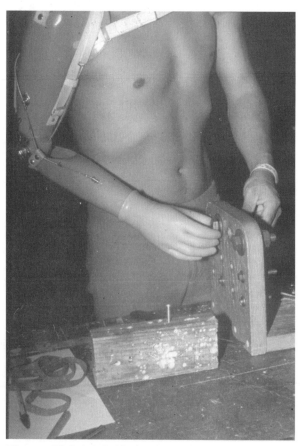

Figure 12.2 A hybrid prosthesis that includes a body-powered elbow and electric hand.

vanced bilateral tasks, such as building a woodworking project with various tools can be attempted later. All persons with an above-elbow prosthesis should be able to achieve complete independence in functional activities of daily living. Case Study 2 describes the management of the person shown in Figure 12.2.

Case Study 2

E. R. is a man 25 years of age from Mexico who sustained a right above-elbow amputation while operating a rice-cleaning machine in 1980. A full-thickness skin graft was taken from his back to cover the end of the residual limb. His preprosthetic program began 2 months after the amputation. During the preprosthetic phase, E. R. was shown a variety of terminal devices and made a very strong request for a myoelectric hand. Because finances were a consideration, the prescription was for a hybrid-type prosthesis; the prosthesis incorporated a myoelectric hand and a body-powered elbow. E. R. was pleased with this combination and agreed to be fitted with a body-powered hook that could be interchanged with the electric hand.

E. R. did extremely well in his occupational therapy program and returned to work full time less than 4 months following his injury. He used his hook at work in the rice factory and his myoelectric hand for social occasions. Three years after his accident, E. R. decided to study engineering in school. He wore and actively used his prosthesis 12 to 14 hours a day. He wears his hook two thirds of the time and his hand approximately one third, and he returns to the Amputee Clinic in Houston on an as-needed basis.

Bilateral Below-Elbow Amputation

The loss of both hands is one of the most traumatic events one can experience. To suddenly become totally dependent on someone else can be a devastating reality. It is extremely important to give these persons some sense of independence and control over their environment before they are fit with prostheses. A universal cuff (an elastic band with a small pocket and a hook-and-loop closure) is ideal to use with a fork or spoon, toothbrush, and pen or pencil. Every opportunity for independence for these persons should be encouraged.

For persons who have lost both hands, body-powered hooks are generally preferred over myoelectric hands. Person who have lost both hands state that they prefer the valuable proprioceptive and kinesthetic feedback they experience when using a body-powered hook. Being able to "feel"

what they are doing, rather than always looking at the task when they wear a myoelectric hand, is a distinct advantage. Wrist flexion units, at least on the dominant side, or perhaps bilaterally, permit midline activities such as shirt buttoning, belt buckling, and toileting. In addition, wrist rotator units, which allow for automatic terminal device positioning, provide for easier bilateral prosthetic use. Special toileting techniques must be taught. Foot skills should also be reviewed, and lower-extremity mobilizing exercises may be performed (Leonard & Meier, 1998).

The progression of prosthetic training for the person with bilateral below-elbow amputations is similar to that for someone with a unilateral amputation. Simple, success-oriented tasks should be introduced early, followed by more advanced bilateral tasks. It is important to stress and reinforce skills in writing, eating, toothbrushing, toileting, bathing, and dressing. These activities reestablish a sense of control and self-esteem. Following mastery of these tasks, vocational, avocational, and recreational activities can be explored.

The person with bilateral below-elbow amputation who uses prostheses can almost always achieve considerable self-reliance with very few, if any, adaptive devices. Those with bilateral below-elbow amputations prove to be the most consistent wearers and users of prostheses. With few exceptions, the prostheses tend to become an essential part of life and body image (Atkins, 1994).

Case Study 3

W. S. is a man 48 years of age who lost both arms below the elbow in 1982, when his hands became entangled in a corn picker. He was hospitalized immediately and rehabilitation followed as soon as his wounds had healed. Before receiving his prostheses, W. S. used a universal cuff for writing, eating, and brushing his teeth. He was extremely motivated to be fit with prostheses and to be independent again. W. S. received his prostheses 1 month after the injury and learned how to use them quickly and proficiently. A release to return to work was written 2 months following the accident. W. S. has no desire for myoelectric hands. He is totally independent in his farming activities, which include driving his tractor (Figure 12.3).

Bilateral Above-Elbow Amputation

The person who loses both arms above the elbow is at a distinct disadvantage when compared to someone with bilateral below-elbow amputations. The value of the human elbow cannot be overempha-

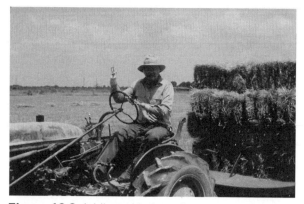

Figure 12.3 A bilateral below-elbow amputee can be independent in vocational activities, such as farming.

sized. When both arms are lost at this level, a prosthesis must provide all motions at the elbow, wrist, and terminal device. Although a great deal of time, effort, and research has been invested in exploring the challenge of perfecting an above-elbow prosthesis, an ideal alternative to the natural arm is far from being achieved.

As previously stated, persons with amputations generally prefer bilateral hook-type terminal devices over myoelectric hands. Moreover, body-powered elbows, versus electric elbows, are the elbows of choice for many of these persons. The issues of weight, cost, repair, and maintenance of electric components often discourage the person with bilateral above-elbow amputations from being a successful wearer of myoelectric hands.

The prosthetic training for a person with bilateral above-elbow amputations may be conducted as a series of staged hospitalizations or outpatient stays. The initial training of basic activities of daily living takes a great deal of time, effort, and motivation on the part of the patient. Often, the basic tasks of writing, eating, tooth brushing, face washing, and dressing (with assistance) are the only goals to be accomplished during the initial hospitalization. A second staged admission to upgrade functional independence may follow to further refine these activities and add others to the daily routine. If the person with bilateral above-elbow amputations shows a strong motivation and desire to become independent, it is possible for this goal to be met, as the following case study demonstrates.

Case Study 4

E. N. is a man 39 years of age from Wyoming who sustained bilateral above-elbow amputations in a high-voltage electrical burn injury in 1983. He was initially fit with bilateral electric elbows, electric hands, and body-powered elbows and hook terminal devices.

Unfortunately, E. N. was never comprehensively trained to use his electric and body-powered prostheses; consequently, 9 months following his injury he remained totally dependent in all activities of daily living. When he was referred to a rehabilitation program in Houston, he was extremely depressed, and his marriage was failing.

The purpose of his rehabilitation hospitalization was to evaluate and upgrade his level of function with and without prostheses. His primary goals included independence in eating, brushing teeth, shaving, showering, toileting, and dressing. Accomplishing his morning activities with his residual limbs had not been explored with E. N. Padding the handle of a toothbrush with foam enabled E. N., during the early days of therapy, to be independent brushing his teeth without the prostheses (see Figure 12.4). He was hospitalized for 4 weeks, during which many of these goals were met through use of adaptive devices, adapted clothing, and custom-made equipment. At the time of discharge, most of E. N.'s rehabilitation goals had been met. These activities were accomplished both with and without his prostheses.

Practice and reinforcement of functional skills were the key elements that enabled E. N. to become independent. Today E. N. is totally independent. He prefers body-powered elbows and hook terminal devices to electric elbows and hands for their superior lightweight, reliability, and ease of operation.

Summary

The opportunity and potential for a person with upper-extremity limb loss is unrestricted. Early fitting, however, is crucial to achieve a successful

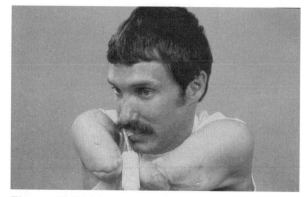

Figure 12.4 Using residual limbs at midline, with a padded toothbrush, a person with a bilateral above-elbow amputation can be independent with brushing teeth.

functional outcome. The motivation and desire to become independent are extremely important to cultivate and reinforce in the person with an upper-extremity amputation. The combined efforts of a skilled rehabilitation physician, prosthetist, and practitioner enable that person to achieve more than previously thought possible. Functional independence should be considered a realistic goal for most persons with upper-extremity amputations. Achievement of that goal results in a truly rewarding experience for the practitioner, the patient, and the entire rehabilitation team. ◆

Study Questions

1. When does a preprosthetic program begin?

2. Describe seven goals of a preprosthetic program.

3. What are some of the important things to consider in a prosthetic training program?

4. What are some of the differences between body-powered and electric prostheses?

5. Ideally, when, from the time one loses an arm, should one be fitted with a prosthesis? Why?

6. Is it possible for a person with a below-elbow amputation to be totally independent? With an above-elbow amputation?

7. What is a hybrid prosthesis?

8. Do most persons with bilateral upper-extremity amputations wear hooks or hands? Why?

9. Can a bilateral below-elbow amputee be independent?

10. Who are the key members of the amputee rehabilitation team and what are their roles?

References

Atkins, D. J. (1989a). Postoperative therapy programs. In D. J. Atkins & R. H. Meier (Eds.), *Comprehensive management of the upper limb amputee* (pp. 11–15). New York: Springer-Verlag.

Atkins, D. J. (1989b). Adult upper limbs prosthetic training. In D. J. Atkins & R. H. Meier (Eds.), *Comprehensive management of the upper limb amputee* (pp. 39–59). New York: Springer-Verlag.

Atkins, D. J. (1994). Managing self-care in adults with upper extremity amputations. In C. Christiansen (Ed.), *Ways of living* (pp. 277–304). Bethesda, MD: American Occupational Therapy Association.

Bennett, J. B., & Alexander, C. B. (1989). Amputation levels and surgical techniques. In D. J. Atkins & R. H. Meier (Eds.), *Comprehensive management of the upper limb amputee* (pp. 1–10). New York: Springer-Verlag.

Burrough, S., & Brook, J. (1985). Patterns of acceptance and rejection of upper limb prostheses. *Orthotics and Prosthetics, 39*, 40–47.

Leonard, J. A., Jr., & Meier, R. H. III. (1998). Upper and lower extremity prosthetics. In J. A. DeLisa & B. M. Gans (Eds.), *Rehabilitation medicine: Principles and practice* (pp. 669–696). Philadelphia: Lippincott-Raven.

Marquardt, E. (1989). The Heidelberg experience. In D. J. Atkins & R. H. Meier (Eds.), *Comprehensive management of the upper limb amputee* (pp. 240–252). New York: Springer-Verlag.

13

Self-Care Strategies After Severe Burns

Sandra Utley Reeves

Sandra Utley Reeves, OTR/L, is Occupational Therapist, Shands Hospital, University of Florida, Gainesville.

Key Terms

full-thickness burn

partial-thickness burn

superficial burn

autograft

hypertrophic scar

keloid scar

scar maturation

boutonnière deformity

boutonnière precautions

heterotopic ossification

total active motion (TAM)

dermis

epidermis

hyperpigmentation

hypopigmentation

split-thickness skin graft

donor site

ectropion

skin appendages

erythema

eschar

excoriation

activities of daily living (ADL)

instrumental activities of daily living (IADL)

Objectives

On completing this chapter, the reader will be able to

1. Recognize and understand the characteristics of the different depths of burn injury.

2. Describe the phases of recovery and the focus of occupational therapy intervention for each phase.

3. Identify factors that increase the potential for scar hypertrophy or contractures.

4. Recognize the relationship between patient–caregiver involvement and education and the potential for long-term compliance with the treatment program.

5. Understand the rationale behind early involvement of burn patients in their own self-care.

6. Recognize the effect that a severe burn has on the life roles, self-image, and values of the patient.

The goal of the burn care team members is long-term functional independence for the patient. However, pain, discomfort, scar contractures, cosmetic disfigurement, and adverse psychological reactions can limit the burn patient's potential for resuming previous life roles and interests. Because the focus of occupational therapy is on returning the burn patient to his or her preinjury lifestyle, ongoing evaluation of the person's physical function, social needs, and psychological status is needed. This evaluation enables effective treatment planning. Understanding and respecting the patient's personal goals and priorities are essential, because they will have a direct effect on adherence to treatment regimens, overall motivation, and functional outcomes.

It takes a coordinated effort by a multidisciplinary team to effectively manage the many medical, functional, and psychosocial problems encountered during burn recovery and rehabilitation. Only through continuous interaction between the patient and members of the burn team can rehabilitation progress efficiently. Ideally, the facility-based burn team should consist of physicians, nurses, occupational and physical therapy practitioners, a social worker, a nutritionist, and a respiratory therapist. A psychiatrist, chaplain, and recreational therapist should also be available to join the team as needed.

Traditionally, a burn patient's recovery was considered successful if he or she survived the injury, returned home, and was able to perform basic self-care tasks including eating, dressing, grooming, toileting, and ambulating. Today, successful burn care is measured by a patient's quality of life once he or she is discharged from the acute care or rehabilitation setting. Functional recovery now includes the burn patient being able to perform complex activities or instrumental activities of daily living (IADL). These abilities allow the patient to resume self-defined roles at home, work, school, and the community, including social and recreational activities.

Factors That Influence Burn Injury Outcomes

The burn team members consider many factors while developing treatment plans and goals for specific patients. They include the depth of the burn, the type of burn, the percentage of total body surface area burned (%TBSA), and the subsequent quality of wound healing and scarring. A patient's age, preinjury health and emotional stability, motiva-tion or compliance with treatment, and family member support are other factors that can have a direct effect on recovery from burn injuries. Potential functional outcomes can be predicted from the analysis of these factors.

Burn Depth

Functional problems encountered during burn recovery can be anticipated, beginning with an assessment of the burn depth. In the past, it was customary to classify burns as first, second, and third degree. However, they are now described as superficial, superficial partial, deep partial, full-thickness, and, in some cases, subdermal. The depth of the burn is estimated from clinical observation of its appearance, sensitivity, and pliability (see Table 13.1).

Superficial and deep partial-thickness burns can usually heal without surgical intervention. Once healed, they tend to be excessively dry, itchy, and vulnerable to injury by shearing forces from rubbing or scratching. These shear forces can cause blisters and, with repeated injury, reduce the skin's ability to remain healthy and unbroken. Partial-thickness and full-thickness burns often result in uneven pigmentation, with combinations of hypopigmentation and hyperpigmentation of the healed scar. Deep partial- and full-thickness burns have a greater potential for thick, hypertrophic scar and contracture formation because of the prolonged period required for healing. This potential is especially true of partial-thickness burns that convert to full-thickness because of infection or repeated trauma. Full-thickness wounds usually require surgical intervention for wound closure, such as skin grafting. Skin graft donor sites usually heal in a way similar to that for superficial partial-thickness burns, with less scarring but uneven pigmentation.

Mechanism of Injury

The severity of a burn injury also depends on the area exposed and the duration and intensity of exposure to heat (thermal exposure). Superficial partial-thickness burns typically occur after a brief contact with hot liquids, hot surfaces, or flames. Deep partial-thickness burns are caused by longer exposure to intense heat, such as with hot water immersion scalds or skin contact with flaming materials and hot surfaces. Full-thickness burns result from prolonged immersion scalds; electrical contact; longer exposure to flames; or contact with hot grease, tar, or chemical agents such as battery acid.

Table 13.1 Burn Wound Characteristics

Burn Depth	Tissue Depth	Clinical Findings	Healing Time	Common Causes	Scar Potential
Superficial (first degree)	Superficial epidermis	Erythema, dry, no blisters; moderate pain	3 to 7 days	Sunburn, brief flash burns, brief exposure to hot liquids or chemicals	No potential for hypertrophic scar or contractures
Superficial partial thickness (superficial second degree) and donor sites	Epidermis, upper dermis	Erythema, wet, blisters; sigsignificant pain	Less than 2 weeks	Severe sunburn or radiation burns, prolonged exposure to hot liquids, brief contact with hot metal objects	Minimal potential for hypertrophy or contractures if no secondary infection or trauma delays healing
Deep partial thickness (deep second degree)	Epidermis and much of dermis nonviable but skin appendages survive, from which skin may regenerate	Erythema; larger, usually broken blisters; on palms and soles of feet, large, possibly intact blisters over beefy red dermis; severe pain to even light touch	Greater than 2 weeks, may convert to full thickness with onset of infection	Flames; firm or prolonged contact with hot metal objets; prolonged contact with hot, viscous liquids	Very high potential for hypertrophic scarring and contractures across joints, web spaces, and facial contours; high risk for boutonnière deformities if dorsal fingers involved
Full thickness (third degree)	Epidermis and dermis; skin appendages and nerve ending are nonviable	Pale, nonblanching, dry, coagulated capillaries may be seen; no sensation to light touch except at deep partial-thickness borders	Larger areas require surgical intervention for wound closure; smaller areas may heal in from borders over extended period of time	Extreme heat or prolonged exposure to heat, hot objects, or chemicals	Extremely high potential for hypertrophic scarring or contractures, depending on the method used for wound closure
Subdermal	Full-thickness burn with damage to underlying tissues	Nonviable surface, may be charred or with exposed fat, tendons, and muscles; electrical injuries may have small external wounds but significant secondary subdermal tissue loss and peripheral nerve damage	Requires surgical intervention for wound closure; may require amputation or significant reconstruction	Electrical burns and severe long duration burns (i.e., house fires, motor vehicle accidents with a passenger trapped in a burning vehicle or under hot exhaust systems), and smoking in bed or alcohol-related burns	Similar to full-thickness except where amputation removes the burn site

Percentage of Total Body Surface Area Involved

The extent of severe burns is measured by estimating the proportion of the body's skin that has been affected. The two most common methods for estimating the % TBSA burned are the "rule of nines" and the Lund and Browder Chart (Solem, 1984).

The *rule of nines* is simple and quick, but relatively inaccurate. It divides the body surface into areas comprising 9%, or multiples of 9%, with the perineum making up the final 1%. The head and neck area is 9%, each upper extremity is 9%, each leg is 18%, and the front and back of the trunk are each 18%. However, the rule of nines applies only to adults. Body proportions vary in children, especially in the head and legs, depending on their age (Carvajal, 1988).

The Lund and Browder Chart provides a more accurate estimate of the total body surface area (Lund & Browder, 1944) and is used in most burn centers. This chart assigns a percentage of surface area to body segments, with adjusted calculations for different age groups. For smaller %TBSA injuries, the therapist can get a quick rough estimate using size of the patient's palm (hand excluding the fingers), which equals approximately 1% of the person's total body surface area.

Severity of Injury

Together, the % TBSA and the depth of the burn serve as primary determinants of burn injury severity. A deep partial-thickness or full-thickness burn to more than 20% TBSA is often the determining factor for admission to a burn intensive care unit. Depending on the patient's age and preinjury health, smaller partial- or full-thickness burn wounds (less than 20% TBSA) can be considered severe burn injuries. For most adults, a deep partial-thickness and full-thickness burn of greater than 40% of total body surface area is considered severe. Children under 5 years of age and adults more than 50 years of age are considered to be at greater survival risk for larger burns, so that a 20% burn can be considered severe for these populations. The presence of associated injuries also contributes to severity; these can include inhalation injury, fractures, or other trauma.

Burns to specific body areas also influence severity, even though the amount of surface area burned is relatively limited. Deep partial-thickness or full-thickness burns of the hands, face, or perineum are usually considered severe (Wachtel, 1985).

Burns of the face, eyes, and neck may interfere with respiration, vision, and feeding and often result in long-term functional and cosmetic impairment. Bilateral hand burns may initially limit the person's self-care ability and can also result in long-term functional disability if not properly managed.

Wound Care and Surgical Intervention

Most burns are treated with some form of antiseptic agent to reduce bacterial counts and the potential for wound infection (Hartford, 1984). If the wound is relatively clean, a biological dressing may be used as a temporary wound covering. Types of biological dressings include homografts, which are processed cadaver skin; xenografts, which are processed pig skin; and synthetic products or artificial skin substitutes. However, the extent and depth of the burn wound determines the need for surgical treatment. When it appears that a deep partial-thickness burn will take more than 2 weeks to heal, surgery may be necessary to accelerate wound healing, shorten hospital length of stay, and reduce the potential for hypertrophic scarring.

Surgical treatment for burn wounds usually consists of cutting away the burned tissue (known as *eschar*) and placing split-thickness skin grafts over the site. These grafts, known as *autografts*, are taken from an unburned area of the patient's body (donor site). If adequate donor sites for autografting are not available, or burn depth or infections create conditions such that the grated tissue will not survive, biological dressings may be used.

Scar Formation

The quality of burn healing is affected by many factors, some of which occur during early phases of care (Helm & Fisher, 1988). The most common burn injury complication that limits function is the development of hypertrophic scars and contractures. Burn scar formation is mainly affected by the time needed for the initial wound to close. Bacterial infections after a burn may delay healing by increasing the body's inflammatory responses. After initial healing, some scars enlarge and rise above the level of the original skin surface and become thick, rigid, and red in surface appearance. These are referred to as *hypertrophic scars*. Hypertrophic scars usually begin developing during the first few months after a deep partial-thickness or full-thickness burn. Infection or trauma at a burn site can result in collagen overgrowth and the development of excess scar tissue that results in hypertrophic scarring. Hypertrophic scars that raise up and also expand horizontally beyond the original borders of the scar are referred to as *keloid scars*.

The raised, firm texture of immature hypertrophic scars results from increased proliferation of blood vessels, cells that produce connective tissue, and collagen (Abston, 1987). A scar's functional or cosmetic significance depends on its anatomical location. Joint motion is limited when a scar complex develops across a joint surface and contracts, creating a restrictive band of scar tissue. This is known as a *contracture*. Such tight or hypertrophic scars on the face can interfere with eating and eye closure, as well as distort facial features.

Regardless of the wound care method used and the time taken for wound closure, scar maturation differs with each person. Superficial partial-thickness, nonhypertrophic scars can mature in 5 to 8 weeks. However, hypertrophic scars can take up to 18 to 24 months, and keloid scars even longer, to mature.

Although it is sometimes possible to predict outcomes from the depth and location of the wound, other factors can affect the results. Race, age, and preexisting health problems, for example, also influence healing and scar formation. Asian, African, and Native American persons seem to have a greater potential for developing hypertrophic scarring and uneven coloring of replaced skin. Elderly patients may heal more slowly but also with less incidence of collagen overgrowth. Small children, however, tend to heal more quickly but have a much higher potential for hypertrophic scarring. Patients with diabetes or other conditions that restrict circulation tend to heal more slowly.

Phases of Recovery

Burn rehabilitation can be divided into three basic phases of recovery: acute care, inpatient rehabilitation, and outpatient rehabilitation. The acute phase begins immediately after injury and usually continues until extensive wound care needs are minimal. During the first few days of this phase, the main focus of the burn team members is on the survival of the patient. During this phase, the burn care team members work to control edema (often by elevating affected extremities) and to ensure that fluid resuscitation is accomplished. Fluid loss because of severe burns can cause burn shock and failure of the kidneys if not managed carefully by the physician. As the medical team members work to stabilize the patient, the occupational therapist should already be anticipating and planning for the patient's rehabilitation needs. This initial evaluation should involve the total patient, not just the burn wound, which means that therapy personnel should learn as much as possible about the patient's preinjury characteristics and lifestyle.

As the patient becomes medically stable, prevention of deformity and loss of function take on more significance. A more extensive evaluation of range of motion (ROM), general strength, and cognitive and overall functional abilities is performed. The therapist then develops and initiates a customized treatment program designed to minimize or prevent long-term loss of independence.

When a burn patient enters the inpatient rehabilitation phase of recovery, independent function and prevention of disability and deformity become the central themes of treatment. Wound care continues, but the patient's active participation increases. Emphasis is placed on general reconditioning (strength, flexibility, and endurance) and scar management as initial steps toward the goal of improving performance with self-care activities (self-feeding, wound and skin care, personal hygiene and grooming skills, and dressing) and social reintegration.

The outpatient rehabilitation phase is an extension of the rehabilitation phase, but patients typically live at home and attend therapy sessions during the day. The focus of care continues to center on minimizing hypertrophic scar and contracture formation; improving flexibility, strength, and endurance; assuring proper skin and scar care techniques; and promoting independence in normal daily activities, including social and recreational pursuits. Community reintegration and socialization issues become more important. A primary objective is to help the patient adjust physically and emotionally to the injury.

Most burn patients discontinue routine outpatient rehabilitation services when they achieve the skills needed to function independently at home and can return to school or work full time. They often reach this point before scar maturation is complete. The total time required before returning to work has been found to be related to the site and severity of the burn, age of the patient, the patient's occupation, and the location of the thermal injury (Bowden, Thomson, & Prasad, 1989; Helm, Walker, & Peyton, 1986). Before discharge from the hospital, follow-up visits to a burn outpatient clinic should be scheduled to monitor the scar maturation process and address unanticipated problems (Petro & Salisbury, 1986).

Occupational Therapy

The role of occupational therapy in the treatment of severe burns is multifaceted and changes as healing progresses and the patient moves through the phases of recovery. It is necessary to maintain or increase ROM, strength, and endurance so that the patient is capable of performing the activities of daily living (ADL) (Trombly, 1995). These goals are essential to preventing contractures and deformities (Parent, 1983).

Systems models of occupational therapy are useful in understanding the effect of a serious burn injury on the life of a patient (Baum & Christiansen, 1997; Kielhofner, 1995; Law et al., 1996). These models help the therapist identify problems and understand the relationships among various aspects of treatment. Such models suggest that restrictions in the ability to move and perform tasks reduce the patient's ability to accomplish necessary roles, which in turn influences his or her views of self as a competent person. Over time, a diminished self-conception can affect interests and values and reduce motivation, resulting in adverse social and emotional consequences.

When persons sustain severe burn injuries, they are unable to complete self-care activities for many reasons, including the severity and location of the wounds; restrictive dressings, medication, and hospital routines; and both pain and anxiety. Restricted abilities, isolation, and dramatic changes in one's usual daily routines seriously alter the patient's previous roles. The new role of *patient* replaces previous roles of worker, student, parent, or spouse (Reilly, 1962).

Psychological affects are a major concern (Fleet, 1992). Changes in motivation may occur at the time of injury and could continue for many years after discharge. Values can change, and self-esteem and confidence may be impaired because of body-image issues. Social and personal interests may be affected, particularly if the injury occurred during a specific social gathering activity or event.

Cheng and Rogers (1989) studied men who had completed rehabilitation for severe burn injuries to determine how their role performance changed in the areas of self-care, leisure, home management, and work. They found that some men experienced minimal role reduction, whereas others managed their self-care requirements but were experiencing role disruption in their leisure, work, and home management. A third pattern seemed to be substantial disruption of all roles. In this study, loss of roles was commonly associated with reduced endurance, the presence of impaired grip strength and upper-extremity skill, and difficulty with walking and standing. Although most of the men studied had achieved independence in self-care within a year after discharge, that achievement did not coincide with role resumption in the areas of home management, work, and leisure.

By viewing the patient within a dynamic conceptual framework of occupation, rehabilitation focuses on the relationship between the injury and the patient as a social being. Within this context, the need to address the emotional as well as the physical dimensions of the injury becomes more apparent, and both assessment and intervention strategies should be planned accordingly.

Assessment: Acute Care Phase

Whenever possible, a patient should be evaluated by an occupational therapist within the first 24 hours after admission to the hospital. A preassessment review of the medical record is needed for obtaining information regarding the mechanism of injury; the %TBSA affected; the depth of the burn; and the patient's age, sex, and medical history. This information should be confirmed and supplemented by communication with the patient or his or her family members.

Ideally, the initial occupational therapy assessment should take place during a dressing change, when the depth and exact location of the burns can be viewed directly and documented carefully. Distinctions should be made between superficial and deep partial-thickness burns, as well as full-thickness burns, by appearance and presence of sensation. The therapist needs to view the wounds as soon as possible after the injury. Burn eschar develops quickly, causing deep partial-thickness burns closely resembling full-thickness burns and making accurate evaluation of burn depth even more difficult. Attention should also be directed to burned joint surface areas and the presence of any circumferential burns. If time allows, an active or active-assistive ROM assessment should be done without dressings to evaluate joint mobility and general strength before serious edema develops or restrictive dressings are applied. The dorsum of the hands should be checked for deep burns over the proximal interphalangeal joints, which could indicate the need to initiate boutonnière deformity precautions or hand splints (see Figure 13.1).

Once the dressings are in place and nursing care is completed, a more comprehensive occupa-

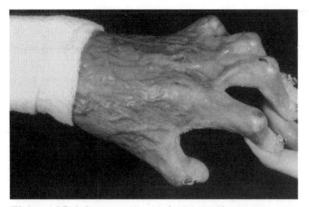

Figure 13.1 Boutonnière deformities, if not prevented in the acute phase, can result in severe deformity and loss of function.

tional therapy assessment can be performed. A careful history is needed from the patient or family members to establish the preburn level of functioning and life roles. This history would include information about the patient's home environment and responsibilities, occupational background and work skills, educational level, hand dominance, and any preexisting conditions (physical, psychological, or social) that would affect the patient's functional performance. Understanding the patient's preinjury roles and level of functioning is important for setting realistic treatment goals but also for establishing a therapeutic relationship with the patient and family members. Patient and caregiver education should be initiated on this first contact and continued as an essential part of therapy throughout the stages of recovery.

During the first few days, acute, diffuse edema develops, limiting the end ranges of affected joints and impairing participation with active ROM. For this reason, formal joint measurement may not be practical. However, the therapist should note any developing joint stiffness not explained by preexisting conditions such as old injuries, congenital abnormalities, or arthritis. Positioning and splinting recommendations should be made, based on the need to reduce edema and preserve joint mobility.

The general rule for positioning or splinting is to keep the extremities elevated above the heart and all joints positioned opposite to the anticipated potential deformity. These recommendations are posted bedside. Passive and active–assistive ROM should be initiated with patients considered to have a high potential for developing contractures. If the patient is able to participate, an active ROM exercise program should be initiated and taught to

the patient and family members. Active exercise programs should be simple, easy to remember, and follow normal patterns of movement. Instructions for exercises should be posted bedside in the form of simple drawings that can be easily seen by the patient and family members.

If loss of active ROM is not promptly regained as acute edema decreases, formal goniometric measurements are needed to formally document changes in joint mobility. Verbal instructions should be given to the patient, and the motion should be demonstrated for clarification. Goniometer measurements should be documented for both involved and uninvolved joints to assist in establishing the patient's personal norms. The extent and the causes of limitations in motion should be determined from both the physical and psychological perspectives. An assessment of active ROM is preferred, but a patient may resist motion because of apprehension, pain, or confusion. If the patient is unresponsive or unable to participate, the therapist should evaluate active–assistive and, in some cases, passive ROM.

An initial assessment of gross strength is easily performed by a manual test of major muscle groups. Because the burn does not initially affect muscle strength, this test can help identify any associated injuries or preexisting conditions that were not reported by other members of the team.

Actual performance of ADL skills should be assessed frequently, beginning in the acute phase and continuing throughout the phases of recovery. Observation of eating and grooming skills is important in determining whether normal or compensatory motions are being used. Adaptive methods are often used by the patient because of interference from dressings, edema, or pain; and they may also be associated with abnormal posturing, which will need to be addressed in treatment planning.

Assessment: Inpatient and Outpatient Rehabilitation Phases

Assessments during both inpatient and outpatient rehabilitation phases include evaluating ROM, strength, endurance, self-care activities, work skills, skin and scar condition, and social and emotional adaptation. Goniometric measurements of ROM deficits using either single joint or total active motion methods should be done weekly, biweekly, or as needed, depending on the frequency of treatment. Muscle strength, dexterity, and endurance can be evaluated by manual muscle testing and other evaluative tools or by using treatment modalities such as a Baltimore Therapeutic Equipment (BTE) Work Simulator®. When the patient has hand burns, dynamometer recordings of grip strength and pinch gauge measures of pinch strength should also documented at regular intervals. Improvement in general strength and endurance can be documented by the patient's performance of self-care activities of increasing physical demand, by duration of participation, and by frequency length of needed rest breaks.

Hypertrophic scars and contractures require close supervision, because they often affect the patient's ability to maintain adequate mobility to perform everyday tasks. It is important to monitor a scar, noticing how it appears, touching it, and observing its effect on single joint or combined joint movements. Tight or hypertrophic scars near joints restrict mobility and cause discomfort as the patient stretches to achieve the end ROM. Tight scarring on the face can result in facial distortion and impaired eating abilities. Early recognition and therapeutic intervention can often stretch out developing contractures and help reduce the likelihood of surgical intervention. However, some scar bands may be unstable and break down during exercise, which would result in further scarring and progressive loss of mobility. Patients with unstable scar bands should be referred to the surgeon for possible release of the scar band and repair of the defect with more durable grafted skin.

Continual assessment of a burn patient's functional skills is a primary objective. The therapist should observe the patient during self-care activities and watch for unnecessary exertion or use of abnormal posturing and movements. Therapy intervention should include instruction and demonstration methods for performing the task in normal movement patterns. For example, a patient with burns involving the trunk and extremities may feel unable to perform any upper-body dressing activities. The patient's ability to integrate correct motions for the activity should be closely monitored, while encouraging creativity in problem solving and task accomplishment.

Awareness of the patient's emotional status is important throughout recovery. Because of pain, fatigue, frustration, and other difficulties encountered with rehabilitation activities, patients may experience extreme anxiety and emotional distress, especially during painful procedures or exercises. The therapist should be aware of a patient's coping abilities and report major difficulties to the team

members. As appropriate, the patient should be encouraged to discuss problems with the burn center's social worker, psychiatrist, or chaplain.

Intervention: Acute Care Phase

During acute care, pain is a primary issue with patients. Most patients with a severe burn injury naturally respond to pain by resisting painful motions or activities. It is also a normal response for most children (and many adults) to regress in their behavior. When this regression occurs, the therapist should be supportive, continually explaining beforehand what is to be done and why, in terms the patient can understand. The patient is usually more interested in whether the procedure will hurt and how long it will last than in technical information. Coordinating treatments with scheduled pain medications is often helpful and highly recommended, especially if active participation is needed. Relaxation techniques such as breathing exercises may be helpful. However, if a patient's anxiety or pain is disproportionate to the treatment, antianxiety medication may be indicated both to relieve anxiety and to increase the effectiveness of pain medication.

Depending on the presence of associated conditions or complications, the patient may be disoriented or unresponsive to verbal cueing and require passive exercise. In this circumstance, it is especially important to continue verbal communication, and full ROM should be attempted during every treatment session (see Figure 13.2). However, time limits on painful treatment sessions should be preset with all cognizant patients and consistently adhered to by the therapist.

Controlling edema is another acute care objective and is frequently achieved through methods that prevent dependent extremity positioning. Many of the positioning techniques used initially are continued throughout recovery. If a patient has hand burns, the upper extremity should be elevated on a pillow incline with the elbow above the heart and the hand above the elbow. For persistent edema, external compression, through use of pressure wraps or compression garments, may be indicated. Patients should be encouraged to actively exercise their hands, especially using the intrinsic muscles. They should also use their hands for eating, grooming, and other functional activities as much as possible. Adolescent and adult patients should be educated regarding the relationship between adequate nutrition for wound healing, so that feedback on calorie and protein intake can be used to foster

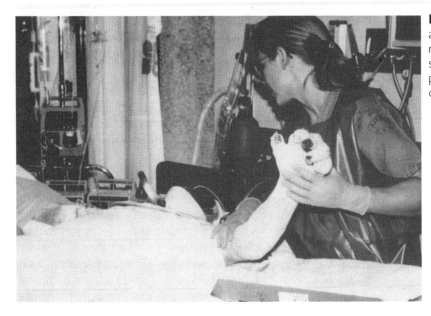

Figure 13.2 Before and during active–assistive or passive range of motion exercises, the therapist should continually reassure the patient and describe what is being done and why.

patient involvement during mealtimes (Mahon & Neufeld, 1984). The combination of exercise, performance of self-care activities, elevation, and elastic bandages not only helps control or decrease hand edema but also promotes normal recovery (see Table 13.2).

Regardless of the education and emotional support provided, some patients perceive their injury as a disability. They experience decreased self-confidence and become increasingly dependent on staff members and family members. When asked to perform a task, their immediate response is to anticipate failure and refuse to even try. Rather than labeling the patient "uncooperative" or "unmotivated," the therapist should grade and carefully select tasks to promote success and increase self-confidence. Feeding oneself is one of the first self-care tasks learned as a child, and the inability to do so carries much significance for a person's self-esteem. Therefore, as soon as a patient is allowed any oral intake, self-feeding—regardless of the assistance required—should be introduced (see Figure 13.3). Early involvement in basic self-care activities, however limited, promotes a sense of efficacy by engaging the patient in goal-directed tasks that focus attention on accomplishment instead of impairment.

When first attempting ADL, the focus should be on accomplishing simple skills, such as holding a spoon with an enlarged handle or getting a cup to the mouth. Initially, self-care tasks should be simplified with adapted aids, as needed, to ensure patient participation and success. As the patient pro-

gresses with ROM, strength, and endurance goals, adapted aids are discontinued and more demanding and complex tasks are reintroduced to the patient's routine. Although considerable time and patience may be involved in this approach, both the patient's general endurance and confidence will be bolstered for later attempts at more complex IADL tasks. When initiating a self-care program with the severely burned patient, it may be advantageous to follow a sequence similar to the sequence of ADL and self-care tasks learned during typical childhood development.

Periods of immobilization after surgical procedures will restrict functional independence. Before surgery, the patient should be informed that a defined period of immobilization will follow the procedure, but that under supervision certain rehabilitation activities will continue. For example, if a patient's hands and forearm burns are surgically excised and autografted, the therapist may still provide shoulder activities at the patient's bedside during the postoperative immobilization period. When a patient's hands are in postoperative dressings, self-feeding may be possible only with adaptive equipment. If adaptations are used for postoperative function, the patient should understand that they are only temporary.

Loss of strength and endurance, and the resulting decrease in daily activity, are frequently a consequence of prolonged bed rest. Severe burns also increase metabolism, placing further demands on the body's general physical condition. To limit deconditioning, acute burn patients should be

Table 13.2 Antideformity Positioning and Exercises

Body Area	Position	Positioning Devices or Splints	Suggested Exercises
Face			
Mouth	Head of bed elevated to decrease facial and head edema	Microstomia prevention appliance (MPA) or thermoplastic splint to preserve oral commissures and size of mouth opening	Early active assistive or passive sustained lateral stretch to mouth with fingers, temperature probe covers, or acrylic straws
Cheeks		Foley catheter placed between molars and inner cheek and inflated to point of slight outer cheek blanching, applied ≤20 minutes	Passive sustained stretch to cheeks and mouth using increasing number of tongue depressors between uncompromised teeth
Eyes		Face mask; ectropion releases usually immobilized with stint dressings, then face mask reapplied post healing	Active eye opening with eyebrows up and mouth open; tight eye closure; passive, sustained lateral eye stretches to help prevent ectropion and eyelid tightness
Nares		Nasal obturators or nasal flange added to facial conformer	Scar massage and manual stretching of nares
Ears	Avoid pressure to the burned ear helix when lying on the side	Foam cutout instead of pillow; thermoplastic ear protectors postop	After healing, massage scar; Otoform or Elastomer conformers under elastic face mask
Neck			
Anterior	No pillows under head; towel roll along thoracic spine to simultaneously extend neck and stretch chest; short mattress	Snug custom-fitted soft foam collar to extend neck or compress scar bands; rigid thermoplastic splint over dressings during the day if contractures develop	Gentle, frequent AROM and sustained passive stretch with massage to stretch scar bands; avoid neck hyperextension in older adults
Posterior	Pillow under head okay		
Shoulders and chest			
Anterior axilla and chest	Shoulders abducted to 100° and slight flexion supported on pillows; towel roll along thoracic spine to stretch chest	Figure 8 wrap around shoulders over axilla pads to protract shoulders and prevent or compress axillary web scar bands; airplane splint postgrafting worn full time, 3 to 5 days, then nights only	Frequent AROM and AAROM of shoulders in all functional planes; sustained stretch with massage and use of modalities to stretch axilla contractures
Posterior axilla and upper back	Shoulders abducted to 90° and 45° horizontal flexion supported on pillows or tray tables	Padded figure 8 wrap around axillas to compress or prevent axillary web scar bands	Frequent AROM and AAROM of shoulders in flexion and horizontal adduction
Elbows			
Anterior	Position with pillows, 0° to 5° flexion, avoid hyperextension	Thermoplastic anterior or posterior elbow splint in position to maintain maximum surface area of site; ≤5° flexion for anterior and ≤90° flexion for posterior elbow burns or grafts	Frequent AROM and self-assisted AAPROM with sustained stretch at end ranges; avoid rigorous PROM if patient has disproportionate pain and evaluate for heterotopic ossification

(continued)

241

Table 13.2 (*continued*)

Body Area	Position	Positioning Devices or Splints	Suggested Exercises
Posterior	Position with pillows in 45° to 90° flexion		
Hands			
Dorsal and volar	Elevate UE on pillow incline with hand above elbow, elbow above heart, and hand roll in palm until initial acute edema resolves	Resting hand splint in antideformity position (MCPs at 75° flexion, IPs at 0°, thumb in combined radial and palmar abduction and wrist at 30° extension) secured over dressings with elastic wraps and well elevated on pillow incline	Boutonnière precautions if greater than or equal to deep partial with no passive flexion of PIP joints or combined MP and IP flexion or fisting; if no deep burns over PIPs, combined IP, MP, and wrist flexion or thumb opposition to give maximum dorsal skin sustained stretch
Volar only	Elevate UE on pillow incline with hand above elbow, elbow above heart, and hand out flat with no hand roll; initiate early palmar stretch splinting and active exercise	Resting hand splint in palmar stretch position worn during all periods of inactivity	Palmar stretch exercises with combined IP and MP extension, finger abduction, thumb radial abduction and extension, and wrist extension to give maximum volar skin sustained stretch
Web spaces	Velfoam strips between fingers wrapped with figure 8 pattern, using Coban® elastic wrap or secured with compression gloves	Conformers under promptly applied custom compression glove	Massage and passive stretch of web spaces, active finger abduction exercises
Trunk			
Anterior and posterior	Keep shoulders aligned with hips at all times when in bed	Keep upright when sitting with pillows or support both arms on tray table	ROM and sustained stretch in trunk flexion, extension, and rotation over bolster
Hips			
Anterior	Use reclining chair and minimize time spent in hip flexion; when supine, keep bed flat as possible, support lateral legs in abduction and neutral rotation; if possible, have patient sleep prone on firm mattress with feet off end of bed	Posterior splint for postop immobilization	Lie supine on firm, flat surface with pillow below buttocks; sit at edge of mat table with feet on floor and lie back slowly until supine to extend hips

(*continued*)

Table 13.2 (*continued*)

Body Area	Position	Positioning Devices or Splints	Suggested Exercises
Posterior	Sit upright with pillows under thighs when supine, head and knees on bed up to allow hip flexion, support lateral legs in abduction and neutral rotation	Splinting usually only needed for postop immobilization in agitated patient	"Knee hugs," squatting, toe touches
Perineum	Sit or lie with legs abducted	Abduction pillow or splint to keep knees apart	"Frog sit" with soles of feet together and slowly pull feet toward body
Knees			
Anterior only	Pillow under knees to allow moderate flexion	Splinting usually only needed for postop immobilization; serial casting for established contracture	"Knee hugs" and squatting
Anterior or posterior	Pillows under distal legs to minimize knee flexion; avoid hyperextension	Thermoplastic posterior knee conformer applied with elastic wrap; serial casting for established contracture	Touch toes with knees bent, then slowly straighten knees; prone with pillow under knee, ankle weights to give slow stretch
Ankles			
Anterior	Pillow under lower leg with heel suspended	Thermoplastic dorsal ankle and toe plantar flexion conformer resting splint	Knee with dorsum of foot flat as possible on mat surface, slowly sit on heels
Posterior	Ankle supported in dorsiflexion with foot-board, blanket roll, or posterior splint	Posterior conformer splint with ankle held in neutral, posterior heel of splint "bubbled out" to avoid excessive pressure to calcaneus and Achilles' tendon	Sustained stretches in dorsiflexion, ambulation, ankle pumps, toe raises with distal foot on 2-in. pad
Toes			
Dorsal	Toes supported in plantar-flexed position with dorsal padding and elastic wraps	Dorsal conforming resting splint to maintain combined ankle and toe plantar flexion	Combined toe and ankle plantar flexion, sustained stretch exercises
Volar	Toes supported in dorsiflexed position with volar padding and elastic wraps	Volar ankle and toe dorsiflexion thermoplastic conformer resting splint, AFO	With knees extended, place wide strap under ball of foot and toes, have patient pull foot dorsally
Web spaces	Velfoam padding strips between toes and secured with figure 8 pattern compression with elastic wrap to preserve webs	Conformers under promptly applied "foot glove" compression garment	Massage and passive stretch of web spaces, active toe abduction exercises

Note. AAROM = active–assistive range of motion; AFO = ankle–foot orthosis; AROM = active range of motion; IP = interphalangeal; MCP = metacarpophalangeal; MP = metaphalangeal; PIP = proximal interphalangeal; PROM = passive range of motion; ROM = range of motion; UE = upper extremity.

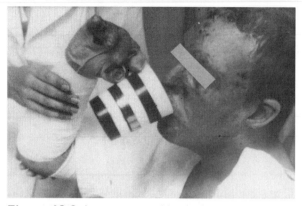

Figure 13.3 As soon as oral intake is allowed, the patient should be encouraged to begin self-feeding regardless of the assistance needed.

involved in active exercise, structured activities, and ambulation throughout the day. A combination of ROM, stretching, and functional activities should be used. A therapist should communicate daily with the burn team members to help determine when to increase or decrease the patient's activity schedule. If the patient is confined to bed, a modified exercise program and ADL activities, such as self-feeding, simple hygiene tasks, or upper-body grooming, could still be performed. Bedside activities such as card or pegboard games, Velcro® darts, or other leisure pastimes can promote upper-extremity flexibility and general strength plus provide opportunities for socialization.

When a patient is medically cleared to ambulate, the treatment program should be adjusted to include out-of-bed exercise and activity. Walking to a chair or standing to do exercises, standing at a sink for grooming tasks, and sitting up in a chair for all meals can help promote conditioning. Patients often complain of fatigue during this phase of increased activity. They will need ongoing support and encouragement to ambulate, perform their exercise program, and complete their self-care tasks independently.

During the transition from dependency on others to self-reliance, patients frequently demonstrate abnormal posturing during exercise or self-care activities. Protective positioning usually begins as a guarding response to avoid pain and discomfort, often in a flexed posture. For example, a patient with a burned arm may hold the extremity close to his side and avoid extending the arm, resulting in a progressive loss of active motion that can eventually cause difficulties with activities such as upper-or lower-extremity dressing and bathing. Use of pre-

ventive or corrective splinting may be needed to preserve long-term joint mobility.

During acute care, a formal schedule may be needed to provide structure, support appropriate patient behaviors, and emphasize treatment objectives. The schedule should include morning and afternoon therapy sessions; dressing changes and nursing procedures; periods for ADL, including ambulation, grooming, eating, and dressing; and free time for visitors and rest periods. The schedule should be developed along with the patient, and the members of the entire burn team should adhere to it. Defining daily expectations in advance will help give the patient a sense of control, reduce anxiety, and foster active involvement in the rehabilitation process.

Treatment: Inpatient Rehabilitation Phase

During the rehabilitation phase, the patient's role in self-care increases as the need for wound care and nursing procedures decreases. The goal is for the patient to complete self-care activities (i.e., feeding, grooming, dressing) as independently and with as little adaptation as possible. Continued patient education stresses the importance of resuming preinjury function, emphasizing the daily routines and habits that will give the patient more control over his or her care. However, decreased ROM, strength, and endurance may interfere with performance of daily living tasks. Decreased joint motion and flexibility may interfere with the more demanding ADL, such as dressing in regular street clothes. Decreased fine-motor control or poor sensation may interfere with the completion of fine-motor tasks, such as fastening clothing, or may put the patient at increased risk for reinjury. Poor strength and decreased general endurance may prevent the patient from performing repetitive activities or completing the task from within acceptable time limits.

To increase ROM and improve strength and endurance, a variety of treatment modalities and activities should be used (Humphrey, Richard, & Staley, 1994). A burn exercise program should include stretching exercises for all extremities, as well as strengthening activities. Flexibility exercises (i.e., slow stretches, alternate toe touches, posture exercises) should be performed in front of a full-length mirror so patients can self-monitor their posture and progress. Endurance can be promoted by encouraging the patient to take part in paced ambulation activities around the hospital, ride a stationary bike, and stand at the sink for hygiene tasks. Equipment such as a BTE Work Simulator® can imitate functional motions to increase upper-body ROM, strength, and endurance, as well as provide written results to monitor patient performance. Other modalities, such as West II and Valpar Work Samples, are also helpful when reproducing functional motions or assessing and simulating work skills (Figure 13.4).

Newly healed skin is extremely fragile and is prone to breakdown. Problems include hypersensitivity and peeling or blisters resulting from friction or even minor trauma. Loss of oil and sweat glands leads to excessive dryness and possible splitting of the skin when it is stretched. Skin-conditioning education and activities should be initiated as wounds heal, addressing the use of massage, application of appropriate moisturizing products, and safe donning of intermediate and custom-made pressure garments. Patients should be taught to massage their skin and apply moisturizers several times a day, whenever it feels tight or dry and before stretching exercises, to desensitize the skin and prevent cracking or splitting.

Compression therapy should be used to provide continuous external vascular support and to

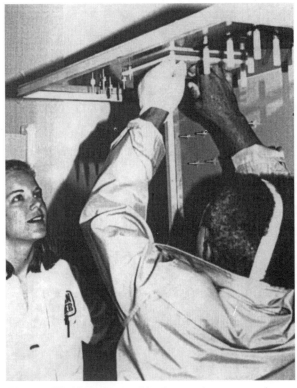

Figure 13.4 Work conditioning equipment can be used to increase active range of motion and general endurance.

reduce the potential for hypertrophic scarring. Poor venous return in burned extremities is evident by the presence of edema in the limb and vascular pooling (as evidenced by skin color). Edema can increase without external venous support or when patients fail to comply with the exercise program. Whenever the patient is out of bed, vascular stockings or elastic wraps should be applied on the lower extremities to aid venous return, especially during ambulation. Because hands are prone to edema, compression wraps or gloves should be worn by persons who have severe hand burns, especially if there is decreased active use.

Early scar compression therapy is provided with a variety of transitional compression techniques and products. For the torso and extremities, these products include elastic bandages, such as Ace® wraps, vascular stockings, or Tubigrip® tubular support bandages. For the hands and digits, compression can be provided with a combination of temporary gloves, such as Isotoner® gloves for lower pressure and Tubigrip® gloves for higher pressure, and digit-sized tubular support bandages such as Tubiton® bandages or self-adherent elastic dressings such as Coban® dressings and Cowrap® dressings.

Special care is needed when applying self-adherent elastic dressings. They should be applied to provide slight tension, using a figure 8 distal to proximal wrapping pattern. To apply a compression wrap to the hand, inch-wide strips of Coban wrap are first placed through the web spaces and attached to a band around the wrist. Silicone gel pads can be used under the Coban wrap to provide added pressure to thicker scars while protecting the skin from irritation. Inch-wide Coban strips are then applied around individual fingers in a distal to proximal manner, and the hand is then wrapped. The fingertips should be slightly exposed, and care should be taken to avoid wrapping too tightly, which is evidenced by poor circulation, blanched or cyanotic fingertips, and the patient's report of discomfort, numbness, or tingling. The self-adherent elastic wraps should include the thumb, all fingers, the web spaces, and the hand, taking the wrap to at least 2 in. above the wrist. Exercises and ADL should be performed with the Coban wrap intact. If the wrap is applied correctly, hand function will not be restricted. For self-feeding, the Coban wrap can be covered with a rubber glove. Persistent edema that does not respond to Coban wraps may be reduced by intermittent compression-pump therapy.

After most wounds are healed, swelling is no longer present, and the patient's weight has stabilized, the patient can be measured for customized scar-compression garments, which should be fitted to the patient before discharge. Compression garments should be worn an average of 23 out of every 24 hours and removed only for bathing and skin care. Face masks and gloves may also be removed for meals and self-feeding. Patients can perform most other ADL tasks without removing the garments. They should be able to participate in most recreational activities and work environments without interference from the garments, although patients may complain of excessive warmth during outside activities in the summer months. Patients should be informed early on, during the acute phase, of the necessity of pressure garments and the need for adhering to the wearing schedule; then, when wound healing allows for garment application, they will be able to recognize scar-compression therapy as a progressive step toward their rehabilitation.

Wearing personal clothing over the scar compression garments should be encouraged to promote a feeling of normalcy and to give the patient practice in donning both compression garments and street clothes (see Figure 13.5). Clothing from home should be casual, loose fitting, comfortable, and made primarily of cotton fiber. To support independent self-care functioning, family members should be asked to bring the patient's clothes and personal grooming items from home early during hospitalization.

Patients who were injured while cooking or bathing may be reluctant to perform related tasks. It is crucial that these fears be identified and addressed. Treatment activities should include education in safety precautions and performance of the fear-provoking tasks with therapist supervision. Safety precautions should be discussed before the treatment session so they can be practiced during the activity.

The rehabilitation phase of burn recovery is greatly influenced by patient habits and routines. Noncompliance with exercise programs often results in contractures, which impair full ROM. When this situation occurs, ADL (habits) cannot be completed without adaptive equipment or compensatory techniques. Poor trunk mobility may inhibit a patient from donning socks and shoes without a sock aid or a long-handled shoehorn. Extended hospitalization or daily outpatient treatment schedules can prevent a patient from resuming familiar roles as family member, student, or provider. It is imperative in this phase that patients recognize their progress and begin to assume previous roles on at least a part-time basis in preparation for discharge.

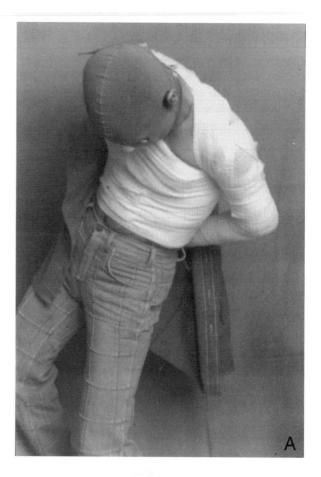

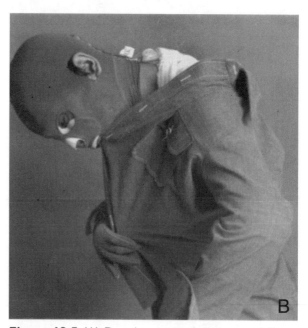

Figure 13.5 (A) Donning street clothes, especially over dressings, can be difficult. (B) Patients should be given the opportunity to problem solve ways to perform tasks independently before adapted equipment is issued.

Burn patients and their family members must be educated about home care activities before discharge from the hospital. Throughout hospitalization, education about what can be expected after discharge can aid the process. Home care booklets, classes, and videotapes are some methods used by burn care facilities to reinforce this information (Adriaenssens, 1988; Mason & Forshaw, 1986; Yurko & Fratianne, 1988). Discharge education and training should involve the members of the whole team and should cover a broad range of topics (Kaplan, 1985).

Before discharge, the patient and caregivers should have opportunities to practice dressing changes, skin care, and application of compression garments and splints. Written instructions should be provided and reviewed regarding:

• wound and skin care;

• use of medications, moisturizers, and sun block lotions;

• sun and trauma precautions;

• home exercise programs (including both therapeutic and recreational activities);

• positioning recommendations;

• use and care of splints;

• self-help devices,

• scar compression garments and conformers; and

• need for environmental modifications (as appropriate).

The patient and family members should demonstrate a thorough understanding of the purpose and content of the home program well before discharge. A list of contacts and phone numbers should also be provided in case questions or concerns arise before the first outpatient appointment.

Intervention: Outpatient Rehabilitation Phase

Current views of occupational therapy practice (e.g., Christiansen, 1991; Kielhofner 1995; Law et al., 1996) recognize the person as constantly changing within a dynamic set of environmental circumstances. Life satisfaction depends on a complex array of conditions, including motivation, experiences, social role expectations, and physical and cognitive capacities. Changes in any of these conditions affect the others.

During the outpatient rehabilitation phase of recovery, burn patients may go through countless physical, functional, and emotional changes, despite continuous and comprehensive patient education. Once home, they truly begin to experience both the functional and social consequences of a burn injury. Changes in self-image, loss of previous work roles, and social relationships have a direct effect on motivation and compliance with therapy recommendations. Although they may eat and dress independently at the end of their hospital stay, they may return unable to even get a spoon to the mouth. Providing adaptive equipment should not be the first response, because many factors could have contributed to this change in functional performance. Identifying the underlying cause of the loss of function is the first step toward developing an appropriate treatment plan. Although scar contracture is the most common cause, other physical and emotional factors can also be contributors to this loss of function. Some patients may suffer from posttraumatic stress disorders (Perry & Difede, 1992), and others must contend with emotional consequences related to preinjury psychological problems (Malt & Ugland, 1989; Tucker, 1986).

Before discharge from the hospital, a patient's strength and endurance may be adequate for self-care independence. Once home, differences between the hospital and home environments may be so great that fatigue may set in before noon. This feeling of fatigue may be functional, but it may also be emotionally based. The normal reaction is to rest instead of participating in home activities and outpatient therapy. The patient may lose his or her momentum and, as a result, strength remains poor or decreases; scars tighten, causing decreased flexibility; and the patient becomes increasingly dependent on others. For this reason, initial outpatient visits should be scheduled to begin shortly after discharge so that patients can receive the physical and emotional support they often need to get them through this difficult adjustment period.

Outpatient treatment plan activities are similar to those used during inpatient rehabilitation, but their intensity and frequency increase. They should include a daily exercise program that emphasizes massage and stretching, followed by flexibility and strengthening activities. Although all these activities should be done frequently throughout the day, scar massage and stretching, especially before self-care activities, can improve a patient's functional skills performance.

Scar contracture is the usual cause of most functional deficits. Where burn scars extend over joint surfaces, there is a progressive loss of functional ROM as the skin shortens. If left untreated, secondary muscle shortening and fibrous contracture of the joint capsule can occur (Abston, 1987). The primary goal of a scar treatment program is to manage scar development so that as scar tissue matures, there is minimal surface distortion or loss of active ROM from tight scar bands, hypertrophic scarring, or adhesions to underlying structures.

Scar compression therapy continues, with the therapist closely monitoring the fit and effectiveness of the compression garments for proper fit, evidence of garment deterioration, and need for underlying conformers and inserts (see Table 13.3). Although pressure garments and conformers are used to minimize scar height and maintain pliability, continuous activity is necessary to oppose the contractile forces of the scar. Splints, serial casting, end-range stretching exercises, and activities that accentuate flexibility also are effective treatments for contractures (Daugherty & Carr-Collins, 1994; Rivers, 1987). There are times when a scar contracture is so strong that prevention of further loss of motion can be the only goal. A scar band may become unstable and tend to break down repeatedly. These types of contractures eventually require surgical intervention to restore functional mobility and scar durability.

Because scar control and remodeling are easier during the early stages of wound maturation, limitations in self-care function can be resolved if appropriate treatments are implemented promptly and the patient participates actively. In addition to other outpatient burn treatment activities, performing basic self-care is an effective, practical, and meaningful way to increase strength, endurance, flexibility, and coordination. Despite the extra time it may take, patients should be encouraged to attempt self-care activities with minimal reliance on compensatory motions or use of adaptive equipment. However, a critical element of success in achieving ADL goals is motivation, which cannot be maintained without task completion. If the patient becomes too frustrated or fatigued to complete the task, he or she may lose motivation and refuse further attempts. This loss of motivation is especially true for small children (see Figure 13.6). As in the acute phase, the therapist should choose self-care tasks that promote not only independence but also self-confidence. If adaptive equipment is needed for task completion, it should be reinforced to the patient that the device should be needed only temporarily. Adapted devices should then be modified or discontinued as active motion increases, and these changes should be presented to the patient as signs of progress.

In some cases, burn depth, extent, and involvement of underlying structures are so major that adaptations are necessary for the patient to function independently. The adaptations should be simple and designed to use all available active ROM (see Figure 13.7). As scars mature and soften, functional skills should gradually improve. Tendon and joint adhesions should also eventually resolve if patients use the motion available and continue with stretching exercises.

Depending on their personalities and coping skills, many burn patients with permanent functional limitations develop their own adaptive methods to accomplish specific tasks (see Figure 13.8). These persons may consider extensive adaptations to be an encumbrance or an embarrassment. If they have to use adaptive equipment, it tends to be

Table 13.3 Insert Materials Used Under Pressure Garments

Material	Applications
Aliplast	Thumb webs, shoe inserts
Aquaplast, $\frac{1}{16}$-in. thick	Facial conformers
Otoform-K silicone elastomer putty	Over thicker, persistent scars and keloid scars
Plastazote	Finger webs, hand dorsum, axillary webs, any firm scar
Silastic elastomer, prosthetic foam	Breast or gluteal cleavage, face, hands
Silicone gel	Hands, face, skin folds, areas of limited friction
Velfoam-2 padding	Any area needing increased compression or protection from garment friction, fabric creases or zippers: finger and axillary webs, anterior neck or clavicular areas

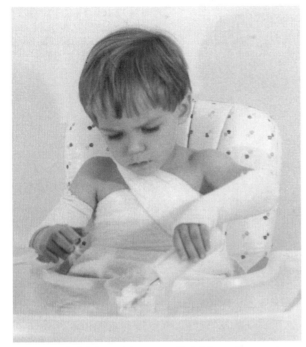

Figure 13.6 Like adults, a small child can be motivated to use his hands if the task is one that holds his interest, such as feeding himself ice cream.

small enough to fit in a pocket or purse, such as a button aid (see Figure 13.9). This positive change of perspective usually occurs during the outpatient rehabilitation phase and is a sign that the patient is adjusting to permanent changes in past roles or is developing new roles.

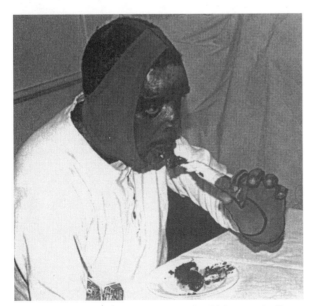

Figure 13.7 Extended handles should be gradually shortened as range of motion improves.

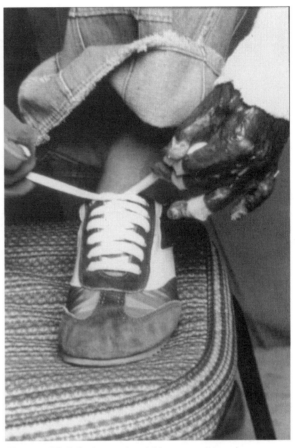

Figure 13.8 Patients should be encouraged to develop strength and dexterity for later task completion.

Early in the outpatient rehabilitation phase, patients may have little interest in self-care because of the emotional effect of the injury. Depression and anxiety are common during recovery and are often manifested in noncompliance or apathy, both of which slow progress toward functional and emotional independence. During this adjustment period, burn patients may receive comfort and encouragement by talking with other burn patients or by attending a burn support group. Talking with a more experienced burn patient facilitates understanding by offering a personal perspective and physical evidence that things will get easier and better with time and continued effort.

During the outpatient rehabilitation phase, therapy should include opportunities to practice work and leisure skills that incorporate past skills and interests related to employment, home management, education, and play. Depending on the patient's length of hospital stay, some of these activities may have already been initiated during the inpatient rehabilitation phase. The patient and

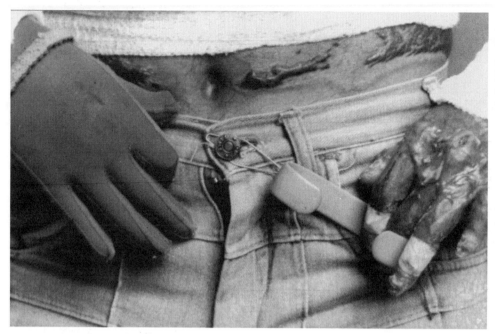

Figure 13.9 This younger patient chose to use a button aid rather than to change his personal preference for snug-fitting jeans.

therapist review current difficulties and address potential adaptations to work or home schedules and environments. Homemakers may practice cooking skills for endurance training and receive safety education to help resolve fear of heat, especially if the burns were house-fire or cooking related. Endurance and fine-motor skills are practiced by imitating specific tasks related to work roles, not just by using a work simulator or traditional exercise equipment (see Figure 13.10). When possible, tools and equipment should be brought to therapy sessions so that the therapist can assist with the analysis of task technique and suggest adaptations, as needed (see Figure 13.11).

Recreational interests and leisure roles should not be neglected during the rehabilitation phases. Leisure activities should be incorporated into therapy routines as early as possible and their positive therapeutic value, both physically and emotionally, acknowledged (see Figure 13.12). If permanent disability precludes resumption of previous work

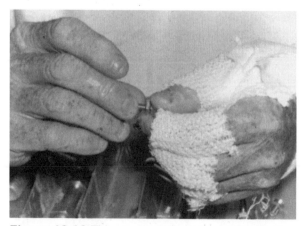

Figure 13.10 This mechanic develops his finger dexterity by working with various sizes of nuts and bolts.

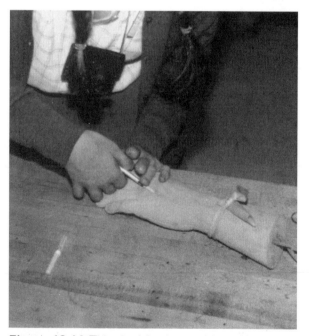

Figure 13.11 This physician is practicing taking blood samples after having lost her distal fingers.

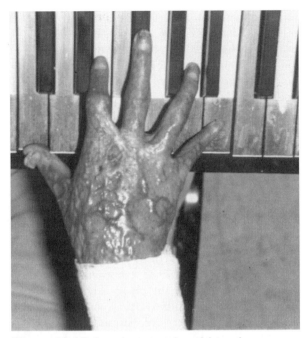

Figure 13.12 A patient stretches tight web spaces and regains a prior leisure skill while practicing on a piano.

roles, leisure roles take on more importance and past interests should be encouraged. An uncomfortable motion may be better tolerated when performed during a leisure activity. However, the therapist should be careful not to suppress the patient's interest by turning the leisure task into an "exercise."

Later, in the outpatient rehabilitation phase, the patient's need for ongoing therapy diminishes. When the patient's return to part-time work or attendance at school will promote occupational recovery, the patient should be weaned from therapy by gradually reducing his or her treatment schedule. A patient who achieves the skills needed to function independently at home and can return to school or work full time should be discharged from ongoing outpatient therapy. However, the patient should be periodically reevaluated to monitor the status of maturing scars, functional skills, and psychosocial adjustment. Because burn scar maturation can take up to 18 months after injury, a patient may still be wearing pressure garments or night splints even after resuming a normal routine, and these also need to be periodically checked and modified when the patient returns to see the burn team members.

Psychosocial adjustment continues during the outpatient phase of burn recovery with the patient examining personal interests and values. The patient must grieve for lost roles and abilities and accept the permanent changes resulting from the burn. These losses often include not only vocational and leisure skills but also the loss of past social roles and identity caused by disfigurement. These issues need to be addressed during outpatient visits.

Facial Scars

Scar contracture and hypertrophy restrict function more than by just limiting ROM. Distortions in facial structures caused by contracting scars can produce severe disfigurement, including altered nasal contours, everted eyelids and lips that expose the conjunctivas and inner lips, contracted oral commissures, or missing features. Eye contractures can produce difficulties in seeing and cause excessive tearing and nasal drainage. Mouth contractures can cause problems with talking, eating, and excessive salivation and interfere with oral hygiene. Any of these conditions can have a devastating effect on the patient's ability to function in society.

There are primarily two treatment choices for compressing facial scarring: a custom-made elastic face mask with underlying conformers or a rigid, total contact, transparent facial orthosis (Rivers, 1987). Elastic face masks are combined with thin, flexible conformers to flatten and shape developing facial and head scars and maintain normal feature contours. The garments are custom made and should be replaced every 6 to 8 weeks to ensure correct compression. They are usually worn with underlying silicone gel, elastomer, or thermoplastic inserts to distribute the pressure over and around facial contours.

A transparent facial orthosis is molded of high-temperature, transparent plastic and is held in place with elastic straps. Fabrication of a transparent facial orthosis involves taking a negative impression of the patient's face, making a positive plaster cast of the impression, heating and stretching the plastic over the cast, finishing the edges, applying adjustable straps, and fitting it to the patient (Rivers, 1984). When fitting the clear orthosis, the therapist can see and check the scars for blanching once it is donned. This blanching is an indication that the scars are getting adequate compression.

Regardless of the method chosen for facial compression, the making of a positive mold early in the healing process, before contractures alter the patient's features, is recommended. This facial mold can be used for fabrication of either the clear orthosis or the face mask conformers and allows for precise fitting or alteration of the devices. It also serves as a three-dimensional model against which facial distortion can be monitored.

Some practitioners and patients prefer a combination of the two techniques, with the clear mask used during the day or social activities and the elastic mask with conformers used at night or when at home. The elastic mask with conformers has the advantage of multidirectional compression and dynamic fit that is less affected by facial movement or changes in position (i.e., upright versus supine). The clear facial orthosis has the advantage of not completely hiding the patient's face, which allows the patient to retain some personal identity.

Regardless of the method chosen, prior education is critical to prepare the patient for the fabrication and fitting process, as well as for long-term compliance with the facial compression and exercise program. Skin-care education should include lubrication and massage, with pressure applied during massage to desensitize scars and to help stretch tight skin. An exercise program to stretch tight facial skin should have already been initiated. To be effective, all compression devices should be applied almost continuously until the scars mature, except during bathing, skin care, exercises, and scar massage. Face masks and gloves should be removed for meals. To avoid misunderstandings with those who are unfamiliar with their condition, adult patients should be advised to remove all facial coverings before entering a store or bank and to carry an identification card that verifies the medical necessity for the mask.

Persons wearing either type of mask often report feelings of self-consciousness, isolation, poor self-esteem, and loss of personal identity (see Figure 13.13). All of these perceptions need to be acknowledged and addressed by those close to the patient. Many patients benefit from counseling and from speaking with someone else who is wearing or has worn a facial mask or orthosis.

Various facial reconstructive procedures are possible to improve both function and appearance. When facial distortion caused by scarring is extensive, scar excision and autografting can usually improve appearance once burn wound maturation is complete. Normal skin appearance (without cosmetics) can never be achieved after a severe burn, but the illusion of normalcy is possible (Salisbury, Petro, & Winski, 1987). When the wounds are mature, the patient should be referred to a cosmetologist who has training in corrective makeup blending for the face or other body areas. Although the appearance of facial scars may be

improved with surgical reconstruction and the use of special camouflaging makeup, the patient will eventually have to realize that he or she will never look the same as before the injury. With the support of others, they can learn to accept their new body image.

Age-Related Considerations

Small children tend to heal and scar differently from older children and adults. Children less than 5 years of age have a higher potential for hypertrophic scarring of both burn and donor sites because of prolonged scar maturation. Smaller muscles, hypermobile joints, and inability to cooperate put them at higher risk for contractures than adults. They are more likely to experience emotional regression, especially during the acute phase. The physical and social restrictions resulting from contractures and disfigurement can interfere with meeting developmental milestones. For this reason, it is helpful to

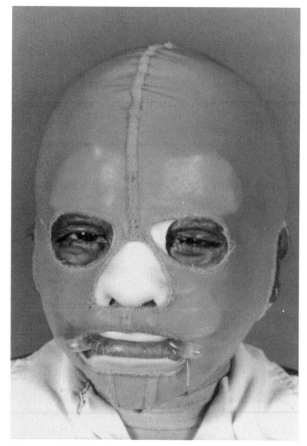

Figure 13.13 Patients with severe facial burns experience a loss of personal identity and must reconcile themselves to a new body image, first with a mask and then without it.

obtain information from parents and family members regarding developmental milestones met by children before the burn, so that if regression occurs, appropriate interventions can be initiated while the patient is still in the hospital.

For school-age children, a school reentry program should be initiated before discharge. With such programming, the teacher, classmates (and in some cases, the school-based therapist) can become well acquainted with the appearance and special needs of the injured child before he or she returns to school (Meyer, Barnett, & Gross, 1987; Rosenstein, 1987). Such foreknowledge helps ease the resumption of the student role for the child and can help improve acceptance by other children who may not otherwise understand the cause of the disfigurement and the need for splints, adapted equipment, and scar-compression garments. Summer camps for burned children, often sponsored by local firefighter organizations, also help the children adjust by placing them in settings where they can socialize with peers who also have been burned.

Elderly persons may not form hypertrophic scars as readily as younger patients, but their scars may stay fragile longer and may heal more slowly. Degenerative joint disease, osteoporosis, cardiopulmonary complications, diabetes, deconditioning, or other preexisting conditions in the elderly person may further complicate the rehabilitative process. Care must be taken during active-assistive or passive ROM exercises not to overstretch joints that may have been restricted even before the burn.

Burn Reconstruction

Throughout rehabilitation and follow-up visits to the burn clinic, the patient's functional skills and emotional adjustment to the injury should be continually reevaluated. When limitations in motion persist or the patient requests reconstruction, the burn team members must assess the specific problems and make recommendations. These recommendations can range from increasing the frequency and intensity of rehabilitation to surgical reconstruction. Early surgical reconstruction is usually indicated when a contracture deformity does not respond to scar treatment techniques and impedes rehabilitation and functional independence. If slow, gradual improvement occurs with therapy and the patient can function independently, the surgeon may delay reconstruction until scars are mature and less likely to recontract.

Various types of surgical procedures are used in burn reconstruction. Most of them are for func-

tional reconstruction; however, some are also used to improve appearance. Scar excision and grafting; advancement, rotation, pedicle, and myocutaneous flaps; steroid injections and dermabrasion; and Z-plasties are a few examples. To gain a better understanding of the procedures, their expected results, and their treatment implications, it is suggested that books dedicated to burn reconstruction be reviewed (e.g., see Achauer, 1991; Salisbury & Bevin, 1981).

Burn reconstruction surgery is usually the last option. Many burn rehabilitation techniques are designed to reduce the need for reconstruction. By providing early and continuous patient education and progressive rehabilitation, many reconstructive surgeries can be prevented. When reconstruction is inevitable, consideration must be given to appropriate timing for reconstruction, the type of procedure, and necessary follow-up treatment.

Summary

To obtain optimal outcomes after severe burns, it is necessary to consider not only the patient's phase of recovery, functional limitations, compliance with treatment, and psychological adjustment but also the patient's personal goals and priorities. It is the therapist's responsibility to anticipate and prevent physical limitations, emotional dependence, and social isolation through prompt therapeutic intervention, psychosocial support, and referral to appropriate ancillary services and community resources. The ultimate goal should be to enable the burn patient to achieve functional independence in his or her preferred lifestyle and chosen roles. ◆

Study Questions

1. How do superficial and deep partial burns vary in regard to scarring potential?

2. How is %TBSA estimated using the rule of nines and the Lund and Browder chart methods?

3. When is patient–caregiver education initiated?

4. What is the general rule for positioning and splinting the burn patient?

5. What is the ADL task that typically carries the most importance for the patient, regardless of age?

6. Who usually develops more hypertrophic scars, burn patients less than 5 years of age or those more than 50 years of age?

7. When should ongoing outpatient burn therapy be discontinued?

References

Abston, S. (1987). Scar reaction after thermal injury and prevention of scars and contractures. In J. Boswick (Ed.), *The art and science of burn care* (pp. 359–371). Gaithersburg, MD: Aspen.

Achauer, B. (1991). *Burn reconstruction.* New York: Thieme Medical Publishers.

Adriaenssens, P. (1988). The video invasion of rehabilitation. *Burns Including Thermal Injuries, 14,* 417–419.

Baum, C. M., & Christiansen, C. H. (1997). Person–environment–occupational performance: A conceptual model for practice. In C. Christiansen & C. Baum (Eds.), *Occupational therapy: Enabling function and well-being* (pp. 48–69). Thorofare, NJ: Slack.

Bowden, M. L., Thomson, P. D., & Prasad, J. K. (1989). Factors influencing return to employment after a burn injury. *Archives of Physical Medicine and Rehabilitation, 70,* 772–775.

Carvajal, H. F. (1988). Resuscitation of the burned child. In H. F. Carvajal & D. H. Parks (Eds.), *Burns in children: Pediatric burn management* (pp. 78–98). Chicago: Year Book Medical Publishers.

Cheng, S., & Rogers, J. C. (1989). Changes in occupational role performance after a severe burn: A retrospective study. *American Journal of Occupational Therapy, 43,* 17–24.

Christiansen, C. (1991). Intervention for life performance. In C. Christiansen & C. Baum (Eds.), *Occupational therapy: Overcoming human performance deficits* (pp. 1–43). Thorofare, NJ: Slack.

Daugherty, M. B., & Carr-Collins, J. A. (1994). Splinting techniques for the burn patient. In R. Richard & M. Staley (Eds.), *Burn care and rehabilitation: Principles and practice* (pp. 242–323). Philadelphia: F. A. Davis.

Fleet, J. (1992). The psychological effects of burn injuries: A literature review. *British Journal of Occupational Therapy, 55,* 198–201.

Hartford, C. (1984). Surgical management. In S. Fisher & P. Helm (Eds.), *Comprehensive rehabilitation of burns* (pp. 28–63). Baltimore: Williams & Wilkins.

Helm, P. A., & Fisher, S. (1988). Rehabilitation of the patient with burns. In J. DeLisa, D. Currie, & B. Gans (Eds.), *Rehabilitation medicine: Principles and practice* (pp. 821–839). Philadelphia: Lippincott.

Helm, P. A., Walker, S. C., & Peyton, S. A. (1986). Return to work following hand burns. *Archives of Physical Medicine and Rehabilitation, 67,* 297–298.

Humphrey, C., Richard, R. L., & Staley, M. J. (1994). Soft tissue management and exercise. In R. Richard & M. Staley (Eds.), *Burn care and rehabilitation: Principles and practice* (pp. 324–360). Philadelphia: F. A. Davis.

Kaplan, S. H. (1985). Patient education techniques used at burn centers. *American Journal of Occupational Therapy, 39,* 655–658.

Kielhofner, G. (1995). *A model of human occupation: Theory and application* (2nd ed.). Baltimore: Williams & Wilkins.

Law, M., Cooper, B., Strong, S., Stewart, D., Rigby, P., & Letts, L. (1996). The Person–Environment–Occupation Model: A transactive approach to occupational performance. *Canadian Journal of Occupational Therapy, 63,* 9–23.

Lund, C., & Browder, N. (1944). The estimation of area of burns. *Surgical Gynecology and Obstetrics, 79,* 352–355.

Mahon, L. M., & Neufeld, N. (1984). The effect of informational feedback on food intake of adult burn patients. *Journal of Applied Behavior Analysis, 17,* 391–396.

Malt, U. F., & Ugland, O. M. (1989). A long term psychosocial follow-up study of burned adults. *Acta Psychiatrica Scandinavia, 80*(Suppl. 355), 94–102.

Mason, S., & Forshaw, A. (1986). Burns after care: A booklet for parents: Your child at home after injury. *Burns Including Thermal Injuries, 12,* 343–350.

Meyer, D. O., Barnett, P. H., & Gross, D. J. (1987). A school reentry program for burned children. Part II: Physical therapy contribution to an existing school reentry program. *Journal of Burn Care and Rehabilitation, 8,* 322–324.

Parent, L. H. (1983). Burns. In C. Trombly (Ed.), *Occupational therapy for physical dysfunction* (2nd ed., pp. 399–408). Baltimore: Williams & Wilkins.

Perry, S., & Difede, J. (1992). Predictors of posttraumatic stress disorder after burn injury. *American Journal of Psychiatry, 149,* 931–935.

Petro, J., & Salisbury, R. (1986). Rehabilitation of the burn patient. *Clinics in Plastic Surgery, 3*(1), 145–149.

Reilly, M. (1962). Occupational therapy can be one of the great ideas of the 20th century. *American Journal of Occupational Therapy, 16,* 1–9.

Rivers, E. (1984). Management of hypertrophic scars. In S. Fisher & P. Helm (Eds.), *Comprehensive rehabilitation of burns* (pp. 177–217). Baltimore: Williams & Wilkins.

Rivers, E. (1987). Rehabilitation management of the burn patient. *Advances in Clinical Rehabilitation, 1,* 177–213.

Rosenstein, D. W. L. (1987). A school reentry program for burned children. Part I: Development and implementation of a school reentry program. *Journal of Burn Care and Rehabilitation, 8,* 319–322.

Salisbury, R., & Bevin, A. (1981). *Atlas of reconstructive burn surgery.* Philadelphia: W. B. Saunders.

Salisbury, R., Petro, J., & Winski, F. (1987). Reconstruction of the burn patient. In J. Boswick (Ed.), *The art and science of burn care* (pp. 353–357). Gaithersburg, MD: Aspen.

Solem, L. (1984). Classification. In S. Fisher & P. Helm (Eds.), *Comprehensive rehabilitation of burns* (pp. 9–15). Baltimore: Williams & Wilkins.

Trombly, C. A. (1995). Theoretical foundation for practice. In C. A. Trombly (Ed.), *Occupational therapy for physical dysfunction* (4th ed., pp. 15–28). Baltimore: Williams & Wilkins.

Tucker, P. (1986). The burn victim: A review of psychosocial issues. *Australian and New Zealand Journal of Psychiatry, 20,* 413–420.

Wachtel, T. (1985). Epidemiology, classification, initial care, and administrative considerations for critically burned patients. In T. Wachtel (Ed.), *Critical care clinics* (pp. 3–26). Philadelphia: W. B. Saunders.

Yurko, L., & Fratianne, R. (1988). Evaluation of burn discharge teaching. *Journal of Burn Care and Rehabilitation, 9,* 643–644.

14

Self-Care Management for Persons With Cognitive Deficits After Alzheimer's Disease and Traumatic Brain Injury

Beatriz C. Abreu

Beatriz C. Abreu, PhD, OTR, FAOTA, is Director, Occupational Therapy, Transitional Learning Community, and Clinical Professor, University of Texas Medical Branch at Galveston, Texas.

The author is grateful to the research and editorial team of Jane Keel and Renee Pearcy for their help with the preparation of this chapter and to Dr. Brent Masel, the Moody Endowment, and the Moody Foundation for their support of this work. The author also acknowledges Mary Hall, Sherida Ryan, and Estella Tse, who coauthored the chapter on cognitive deficits in the first edition.

Key Terms

Alzheimer's disease

cognitive deficits

cognitive rehabilitation

flat affect

functional training

self-care management

traumatic brain injury

Objectives

On completing this chapter, the reader will be able to

1. Identify major types of cognitive dysfunction.

2. Identify major brain structures and the typical cognitive deficits that result when disorders occur within them.

3. Describe the clinical features and functional consequences of Alzheimer's disease.

4. Describe the clinical features and functional consequences of traumatic brain injury.

5. Distinguish between the clinical features of Alzheimer's disease and traumatic brain injury and appreciate how these differences influence intervention planning.

6. Plan appropriate assessments and interventions to use with clients with cognitive deficits, with particular attention to the self-care needs of persons with these conditions.

The purpose of this chapter is to present an approach for the evaluation and treatment of cognitive and self-care skills for persons who have been affected by Alzheimer's disease and traumatic brain injury (TBI). The chapter begins with a review of general behavioral changes because of cognitive deficits, followed by a brief summary of the functions of the brain. Also addressed are specific changes in cognition and self-care management after Alzheimer's disease and TBI. General evaluation and treatment strategies for both conditions are reviewed and measurement treatment outcomes are discussed.

Alzheimer's Disease and TBI

In most countries, there is a large and increasing population of persons who are affected by cognitive deficits after Alzheimer's disease and TBI (Horn & Zasler, 1996; Van Duijn, 1996). In the United States, about 4 million people have Alzheimer's disease (BIOTA, 1998), and each year more than 2 million people incur head injuries (Horn & Zasler, 1996). Cognitive deficits caused by Alzheimer's disease and TBI influence a person's self-care independence and increase the need for occupational therapy services in both institutional and home settings. In addition, occupational therapy practitioners are being asked to work with other diagnoses, such as schizophrenia, stroke, brain tumors, and cerebral palsy, which also involve cognitive deficits and self-care management issues. Given this increased demand for service, occupational therapy practitioners need to understand more fully the effect of such cognitive impairments on self-care management to provide effective evaluation and treatment strategies.

The relationship between cognition and self-care management for clients with cognitive deficits is complex, dynamic, and difficult to comprehend. Although there are no simple answers when dealing with Alzheimer's disease and TBI, the practical approach for evaluation and treatment presented in this chapter might prove useful. One general and perhaps obvious principle that may be applied to the relationship between cognition and self-care management is that the more severe the cognitive deficit, the more dependent the person will be in self-care. There is extensive information about cognition and cognitive impairments in both the cognitive psychology and neuropsychology literature, but a review of this knowledge is beyond the scope

of this chapter. The following section offers a brief description of the effect of Alzheimer's disease and TBI on clients as well as their caregivers.

Behavioral Changes Caused by Cognitive Deficits

When cognitive changes that are attributable to Alzheimer's disease and TBI first appear, the clients and their family members may not fully realize the scope and devastating effect that these conditions will have on their entire social support system (Corcoran, 1994). The behavioral changes caused by such deficits extend far beyond the person with the disability. Family members, friends, and others will spend a tremendous amount of time assisting persons with cognitive impairments with self-care management. These persons must become caregivers, and they frequently become overworked and stressed when faced with these new role responsibilities (Frosch et al., 1997). As a result, the emotional state of the group members is adversely affected and they themselves become candidates for counseling and guidance. Through retraining and compensatory strategies, occupational therapy practitioners, as part of a multidisciplinary health care team, may be able to use purposeful activity and ordinary occupation to promote health and achieve functional outcomes for both clients and family members.

Two of the most common cognitive deficits associated with Alzheimer's disease and TBI are the impairment of memory and the lack of awareness of disability. These deficits often lead to unsafe personal behaviors that create additional stressors for family members. Practitioners and other members of the health care team also may become burned out with the chronicity, decline, and maladaptive behaviors that are prevalent with such diagnoses. Cognitive deficits, whether minimal, moderate, or severe, have far-reaching consequences on the total social support network.

Alzheimer's disease and TBI are two acquired, persistent impairments that affect multiple areas of cognitive function. The illness trajectories followed by Alzheimer's disease and TBI are quite different. In Alzheimer's disease, clients show deterioration in thinking, behavior, and functional ability over time. In TBI, clients show recovery, followed by a plateau in thinking, behavior, and functional ability over time. Rehabilitation for both Alzheimer's disease and TBI includes the use of retraining and compensatory strategies. The primary focus for Alzheimer's disease is on compensatory strategies, whereas the emphasis for TBI includes both retraining and compensatory strategies. Specific changes in the behavior of clients after Alzheimer's disease are addressed by retraining and compensatory strategies.

All functional behavior is controlled by the nervous system and, in particular, the brain. The nervous system is an organized group of nerve and other nonneural cells that function to receive, integrate, and transmit information. The brain is the part of the nervous system that is most notably damaged by Alzheimer's disease and TBI. Four major structures of the brain that are commonly affected by Alzheimer's disease and TBI are the frontal, parietal, temporal, and occipital lobes (see Figure 14.1). Brief descriptions of the roles in cognition played by each of these four brain structures follows.

Frontal Lobes

The frontal lobes are located in the most forward section of the brain, one on each side of the mid-line. Damage to the frontal lobes causes both cognitive and motor dysfunction. Cognitive impairment may be noted by such symptoms as the lack of alertness and motivation, poor judgment, flat affect, and, possibly, memory problems. Broca's aphasia may also occur with damage to the lower portion of the lobe, resulting in the inability to speak or understand spoken or written language. Decline in the function of the frontal lobes may result in a decreased concern for personal hygiene, poor insight, difficulty in problem solving, emotional dullness, and social withdrawal. In addition, certain pathological motor responses, such as grasp reflex and groping responses with the hands, may occur.

Parietal Lobes

The parietal lobes are located between the frontal and the occipital lobes. Damage to the parietal lobes may result in a decreased ability to engage in and disengage from tasks. In addition, there may be a reduction in the ability to detect spatial orientation. Clients may have difficulty determining the

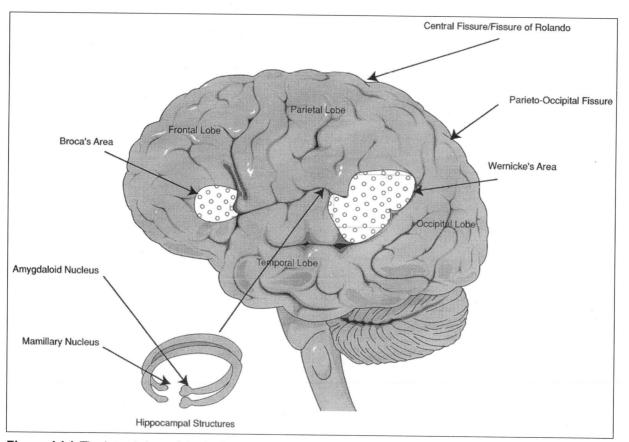

Figure 14.1 The lateral view of the brain, showing the locations of the structures affected by Alzheimer's disease and traumatic brain injury.

location of places and objects and distance between them and may also lose perspective of their own spatial qualities. Tactile memory may be impaired, and clients may not be able to recognize objects by touch.

Temporal Lobes

The temporal lobes are located below the frontal and parietal lobes. Damage to the temporal lobes can result in decreased visual and auditory memory and impairment of emotional memories. This is especially true when there is damage to the hippocampus or to the amygdala, both of which are located within the temporal lobes. A second area in the posterior portion of the left frontal lobe, the Wernicke's area, affects speech and language. Damage to this area can result in *Wernicke's aphasia*, or loss of comprehension of the spoken and often the written word. Although clients can speak, their speech may be disorganized, illogical, and without content.

Occipital Lobes

The occipital lobes are located behind the parietal and temporal lobes. Damage to the occipital lobes may cause impairment in the visual field and problems with spatial memory and object identification. Clients may be able to see, but their level of pattern recognition and visual memory may be impaired.

Specific Changes in Cognition and Self-Care Management After Alzheimer's Disease

Alzheimer's disease is a progressive, degenerative disease of uncertain causes that manifests itself in damage to the brain. Researchers have proposed various causes for Alzheimer's disease including neurochemical, immunological, toxic, viral, abnormal proteins, and genetic factors (Glickstein, 1997). Alzheimer's disease is named after Dr. Alois Alzheimer, who first described the condition in 1907. Alzheimer's disease is the fourth leading cause of death in persons more than 65 years of age, and the incidence increases in persons more than 85 years of age. Alzheimer's disease is marked by a loss of cognitive abilities that is not considered a part of the normal aging process. *Dementia* has been classified according to the area of damage: (a) cortical damage, including Alzheimer's and Pick's disease; (b) subcortical damage secondary to Huntington's or

Parkinson's disease; and (c) a mixed type, such as multi-infarct dementia. Readers should refer to the *Diagnostic and Statistical Manual* (4th ed.) for a more elaborate classification of dementia (American Psychiatric Association, 1994).

There are three specific stages used to address cognition and self-care management issues associated with Alzheimer's disease: mild, moderate, and severe (Reisburg, 1984; Reisburg, Ferris, De Leon, & Crook, 1982). The three stages used to describe and predict the behaviors that are expected to emerge during the course of the disease are not rigidly defined. Unfortunately, they portray a grim picture of dementia. Practitioners may develop a clearer understanding of the complexities involved in treating Alzheimer's disease when they better understand the following social issues associated with the disease.

- There is social stigma attached to dementia.
- The diagnostic process is frequently based on subjective factors.
- Clients with Alzheimer's disease are sometimes treated in a dehumanizing manner once a diagnosis is made.
- Some disruptive behaviors observed in clients may be viewed as normal reactions to increased anxiety (Herskovits, 1995; Ronch, 1996).

Because of these social phenomena associated with Alzheimer's disease, occupational therapy practitioners should seek to understand the factors that contribute to caregiving and strive to promote the preservation of compassion and the client's personal identity.

First Stage of Alzheimer's Disease—Mild

The first stage of Alzheimer's disease begins with the appearance of symptoms such as forgetfulness, repetition of questions, and difficulty in using words. Forgetfulness includes the inability to recall information after brief (short-term memory) or extended (long-term memory) periods of time. An example of forgetfulness would be the inability to remember names and to recall recent events, conversations, or object placements. Please note that age or stress-related forgetfulness does not indicate the presence of Alzheimer's disease and does not, like Alzheimer's disease, interfere with daily living.

During the first stage of Alzheimer's disease, most clients encounter difficulties with the initiation, speed, amount, and quality of performance of self-care and begin to require assistance and supervision. They become forgetful, which begins to affect their job performance. Clients get confused about travel directions and begin to miss appointments. Judgment and problem-solving skills are impaired, and money-management problems begin to arise. As the clients become more passive and forgetful, family members notice personality and behavioral changes. This stage may last from 2 to 4 years, during which clients usually reside at home.

Second Stage of Alzheimer's Disease—Moderate

During the second stage, which lasts from 2 to 10 years, the symptoms worsen and the necessity for supervision and assistance by caregivers increases. Symptoms include difficulty with short- and long-term memory, leading to confabulation. Clients invent stories to fill in the blanks of memory loss. In addition, clients encounter difficulty in recognizing family members and friends, as well as in remembering their visits. Difficulties with finding words to express themselves increases, and clients exhibit a decreased ability to read, write, and perform mathematical calculations. They may be unable to dress and bathe independently, and supervision for mobility and travel is required. The client tends to sleep often and becomes restless and suspicious; changes in body weight occur. At this stage, many persons with Alzheimer's disease are unable to maintain jobs. The caregivers must offer moderate but constant supervision so that the person can safely perform daily activities.

Third Stage of Alzheimer's Disease—Severe

In the final stage of Alzheimer's disease, there is a global decline of all daily functions and a complete loss of judgment. In this stage, clients are unable to judge right from wrong and are dependent on 24-hour supervision and maximal assistance. This severe stage may last from 1 to 3 years. Clients have little capacity for self-care; become incontinent; and require help with eating, dressing, bathing, and toileting. They sleep more frequently and for longer periods of time. They may groan and scream and become disoriented. Clients are unable to recognize family members, friends, and even themselves. Some suffer a marked weight loss. Many family members are forced to place their loved ones in nursing homes or long-term care institutions where they can receive the most effective care and treatment.

Clients with Alzheimer's disease who have lost their self-identity and self-care management skills still maintain the capacity for love, affection, satisfaction, joy, pain, fear, and anxiety. Therefore, practitioners need to devise management and coping strategies that will allow the clients and their family members to gain some relief.

Specific Changes in Cognition and Self-Care Management After TBI

TBI is nonprogressive, persistent damage to the brain. TBI is usually caused by a blow to the head, either from an external object or from the impact of internal forces caused by high-speed acceleration or deceleration. In the United States more than half of all traumatic brain injuries are caused by motor vehicle accidents. Many of these are alcohol related. The remainder are accounted for by falls, assaults, and sports injuries (Brain Injury Association, 1998). More than two thirds of TBI cases are diagnosed in persons under 30 years of age. Young males between 14 and 24 years of age have the highest rate of injury. The immediate or primary brain injuries after head trauma are classified as *closed* or *penetrating:* a closed head injury is one that does not involve penetration of the brain by a foreign object; a penetrating head injury involves just such a violation. TBI may include brain contusions, vascular damage, and intracranial pressure changes (Scott & Dow, 1995). These injuries can be localized or diffuse. Localized injuries are specific to certain areas of the brain, such as damage to the frontal lobe. With diffuse injuries, there is a more generalized affect, and many structures are involved. TBI is a complex diagnosis and, for the purposes of discussion, three stages of cognitive function will be used to describe the recovery of abilities as well as the progression and plateauing (leveling off) of thinking and behavior.

Stages of Recovery After TBI

In TBI, the trajectory of recovery generally depicts an upward progression as opposed to the regression shown in Alzheimer's disease. TBI clients may advance from severe, to moderate, to mild. Some of the symptoms may diminish over time, but others may be more persistent.

Two of the most common scales used to characterize particular aspects of recovery after TBI are the Glasgow Coma Scale (GCS) and the Post-

Traumatic Amnesia (PTA) measures (Giacino, Kezmarsky, DeLuca, & Cicerone, 1991; Teasdale & Jennett, 1974). The GCS is based on the duration of prolonged unconsciousness or deep sleep, whereas the PTA is based on the duration of memory loss of the period preceding the injury. The duration of memory loss is also called *retrograde amnesia*. These scales can be used to categorize and predict clients' functional outcome.

The GCS consists of a 15-point scale used to rate eye opening and motor and verbal responses. The PTA is a measurement obtained by estimating the duration of the memory loss from the moment of trauma to the time of evaluation, at which point clients are able to demonstrate the ability to communicate about memory.

The GCS and PTA are used to classify TBI clients into five categories. In general, lower scores on the GCS and a greater PTA duration indicate a more severe injury. The five classifications of TBI are mild, moderate, severe, very severe, and extremely severe. The mild category includes those clients who may not have been rendered unconscious, who achieved GCS scores ranging from 13 to 15, and whose memory loss after trauma lasted from 5 minutes to 1 hour as measured by the PTA. The moderate category refers to clients who endured a period of unconsciousness and achieved a GCS score of from 9 to 12 and a PTA duration of less than 24 hours. The severe classification comprises clients who were in a coma, with GCS scores below 8 and a PTA duration of more than 24 hours. The very severe classification includes clients who were in a coma and had a GCS score of 5 points and a PTA duration of 4 weeks. Finally, the extremely severe category includes those with sustained coma, a GCS below 5 points, and a PTA of more than 4 weeks.

The five TBI classifications are also used to predict functional outcomes. Although the outcomes for the very severe and extremely severe are projected to be poor, many such clients have nonetheless regained functional self-care and some productive employment. The classifications of TBI outcomes using the GCS and PTA should not be confused with the stages of recovery described in the following section.

First Recovery Stage—Severe

Damage from TBI varies according to the nature of the blow or forces applied to the head and brain. Many clients with TBI incur severe damage and begin their recovery in this first stage. Some clients may have survived only because of advances in medical technology (Horn & Zasler, 1996). As a result, their families must confront the ethical challenge of prolonged life in a coma or vegetative state. Although many of these family groups hope for functional improvement, some clients will remain totally dependent.

There are three levels within the first stage of recovery: (a) coma, (b) persistent vegetative state, and (c) reactive level. During coma, persons are bedridden, with no meaningful interaction with people and the environment. These clients do have a sleep–wake pattern, and they may be able to move reflexively, exhibiting grasping, chewing, sucking, and postural reflexes. During this period, clients are totally dependent in self-care management. From coma, clients may move to a persistent vegetative level, at which they are able to control respiration, blood pressure, and digestive and excretory functions, but they are still totally dependent on others for self-care management. After the vegetative state, the clients may progress to the final level of the first stage, where they become more responsive and begin to interact with the environment. The range of physical and cognitive skills among clients in this stage may vary greatly. The rate of recovery of physical skills does not necessarily correlate to the rate of recovery of cognitive skills. Clients may exhibit the physical capability to perform self-care, but they are unable to do so because of low arousal, severe impairment in awareness of disability, poor judgment, and limited problem-solving skills. Regardless of their apparent physical recovery, clients may be confused and agitated and unable to take care of themselves safely. These clients may need help with bathing, dressing, eating, and going to the toilet; they may also require assistance with mobility. Clients may be able to talk, yet have communication problems because they are disoriented in time, person, and place. Many of these symptoms are reversible, and many clients advance to the second stage of recovery.

Second Recovery Stage—Moderate

In the second stage of recovery, clients may increase their cognitive and physical capabilities and require less assistance and supervision. As in the first stage, recovery of cognitive capabilities does not proceed hand-in-hand with that of physical capabilities. Some clients may show moderate cognitive improvement but minimal physical or motor recovery. In the second stage, clients are more purposeful and interact more appropriately with the environment, but they may demonstrate difficulty with detecting, processing, and responding to stimuli. Their behaviors have been characterized as distractible, impulsive or slow, hyperactive or hypoactive, and repetitive (perseveration). They may have difficulty with short-and long-term memory, including the recall and recognition of names, faces, objects, and locations. Clients may also be unable to remember family members and friends, when they ate, when or whether they took a shower, or whether they had traveled. They may have problems reading, writing, and doing simple math. Many can perform cash transactions independently but require supervision in budgeting and banking.

Clients in this stage often exhibit emotional changes that affect their relationships with others. They may become irritable, short-tempered, and disinhibited, leading to cursing and sexually inappropriate behavior. In general, clients with TBI are more apt than they were before injury to express emotional distress and have sleep disturbances. They may have both verbal and nonverbal speech and language problems. These language problems can take the form of responses that are inappropriate to the situation, are irrelevant, are incoherent, or demonstrate misunderstanding of the intentions of others. Some clients experience difficulty with intonation and gestures. Their speech may not have the inflection necessary to communicate meaning, making them sound robotic.

During this stage, caregivers must provide constant supervision to provide a safe environment for self-care. Clients may not regain their former employment status, but they may be able to perform other productive activities. Some persons with TBI progress to the third stage of recovery, although others remain fixed at this level for the rest of their lives.

Third Recovery Stage—Mild

Those clients who have successfully moved through stage two and those persons with a mild, closed head injury enter the third stage of recovery. Clients who sustain mild TBI may not experience coma, and, if they have posttraumatic memory loss, it is of brief duration. Clients who reach this stage may have persistent mild chronic symptoms, may experience reversal of some of the symptoms, or may achieve total recovery. In this final stage, there is global improvement of cognition and self-care management. Clients may be distractible and mildly forgetful and may still need assistance with organization and structure. They may also complain about

headaches, sensitivity to light and sound, lack of sleep, and sexual disturbances. Some clients appear fatigued, apathetic, passive, and indifferent. Others may have loss of role identity or reduced interest in leisure activities, and may become socially isolated, withdrawn, and depressed. Many are able to walk, talk, and perform basic self-care management independently. In addition, with the use of compensatory strategies, many are able to shop, clean, cook, and go to school. Most are able to regain productive employment and reshape and simplify their responsibilities. Some are able to reconstruct and find more meaning in their lives. Often, clients turn to religion, become active in the community, or advocate for brain injury awareness.

The three stages described above are intended to provide general guidelines that may help practitioners describe and predict the behaviors that emerge during recovery. The stages are not homogeneous across or within cognitive or functional areas. For example, the recovery of short- and long-term memory may not be the same for any two clients. In addition, clients may not achieve the same levels of proficiency in feeding and bathing.

These stages describe a hopeful picture for TBI clients. As practitioners consider the persistent nature of symptoms and their effect on the client's self-image and support system, they should better appreciate the psychological and social consequences of TBI on clients and their family members.

Evaluation of Cognition and Self-Care Management

One objective of occupational therapy evaluation is to gather information that can guide intervention, whether it be remedial or compensatory. Both standardized and nonstandardized tests are used. In evaluating cognition and self-care function, practitioners should administer assessments frequently to discover how clients respond to cues and repetition. When interpreting results, a client's improvement in responding to cues and repetition will have more clinical significance than a change in the client's standardized norm scores. Observed changes in cognition and self-care may be used in the development of intervention strategies.

General Evaluation Strategies

The use of standardized and nonstandardized measurements for the evaluation of cognition and self-care management is common in the rehabilitation process. Measurement strategies are used to describe, classify, and assign numbers to behaviors to establish a baseline for treatment, to monitor changes, and to provide information useful for discharge planning. Two perspectives, one a "bottom up" and the other "top down," are useful for evaluation (Abreu, 1998, in press). The bottom-up (micro) perspective is used to measure specific impairment within particular performance components, such as cognition. The top-down (macro) perspective is used to measure and describe function and ordinary day-to-day occupations. Successful rehabilitation results from a confluent, free-flowing application of both perspectives. In therapeutic practice, *confluence* denotes a fluid movement back and forth between perspectives (Peloquin, 1996), which results in attention being given simultaneously to both cognition and self-care management. This evaluation model balances an understanding of the specific nature of impairments with an understanding of people as occupational beings. It rejects the commonplace assumption that practitioners must choose between holism and reductionism and promotes the use of both related perspectives (Abreu, 1998). No causality or directional relationship is implied or necessary for this model to be effective (Wood, Abreu, Duval, & Gerber, 1994).

During evaluation, practitioners must analyze the processing strategies employed by clients during task performance. In addition, they must examine the conditions that can affect the performance positively or negatively, including the use of cues and test repetition (Abreu & Toglia, 1987; Toglia, 1991). This evaluation can be accomplished by using a process-oriented approach to probe clients and analyze their ability to change with practice and to benefit from instructions and cues.

Identifying Cognitive Impairments

Practitioners can use standardized and nonstandardized tests to identify cognitive impairments and determine the degree of change in performance. Examples of evaluation strategies used in this approach are test repetition, external cueing, and environment modifications. Practitioners using these strategies can measure the client's cognitive deficits and can determine the conditions that improve or cause deterioration in performance (Abreu & Toglia, 1987). Standardized tests use scores to indicate how well the client performed on the test relative to norms. In contrast, nonstandardized

tests do not incorporate norms. Tables 14.1, 14.2, and 14.3 list assessments used for both Alzheimer's disease and TBI.

Practitioners should select various standardized and nonstandardized measurement tools to survey at least four different performance components. The first component is *cognitive function*, or the manner in which clients gather information from the environment. This component includes attention, memory, and problem-solving capabilities. Practitioners may use a cancellation test to evaluate attention, memory can be tested with a simple recall schema for auditory and visual memory, and simple mathematics problems may be used for problem solving. The second component is the awareness of disability, which may be tested through an interview. Practitioners may ask whether clients are aware of any problems, determine whether they recognize errors, and find out whether they predict that they are going to have any problems. The third cognitive performance component includes movement and postural control, which may be tested as practitioners observe clients performing arts, crafts, or other activities. The fourth component includes the client's body alignment, examined through observation while the body is in action and at rest. The evaluation of both cognitive and motor components is essential, because motor performance is a reflection of the cognitive process.

Evaluating Daily Living Skills

The evaluation of daily living skills is designed to identify and describe the client's level of disability and his or her subjective sense of satisfaction with performance after brain injury. Evaluation from this perspective assumes a humanistic orientation, whereby practitioners become active observers, recorders, and collaborators. Practitioners use narrative and functional analysis to explain and predict behavior, based on four characteristics: lifestyle status, life stages, health status, and level of disadvantage. Practitioners interview clients and family members, asking questions about each area.

Questions on lifestyle focus on communication, work, and day-to-day operations, including personal characteristics and the use of economic resources. A sample question might be: "How would you describe your lifestyle before your accident?" Life stages status is examined by asking for a description of the physical, emotional, and spiritual characteristics; for example, "What was your latest accomplishment?" Relevant factors include age, marital status, accom-

Table 14.1 Global Deterioration Scale (GDS)

GDS Scale	Cognitive Function	Clinical Phase and Characteristics
1	No cognitive decline	Normal phase. No subjective memory complaints.
2	Very mild decline	Forgetfulness phase. Subjective memory complaints such as forgetting where common objects have been placed or forgetting names of personal acquaintances.
3	Mild decline	Early confusional phase. First explicit evidence of cognitive disturbance. Decreased retention and concentration, misplaces objects, and exhibits anomia. Performance decreases when placed in stressful employment or social settings. Denial and mild-to-moderate anxiety is observed.
4	Moderate decline	Late confusional phase. Topographical apraxia, decreased knowledge about current and recent events, possibly decreased memory in relation to personal history, and isunable to perform complex tasks. Orientation to person and place or recognizing familiar faces or persons may not be disturbed. Displays a flattened affect and tends to withdraw from stressful or challenging situations.
5	Moderately severe decline	Early dementia phase. Dependent on others to survive. Disoriented. Independent in toileting and eating but has difficulty dressing self. Able to retain major personal and family facts.
6	Severe decline	Middle dementia phase. Requires moderate-to-maximal assistance with ADL tasks, disoriented, may become incontinent, and begins to display behavioral and psychological deficits such as paranoia, obsessive-compulsive behaviors, anxiety, agitation, or cognitive abulia.
7	Very severe decline	Late dementia phase. Unable to verbally communicate, ADL dependent, loss of psychomotor skills, and may display generalized cortical or focal neurologic signs symtomatology.

Note: ADL = activities of daily living. From "The Global Deterioration Scale for Assessment of Primary Degenerative Dementia," by B. Reisberg, S. H. Ferris, M. J. DeLeon, & T. Crook, 1982, *American Journal of Psychiatry, 139,* 1136–1139. Adapted with permission.

plishments, and losses. Practitioners survey the client's health status, including premorbid conditions and changes in behavior or condition after the accident or illness: "How was your health before the illness?" To determine the level of disadvantage experienced by the client, practitioners investigate the degree of personal and social restrictions. Examples might be a client's inability to attend movies, shop, cook, or provide in any way for family members or others. "What support system does your community offer to persons with brain injury?" is a useful question.

Practitioners evaluate the client's motivation, goals, actions, and capacity through an analysis of ordinary occupations and functional tasks. Practitioners use both standardized and nonstandardized tests to establish the client's ability in self-care. Such tests are based on a performance level of

Table 14.2 Assessments for Alzheimer's Disease

Test	Purpose	Reference
Alzheimer Home Assessment	To evaluate the home environment to ensure safety	Painter, J. (1996). Home environment considerations for people with Alzheimer's disease. *Occupational Therapy in Healthcare, 10,* 45–63.
Cleveland Scale of Daily Living (CSADL)	To measure physical, instrumental activities of daily living, communication skills, and social behaviors	Patterson, M. B., Mack, J. L., Neundorfer, M. M., Martin, R. J., Smyth, K. A., & Whitehouse, P. J. (1992). Assessment of functional ability in Alzheimer's disease: A review and a preliminary report on the Cleveland scale of activities of daily living. *Alzheimer's Disease and Associated Disorders, 6,* 145–163.
Clifton Assessment Procedures for the Elderly (CAPE)	To measure physical disability, apathy, communication, and social disturbances	Pattie, A. H., & Gilleard, C. J. (1979). *Clifton assessment procedures for the elderly (CAPE).* Sevenoaks, Kent: Hodder & Stoughton.
Clinical Dementia Rating (CDR)	To measure and follow the natural history (i.e., irrespective of intervention) of senile dementia of the Alzheimer's type (SDAT)	Morris, J. C. (1993). The clinical dementia rating (CDR): Current version and scoring rules. *Neurology, 43*(11), 2412–2414.
Echelle Comportment et Adaption (ECA)	To measure physical independence, social integration, occupation, orientation, mobility, and language	Ritchie, K., & Ledesert, B. (1991). The measurement of incapacity in the severely demented elderly: The validation of a behavioral assessment scale. *International Journal of Geriatric Psychiatry, 6,* 217–226.
Global Deterioration Scale (GDS)	To assess the clinically identifiable and ratable stages of primary degenerative dementia and age-associated memory impairment	Reisberg, B., Ferris, S. H., De Leon, M. J., & Crook, T. (1982). The global deterioration scale for assessment of primary degenerative dementia. *American Journal of Psychiatry, 139,* 1136–1139.
Kitchen Task Assessment (KTA)	A functional measure that records the level of cognitive support required by a person with Alzheimer's disease	Baum, C. & Edwards, D. F. (1993). Cognitive performance in senile dementia of Alzheimer's type: The kitchen task assessment. *American Journal of Occupational Therapy, 47,* 431–436.
London Psychogeriatric Rating Scale (LPRS)	To measure mental disorganization, confusion, physical disability, socially irritating behavior, and disengagement	Hersch, E. L., Kral, V. A., & Palmer, R. B. (1978). Clinical value of the London psychogeriatric rating scale. *Journal of American Geriatrics Society, 26,* 348–354.
Structured Assessment of Independent Living Skills (SAILS)	To measure language, orientation, money-related skills, instrumental activities, and social interaction	Mahurin, R. K., De Bettignes, B. H., & Pirozzolo, F. J. (1991). Structured assessment of independent living skills: Preliminary report of a performance measure of functional abilities in dementia. *Journal of Gerontology: Psychological Sciences, 46,* 48–66.

Table 14.3 Assessments for Traumatic Brain Injury

Test	Purpose	Reference
Coma/Near Coma Scale (CNC)	Monitors responsivity to stimulation, indicating the severity of sensory, perceptual, and primitive response deficits at the coma level	Rappaport M., Doughtery, A. M., & Kelting D. L. (1992). Evaluation of coma and vegetative states. *Archives of Physical Medicine and Rehabilitation, 73,* 628–634.
Coma Recovery Scale (CRS)	Monitors responsivity to stimulation, indicating the severity of sensory, perceptual, and primitive response deficits at the coma level	Giacino, J. T., Kezmarsky, M. A., DeLuca, J., & Cicerone, K. D. (1991). Monitoring rate of recovery to predict outcome in minimally responsive patients. *Archives of Physical Medicine and Rehabilitation, 72,* 897–900.
Sensory Stimulation Assessment Measure (SSAM)	Monitors responsivity to stimulation, indicating the severity of sensory, perceptual, and primitive response deficits at the coma level	Rader, M. A., Alston, J. B., & Ellis, D. W. (1989). Sensory stimulation of severely brain-injured patients. *Brain Injury, 3,* 141–147.
Western Sensory Stimulation Profile (WNSSP)	Monitors responsivity to stimulation, indicating the severity of sensory, sensory stimulation perceptual, and primitive response deficits at the coma level	Ansell, B. J., Keenan, J. E. (1989). The western neuro profile: A tool for assessing slow-to-recover head injury patients. *Archives of Physical Medicine and Rehabilitation, 70,* 104–108.
Awareness Questionnaire	Measures cognitive, behavioral/affective, and motor/sensory factors	Sherer, M., Bergloff, P., Boake, C., High, W., Jr., & Levin, E. (1998). The awareness questionnaire: Factor structure and internal consistency. *Brain Injury, 12,* 63–68.
Self-Awareness Deficits Interview	Qualitative methods to evaluate self-awareness	Fleming, J. M., Strong, J., & Ashton, R. (1996). Self-awareness of deficits in adults with traumatic brain injury: How best to measure? *Brain Injury, 10,* 1–15.
Community Integration Questionnaire (CQI)	Measures handicap in homelike setting, social network, and integration into productive activities	Willer B., Ottenbacher, K. J., & Coad, M. L. (1994). The community integration questionnaire: A comparative examination. *Archives of Physical Medicine and Rehabilitation, 73,* 103–111.
Functional Independence Measure (FIM)	Measures disability, using average daily minutes of assistance needed from another person	Corrigan, J., Smith-Knapp, K., & Granger, C. V. (1997). Validity of the functional independence measure for persons with traumatic brain injury. *Archives of Physical Medicine and Rehabilitation, 78,* 828–834.
Head Injury Symptom Checklist	Measures impairment in mild traumatic brain injury	McLean, A., Dikmen, S., Temkin, N., Wyler, A. R., & Gale, J. I. (1984). Psychosocial functioning at one month after injury. *Neurosurgery 14,* 393–399.
Medical Outcome Study, SF-36	Measures physical health and role limitations	Ware, J. E. (1993). *SF-36 health survey manual and interpretation guide.* Boston: Health Institute, England Medical Center.
Assessment of Motor and Process Skills	To evaluate household task performances	Darragh, A. R., Sample, P. L., & Fisher, A. G. (1998). Environment effect of functional task performance in adults with acquired brain injuries: Use of the assessment of motor and process skills. *Archives of Physical Medicine and Rehabilitation, 79,* 418–423.

100%. Clients are classified as independent or requiring mild, moderate, or maximum assistance.

Intervention for Cognition and Self-Care Management

Treatment alternatives for persons with cognitive deficits are varied and complex. The goals are (a) to maintain, restore, and improve self-care; (b) to promote health; and (c) to ease caregiving (American Occupational Therapy Association, 1991, 1994). The use of cueing and the repetition of tasks continue as a basic theme in the treatment of cognition and self-care, whether the treatment is for remediation or compensation. Cues and repetition are used to determine the most efficient methods for instruction and training.

General Treatment Strategies

Presented below are four dynamically inter-related intervention strategies that are used for both Alzheimer's disease and TBI (see Figure 14.2). These strategies are drugs and medications, cogni-

tive rehabilitation, human connection, and caregiver education.

Drugs and medications. Drugs and medications may be used to calm clients, increase their attention span, and foster the success of their cognitive rehabilitation. They are used to reduce symptoms and enhance function for clients with Alzheimer's disease and TBI (Parenté & Herrmann, 1996; Wolf-Klein, 1993). Hidergine, vasopressin, and Cognex are used to increase cognitive function; Prozac and Zoloft to calm agitated and depressed clients; Xanax for anxiety and agitation; and Haldol for paranoia and hallucinations. In addition, some investigators advocate the use of herbs, including ginseng and ginkgo biloba, for treatment. These drug interventions may assist in the improvement or retainment of self-care skills.

Cognitive rehabilitation. Cognitive rehabilitation approaches are designed to remediate or compensate for cognitive deficits. Practitioners use cognitive and behavioral learning strategies to design programs for clients with Alzheimer's disease and TBI (Katz, 1998).

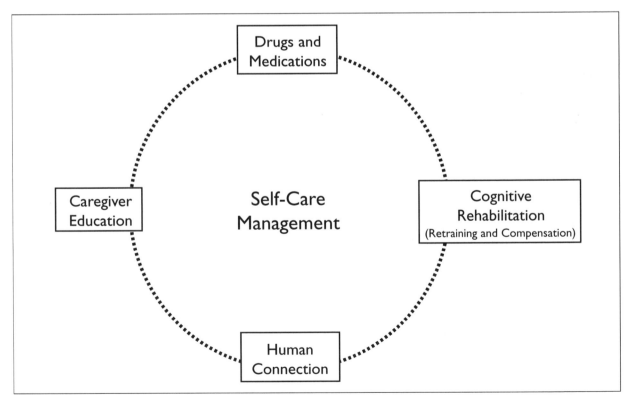

Figure 14.2 Four treatment strategies as they relate to self-care management. From *The Quadraphonic Approach: Evaluation and Treatment of the Brain Injured Patient,* by B. C. Abreu, 1990, New York: Therapeutic Service Systems. Copyright 1990 by Therapeutic Service Systems. Adapted with permission.

Cognitive learning strategies, based on cognitive psychology, are used to treat deficits that cannot be directly observed, such as memory and problem solving. Using these strategies, practitioners teach clients to process, structure, and modify information from the environment to improve self-care management skills. Practitioners prescribe specific tasks, situations, and rules of behavior for clients and teach them to use imagery, conscious awareness, and self-monitoring techniques. The assumption when using cognitive strategies is that the client's motivation in self-care lies in his or her desire to master competency and enjoy independence. The success of cognitive learning strategies depends on the client's ability to use conscious awareness and self-monitoring techniques.

Behavioral learning strategies are based on behavior modification (Giles & Clark-Wilson, 1993; Jacobs, 1993). Practitioners use behavioral learning strategies to treat deficits that can be observed directly, such as activities of daily living. Practitioners identify possible functional relationships of cause and effect, such as reward and punishment, to shape specified behaviors. The assumption is that clients are motivated to perform self-care by their positive or negative environmental reinforcements. Behavioral learning strategies are limited by the fact that they require a very rigorous program involving the entire health care team. Most practitioners use a combination of cognitive and behavioral learning strategies, several of which are shown in Table 14.4.

Human connection. Human connection strategies are based on universal principles of wellness, social science, and occupational science. They are used to regain or preserve the client's meaningful and emotional experiences (Wilcock, 1998; Zemke & Clark, 1996). Practitioners need to use human connection strategies for self-care management, because these emotional experiences are essential to holistic treatment. Practitioners must recognize that clients are meaningfully connected within society and that they can maintain a sense of well-being regardless of their cognitive deficits (Abreu, 1998; Hasselkus, 1998; Herskovits, 1995). Practitioners must try to understand the experience of disability, the trajectory of illness, the loss of well-being, and the disruption of self. Examples of human connection strategies are empathic communication, caring touch, and reconstruction of rituals and habits (Clark, 1993; Crepeau, 1995; Peloquin, 1995; Zemke, 1995).

Caregiver education. Caregiver education strategies include the identification and description of the needs and characteristics of clients for the family members. These strategies are used to prepare the caregivers for their new role. Although there are many reports on family-focused intervention, there are few guidelines for these strategies. Practitioners must consider cultural differences and use sociological principles to develop an approach to caregiving. Haley and others (1996) have shown that African-American caregivers often report less depression than white caregivers in assisting clients with Alzheimer's disease. Other studies suggest that Hispanic caregivers are strongly governed by familial relationships, values, and norms (Cox & Monk, 1993).

For Alzheimer's disease, practitioners must educate family members about how to deal with fear of genetic linkages, puzzlement, and the responsibilities of caregiving for a person with substantial cognitive deficits. In addition, practitioners must inform caregivers about the need for respite services and support groups. In the later stages of dementia, caregivers must be prepared to deal with nursing care decisions, guardianship, and informed consent.

For TBI, practitioners must educate family members about confusion, awareness of disability, and other effects of cognitive impairment. Practitioners should inform clients and family members about community resources and support groups. In cases involving chronic and severe impairment, placement, guardianship, and informed consent should be addressed. Many caregivers become advocates for their significant others who have Alzheimer's disease or TBI.

Intervention Phases

Most treatment involves three phases: preparation, performance, and review. To be effective, each phase requires collaboration among practitioners, clients, and family members.

Preparation phase. In the first phase, practitioners work with clients and family members to establish emotional and social connections and to have the clients express their goals. There are three parts to the preparation phase. First, the practitioners, clients, and family members establish a trusting and relaxed rapport through conversation and stress reduction and meditation techniques. Practitioners then help clients become aware of and focus their attention on the goals and projected outcomes of intervention. Practitioners may use instruction and cueing with multiple senses to increase the awareness of treatment; they may, for example, present

Table 14.4 Treatment Strategies for Self-Care Management

Action	Retraining for Mild Cognitive Impairment	Compensation for Moderate Cognitive Impairment	Total Caregiving for Severe Cognitive Impairment
Personal hygiene			
Unable to brush hair	Clients are taught to simplify and organize task in parts: right side, left side, and front. Therapists' cues match clients' most beneficial sensory modality (auditory, visual, tactile, or kinesthetic). Clients are taught to say steps aloud before and during task.	Clients are given checklist with steps and sequences. Clients are taught one-handed techniques. Therapists appropriately modify brushes: larger or smaller; heavier or lighter; bright colors. Therapists appropriately modify location of brush: constant, nonrotated location to match any perceptual or cognitive loss. Therapists appropriately modify mirror location and size.	Use caregiver assistance for part or whole task.
Unable to perform oral hygiene	Clients are taught to use toothbrush and floss in parts: front teeth first, followed by left, right, and back teeth.	Battery-operated toothbrushes, one-handed flossing.	Use caregiver assistance for part or whole task.
Unable to bathe and shower	Clients are taught to simplify and organize task in steps: Temperature control (cold water before hot) regulation, remember to clean critical body areas.	Clients are given checklist with steps and sequences. Clients are given bathtub and shower seats, adapter shower handles, soap on a rope, rubber mats, and handrails.	Use caregiver assistance for part or whole task.
Dressing			
Unable to perform upper-extremity/ dressing	Clients are taught to arrange garments in a specific order and dress in a specific sequence. Clients are taught to say steps aloud before and during task.	Clients are given checklist with correct steps and sequences. Clients are given pictures or photos of correct steps as cues. Clients are taught one-handed techniques. Therapists appropriately modify clothing: larger sizes, Velcro® snaps, button aids, zipper aids.	Use caregiver assistance for part or whole task.

(continued)

271

Table 14.4 (*continued*)

Action	Retraining for Mild Cognitive Impairment	Compensation for Moderate Cognitive Impairment	Total Caregiving for Severe Cognitive Impairment
Unable to perform lower-extremity dressing (i.e., unable to put shoes on feet; unable to put on prosthetic devices)	Clients are taught to arrange garments in a specific order and dress in a specific sequence; in addition postural control training in bed, sitting on a chair, or standing. Clients are taught to say steps aloud before and during task.	Clients are given checklist with correct steps and sequences. Clients are given pictures or photos of correct steps as cues. Clients are taught one-handed techniques. Therapists appropriately modify clothing: elastic pants, Velcro® snaps, button aids, zipper aids, long-handled shoehorns, shoe aids, stocking aids.	Use caregiver assistance for part or whole task.
Eating			
Unable to indicate food needs	Clients are taught to remember the specific time schedule.	Clients are taught to set alarm clocks to remember schedules. Clients are taught to use a memory notebook or visual aids to point out needs to others.	Use caregiver assistance for part or whole task.
Unable to get or set up food	Clients are taught mobility techniques to get food within reach. Clients are taught to organize and arrange utensils within their visual field and easy reach (low placement).	Clients are taught appropriate techniques: use a one-handed technique, switch handedness, or use two hands in a specific way. Therapists set up food location to help client.	Use caregiver assistance for part or whole task.
Unable to select or use utensils	Clients are taught to organize and arrange utensils within their visual field and easy reach before starting to eat. Clients are taught to look over the entire place setting to locate utensils before starting to eat.	Therapists set up utensil location to help clients. Therapists arrange kitchen drawers with utensil facing open end of drawer and handles pointing toward rear. Therapists appropriately modify utensils: large or small handles, heavier or lighter, colorful. Clients are provided one-handed knives.	Use caregiver assistance for part or whole task.

Table 14.4 (continued)

Action	Retraining for Mild Cognitive Impairment	Compensation for Moderate Cognitive Impairment	Total Caregiving for Severe Cognitive Impairment
Unable to eat or drink	Clients are taught oral–motor retraining. Clients are taught swallowing retraining. Clients are taught to take small bites and to drink fluids to encourage swallowing (refer to neurodevelopmental motor techniques).	Therapists appropriately modify consistencies: make thicker consistencies liquid, use straws. Therapists appropriately modify drinking cups: larger, smaller, heavier, lighter, colorful, personalized with picture or name. Therapists appropriately modify use of napkins as bibs. Modify for motor incoordination: scoop dish, plate guard, nonskid mat.	Use caregiver assistance for part or whole task.
Unable to finish eating in a timely manner	Clients are taught self-monitoring: estimating time and speed of eating routine to slow down or speed up the process. Clients are taught to self-question: "Am I eating slow enough?" "Am I eating fast enough?"	Clients are taught to set alarm clocks to remember timing. Clients are taught to keep a log of when they started eating and at what time they finished eating.	Use caregiver assistance for part or whole task.

273

instructions visually and auditorily. Finally, practitioners and clients develop strategies to maximize the ability to organize and process information during preparation for self-care. The instructional information may have to be broken down into small bites to make it more understandable.

Performance phase. In the performance phase, the goal is (a) to improve or compensate for the client's impaired memory and learning ability and (b) to increase the client's satisfaction. The process involves practice, feedback, and environmental modification, based on the client's evaluation and goals. Practitioners, clients, tasks, exercises, and occupations all contribute to environmental change or contextual modification during treatment (see Figure 14.3).

Practice consists of planned repetition of clients' actions and behaviors at a predetermined frequency for a predetermined duration. For example, clients might be asked to repeat the action of putting on a sweater three times in a half-hour, three times a week.

Practitioners and caregivers use feedback to provide helpful responses to clients during practice. The frequency varies depending on the clients' cognitive and physical recovery level, which is determined through the use of performance tests. Clients may be independent or require mild, moderate, or maximum assistance. If the baseline performance is established at less than 50% of optimum performance, practitioners will employ constant feedback. If the baseline is established above the 50% level, the frequency of feedback will be less and will decline as the client improves.

Environmental modifications include adaptation by clients, practitioners, and family members to the surroundings and the changing of the objects within that environment. There are two types of environments. A *congruent environment* is one that is simple and familiar, requiring minimal cognitive processing demands. For example, making soup from a can in the client's home kitchen with no time constraints is an activity taking place in a congruent environment. A *contextual interference environment* is a complex one that requires maximal processing demands. An example of an activity in this sort of environment would be making a full-course meal in an unfamiliar kitchen with a time limit. Contextual interference makes the immediate treatment goal more difficult to achieve, but, if used properly, it can strengthen the learning pattern. Such an environment is used for those clients whose performance requires mild assistance. A congruent environment is

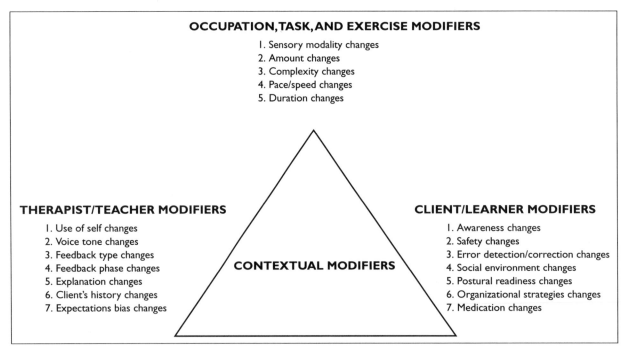

Figure 14.3 Sources of environmental change. From *The Quadraphonic Approach: Evaluation and Treatment of the Brain Injured Patient,* by B. C. Abreu, 1990, New York: Therapeutic Service Systems. Copyright 1990 by Therapeutic Service Systems. Adapted with permission.

used for clients requiring moderate and maximum assistance.

Review phase. At the end of each treatment session, practitioners bring closure by reevaluating and documenting the client's progress. Practitioners compare current performance to prior results. On the basis of this constant reevaluation, practitioners, clients, and family members readjust goals and timetables. It is important to note that clients with chronic symptoms who are maximally dependent in self-care may not achieve major functional progress. With these clients, the focus must be on humanistic connection and well-being. Examples of strategies used in each phase are given in Table 14.5. Tables 14.6 and 14.7 list examples of treatment strategies for clients with Alzheimer's disease and TBI.

Measuring Treatment Outcomes

Outcome measurement is an attempt to quantify the quality of therapeutic services in terms of effectiveness, or achievement of goals; efficiency, or optimal rate of progress; and value, or cost containment (Foto, 1996). Both standardized and nonstandardized measures are used to quantify results. Clients with Alzheimer's disease and TBI in the severe phase may not be able to achieve functional improvement, so the measurement of functional outcomes may not be appropriate. In these cases, the critical outcome is physical, mental, and spiritual wellness.

Conclusion

Management of Alzheimer's disease and TBI is a collaborative effort requiring the coordinated efforts of the entire rehabilitation team, the client, and family members. This collaboration allows constant monitoring of self-care skills and enrichment through cultural diversity. Health is more than the absence of illness: it also includes social and cultural factors, such as community awareness integration. Such integration provides an opportunity to develop healthy lifestyles for clients and family members (Wilcock, 1998). The treatment interventions can enable clients to heighten their sense of connection with others, sense of power, self-control, self-reconstruction, and meaningful occupations. Self-care management for those with cognitive deficits after Alzheimer's disease and TBI remains both an art and a science. ◆

Study Questions

1. What are the possible practical applications for occupational therapy of understanding the human nervous system?

2. What are the similarities and differences of Alzheimer's disease and TBI?

3. What are the differences between the "micro" and "macro" perspectives?

4. How is wellness a part of occupational therapy intervention?

Table 14.5 Treatment Phases

Preparation Phase	Performance Phase	Review Phase
Identify language regulators • Verbal instructions: language used, level, volume, speed, inflections, concreteness, complexity, general cues, specific cues, give-away cues, hierarchy • Written instructions: language used, level, speed of presentation, size, concreteness, complexity, general cues, specific cues, give-away cues • Gestural instructions: language used, speed, concreteness, general cues, specific cues, give-away cues	List goals by common denominator Analyze underlying skills for each goal Analyze pretreatment, concurrent, and post-treatment practice strategies Bottom-up (micro) goals • Able to orient eyes, head, and neck 100% of the time during a variety of postures in 1 week • Able to realign and adjust to self-initiated postural control during dressing tasks 75% of the time in 2 weeks	Performance tested after interval long enough to have practice effects dissipated Question client or family about their satisfaction with the results of the treatment session Question client or family about their dissatisfaction with the results of the treatment session Adjust, expand goals in an interdisciplinary context

(continued)

Table 14.5 (*continued*)

Preparation Phase	Performance Phase	Review Phase
• Pictorial instructions: line drawings, black and white pictures, color pictures, two-dimensional, three-dimensional • Tactile or kinesthetic instructions: amount of hand guidance, tactile proprioceptive pressure used, speed of movement, general cues, specific cues, give-away cues Identify sociocultural regulators: client's value judgment on the meaningfulness of the skill Identify physical regulators: physical attributes that control actions of that skill, such as temporal and spatial attributes (location and target speed) Identify physical appearances: physical affordances and attributes that may or may not control action; they can conceal or make the goal of the skill more salient, such as color, texture, size Schedule practice location: the practice setting; real-life or simulated environments (client's room, gym, unit kitchen, bathroom, gift shops) Schedule practice frequency and intensity: amount of repetition of specific skill and time of analysis dedicated to the practice of each skill in one training session Identify the nature of feedback: verbal, nonverbal, general, specific, give-away, or face-saving hierarchy Schedule feedback frequency and intensity: constant, immediate, delayed, infrequent (e.g., 100% feedback = every trial, 50% = 5 times out of every trial	• Able to realign and adjust to externally initiated postural control during dressing tasks 75% of the time in 3 weeks • Able to increase body response during self-care from 12 seconds to 7 seconds in 1 week Top-down (macro) goals • Client is able to perform favorite occupation safely in 3 weeks, while standing. • Client is able to perform more than one activity, task, or role safely in 2 weeks. • Client is able to engage in favorite social recreation (e.g., dancing) in 2 weeks. Example • Orienting activities and tasks that elicit eye, head, and neck movement in a variety of positions and locations General Rules • Instruct learners on the importance of practice as it relates to posture (i.e., home, institution, and community safety). • Involve family during practice; they can help you validate responses. • During the initial trial, allow client to respond without modification; then adapt the modification strategies during the next trials. • Notice and recognize improvement from gross to subtle changes in visual, auditory, vestibular, and proprioceptive stimuli.	Determine the performance effect of random, variable, and blocked practice

Table 14.6 Treatment Strategies for Alzheimer's Disease

Strategy	Purpose	Resource
Cognitive and behavioral strategies	Establish cognitive disability perspective	Levy, L. L. (1986). A practical guide to the care of the Alzheimer's disease victim: The cognitive disability perspective. *Topics in Geriatric Rehabilitation, 1,* 16–26.
Behavioral strategies	Regain and retain meaningful life skills Assess motor and process skills	Josephsson, S., Bäckman, L., Borell, L., Nygård, L., & Berspång, B. (1995). Effectiveness of an intervention to improve occupational to improve occupational performance in dementia. *Occupational Therapy Journal of Research, 15,* 36–49.
	Use morning bright light for disturbed sleep and behavior disorders	Van Someren, E. J., Kessler, A., Mirmiran, M., & Swaab, D. F. (1997). Indirect bright light improves circadian rest-activity rhythm disturbances in demented patients. *Biological Psychiatry, 41,* 955–963.
		Mishima, K., Okawa, M., Hishikawa, Y., Hozumi, S., Hori, H., & Takahashi, K. (1994). Morning bright light therapy for sleep and behavior disorders in elderly patients with dementia. *Acta Psychiatrica Scandinavica, 89,* 1–7.
	Address cognitive deficits	Bellus, S. B., Kost, P. P., Vergo, J. G., & Dinezza, G. J. (1998). Improvements in cognitive functioning following intensive behavioral rehabilitation. *Brain Injury, 12*(2), 139–145.
	Strengthen physical and social cues in the environment Preserve stability in physical and social environment	Roberts, B. L., & Algase, D. L. (1988). Victims of Alzheimer's disease and the environment. *Nursing Clinics of North America, 23,* 83–93.
Cognitive strategies	Use memory wallets to prompt factual information during prompted conversations	Zanetti, O., Binetti, G., Magni, E., Rozzini, L. Bianchetti, A., & Trabucchi, M. (1997). Procedural memory stimulation in Alzheimer's disease: Impact of a training programme. *Acta Neurologica Scandinavica, 95,* 152–157.
		Bourgeois, M. S. (1992). Evaluating memory wallets in conversations with persons with dementia. *Journal of Speech and Hearing Research, 35,* 1344–1357.
	During group therapy for orientation, employ strategies for reminiscence through recollection; strategies for reality orientation through time, place, and person; and strategies for remotivation through discussion, thought, and deduction	Zanetti, O., Frisoni, G. B., De Leo, D., Dello Buono, M., Bianchetti, A., & Trabucchi, M. (1995). Reality orientation therapy in Alzheimer disease: Useful or not? A controlled study. *Alzheimer Disease and Associated Disorders, 9,* 132–138.
		Koh, K., Ray, R., Lee, J., Nair, A., Ho, T., Ang, P.C. (1994). Dementia in elderly patients: Can the 3R mental stimulation programme improve mental status? *Age and Ageing, 23,* 195–196.
Human connection strategies	Promote calmness by playing classical music an the favorite music of the patient	Casby, J. A., & Holm, M. B. (1994). The effect of music on repetitive disruptive vocalizations of persons with dementia. *American Journal of Occupational Therapy, 48,* 883–889.
	Understand the style and preference of the caregiver through qualitative analysis	Corcoran, M. A. (1994). Management decisions made by caregiver spouses of persons with Alzheimer's disease. *American Journal of Occupational Therapy, 48,* 38–45.

Table 14.7 Treatment Strategies for Traumatic Brain Injury (TBI)

Strategy	Purpose	Resource
Cognitive retraining	Attentional retraining using microcomputers to assist TBI clients in a hospital	Gray, J. M., Robertson, I., Pentland, B., & Anderson, S. (1992). Microcomputer based attentional retraining after brain damage: A randomized group controlled trial. *Neuropsychological Rehabilitation, 2,* 97–115.
	Changing physical traits and using clients' communication skills and self-awareness of brain injury clients	Toglia, J. P. (1991). Generalization of treatment: A multi-context approach to cognitive perceptual impairment in adults with brain injury. *American Journal of Occupational Therapy, 45,* 505–516.
	Metacognitive training	Abreu, B. C., & Toglia, J. P. (1987). Cognitive rehabilitation: A model for occupational therapy. *American Journal of Occupational Therapy, 41,* 439–448.
	Compensatory strategies checklist and phone calls to assist clients with TBI in home settings	Schwartz, S. M. (1994). Adults with traumatic brain injury: Three case studies of cognitive rehabilitation in home setting. *American Journal of Occupational Therapy, 49,* 655–667.
	Verbal information retraining using mnemonic strategy	Gasquoine, P. G. (1991). Learning in post-traumatic amnesia following extremely severe closed head injury. *Brain Injury 5,* 156–175.
		Neistadt, M. E. (1994). Perceptual retraining for adults with diffuse brain injury. *American Journal of Occupational Therapy, 48,* 225–233.
	Reaction time training after TBI using feedback	Deacon, D., & Campbell, K. B. (1991). Decision making following closed-head injury: Can response speed be re-trained? *Journal of Clinical and Experimental Neuropsychology 13,* 639–651.
	Scaffolding: previous skills used serve as a platform for the acquisition of new skills (e.g., scanning training leads to wheelchair use) Metacognition: personal control use, introspection, talking aloud to self-monitor; awareness training	Ben-Yishay, Y., & Diller, L. (1993). Cognitive remediation in traumatic brain injury: Update and issues. *Archives of Physical Medicine and Rehabilitation, 74,* 204–213.
	Self-monitoring instructions to increase interpersonal skills	Schloss, P. J., Thompson, C. K., Gajar, A. H., & Schloss, C. (1985). Influence of self-monitoring on heterosexual conversational behaviors of head trauma youth. *Applied Research in Mental Retardation, 6,* 269–282.
	Postural control training for vestibular pathologies after TBI	Shumway-Cook, A. (1994). Vestibular rehabilitation in traumatic brain injury. In S. J. Herdman (Ed.), *Vestibular rehabilitation* (pp. 347–359). Philadelphia: F. A. Davis.

(continued)

Table 14.7 (*continued*)

Strategy	Purpose	Resource
Cognitive retraining and human connection	Information processing, teach/learning, neurodevelopmental, biomechanical strategies for cognitive and postural control training Narrative, storytelling for personalized and meaningful training	Abreu, B. C. (1998). The quadraphonic approach: Holistic rehabilitation for brain injury. In N. Katz (Ed.), *Cognition and occupation in rehabilitation: Cognitive models for intervention in occupational therapy* (pp. 51–97). Rockville, MD: American Occupational Therapy Association. Abreu, B. C. (in press). The reasoning behind assessment and treatment of memory and learning. In C. Unsworth (Ed.), *Cognitive and perceptual dysfunction: A clinical reasoning approach to assessment and treatment.* Philadelphia: F. A. Davis.
Human connection	Structuring of the volunteer role, structured failure experiences videotaped and replayed for reinforcement Family and client education to develop a new identity rather than reproducing the old identity	Krefting, L. (1989). Reintegration into the community after head injury: The results of an ethnographic study. *Occupational Therapy Journal of Research, 9,* 67–83.
	Peer group experiences to assist clients with TBI, provide support, self-advocacy, and fellowship network with other clients with TBI	Schwartzberg, S. L. (1994). Helping factors in a peer-developed support group for persons with head injury. Part 1: Participant observer perspective. *American Journal of Occupational Therapy, 48,* 297–304. Schollz, C. H. (1994). Helping factors in a peer-developed support group for persons with head injury. Part 2: Survivor interview perspective. *American Journal of Occupational Therapy, 48,* 305–309.
Behavioral	Washing and dressing retraining	Giles, G. M., Ridley, J. E., Dill, A., & Frye, S. (1997). A consecutive series of adults with brain injury treated with a washing and dressing retraining program. *American Journal of Occupational Therapy, 51,* 256–266.
	Repetition, multisensory input, and human connection	Zencius, A. H., Wesolowski, M. D., & Rodriguez, I. M. (1998). Improving orientation in head injured adults by repeated practice, multi-sensory input, and peer participation. *Brain Injury, 12,* 53–61.
Sensory stimulation	Uncertain evidence for effectiveness of sensory stimulation to promote recovery from coma	Giacino, J. T. (1996). Sensory stimulation: Theoretical perspectives and the evidence for effectiveness. *Neurorehabilitation, 6,* 69–78.

References

Abreu, B. C. (1998). The quadraphonic approach: Holistic rehabilitation for brain injury. In N. Katz (Ed.), *Cognition and occupation in rehabilitation* (pp. 51–97). Bethesda, MD: American Occupational Therapy Association.

Abreu, B. C. (in press). The reasoning behind assessment and treatment of memory and learning. In C. Unsworth (Ed.), *Cognitive and perceptual dysfunction: A clinical reasoning approach to assessment and treatment.* Philadelphia: F. A. Davis.

Abreu, B. C., & Toglia, J. P. (1987). Cognitive rehabilitation: A model for occupational therapy. *American Journal of Occupational Therapy, 41,* 439–448.

American Occupational Therapy Association. (1991). Statement: Occupational therapy services management of persons with cognitive impairments. *American Journal of Occupational Therapy, 45,* 1067–1068.

American Occupational Therapy Association. (1994). Statement: Occupational therapy services for persons with Alzheimer's disease and other dementias. *American Journal of Occupational Therapy, 48,* 1029–1031.

American Psychiatric Association. (1994). *Diagnostic and statistical manual of mental disorders* (4th ed.). Washington, DC: American Psychiatric Association.

BIOTA. (1998). *Fact sheet: Alzheimer's disease* [On-line]. Available: http://www.biota.com.au/alzfact.htm

Brain Injury Association, Inc. (1998). Brain injury fact sheet (national): About OVC [On-line]. Available: http://205.182.14.25/about/projects/1.1/natstats.html

Clark, F. (1993). Occupation embedded in real life: Interweaving occupational science and occupational therapy. 1993 Eleanor Clark Slagle lecture. *American Journal of Occupational Therapy, 47,* 1067–1068.

Corcoran, M. A. (1994). Management decisions made by caregiver spouses of persons with Alzheimer's disease. *American Journal of Occupational Therapy, 48,* 38–45.

Cox, C., & Monk, A. (1993). Hispanic culture and family care of Alzheimer's patients. *Health and Social Work, 18*(2), 92–100.

Crepeau, E. B. (1995). The practice of the future: Putting occupation back into therapy. In C. B. Royeen (Ed.), *AOTA self-study series: Rituals.* Bethesda, MD: American Occupational Therapy Association.

Foto, M. (1996). Nationally Speaking—Outcome studies: The what, why, how, and when. *American Journal of Occupational Therapy, 50*(2), 87–88.

Frosch, S., Gruber, A., Jones, C., Noel, E., Westerlund, A., & Zavisin, T. (1997). The long-term effects of traumatic brain injury on the roles of caregivers. *Brain Injury, 11*(12), 891–906.

Giacino, J. T., Kezmarsky, M. A., DeLuca, J., & Cicerone, K. D. (1991). Monitoring rate of recovery to predict outcome in minimally responsive patients. *Archives of Physical Medicine and Rehabilitation, 72,* 897–900.

Giles, G. M., & Clark-Wilson, J. (1993). *Brain injury rehabilitation: A neurofunctional approach.* San Diego, CA: Singular Publishing Group.

Glickstein, J. K. (1997). *Therapeutic interventions in Alzheimer's disease* (2nd ed.). Gaithersburg, MD: Aspen.

Haley, W. E., Roth, D. L., Coleton, M. I., Ford, G. R., West, C. A. C., Collins, R. P., & Isobe, T. (1996). Appraisal, coping, and social support as mediators of well-being in black and white family caregivers of patients with Alzheimer's disease. *Journal of Consulting and Clinical Psychology, 64,* 121–129.

Hasselkus, B. R. (1998). Occupation and well-being in dementia: The experience of day-care staff. *American Journal of Occupational Therapy, 52,* 423–434.

Herskovits, E. (1995). Struggling over subjectivity: Debates about "self" and Alzheimer's disease. *Medical Anthropology Quarterly, 9,* 146–164.

Horn, L. J., & Zasler, N. D. (Eds.). (1996). *Medical rehabilitation of traumatic brain injury.* St. Louis, MO: Mosby.

Jacobs, H. E. (1993). Behavior analysis guidelines and brain injury rehabilitation: Peoples, principles, and programs. Gaithersburg, MD: Aspen.

Katz, N. (Ed.). (1998). *Cognition and occupation in rehabilitation: Cognitive models for intervention in occupational therapy.* Bethesda, MD: American Occupational Therapy Association.

Parenté, R., & Herrmann, D. (1996). *Retraining cognition: techniques and applications.* Gaithersburg, MD: Aspen.

Peloquin, S. M. (1995). The fullness of empathy reflections and illustrations. *American Journal of Occupational Therapy, 49,* 24–31.

Peloquin, S. M. (1996). Using the arts to enhance confluent learning. *American Journal of Occupational Therapy, 50,* 148–151.

Reisberg, B. (1984). Alzheimer's disease: Stages of cognitive decline. *American Journal of Nursing, 84*(2), 225–228, 232.

Reisberg, B., Ferris, S. H., De Leon, M. J., & Crook, T. (1982). The global deterioration scale for assessment of primary degenerative dementia. *American Journal of Psychiatry, 139,* 1136–1139.

Ronch, J. L. (1996). Assessment of quality of life: Preservation of the self. *International Psychogeriatrics, 8,* 267–275.

Scott, A. D., & Dow, P. W. (1995). Traumatic brain injury. In C. A. Trombly (Ed.), *Occupational therapy for physical dysfunction* (4th ed., pp. 705–731). Baltimore: Williams & Wilkins.

Teasdale, G., & Jennett, B. (1974). Assessment of coma and impaired consciousness: A practical scale. *Lancet, 2*, 81–84.

Toglia, J. P. (1991). Generalization of treatment: A multicontext approach to cognitive perceptual impairment in adults with brain injury. *American Journal of Occupational Therapy, 45*, 505–516.

Van Duijn, C. M. (1996). Epidemiology of the dementias: Recent developments and new approaches. *Journal of Neurology, Neurosurgery, and Psychiatry, 60*, 478–488.

Wilcock, A. A. (1998). *An occupational perspective of health.* Thorofare, NJ: Slack.

Wolf-Klein, G. P. (1993). New Alzheimer's drug expands your options in symptom management. *Geriatrics, 48*(8), 26–36.

Wood, W., Abreu, B., Duval, M., & Gerber, D. (1994). Occupational performance and the functional approach. In C. B. Royeen (Ed.), *AOTA self-study series: Cognitive rehabilitation.* Bethesda, MD: American Occupational Therapy Association.

Zemke, R. (1995). Habits. In C. B. Royeen (Ed.), *AOTA self-study series: The practice of the future: Putting occupation back into therapy.* Bethesda, MD: American Occupational Therapy Association.

Zemke, R., & Clark, F. (Eds.). (1996). Occupational science: The evolving discipline. Philadelphia: F. A. Davis.

15

Meeting Self-Care Needs of Persons With Psychiatric Disabilities

Carol A. Haertlein
Virginia C. Stoffel

Carol A. Haertlein, PhD, OT, FAOTA, is Associate Professor, Occupational Therapy Program, Department of Health Sciences, University of Wisconsin–Milwaukee.

Virginia C. Stoffel, MS, OT, FAOTA, is Associate Professor, Occupational Therapy Program, Department of Health Sciences, University of Wisconsin–Milwaukee.

Key Terms

assertive community treatment

case management

community supports

mood disorders

personality disorders

psychiatric impairments and disorders

psychiatric rehabilitation

psychoeducational models

schizophrenia

self-care assessments

self-care strategies

substance abuse and dependence

Objectives

On completing this chapter, the reader will be able to

1. Describe the scope of occupational therapy services for persons with psychiatric disabilities.

2. Identify the effect of environment and context on self-care activities.

3. Explain how psychiatric disorders can affect self-care routines.

4. Identify useful evaluation strategies in self-care.

5. Identify strategies that enable success in self-care routines, including the psychoeducational approach, case management, assertive community treatment, psychiatric rehabilitation, and building community supports.

Speaking of fantasies, I once had one: that I was one of millions of mental health clients who all lived in the communities of our choice, in our own places, with our own kitchens, our own furniture, our own bathrooms, our own food and clothing. . . . We shared our communities with all kinds of people . . . we did things together, helped each other, and laughed and cried with each other . . . we all had decently paying, fulfilling jobs. (*Howie the Harp, 1995, p. xiii*)

The above quote reflects the hopes and dreams of dozens of persons that we serve every day. We (the authors of this chapter) are currently university professors, and the persons with whom we work are university students. Their aspirations are not much different from the hundreds of persons with psychiatric disorders with whom we have worked over the past 2 decades. Just as we strive to help our students reach their goals, how can we, as occupational therapy practitioners, support the millions of persons with psychiatric disorders to reach those same goals?

Focus of Self-Care Services

Occupational therapy practitioners can provide a wide range of self-care services for persons with psychiatric disabilities (also referred to as consumers). Occupational therapy services are typically designed to address occupational behaviors (i.e., self-maintenance, work, play), performance components, and performance contexts. The focus of services for persons with psychiatric disabilities may center on one or more of these areas. Emphasis may be on the evaluation and development of the neuromotor, cognitive, psychological, and social abilities (performance components) underlying the occupational behaviors, or the therapist may directly address the skills necessary to complete self-maintenance, work, and play tasks. The context in which the consumer is served is often overlooked, but it may be the most critical aspect of providing meaningful occupational therapy services.

The following case study illustrates how occupational behaviors, performance components, and performance contexts all interact to determine and effect quality occupational therapy services for one consumer.

> B. T. is a man 40 years of age with a 22-year history of mental illness, specifically chronic schizophrenia and dependent personality disorder. B. T. had his first psychotic incident during exam week of his first semester in college. Following a hospitalization of several months, he returned to the university to continue his education. For about 3 years he was able to live independently and attend classes with the help of two roommates and his mother.
>
> As the time approached to make an employment decision, and when his roommates graduated and moved away, B. T. experienced another psychotic episode, with severe depression. This hospitalization was for a longer period, extended by his setbacks any time he was given a trial discharge or extended home pass.
>
> The intervening years, from this point until age 37, consisted of several hospitalizations, group home placements, and brief periods of living with his mother. Each of these settings seemed only to increase his dependency and his belief that he was unable to meet his most basic self-care needs.
>
> At age 37, B. T. was admitted to a community support program (CSP) and initially attended groups in a day treatment setting. These groups focused on learning the skills that would lead to independent living (i.e., personal hygiene, meal planning, grocery shopping, cooking, budgeting, home care). Once he found an apartment, with the help of his occupational therapist and case manager, he began the process of doing those activities independently.
>
> An occupational therapy practitioner now meets with B. T. every other week to help him with his grocery shopping. He prepares his own meal plan and shopping list before the trip. The practitioner reports that B. T. is independent in most tasks but needs some encouragement and support to deal with difficult situations, such as dealing with the crowds at the grocery store or confronting the landlord about repairs.
>
> B. T. credits the one-on-one feedback and the constant encouragement from his occupational therapy practitioner and case manager and other CSP staff members with his ability to live independently for the past 3 years. "I thought I took care of myself before, but I really didn't know how. I only knew how to get others to take care of me. With the help of my occupational therapist, I now know that I can take care of myself and my apartment. I'm even budgeting my money so I can take a trip soon!"
>
> As B. T. acquired the knowledge and skills necessary for independent living, his self-esteem and motivation increased to the point where he was willing to engage in the necessary occupational behaviors. ∎

This chapter focuses on strategies for meeting self-care needs for persons with a psychiatric disability. Specific attention is devoted to serious mental illnesses, particularly schizophrenia. Other conditions, such as mood disorders, personality disorders, and substance abuse, will be addressed briefly. It is our belief that self-care services should be primarily targeted to the level of occupational behaviors within the context (communities) in which consumers are functioning.

Psychiatric Impairments and Self-Care Activities

Performing self-care activities is a highly complex process that may include the person's own abilities and skills, the environment, societal norms, and other persons. Performing a self-care activity, such as bathing, is associated with knowledge of hygiene and healthy behavior, knowledge to use the supplies and equipment necessary for safe bathing, the motivation to respond to sociocultural norms of acceptable cleanliness, and the ability to recognize and respond to feedback from others regarding the practice of adequate bathing routines, among others. It also requires adequate manual dexterity to manipulate faucets and shampoo bottles; strength, flexibility, and balance to enter and exit the tub; tactile sensitivity to regulate water temperature; kinesthetic awareness to wash all body parts; and information-ordering ability to organize bathing tasks.

A person with a psychiatric disorder is unlikely to bathe if he or she is indifferent to sociocultural expectations and feedback from others, lacks sufficient self-esteem to maintain his or her own health, lacks the knowledge or physical skills to use equipment and supplies in a particular environment, or cannot cognitively process the task demands of bathing. Difficulty with carrying out self-care tasks may be increased by impairment in daily habits and interpersonal skills (seeking help) and lack of meaningful life roles.

Impairment in self-care activities may appear as total lack of performance of self-care activities, partial or incomplete performance, performance that does not meet the socially accepted standards, or performance that is insufficient to meet the person's needs. These same signs of disability may be present in the other areas of occupational performance of work and leisure. But the effect of impaired performance of self-care activities is very different. Self-care activities include the very essence of survival on a daily basis and the foundation skills—acceptable hygiene, adequate nourishment, communication, and medication management—needed to be successful in work and leisure occupations.

Schizophrenia

Schizophrenia is a pervasive and usually chronic disorder that is diagnosed when a person shows deterioration from a previous level of function in work, self-care, or interpersonal relations. A wide range of characteristics is present in schizophrenia, not all of which are found in all persons diagnosed with the condition. Typically, disturbances are seen in affect and mood, behavior, and thought (both in content and form). Mood impairment is seen as blunted, flat, and emotionless; inappropriate (e.g., laughter at sad news) or fluctuating (labile); and apathetic but alert. Behavior changes include social withdrawal and isolation, peculiar conduct, psychomotor manifestations (e.g., retardation, twitching), and impairment in function at work, school, and home. Thought disturbances are especially profound and appear as delusional ideation (e.g., mind control), hallucinations (e.g., visual, auditory), incoherence, looseness of associations, changes in speech patterns, and odd beliefs or magical thinking (Bonder, 1995).

Care for persons with this debilitating disease has improved over the past 30 years, so the most debilitating symptoms (i.e., delusions, hallucinations, behaviors) can now be controlled successfully with medication. However, it is worth noting that symptom relapse is not unusual, even with the effective use of medication. Moreover, some consumers may have the damaging side effect of *tardive dyskinesia* from long-term medication use (injury to the nervous system causing involuntary movements). Other ways of assisting those with this disease include social skills training, psychoeducational approaches for self-care skills, family member support and intervention, and CSPs. Several of these methods are described later in this chapter.

The course of schizophrenia often begins with an acute episode of up to 6 months' duration, occurring in late adolescence or early adulthood, with fluctuating remissions and exacerbations for the next several years. The most deterioration occurs in the first 5 years of the illness. Severity of symptoms is not always a good indicator of the outcome, with 20% to 25% of those stricken able to avoid severe and chronic behavior deterioration (Bonder, 1995). The prognosis improves with acute onset at a later age, the presence of a clear precipitating factor, no family history, a normal IQ, and good premorbid adjustment. But the majority of persons with schizophrenia have chronic disability and function marginally in all aspects of occupational performance throughout their lives.

Dysfunction in self-care. Changes in self-care appear as one of the most noticeable early symptoms of schizophrenia. The stricken person ceases or changes personal care habits of bathing, shaving, hair care, and so forth. Women may adopt inappropriate and attention-seeking uses of makeup (e.g., excessive eye shadow and liner, unusual lipstick color and application). Changes in dress are common, and the person often becomes unkempt, slovenly, or dirty. Inappropriate attire is often seen; for example, clothes that are either too casual or dressy for the occasion or inappropriate for the weather, especially for persons with a long history of the disease. This sometimes occurs in response to hallucinations or delusional thinking, as described below.

> R. F., a man 40 years of age diagnosed with chronic paranoid schizophrenia, always wears a long-sleeved shirt, and often a sweater or jacket too, even in very warm weather. He feels he must do this to keep the panther, tattooed on his forearm, from biting him or from coming alive and attacking someone else.

A typical secondary effect of deterioration in personal care habits is the adverse responses of others. Family members and friends may react with concern or denial, but strangers will almost always respond with avoidance, contributing to the person's delusional thought processes, social withdrawal, or other symptomatic behavior. The interaction of declining self-care and interpersonal rejection becomes a self-perpetuating, downward cycle.

Eating habits of persons with schizophrenia may deteriorate, and they may have a total disregard for good nutrition. They may start to overeat at meals, eat junk food in excess, or avoid certain foods or meals in conjunction with other bizarre behaviors. Daily medication management is often very difficult and usually has to be supervised by someone else. Reminders of appointments for medication checkups or reviews may also be needed. There is a noticeable change in interpersonal communication, which lacks both responsiveness and initiative. This behavior, coupled with a tendency toward social isolation and emotionless expression, interferes with functional communication and, consequently, getting need fulfillment at several levels. For example, even though they experience hunger, persons with schizophrenia may not seek information from others regarding the time of the next meal. Their lack of responsiveness may cause them to miss the call or reminder for that meal. At this point, they are still hungry and will typically manage to find their way to the area vending machine, where they fill up on junk food.

In early signs of the illness (late adolescence through early adulthood), persons may have never developed the abilities that facilitate good self-care (i.e., organizational skills, awareness of socially accepted standards). More often, those who have had frequent or long-term hospitalizations lose skills and abilities (Bonder, 1995), lose motivation and interest in maintaining self-care routines, and stop responding to external cues in the environment (i.e., time, events, temperature). The most socially debilitating effects of schizophrenia may be the functional impairments that usually occur when symptoms are managed with medications, for example foot tapping and pin rolling finger motions that may bring embarrassing attention from others (Bonder, 1995). Even when self-care habits and social standards are not affected, persons with schizophrenia may be unable to manage the more complex self-maintenance skills of meal planning and preparation, money management, clothing care, and transportation in the community.

In summary, persons with schizophrenia often have the following problems in self-care:

- A decline or change in personal hygiene habits (bathing, shaving, teeth care, hair care)
- Unkempt or inappropriate clothing
- Poor eating habits and neglect of nutrition
- Inability to manage medications
- Lack of responsiveness and initiation in interpersonal relationships, even when basic needs are not met

Mood Disorders

Mood, or affective, disorders include a wide range of conditions, from sadness and grief to the more severe bipolar disorders and major depression. Self-care is more likely to be affected by depression than by a manic condition.

Major depression and the depressive condition of bipolar disorder are characterized by a depressed mood, feelings of worthlessness, and loss of interest or pleasure in most activities (Bonder, 1995; Ward, 1998). For example, S. T., a 35-year-old woman diagnosed with a bipolar disorder, was depressed and had difficulty recognizing such simple pleasures as the feeling of a warm bath or the taste of a hot cup of coffee on a cold day. Behavior manifestations of a depressive disorder include changes in appetite and sleep patterns, as well as lethargy or agitation. Thought disturbances are seen in decreased ability to concentrate, delusions, and suicidal ideation (thoughts).

Treating persons with depression using medication is usually effective, although it is generally accepted that most depressive episodes will resolve themselves with or without treatment in about 6 months (Bonder, 1995). Psychotherapy is usually considered to be helpful for persons with depression as well and can take many forms, including cognitive therapy, self-monitoring behavioral approaches, psychoanalysis, and social learning-based treatment. Electroconvulsive treatment is sometimes used and is considered to be effective for specific symptoms, including suicidal tendencies, severe delusional thinking, and nonresponsiveness to drug therapy.

The course of a depressive episode varies, but most persons experience depressed mood and loss of interest, as well as some of the symptoms named above. Onset may be sudden or gradual over several weeks. Recurrence is seen in about half of those afflicted, with the recurring episode coming within 2 years of the first. Suicide attempts occur in about 30% of those diagnosed with depression (Bonder, 1995).

Dysfunction in self-care. The range of self-care dysfunction in persons with depressive disorders is wide, from no self-care dysfunction to the person who is unable to get out of bed and engage in any occupational behaviors. The deficits in self-care are not from loss of skills or undeveloped abilities, as found in schizophrenia, but as secondary symptoms of the altered mood and the behavioral and thought disturbances. However, because of the habitual nature of the performance of most self-care activities, direct intervention at the performance level not only reestablishes routines but also alters self-perceptions and cognition at the same time.

A fairly common behavioral change in self-care habits for persons with depression is altered appetite. This change may appear as decreased eating, which results in weight loss and potentially inadequate nutrition, or increased appetite secondary to agitation with subsequent weight gain. Personal hygiene may be neglected because of the depressed mood, loss of interest, impaired concentration, and lethargy. Managing daily medications may be impaired by lowered concentration. Dressing and appearance of clothes may suffer as a result of loss of interest and depressed mood. Functional communication may be impaired, as the depressed mood, loss of interest, and behavioral manifestations elicit negative reactions and avoidance responses from others. In addition to these self-care deficits, the more complex occupations of self-maintenance or the instrumental activities of daily living may be impaired.

In summary, persons with depression experience self-care difficulties in the following:

- Eating, resulting in weight loss or gain with potential nutritional compromise
- Personal hygiene, including dressing
- Managing medications or other tasks of organization
- The ability to express needs to others

Personality Disorders

Persons with personality disorders have exaggerations of traits found in persons without psychiatric disturbances, such as limited or unstable emotional responses (schizoid or borderline), self-absorption (narcissistic), or fearfulness (dependent) (Bonder, 1995). Persons with personality disorders typically have long-term behavioral patterns that are dysfunctional throughout life, in which the affected person learns little or nothing from life experiences. It is only when the personality decompensates in the face of crisis, or the person seeks help for another psychiatric condition, that the disorder is diagnosed.

Treating persons with personality disorders is difficult at best. Interventions may include medications, skill training, behavioral interventions, hospitalization, and psychotherapy, depending on the manifestation of symptoms (Bonder, 1995). Personality patterns tend to be stable and often are not problematic if the person learns effective stress management techniques as a way of preventing crises.

Dysfunction in self-care. Although the potential exists for persons with different classifications of personality disorder to have impairment in self-care skills, typically this is not the case. Occupational function is more often problematic at the level of work and leisure behaviors because of the interpersonal interactions often expected in those performance areas. Dysfunction in self-care, when present, does not represent a deficit in skills but rather is a symptom of the disorder. For example, the person with schizoid personality disorder may exhibit unkempt dressing because of a lack of interpersonal feedback resulting from social isolation. The person with a narcissistic personality disorder may use excessive makeup and dress seductively as part of the attention-seeking behavior (Bonder, 1995). The impulsivity of the person with borderline personality disorder may lead to abandonment of hygiene and eating routines as value systems fluctuate, relationships waiver, and a steady stream of inconsistencies is exhibited. There is potential for dysfunction in the more complex self-maintenance activities for many persons with personality disorders, particularly in money management and care of the home, clothing, and others. A common feature among persons with personality disorders is impaired interpersonal relationships. All self-maintenance activities that affect interactions with others are impaired in persons with personality disorders.

In summary, persons with personality disorders have difficulties in self-care that are seen as manifestations of the exaggerated human trait that characterizes the particular disorder (e.g., unkempt appearance in the person with socially isolated schizoid personality) and impairment in all self-care and self-maintenance activities that involve human interactions.

Substance Abuse and Dependence

Persons who have histories of substance abuse and dependence often have other psychiatric diagnoses (e.g., the person with depression who drinks to avoid feelings of hopelessness) or have situational responses to a physical condition (e.g., the persons who abuses prescription drugs to cope with pain and develops a physical and psychological dependence on them). *Abuse* is defined as the regular intake of a substance that may or may not be intoxicating but interferes with some aspect of function (Ward, 1998). *Dependence* is more severe and interferes with most aspects of function, increases tolerance for the substance, elicits withdrawal symptoms, and renders efforts to decrease the use of the substance unsuccessful (Bonder, 1995) . Familiar substances that are abused and considered to be more psychologically than physically addictive are caffeine and cocaine. The substances that are more likely to create physical and psychological dependence are alcohol, nicotine, amphetamines, and barbiturates.

Changes in a person's mood, behavior, and thought can occur when substance abuse or dependence is present. Mood changes range from lethargy (related to alcohol and barbiturate use) to excitability and elation (related to cocaine and heroin use). Behavior usually becomes erratic and unpredictable in response to the chemical effects of the substances. With a physical or psychological addiction, behavior becomes focused on obtaining the substance rather than on involvement in meaningful occupational behaviors. Lifestyle changes evolve from these altered behaviors (e.g., loss of job, changes in leisure activities). Interpersonal relationships are almost always affected, as persons with similar lifestyles and behaviors are more accepting of and

acceptable to others with abuse or dependence problems. Impaired judgment and concentration appear as the addictive characteristics of the substance increase. The person becomes preoccupied with thoughts of seeking and using the addictive substance.

The management and course of substance abuse and dependence vary with the underlying causes (e.g., situational response to physical pain, socioeconomic forces, simultaneous psychoses). For most addictions, recognition of the problem and willingness to do something about it are important first steps (Bonder, 1995; Ward, 1998). Behavioral interventions, self-help groups, medications for physiological withdrawals, cognitive therapies, and other psychotherapeutic interventions have all met with varying success.

Dysfunction in self-care. The potential for dysfunction in all areas of occupation is substantial for persons with substance abuse or dependence. Work and leisure are commonly affected, with work being neglected and leisure focusing on obtaining and using the substance. Self-care is impaired when persons lose interest in eating, hygiene, and other personal care habits as the need for the substance supersedes all other occupations. Central nervous system changes are most apparent during intoxication but may persist and increase if abuse continues, causing impaired judgment, altered motor activity, and forgetfulness. These changes may manifest themselves as loss of skills in self-care activities and in more complex self-maintenance activities such as money management and shopping.

In summary, the problems in self-care for persons with substance abuse and dependence include neglect of self-care activities, as obtaining and using the substance supersede all other occupations, and loss of self-care and self-maintenance skills, as ongoing substance use causes central nervous system damage.

Self-Care Evaluation for Persons With Psychiatric Disorders

The first consideration in evaluation of the self-care needs of someone with a psychiatric disability is deciding just what to evaluate—occupational behaviors in self-care, performance components underlying the skills, or the context in which self-care will occur. As stated earlier, the emphasis will likely focus on the occupational behaviors at the level of performance.

The underlying components affecting self-care function may be cognitive (lack of knowledge or impaired intellect or judgment) or psychosocial (decreased motivation or lowered self-esteem). These components can often be analyzed simultaneously with occupational behaviors. Evaluation should begin at the level of performance; then performance components can be considered as necessary. This perspective allows the therapist to assist someone with psychiatric disabilities to focus on what is "necessary and fulfilling" (Bonder, 1993, p. 214) to be able to perform meaningful self-care activities, not on whether he or she is depressed or isolated. It may be helpful at some level of evaluation and treatment to identify the relationship between the person's social isolation and depression. But it is probably more meaningful to assist in developing budget and money-management skills so that the person can afford to eat one meal a day at the local coffee shop and, in so doing, meet his or her social needs.

Assessments that are designed for direct observation of the performance of self-care activities under standardized conditions are usually considered the most valid and reliable, although they are the most costly in time and rely on the knowledge level of the evaluator (Christiansen, 1991). Because self-report (including questionnaires and interviews) of self-care levels has been identified as generally unreliable in persons with psychiatric disorders, especially among persons with schizophrenia, the trade-off of higher costs for meaningful

information is worthwhile. A discussion of self-care assessments specifically developed for persons with psychiatric disabilities is presented elsewhere in this book. Some assessments use direct observation of self-care activities more than others, although not necessarily under standardized conditions. However, all assessments incorporate direct observation to some extent.

Two assessments found in the occupational therapy literature include activities of self-care and rely primarily on observation of skill. They are the Routine Task Inventory (RTI-2; Allen, 1992) and the Comprehensive Occupational Therapy Evaluation (COTE; Brayman & Kirby, 1982). The RTI-2 is designed for use with persons with cognitive impairment, which can include psychiatric disorders. The COTE is designed for use with persons with psychiatric disorders, but it does not break down the category of self-care into specific activities (i.e., bathing, dressing). Both are mentioned here because of their availability and their potential contribution to meeting the self-care needs of persons with psychiatric disorders. Table 15.1 lists the specific self-care activities that can be evaluated with the assessments currently found in the occupational therapy literature (Asher, 1996). Readers are urged to evaluate the validity, reliability, assessment protocols, clinical applications, and other supporting information for each instrument before using it in a clinical setting.

Other dimensions of function that might influence engagement in self-care activities for persons with psychiatric disorders include the person's life

Table 15.1 Activities Included in Self-Care Assessments

Assessment	Self-Care Activities
Routine Task Inventory (RTI-2) (Allen, 1992)	Grooming, dressing, bathing, feeding, tioleting, taking medication, using telephone, communicating
Comprehensive Occupational Therapy Evaluation (COTE) (Brayman & Kirby, 1982)	Appearance: clean skin, clean hair, hair combed, clean clothes, clothes ironed, clothes suitable for occasion)
Scorable Self-Care Evaluation (Revised) (Clark & Peters, 1993)	Personal care: appearance, hygiene (frequency), emergency communication, first aid
Milwaukee Evaluation of Daily Living Skills (MEDLS) (Leonardelli, 1988)	Basic communication, bathing, brushing teeth, denture care, dressing, eating, eyeglass care, hair care, makeup use, medication management, nail care, personal health care, shaving, telephone use
Kohlman Evaluation of Living Skills (KELS) (Thomson, 1993)	Appearance, frequency of self-care, safety and health (telephone, emergency, danger in home, first aid, dental and medical facilities)

roles, use of time, and perceived quality of life. Instruments useful for evaluation of function in these areas include the Role Checklist (Oakley, Kielhofner, Barris, & Reichler, 1986), Occupational Questionnaire (Smith, 1993), and the Wisconsin Quality of Life Index (Becker, Diamond, & Sainfort, 1993). The Wisconsin Quality of Life Index includes items such as housing, neighborhood, access to transportation, physical health status, money, and personal safety. These dimensions of daily life may affect the ability to satisfy self-care needs and should be considered when working with persons with psychiatric disorders.

Self-Care Strategies

Assisting persons with psychiatric disorders to develop strategies to manage self-care needs can take on many forms, including psychoeducational approaches, case management, assertive community treatment, psychiatric rehabilitation, and building community supports. Most of the programs found in the occupational therapy literature use an academic or educational model (psychoeducational) to address self-care needs for persons with psychiatric disorders (Fike, 1990; Friedlob, Janis, & Deets-Aron, 1986; Neistadt & Cohn, 1990). Psychoeducational models are certainly found outside of the occupational therapy literature and are usually described in conjunction with the other strategies mentioned above that are helpful to consumers.

Psychoeducational Models

The concept that therapists can use educational approaches to change the self-care habits, routines, and skills of the persons we serve is grounded in the belief that therapy is learning. This is not a new concept in occupational therapy; references to teaching and learning in therapy have appeared in the occupational therapy literature since the 1960s. In chapter 5, Snell and Vogtle present an overview of principles for behavioral and cognitive approaches and suggest guidelines useful for planning self-care strategies.

Educational guidelines. Behavioral approaches (cause–effect associations, shaping, reinforcement, behavior modification, habituation, and sensitization) are most effective for persons with psychiatric disorders whose cognitive abilities are impaired by psychoses (e.g., acute schizophrenia, severe depression), those with normal attention span and memory abilities (e.g., personality disorders), and those in situations where the environment is unchanging and responses require little or no judgment in determining what to

do (e.g., persons living in group homes). Cognitive approaches (teaching how learning occurs, transferring learning, role-playing, rehearsal, imagery, and memory enhancement techniques) are best used when the person must learn to do situational problem solving (e.g., select appropriate clothing for weather conditions), when the persons has deficits in attention span, memory, or other cognitive abilities (e.g., a person with central nervous system damage such as someone with a long history of substance use), or when the skills being learned need to be generalized or transferred to other situations (e.g., using acceptable eating behaviors in a restaurant).

The following case study demonstrates how behavioral and cognitive approaches were combined when assisting a client to develop socially acceptable standards of personal hygiene.

> The format of an activities of daily living (ADL) skills group at a community day treatment setting is open ended and addresses the needs of persons as determined by members on a day-to-day basis. All consumers in the treatment program attend the ADL group. Consequently, the group's focus varies, depending on whose issues are being dealt with on a given day. Group members assume a supportive peer role and give feedback to each other about how to accomplish their goals. For some consumers, this need may be to learn how to plan and cook a nutritious meal. For others, it may be to learn how to shop in a grocery store and make appropriate, cost-effective purchase decisions. Still others need feedback on a more basic level.
>
> T. R. joined the program and initially remained a quiet, background participant in most of the activities. Some of the staff members and consumers had difficulty approaching T. R. because of his obvious body odor and disheveled appearance. In the context of the ADL group, his peers were able to share with T. R. the effect he had on others and how that effect was keeping others from approaching and getting to know him. The group used role-playing and rehearsal (cognitive techniques) to help T. R. improve his personal hygiene and to learn how to use the machines at the laundromat. A group shopping trip helped him to begin to overcome his anxiety about being in crowds and having a store clerk approach him. After a few weeks, he was attending the group in clean clothes and had a more pleasing odor, as he used the aftershave cologne a fellow group member had given to him as a present (reinforcement—a behavioral technique).

Strategies and characteristics of the psychoeducational approach. Specific strategies common to psychoeducational programs include verbal, written, visual, and experiential learning in various areas of daily living, including technology-based learning; community outings to relate learning to real-life experiences and apply the new skills to the real environment, and role-playing, rehearsal, and education games. Characteristics suggested for a consumer's successful involvement in a psychoeducational program include the following:

- The person is able to learn
- Enrollment in the program is voluntary
- Participants in the program are students and instructors, not patients or clients and staff members
- Students set their own goals for learning
- Involvement in the program is time limited (imparts a sense of urgency to acquire skills or knowledge)
- There is some financial cost to the students (Bakker & Armstrong, 1976; Lillie & Armstrong, 1982)

When implementing the psychoeducational approach, it is important to take the mystique out of learning; that is, it is important to tell learners that behavior patterns are learned, everyone goes through essentially the same learning process, and behavior can be acquired or changed. As Lamb (1976) stated when describing a psychoeducational model for persons with long-term psychiatric disorders, it is crucial to help consumers "realize that the basic skills of everyday living are learned skills" (p. 877). The key principle to success is consumer involvement—in establishing the goals for learning, in establishing the curriculum, and in taking some responsibility for its implementation. Another key factor is conducting the program away from the site of mental health treatment, if possible. By doing so, the consumer can acquire

> a new identity, that of student, and feels he [or she] can participate in activities outside of mental health centers just like other people in the community. That, plus the information imparted to him [or her] in the course, helps the student move beyond the mental health system. (Lamb, 1976, p. 877)

The adoption of psychoeducational strategies into occupational therapy services for persons with psychiatric disorders is described by Crist (1986), Kielhofner & Brinson (1989), Neistadt and Marques (1984), and Weissenberg and Giladi (1989), among others. For the most part, these programs emphasize the more complex self-maintenance activities

of daily living; however, the format and approaches they use are easily extended to self-care skills.

Case Management

Case management is defined as a "service which assists clients in negotiating for services that they both need and want" (Cohen & Nemec, 1988, p. 27). Extensive literature is available about case-management approaches and strategies to assist persons with psychiatric disorders. One study reported that consumers involved in intensive case management over a 2-year period had fewer emergency visits and increased social networks, and that their family members had a reduced burden of care (Aberg-Wistedt, Cressell, Lidberg, Liljenberg, & Osby, 1995).

Four models of case management are usually described in the literature—full support, personal strengths, rehabilitation, and expanded broker or generalist (Solomon, 1992). Although there are subtle distinctions among them, for the most part they have the following characteristics in common: establishing a close relationship with the consumer; working with the consumer in his or her own environment; evaluating skills and training in areas such as self-care, symptom management, and money management; linking consumers to preferred service providers; and advocating for service improvement (Cohen, Nemec, Farkas, & Forbess, 1988). Services may be provided by teams or individuals.

The National Association of Case Management (1997) has developed practice guidelines for case management and identified three levels of intensity for case managers based on the individualized needs of the mental health consumer. Levels I and II case management involve having the case manager teach independent living skills in the person's natural environment, whereas Level III is primarily directed toward finding the community resources matched to the person's needs.

Occupational therapy practitioners are well suited to the responsibilities associated with case management to assist persons with psychiatric disorders. The focus on the occupational behaviors of self-care, work, and leisure encompasses all the activities of a consumer's total day. The occupational therapy practitioner's knowledge of activity analysis, therapeutic use of self, self-care, and interdisciplinary team approaches provides a solid foundation for the case-manager role. Additional preparation in accessing community agencies and advocacy could be sought from programs mentioned later in the chapter.

Assertive Community Treatment

The assertive community treatment (ACT) program was developed by Drs. Leonard Stein, Mary Ann Test, and Arnold Marx in the early 1970s at Mendota Mental Health Institute in Madison, Wisconsin (Stein & Santos, 1998). This comprehensive, multidisciplinary program offers full-support case management services in the community with a team of staff members whose expertise informs the group decision making. By working collaboratively with the community and family members, the model ACT program has had success in achieving goals related to community living and employment.

Occupational therapy practitioners can offer the ACT team concrete expertise in the area of self-care evaluation and training. The standard evaluation used by the ACT includes an activities of daily living assessment that includes food and nutrition skills, maintenance and housekeeping skills, personal hygiene and grooming skills, mobility skills, recreation or leisure skills, social skills, communication skills, interpersonal relationships, money management and banking skills, time management, problem-solving and decision-making skills, and safety skills (Stein & Santos, 1998). Occupational therapy practitioners are skilled in the evaluation of the person's capacity for self-care, as well as evaluating the needed environment to support each person's optimal function. In addition, the occupational therapist can serve as the vocational specialist to facilitate the work experiences of the consumer.

Psychiatric Rehabilitation

The literature on psychiatric rehabilitation has become rich with principles and outcomes supporting persons with psychiatric disabilities living full lives in their community of choice. The emphasis on rehabilitation over treatment focuses on improved functioning and life satisfaction, assessing present and needed skills and supports, teaching skills, and coordinating and modifying resources versus the treatment focus on "cure," symptomology, and medications (Anthony, Cohen, & Farkas, 1990). Occupational therapy practitioners are seen as one of several professionals who contribute to the rehabilitation process.

The basic principles of psychiatric rehabilitation include a focus on competencies, the consumer's environment, the eclectic use of techniques, vocational outcomes, instilling hope, and the active involvement of the client in the rehabilitation process. These principles have been applied by the State of Wisconsin's Blue Ribbon Commission on Mental Health (1997) to their reorganization of the state mental health program. Shifting the paradigm of care from treatment to rehabilitation to recovery has been advocated by the Wisconsin Blue Ribbon Commission. A vision of recovery includes the goal of attaining a productive and fulfilling life regardless of mental illness. Occupational therapy practitioners will focus on self-care skills in the context of helping persons build meaningful life roles in their community of choice.

Building Community Supports

The integration of persons with psychiatric disorders into the community is a challenge to all persons with an interest in community mental health, such as consumers, family members, mental health professionals, policymakers, housing professionals, and employers. Carling (1975) and his colleagues at the Center for Community Change have identified several principles that underlie successful integration. They call for a radical shift in thinking about the needs of persons with psychiatric disorders and how they are met. These principles are consistent with those of a client-centered approach for occupational therapy as described by Law (1998). A summary of the principles proposed by Carling (1975) includes the following:

- All persons, regardless of any differences, belong in a community.
- Persons with differences can be integrated into typical neighborhoods, work situations, and community social situations.
- Support is necessary for *all* persons and their family members (not just those who are different) and should be offered in regular places in the community.
- The development of relationships between persons with and without labels is crucial; each has much to teach the other.
- Clients and their family members should be involved in the design, operation, and monitoring of all services and should have the power to hold services accountable.
- Success in housing, work, and social relationships is primarily a function of whether a person has the skills and supports that are relevant to that environment or relationship.
- Person's needs and relationships change over time; services and supports should be available at varying levels for as long as a person needs them (Bonder, 1995).

Issues that must be addressed in communities for full integration of persons with psychiatric disabilities include access to and support in housing, employment, education, health and dental care, and resocialization. Occupational therapy practitioners are well suited to address these needs for mental health consumers. They must position themselves in community agencies, work to establish informal networks for clients, and empower consumers to help themselves. ◆

Study Questions

1. What are the factors that contribute to poor self-care skills among persons with psychiatric disorders?

2. Identify the behavioral characteristics of persons with schizophrenia. Describe the course of the disease and the problems with self-care.

3. Describe depression and the range of self-care dysfunction in persons with this disorder.

4. Compare and contrast the self-care difficulties of persons with personality disorders and persons with a diagnosis of schizophrenia.

5. What conditions are most likely to resolve with medication?

6. List three assessments designed to measure self-care function in persons with psychosocial conditions.

7. Describe psychoeducational models of intervention. List the characteristics necessary for a client's successful involvement in such a program.

8. Describe the principles for integrating persons with psychiatric conditions within the community.

References

Aberg-Wistedt, A., Cressell, T., Lidberg, Y., Liljenberg, B., & Osbey, U. (1995). Two-year outcome of team-based intensive case management for patients with schizophrenia. *Psychiatric Services, 46*, 1263–1266.

Allen, C. K. (1992). Routine Task Inventory (RTI-2). In C. K. Allen, C. A. Earhart, & T. Blue (Eds.), *Occupational therapy treatment goals for the physically and cognitively disabled* (pp. 54–68). Rockville, MD: American Occupational Therapy Association.

Anthony, W., Cohen, M., & Farkas, M. (1990). *Psychiatric rehabilitation*. Boston: Center for Psychiatric Rehabilitation.

Asher, I. E. (1996). *Occupational therapy assessment tools: An annotated index* (2nd ed.). Bethesda, MD: American Occupational Therapy Association.

Bakker, C. B., & Armstrong, H. E. (1976). The adult development program: An educational approach to the delivery of mental health services. *Hospital and Community Psychiatry, 27*, 330–334.

Becker, M., Diamond, R., & Sainfort, F. (1993). A new patient focused index for measuring quality of life in persons with severe and persistent mental illness. *Quality of Life Research, 2*, 239–251.

Bonder, B. (1993). Issues in assessment of psychosocial components of function. *American Journal of Occupational Therapy, 47*, 211–216.

Bonder, B. (1995). *Psychopathology and function* (2nd ed.). Thorofare, NJ: Slack.

Brayman, S., & Kirby, T. (1982). The comprehensive occupational therapy evaluation. In B. J. Hemphill (Ed.), *The evaluation process in psychiatric occupational therapy* (pp. 221–226). Thorofare, NJ: Slack.

Carling, P. J. (1975). *Return to community: Building support systems for people with psychiatric disabilities*. New York: Guilford Press.

Christiansen, C. (1991). Occupational performance assessment. In C. Christiansen & C. Baum (Eds.), *Occupational therapy: Overcoming human performance deficits* (pp. 375–421). Thorofare, NJ: Slack.

Clark, E. N., & Peters, M. (1993). *Scorable Self-Care Evaluation* (Revised). San Antonio, TX: Therapy Skill Builders.

Cohen, M., & Nemec, P. (1988). Trainer orientation. In M. Cohen, P. Nemec, & M. Farkas (Eds.), *Case management training technology*. Boston: Center for Psychiatric Rehabilitation, Boston University.

Cohen, M., Nemec, P., Farkas, M., & Forbess, R. (1988). Training module: Introduction. In M. Cohen, P. Nemec, & M. Farkas (Eds.), *Case management training technology*. Boston: Center for Psychiatric Rehabilitation, Boston University.

Crist, P. H. (1986). Community living skills: A psychoeducational community-based program. *Occupational Therapy in Mental Health, 6*(2), 51–64.

Fike, M. L. (1990). Considerations and techniques in the treatment of multiple personality disorder. *American Journal of Occupational Therapy, 44*, 984–990.

Friedlob, S. A., Janis, G. A., & Deets-Aron, C. (1986). A hospital-connected halfway house program for individuals with long-term neuropsychiatric disabilities. *American Journal of Occupational Therapy, 40*, 271–277.

Howie the Harp. (1995). Preface. In P. J. Carling (Ed.), *Return to community: Building support systems for people with psychiatric disabilities* (pp. xiii–xvii). New York: Guilford Press.

Kielhofner, G., & Brinson, M. (1989). Development and evaluation of an aftercare program for young chronic psychiatrically disabled adults. *Occupational Therapy in Mental Health, 9*(2), 1–25.

Lamb, H. R. (1976). An educational model for teaching skills to long-term patients. *Hospital and Community Psychiatry, 27,* 875–877.

Law, M. (Ed.). (1998). *Client-centered occupational therapy.* Thorofare, NJ: Slack.

Leonardelli, C. A. (1988). *The Milwaukee Evaluation of Daily Living Skills: Evaluation in long-term psychiatric care.* Thorofare, NJ: Slack.

Lillie, M. D., & Armstrong, H. E. (1982). Contributions to the development of psychoeducational approaches to mental health service. *American Journal of Occupational Therapy, 36,* 438–443.

National Association of Case Management & The Community Support Program, Division of Knowledge Development and Systems Change, Center for Mental Health Services, Substance Abuse and Mental Health Services Administration. (1997). *Case management practice guidelines for adults with severe and persistent mental illness.* Ocean Ridge, FL: National Association of Case Management.

Neistadt, M. E., & Cohn, E. S. (1990). *An independent living skills model for Level I fieldwork.* Rockville, MD: American Occupational Therapy Association.

Neistadt, M. E., & Marques, K. (1984). An independent living skills training program. *American Journal of Occupational Therapy, 38,* 671–676.

Oakley, F., Kielhofner, G., Barris, R., & Reichler, R. K. (1986). The role checklist: Development and empirical assessment of reliability. *Occupational Therapy Journal of Research, 6*(3), 157–169.

Smith, N. R. (1993). *Occupational questionnaire.* Chicago: The Model of Human Occupational Clearinghouse, The University of Illinois at Chicago.

Solomon, P. (1992). The efficacy of case management services for severely mentally disabled clients. *Community Mental Health Journal, 28,* 163–180.

Stein, L. I., & Santos, A. B. (1998). *Assertive community treatment of persons with severe mental illness.* New York: W. W. Norton.

Thomson, L. K. (1992). *Kohlman Evaluation of Living Skills (KELS).* Rockville, MD: American Occupational Therapy Association.

Ward, J. D. (1998). Psychological dysfunction in adults. In M. E. Neistadt & E. B. Crepeau (Eds.), *Willard and Spackman's occupational therapy* (9th ed., pp.716–740). Philadelphia: Lippincott.

Weissenberg, R., & Giladi, N. (1989). Home economics day: A program for disturbed adolescents to promote acquisition of habits and skills. *Occupational Therapy in Mental Health, 9,* 89–103.

Wisconsin Blue Ribbon Commission on Mental Health. (1997). *The Blue Ribbon Commission on Mental Health: Final report.* Madison, WI: Office of the Governor Tommy G. Thompson.

16

Living With Vision Loss

Don Golembiewski

Don Golembiewski, MA, is Coordinator, Independent Living Services for Older Blind Individuals, Madison, Wisconsin.

Key Terms

counts fingers (CF) or finger counting (FC)

hand movement (HM)

legal blindness

light perception (LP)

light projection (L. Proj.)

no light perception (NLP)

severe visual impairment

sighted guide technique

Objectives

On completing this chapter, the reader will be able to

1. Describe the major age-related eye conditions.

2. Understand the functional characteristics resulting from the different age-related eye conditions.

3. Describe the terms used to classify the levels of vision loss.

4. Describe the phases of adjustment to a severe loss of vision.

5. Identify the factors that increase the potential for increased independence in daily living skills.

6. Describe the effect that lighting has on the functional abilities of persons with severe visual impairments.

7. Describe the importance of texture and color contrast in the successful completion of activities of daily living.

8. Understand the rationale behind the early involvement of clients with a severe vision loss.

This chapter describes the visual impairments, short of total blindness, most commonly associated with aging. It details strategies that allow persons with these conditions to function with confidence and independence. Many of the strategies, tools, and approaches also apply to younger persons and those who are congenitally blind. Persons who are younger or congenitally blind make up a relatively small percentage of the population having difficulty seeing (Kirchner & Schmeidler, 1997).

A severe vision loss will negatively affect virtually all daily living activities of persons living with low vision (Carroll, 1961). This functional effect will be different for each person and will vary in an intensity that may not be in proportion to the severity of the loss. Thus, it is understandable why the information presented in this chapter only touches on the full range of adaptive strategies and aids available to this highly diverse population. Attention will focus on the crucial deficit areas of communication skills, mobility skills, personal management, and household or environmental modifications. Information in the following section is presented to establish a foundation for the ocular conditions and coping strategies that are discussed.

Definitions of Visual Acuity

Visual acuity levels are reported by eye care providers (ophthalmologists and optometrists) with the following designations (Jose, 1983):

- *No light perception* (NLP) is the designation meaning total blindness.
- *Light perception* (LP) designates the ability to perceive light only.
- *Light projection* (L. Proj.) is the ability not only to see light but also to determine the direction of the source.
- *Hand movement* (HM) is used to designate the ability to see movement or gross forms.
- *Counts fingers* (CF) or finger counting (FC), often used in conjunction with "at 2 feet," or another distance, is an unreliable and seldom used designation of vision. This designation is neither truly objective nor exact but may occasionally still be seen on medical reports.

Snellen Notation is the tested level of vision that coincides with each line of progressively smaller print letters a client is able to read on a Snellen chart. The use of the Snellen eye chart with the familiar large capital "E" or "O" on the top line is the standard tool for the measurement of distance acuity. Depending on the chart, the top line with large type may measure vision of 20/400 or 20/200. As each line of type decreases in size, the acuity level increases. The bottom line on most charts represents vision of 20/15.

Legal Blindness and Severe Visual Impairment

Clinical legal blindness is defined as having vision of 20/200 (20 over 200) or less (using the Snellen eye chart measurement) in the better eye with best standard eyeglass correction, or having a visual field that encompasses or subtends an angle of 20° or less. The first part of this definition states how clearly one can see (acuity), and the second part states how much area of the potential visual field one sees. For example, 20/200 means the person sees at 20 feet what someone with 20/20 or normal or perfect vision sees at 200 feet. The normal visual field with both eyes (binocular) will approach 180° (Jose, 1983). The National Center for Health Statistics defines severe visual impairment as a self- or proxy-reported inability to read standard newsprint (Nelson & Dimitrova, 1993).

Statistics on Severe Visual Impairment and Blindness

The estimated prevalence in 1991–1992 of persons who have a functional visual limitation or a severe functional visual limitation is 9.7 million among persons in the United States 15 years of age or older and who are not institutionalized (Kirchner & Schmeidler, 1997). The estimated prevalence in 1990 of persons in the United States 15 years of age or older who are not institutionalized and are legally blind is 1.1 million (Kirchner & Schmeidler, 1997). Relatively few young persons are blind. It is estimated that two thirds of the severely visually impaired or legally blind population are more than 65 years of age (Ponchillia & Ponchillia, 1996).

Regardless of the language or numbers seen on medical reports, persons with serious eye conditions cannot routinely expect their vision to remain stable. For most persons, vision will likely change very gradually over time. For some persons, vision may fluctuate on a daily or even an hourly basis. Ophthalmologic reports often will not tell the entire story of how well one functions visually.

Visual Acuity and Function

While total blindness is a condition readily comprehended, visual acuity in persons who are severely visually impaired is often misunderstood (Tuttle & Tuttle, 1996). Just as each person has different physical abilities, each person with low vision can be expected to have a unique ability to see. Approximately 80% to 85% of all persons who are legally blind have some level of useful vision (Flax, Golembiewski, & McCaulley, 1993). Therefore, most persons have the ability to see something, such as large print, the shapes of houses or furniture, trees or people, the action on television, or simply light and dark, and they are able to use their sight for purposeful activities. To complicate matters, however, many persons with severe vision loss have visual abilities that fluctuate and are unpredictable. Fatigue, poor lighting, glare, motivation, and other factors affect the ability to see. This uncertainty and variability can make service delivery challenging.

Each major eye condition causes a typical vision loss. Age, age at onset of condition, duration of condition, other eye conditions, other health concerns, personal motivation, and environmental factors can affect how well and how much each person sees and how he or she is able to use or process what they see. Regardless of the condition, however, a person with any severe visual impairment may experience feelings of isolation, depression, inadequacy, and self-doubt.

Common Eye Conditions

Macular degeneration, diabetic retinopathy, glaucoma, and cataracts are the leading causes of age-related vision loss in the United States (Flax et al., 1993). Each of these conditions is described in the following sections.

Macular Degeneration

Macular degeneration or age-related macular degeneration (AMD) is a condition that affects the central visual acuity, primarily in those persons more than 50 years of age. The vision loss may begin in one eye and progress to the other. Some major concerns of clients with AMD include their inability to read small print, drive a car, see their grandchildren's faces, set their thermostat or stove dials, or see themselves in a mirror.

Many persons with AMD find that the use of optical aids such as magnifiers, telescopes, and video magnifiers or closed circuit televisions enable them to read and function at a much more satisfactory level. The use of eccentric viewing exercises and techniques may also help persons with AMD to use the viable area of their visual field (Flax et al., 1993).

Diabetic Retinopathy

Diabetic retinopathy is a condition that affects the retinas of some persons who are diabetic. The retina, or innermost layer of the eye, receives images transmitted through the cornea and contains the rods and cones, which are sensory receptors. Diabetes may cause hemorrhages or blood vessel changes that affect the retina and thus interfere with vision. The entire visual field may become involved, causing severe functional limitations often characterized by highly fluctuating vision.

Glaucoma

Glaucoma is another leading cause of blindness in the United States. Glaucoma damage is the result of a buildup of pressure within the eye that damages the optic nerve. This increased pressure causes a decrease of vision in the peripheral field, commonly known as tunnel vision. As the term suggests, persons with tunnel vision cannot see things on either side without turning their head. A person with glaucoma may have 20/20 vision in the central part of the visual field; however, that area of vision may only be 10° in size. Persons with glaucoma may find their reading ability relatively unchanged. Their ability to use their peripheral vision to negotiate steps or icy sidewalks, or to use their vision under dimly lit circumstances, however, is greatly diminished.

Cataracts

Cataracts are another common condition affecting the older population. A cataract is an opacity, or cloudiness, of the normally clear lens inside the eye. The lens is responsible for focusing light onto the retina. Because of the aging process, disease, trauma, or other factors, cataracts may occur, causing a person to have vision that is often described as "looking through a dirty windshield or a gauze curtain." The medical treatment for cataracts is surgery and most often the implantation of an artificial lens. Often persons who have cataracts function well with optical aids, and they may also benefit from wearing special optical filter sunglasses (absorptive lenses) or broad-brimmed hats to reduce glare.

Presbyopia

Presbyopia is the reduction in accommodative ability that occurs with age (Jose, 1983). Accommodation refers to the ability of the eyes to adjust or focus. This condition, commonly beginning between 42 and 45 years of age, is characterized by the inability to focus on near objects, such as fine print in a book. Presbyopia is a normal consequence of aging and is not a cause for alarm. It does cause functional complications, especially when combined with other serious eye conditions.

Functional Consequences of Eye Conditions

For rehabilitation practitioners, the functional consequences of eye conditions are of most concern. In the following sections, visual deficits resulting from central vision loss, loss of peripheral vision, and overall or general vision loss are described. Case studies are presented to illustrate how these conditions were experienced by selected persons and how they adapted to their visual deficit. Figure 16.1 depicts a scene as viewed by someone with normal vision.

Central Vision Loss

Central vision is often referred to as the identification or fine detail vision, as it is what we use to tell us what we are looking at. Central vision loss (CVL) will therefore cause a person to lose central or fine detailed vision. Color discrimination, located centrally on the retina, will also be severely affected. A simple yet useful analogy is to consider the normal circular visual field as a donut complete with donut hole. Persons with CVL will see the donut but not the hole. Without the benefit of fine detailed vision,

the client will see better using his or her eccentric or peripheral vision. As one turns one's eyes, the scotoma or blind spot moves with the visual field. To make best use of the remaining useful portion of the visual field, the client must not look directly at the object of concern, but rather to his or her best area of the peripheral field (eccentric viewing). It is not unusual for a client with CVL to be unable to read newspaper headlines from inches away while being able to see a fly in the corner of the ceiling or a bit of paper on the floor. Further, the person with CVL will often complain of not being able to see photographs of grandchildren or recognize faces from across the table but may be able to see whether that person's shoes are shined. Figure 16.2 shows the same scene as perceived by someone with CVL.

Case Study: Age-Related Macular Degeneration

R. L. is a man 83 years of age with a confirmed diagnosis of AMD. His wife was concerned about his vision and how it is limiting him. He was unable to see newspaper headlines and contended he could not see well enough to do certain household chores. She lost a sewing needle in a shag carpet and was unable to locate it. After R. L. found it visually, his wife became very confused about his vision. Why couldn't he see well enough to help her, but yet could see to find a very small item for which she had searched at length? After the functional limitations of AMD were explained to her, she understood his inability to see fine detail, while maintaining his ability to see peripherally. As doing dishes is a tactual job, we worked out a new compromise. While he did do more housework, she would be responsible for more of the visual tasks, such as balancing the checkbook.

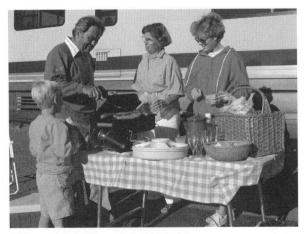

Figure 16.1 Clear or normal vision.

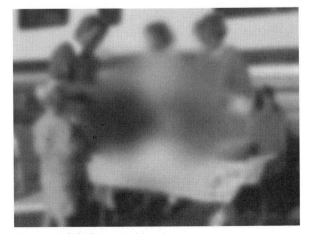

Figure 16.2 Central vision loss.

Case Study: Age-Related Macular Degeneration

M. M. has AMD and misses seeing photographs of her grandchildren. She generally sees shapes of persons sitting in front of her but cannot recognize them. Looking directly at someone's face, she can see rings on their fingers but cannot see whether they are wearing glasses or makeup. One concern is that friends do not understand the effect of AMD. She can walk to the nearby grocery store and independently do her shopping with the assistance of a small lighted magnifier, but she does not recognize or even see well enough to acknowledge friendly waves from across the street. In her neighborhood, this snub is considered serious and not taken lightly. M. M. was encouraged to inform her friends of her inability to recognize persons from a distance and to carry a white cane for identification purposes. She routinely offers friends a copy of a brochure on AMD she picked up from her ophthalmologist's office.

Peripheral Vision Loss

Peripheral vision loss (PVL) will limit activities where peripheral or side vision is necessary. The client with PVL will have limitations with independent mobility, especially in low-light situations. With a narrow visual field, the client with PVL must continually scan his or her environment to view, in series, what the person with a normal field sees instantly. If an object is not immediately in the center field of vision, it appears as if it does not exist. Often low-lying objects, such as coffee tables, steps, rugs, or uneven pavement, cause serious difficulties.

Peripheral vision is sometimes referred to as the orientation vision, as it is most relied upon to tell us where we are in relation to objects in our environment. It is also the area of best vision in low-light environments. Many persons with PVL function best when adequate task lighting, color contrasting background, and centrally presented objectives are available. Figure 16.3 depicts the same scene as viewed by a person with PVL.

Case Study: Glaucoma

P. T. has advanced glaucoma. He lives alone in a very small home in a rural area. He has a strong network of natural supports on which he relies. His visual field is 10° in his left eye and no light perception in the right. His acuity is unknown. He is able to read some print quite slowly, usually one letter at a time when extremely bright

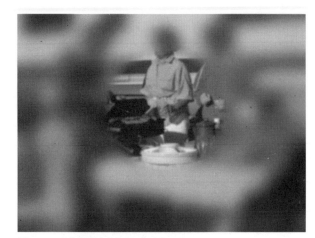

Figure 16.3 Peripheral vision loss.

task lighting is available. He has given up trying to walk alone outside except in very bright sunlight, for which he uses sunglasses.

P. T. experienced his vision loss at least in part because he refused to follow his medication regimen. He explained that his uncle had glaucoma and lost all vision over a 10-year span despite taking drops to relieve the pressure. Because he refused to take the proper medication, he had permanently lost his vision to glaucoma much faster.

Overall or General Vision Loss

A person with this type of loss may have a loss of vision in any or the entire field of vision. Cataracts or diabetic retinopathy may cause this general type of loss. Any portion of the visual field may be affected and any types of visual limitations may be present. The vision of a person with general vision loss is shown in Figure 16.4.

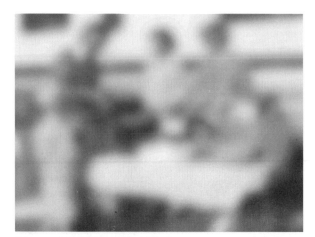

Figure 16.4 General vision loss.

Case Study: Diabetic Retinopathy

B. A. is diabetic with greatly fluctuating vision. Her vision in the morning is very cloudy with everything appearing dark. Turning on bright lights helps, but then she sometimes needs to control the indoor glare by wearing optical filter sunglasses. When she reads, she tries to look around or past her numerous hemorrhages and retinal scars that seem to move about. By midmorning, her vision seems to clear, so she tries to do her reading then with her back to the brightest window. Later her vision may become cloudy for a period before getting relatively clear again during the evening hours. Figure 16.5 depicts the view of a person with diabetic retinopathy.

Adjustment to Low Vision

Blindness shares much with other disabling conditions in the stages of the adjustment process. There are seven phases of adjusting to life with blindness (Tuttle & Tuttle, 1996). These phases include (a) trauma, (b) shock and denial, (c) mourning and withdrawal, (d) succumbing and depression, (e) reassessment and reaffirmation, (f) coping and mobilization, and (g) self-acceptance and self-esteem.

Each person will feel the effects of blindness or low vision differently. For example, a person who has been highly active, has driven trucks for a living, or has been an outdoor enthusiast may have difficulty with a perceived need to adopt a more sedentary lifestyle. By the same token, an avid reader who develops AMD may feel a major loss that may be just an annoying inconvenience to another who has never enjoyed reading.

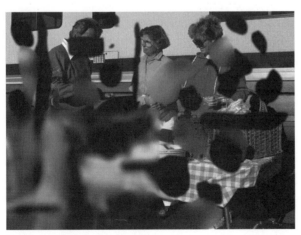

Figure 16.5 Diabetic retinopathy.

Social factors must be considered as an important part of adjusting to blindness. Because blindness limits the ease of mobility, such as driving across town or walking to the corner coffee shop, persons who have lost vision will not have the same freedom of movement they enjoyed previously. To avoid feelings of isolation, social contacts should be continued and new ones explored as well.

Case Study: Severe Vision Loss

K. T. was despondent over his severe vision loss. The biggest effect on him was a self-imposed withdrawal from the coffee club group of fellow retirees at the nearby café. All were long-time friends who shared similar life experiences, sports allegiances, and community connections. After his vision declined, he felt the others were now being overly protective and treating him like a blind person, not as good old K. T. One friend apologized profusely after asking if everyone had seen the recent football game. A painful silence made everyone feel uncomfortable. K. T. didn't feel they understood him at all, so he gave up his coffee group. Eventually, K. T. heard of a support group for persons with vision loss that met every month at the local senior center. Everyone was welcome, although most attendees were more than 70 years of age. No dues were collected and the aging office provided transportation. After a few meetings that included discussions of dealing with the sighted world and living as a blind person, K. T. began to accept his vision loss and was able to better understand how he was misinterpreting his friends' comments. He then resumed meeting with his coffee buddies and was able to Monday-morning quarterback as he always had. He even told a joke about a dog guide for the blind that easily and permanently broke the ice.

Evaluation of Independent Living Needs

Because of the individualized nature of visual abilities, an evaluation format is necessary to help target service needs. Two assessments are described here. The first instrument, *Assessment for Vision Rehabilitation Services* (Golembiewski, 1998), is verbally administered to screen potential recipients of vision rehabilitation services. It is designed for ease of use by professionals and nonprofessionals alike. Each of the functional areas is queried in three steps. Can you accomplish the task? If not, is it due to a vision loss? Do you want assistance with the visually restricting task? Although assessments that are not performance based have limitations, this tool is meant as a simple means of identifying those who are truly appropriate for vision rehabilitation services. It is intended as a basis for formulating a plan of service (see Appendix).

The second assessment is meant to be administered functionally either in the client's home or in an institutional facility. This assessment, which is not standardized, identifies the need for adaptive aids and techniques that can be recommended by a person qualified to provide rehabilitation services for persons with blindness or low vision. The need areas identified will form the basis for the individualized plan for services developed for the client. Items included in this performance-based assessment are listed in Table 16.1.

Assisting Persons With Vision Loss

Intervention options for persons with vision loss can be organized according to the standard categories outlined in chapter 4. These include *remediation* (teaching and training), *compensation* (changing the task or environment), *disability prevention* (encouraging the performance of tasks that prevent health problems and encouraging safe task methods), and *health promotion* (encouraging engagement in meaningful, balanced, and healthy occupations and environmental interactions). In this chapter, specific attention will be paid to compensatory strategies that permit accomplishment of activities of daily living, including environmental modifications as well as specific procedures and techniques for accomplish-

Table 16.1 Items Included in Performance-Based Assessments of Persons Who Are Blind or Visually Impaired

Low Vision
  Near vision
  Intermediate vision
  Distance vision
  Current optical aid use
  Illumination
  Absorptive lenses
  Clinical low vision exam

Communications
  Braille
  Script writing
  Typing
  Telephone use
  Tape recorder
  Telling time
  Library service

Food Preparation
  Safety
  Labeling
  Recipes
  Shopping
  Timing
  Pouring and measuring
  Cutting, peeling, slicing, and spreading
  Appliance use
  Dietary and nutritional concerns

Personal Management
  Grooming and hygiene
  Clothing care and identification
  Money handling
  Table etiquette
  Diabetic concerns
  Medication management
  Knowledge of eye disease
  Acceptance of eye condition

Home Management
  Cleaning
  Laundry
  Household organization
  Minor repairs and tool use
  Safety

Leisure Time Activities
  Social and support groups
  Crafts and hobbies
  Table games
  Sewing

Orientation and Movement
  Sighted guide
  Self-protective techniques
  Doorways
  Indoor travel
  Room familiarization
  Outdoor travel
  Automobiles
  Searching techniques
  Cane
  Orientation and mobility specialist

Community Resources
  Aging network

ing tasks using other sensory cues. The following sections describe lighting and color contrast changes in the environment, orientation and mobility, communication, household organization, food preparation, and personal management.

Environmental Lighting

Proper lighting is critical for a person with vision loss to make the best use of residual vision (Jose, 1983). Too much, too little, or poorly directed light will hinder the ability to perform daily living tasks (Tuttle & Tuttle, 1996). The need for or tolerance of certain light levels is highly individual and needs to be evaluated. Functional trials with various light levels are needed to establish the optimum visual environment that will improve performance and avoid fatigue.

Any work area should be illuminated with a general light source, adding focused task lighting as needed. The light source must be kept below eye level or be positioned behind or to the side of the person. Halogen stand lamps, gooseneck lamps, or other types of flexible and portable lighting are ideal sources of extremely bright task lighting. Some lamps are available in portable models. Lampshades should be used to help eliminate glare and to direct light to the targeted work area. Improving household lighting is perhaps the least expensive but most beneficial of all adaptations that a person with visual impairments can make. Many persons use flashlights with ultra bright krypton or halogen bulbs for portable task lighting. These are useful for setting stove and laundry dials as well as thermostats, and for seeing in dark areas of closets, drawers, or hallways.

Environmental light can be more useful if the work area is adjusted so that the light streams from the back or side of the task area. Rotating the task area or work surface from facing toward a window to a position facing away from a bright light source can often increase functional vision. Adjusting window shades or blinds will also minimize glare.

Case Study: Advanced Glaucoma

M. L. is a man 18 years of age with Down syndrome and advanced glaucoma. The visual acuity report is unreliable because of the communication limitations and questionable responses to standard tests. The special education teacher knew that glaucoma could cause night blindness and that additional light may be useful for his student. The teacher contacted the vision rehabilitation specialist for a consultation on a seemingly drastic and sudden functional decrease. When the classroom environment was reviewed, M. L.'s desk had been rotated so that he could look out of a large bank of windows facing an open area covered with snow. The teacher learned that turning the desk toward the light not only did not help, but it caused severe problems with glare and photophobia. With his desk rotated, M. L. had his back to the windows and he was able to resume visual tasks as before.

If glare is a problem, wearing sunglasses that block infrared and ultraviolet light is an option. They may be referred to as absorptive lenses or optical filters. Sunglasses that control glare and absorb irritating light are available in differing colors, shades, and percentages of light transmission. Many persons with photophobia or unstable conditions need different lenses for indoor and outdoor conditions.

Case Study: Photophobia

C. D. had a combination of eye conditions and severe photophobia. She had trouble in bright outdoor conditions, on overcast days, and even indoors. After a few trials with optical filters that block infrared and ultraviolet light, she realized that all three situations required different levels of light transmission and tints for her to be most comfortable. A high light transmission (40%) amber lens allowed her to use her vision best indoors for some reading, a medium level (10%) gray was best for overcast days, and a dark green low transmission (2%) was necessary on bright days. The best environment for her to read print was in natural light, so she positioned her reading desk by the brightest window available. As the light was also irritating, she used the 40% light transmission amber filters for reading.

Color Contrast

To enhance visual abilities for accomplishing daily living tasks, the practical use of color contrast should be widely incorporated into all environmental features. The use of light dishware that stands out more clearly against dark solid color tables or tablecloths is recommended. Two cutting boards should be available—a light-colored one for dark foods and a dark one for light foods. Contrasting or brightly colored items should be strategically placed to help locate furniture such as coffee tables and the backs or arms of chairs. Colored tape strips can be added to countertop edges, door sills, and steps to improve contrast. High contrast electrical outlet switch plate covers and cabinet handles can make them easier to find. Contrasting or bright fluorescent tape added to tool handles will make them easier to locate on dark work surfaces.

As some persons have a decreased ability to distinguish color, especially in low-light conditions, high contrast is especially important as environmental landmarks. A simple cafeteria tray can be used not only to keep craft supplies from rolling away but also as a means of increasing color contrast. If possible, a dark and a light tray should be available to contrast with the predominant color of the current supplies. If only dark trays are available, white or light contact paper or electrical tape can be applied to one side to provide better contrast as needed.

In most instances, solid colors are best for background surfaces. Floral or festive holiday patterns, or other busy backgrounds for tablecloths or other work surfaces, act as camouflage. The use of boldly patterned wallpaper or tabletop work surfaces should be avoided. Electric outlets, eating utensils, and tools are very difficult to locate on this type of background (see Figure 16.6).

Orientation and Mobility

Orientation is a term for knowing where you are, where you are going, and how you are going to get there. *Mobility* is the means of the actual travel of getting there.

Sighted guide techniques. The most comfortable, widely used, safe, and efficient way to assist a blind person in traveling is to serve as a sighted guide. In this position, the blind person holds the arm of the guide just above the elbow. The blind person will be a half-step behind and to the side of the sighted guide. In this position, a blind person can safely follow the guide's body movements as they walk. Figures 16.7 and 16.8 show the best approach that a sighted guide can use to assist a blind person in traveling.

To begin the sighted guide technique, the guide and the blind person will first make contact with their arms. The guide will verbally offer assistance. The person needing sighted assistance will move his or her hand up above the guide's elbow, keeping the thumb on the outside of the guide's arm. The four fingers should be on the medial side of the guide's arm, maintaining a firm and comfortable grip. In this position, the blind person is a half-step behind and to the side of the guide. The opposite shoulders of the traveling partners should be in alignment (Hill & Ponder, 1976).

Narrow spaces. To negotiate narrow spaces, the guide will move his or her arm to the middle of the blind person's back as a sign that he or she should walk directly behind the guide. Extending the arm will increase the space between them and will prevent the follower from walking on the heels of the guide, as well as allow single file travel through narrow or congested areas.

The question of which side is best for the guide is based on a number of factors, most notably personal preference. Strength, hand dominance, the need for a support cane, hearing losses, the need to carry a package or purse, and other factors affect this decision. Most experienced travelers find they are able to travel equally well on either side of a sighted guide. Also, with experience, most sighted guide partnerships require less verbal input about the

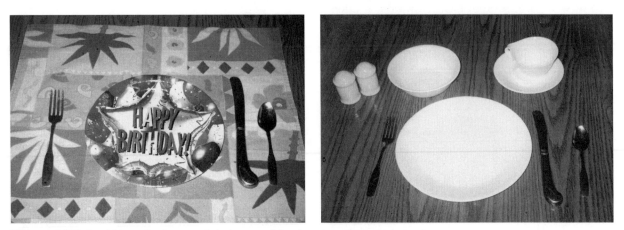

Figure 16.6 Avoid busy backgrounds but use solid colors to enhance contrast.

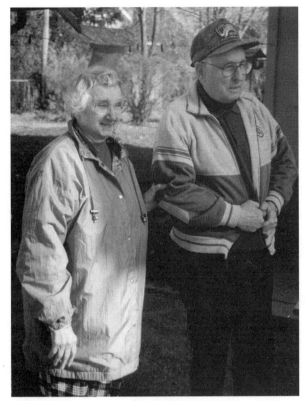

Figure 16.7 Sighted guide technique.

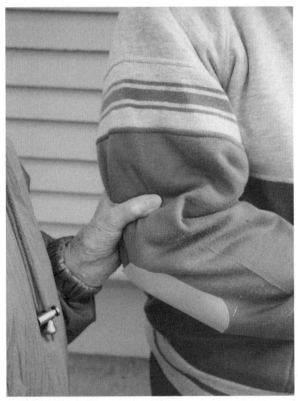

Figure 16.8 The proper grip of the sighted guide technique.

travel environment. Travel companions can safely carry on conversations just as other friends do.

Curbs and stairs. At each change of elevation, whether at a curb or a flight of stairs, the sighted guide will pause and verbally describe the change. It is generally safer to keep the person's weight forward when ascending and backward when descending.

Seating. The sighted guide should lead a blind person to the chair so that his or her body comes in contact with the chair. Placing the person's hand on the back of the chair provides a reference point.

Doorways. After describing in which direction the door opens (toward the person or away) and on which side it is hinged, the sighted guide should always go through doorways first. Revolving doors may cause problems for some slow-walking travelers. Use another door or practice using revolving doors during less busy times.

Automobiles. The sighted guide should verbally explain the direction in which the vehicle is pointing. After the passenger door is opened, the guide should place one of the blind person's hands on the roof and one on the top edge of the open door. It is neither safe nor efficient to attempt to guide a blind person by pushing from behind. In this position, the guide will not readily see uneven pavement, patches of ice, water, or otherwise slippery surfaces. In addition, sudden noises or safety concerns may cause a clumsy resistance to the guide's efforts. Finally, no one is in front of the blind person to act as a buffer or stabilizer should a stumble occur or an immediate stop become necessary.

Self-protection techniques. Self-protection techniques are necessary even in a familiar home environment. This technique involves holding one arm (usually the nondominant one) at shoulder height, palm out with the hand just below eye level. The dominant hand is held diagonally across the body, palm inward, in front of the opposite upper thigh. This positioning in front of the face and across the torso will provide safe coverage from open cupboards, closet doors, and narrow poles. Figure 16.9 shows two self-protection techniques.

Room familiarization. Room familiarization begins at the primary entrance to a room. A person should be guided around the perimeter of the room, with special emphasis placed on locating all permanent or semipermanent landmarks, such as light switches and outlets, windows, furniture, closet doors, hanging plants, and the like.

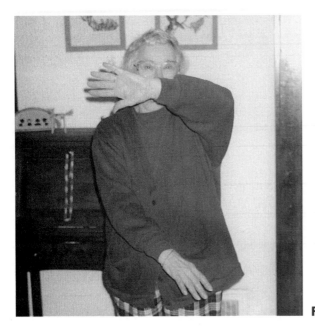

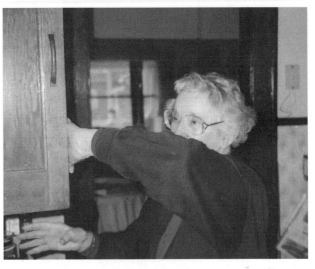

Figure 16.9 Two examples of self-protection techniques.

For outdoor or more advanced independent travel, persons may require instruction in the use of telescopic aids, a white cane, electronic mobility devices, or a dog guide. The state agency for the blind or a private agency for the blind can be contacted for more information on the white cane safety law and the regulations governing the legal use of a white cane.

A certified orientation and mobility specialist is a professional trained in providing travel instruction to blind persons. The state agency for the blind or a private organization for the blind can provide information on obtaining these services.

Case Study: Glaucoma

M. T. is a widower living alone on the farm he has called home for more than 40 years. Despite his vision impairment, he thoroughly enjoyed going to his workshop in one of his outbuildings. He found that glaucoma had reduced his visual field to a small tunnel and that his remaining vision did not work very well in low-light conditions. He placed a wind chime near his back doorway and strung a thin rope on posts from his house to the outbuilding. The rope allows him the guidance needed and the wind chime, given the right breeze, helps him locate the back door when he is elsewhere on his property. M. T. also has used a radio at his back door to provide an audible directional beacon for which to aim. In his barn, M. T. must negotiate around a few low beams. He strategically placed lengths of bailing twine

about 3 feet in front of all low obstructions. These soft warning signs alert him and have saved more than a few bumps on the head.

Case Study: Orientation

A stroke caused S. L. to become confused about her location even while in her own home. Her husband was concerned about helping her determine her location and the direction she must travel. A cuckoo clock with its audible tick-tock provides the orientation to her current location and to the direction of the other rooms in her home.

Systematic searching patterns. Persons with vision loss will find it useful to search for dropped objects in an organized or patterned way. For example, when searching for a dropped object, the person should listen for the sound of the object hitting the floor, turn to face that location, and then search for it in that direction. Either a circular pattern with gradually increasing concentric circles radiating outward or an up–over–back grid-like pattern can be tried. In all instances, a methodical pattern will ensure complete coverage and be less frustrating.

Communication

As with other types of disabilities, such as hearing loss, persons with blindness and vision loss are sometimes treated inappropriately by persons who do not understand their conditions. The following guidelines provide useful suggestions for polite, respectful, and appropriate interactions with persons who have vision loss.

- When you offer assistance, speak in a normal tone of voice unless you know of a hearing loss. Also, speak directly to a blind person, not through a sighted interpreter.

- Always introduce yourself as you approach a blind person. Voice recognition is not always reliable, especially in a crowded or noisy environment.

- Inform the blind person when you leave. No one wants to appear foolish by starting to talk to oneself.

- Use words like "look" and "see" as you do in everyday conversations because attempts to use substitutes are usually awkward and may make everyone less comfortable.

- When dining, use the "face of the clock" method of orientation to describe the location of food. The peas are at two o'clock, the meat is at six, and the french fries are at ten. The same method can be used for locating utensils, condiments, and other items.

- Be verbally specific when giving directions. Use right and left, behind or in front. Avoid gestures, pointing, and nonspecific terms such as "over there" and "that way." Rather than saying "It is right there," say, "The blue candy dish is in front of you and to the right" or "It is at two o'clock." Figure 16.10 portrays the appropriate table setting for persons with vision loss.

- Never move furniture without informing the blind person who is familiar with a particular arrangement.

Print size and type. Whenever possible, print size should be large using clear block letters and should be black on either white or yellow, or vice versa. It is best to avoid ornate, serif, and condensed typefaces. Most colored or patterned paper should also be avoided. As some persons find that yellow paper offers better contrast for reading print, an alternative approach is to use a sheet of yellow acetate or a report cover over black print on white paper. Announcements and other notices should be posted in large print on bulletin boards in public places. One strategy used in senior centers is to post all headlines in very large type, thereby allowing persons with low vision to see the subject of the posting and read the document with optical aids or to request further assistance when indicated.

The primary concerns with cursive writing include the inability to stay on the line, writing uphill or down, not crossing "t"s or dotting "i"s, and being uncertain of the need to correct mistakes.

The most basic handwriting task is that of signing one's name. For some, it can be the single most important aspect of achieving a better sense of well-being and confidence. Everyone should be encouraged to sign his or her own name. Darkening the signature line with a bold pen can provide enough of a barrier for a person with low vision to sign his or her name. Signature guides can be as simple as a credit card-sized piece of thin cardboard or plastic, usually black with a rectangular window cut out. Other guides are metal and some have an elastic band, allowing the writer to easily make the tails of letters below the line. The guide is placed over the signature space, creating a structurally rigid barrier or frame. With practice and encouragement, persons can sign their name. One can also suggest using natural motions or use "auto pilot." Often the faster one signs his or her name after a lengthy nonwriting period, the better it looks. A signature guide is shown in Figure 16.11.

For persons with relatively good vision, the first option is to use bold-lined paper in various sizes. This bold-lined and wide-spaced writing paper

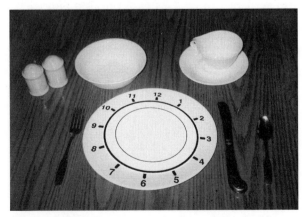

Figure 16.10 Orientation via "face of the clock."

Figure 16.11 Black plastic signature guide.

makes it easier to stay on the line. This paper is available in different width spacing and in different boldness of the lines. Some persons use different sizes of bold-lined paper for different purposes. Relatively narrow-lined paper is suitable for writing personal letters that do not necessarily need to be reread. Very bold-lined paper is more useful for writing that will be later referenced, such as an address book, a recipe, or a shopping list.

A black script writing template of plastic or cardboard may be even more helpful for persons with less vision. These templates force the writing to conform to the space available and assure parallel lines. Paper clips hold the writing paper firmly. Using the various types of bold line pens makes seeing where the writing starts and stops much easier.

A Marks writing guide is a clipboard-type device that holds writing paper in place and uses a line-sized frame that is moved down the page. As the end of each line is reached, the frame is moved down to the next line (see Figure 16.12). Envelopes can also be addressed using this type of guide, or envelope templates are available with windows cut out for each line of the address. Writing paper that is embossed with raised lines is available in 50-sheet pads.

Case Study: AMD

L. B. moved from her small town in South Carolina to northern Wisconsin to die. She came to live with her daughter because of an inoperable condition that caused her physician to predict only a 2-month life expectancy. When seen by the local rehabilitation teacher from the state services for the blind, she agreed to enroll in the talking book program to help pass the time. As a signature is required for services for the blind, she responded that she had been unable to sign her name for a few years because of AMD. She was shown a black plastic signature template and assigned a practice regimen. With time and encouragement, she progressed to writing letters to her relatives and friends in South Carolina. After more practice, she was able to write telephone messages for her daughter's home-based business. This saved the cost of call forwarding and boosted her self-confidence as well. Because of her charming personality and wonderful South Carolina accent, she was a true asset to the business.

Braille. Braille is a system of reading and writing using a configuration of six raised dots in a rectangular pattern resembling a muffin pan (Ashcroft & Henderson, 1963). Louis Braille, a blind Frenchman, developed the system for his own use. Before the development of braille, other systems of tactual reading were tried, but not until braille was developed did the blind have the ability to become truly literate by writing in addition to reading raised symbols (see Figure 16.13).

Braille need not be used just for reading and writing text, it can also be used for labeling items such as medicines, canned goods, or playing cards. The Library of Congress (Ashcroft & Henderson, 1963) publishes an instructional manual on learning the full braille code. Braille can be written with a Perkins brailler, which looks somewhat like an antique typewriter, or with a portable slate and stylus.

Telephone use. Many styles of large print telephones are available. Some have raised numbers in bold print, allowing easier location of each number. Some models also have volume controls for persons with a hearing loss. Voice recognition telephones are also available for persons with physical limitations

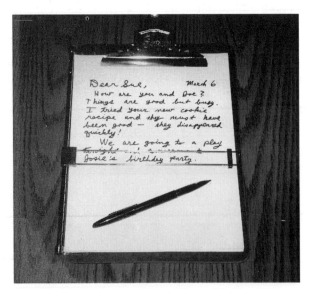

Figure 16.12 Marks script writing guide.

1	2	3	4	5	6	7	8	9	0
a	b	c	d	e	f	g	h	i	j
k	l	m	n	o	p	q	r	s	t
u	v	x	y	z		w			

Figure 16.13 The braille alphabet.

in addition to vision loss. Many telephones have speed dial buttons that can be tactually or visually marked for easy location. It is possible to adapt rotary telephones with large print dial overlays, and large print push-button adapters can be applied to standard push button telephones.

Rotary telephones can be marked with a small strip of masking tape; with Hi-Marks, a bright orange glue-like material that comes in a tube; or with other tactual aids. Normally, a mark at the "5" will act as a landmark from which the other numbers can be counted. Standard push-button telephones can be dialed using three fingers that cover each row of numbers. The pointer finger pushes the one, the index finger pushes the two, and the ring finger pushes the three. To reach the second row of four through six, one simply moves the three fingers down one row and so forth.

Many telephone companies offer exemptions from directory assistance charges for assistance calls made by persons who are blind or visually impaired. Each company may have different regulations and eligibility policies. It is best to check with local providers.

Cassette tape recording. Cassette tape recording is another option for the storage and retrieval of information. Persons can mail taped letters to friends using special cassette mailers, while qualifying for "Free Matter for the Blind" mailing privileges. A letter is recorded, placed in a special mailer, and put in a mailbox. Most of these mailers have double from and to labels. The from and to addresses are reversed on each side, and are designed for repeated round-trip use. Other mailers contain a reversible postcard-like label that is placed in a clear window.

Volunteer reader services. Perhaps the single most frequently used means of reading is to secure the services of a sighted volunteer or paid reader. Volunteers may be coordinated through religious organizations, aging units, government offices, and private agencies.

Household Organization

Organization is especially important for persons with vision loss. Every household item should have its place and should be in it when not in use. Cleaning supplies or toxic substances in similarly shaped containers must be labeled in large print or by tactual means.

The standard array of commercially available organizational aids, including assorted bins, pocket folders, files, and large-print or tactual labels, can all be used to put and keep household items in their place. Textures, smells, colors, shapes, sizes, sounds, and other properties of objects can all be incorporated into a discussion of organization techniques.

Marking and labeling. A wide variety of marking and labeling aids are available for persons with vision loss. Textures, bright colors, high contrast markings, and various shapes can be used to mark and distinguish like-shaped items, dial settings, controls, clothing, tools, and other items. A sampling of available aids follows:

- Hi-Marks is a bright orange, glue-like material that comes in a tube. Dots, bumps, letters, and lines can be drawn to provide both a visual and a tactual mark. Stoves, thermostats, microwave ovens, laundry equipment, radios, and virtually any dial on any appliance can be easily marked.
- Spot-N-Line is a similar tactual marking aid available in black or white. Both materials are durable and inexpensive, but they may be difficult for a persons who is blind or severely visually impaired to apply independently.
- Bump Dots in black or white are soft foam dots with sticky backing used for marking various items.
- Beads can also be glued in place as tactual landmarks. Bright nail polish can be used for marking dials.
- Bold felt tip pens are ideal for labeling purposes. For reusable labels, index cards can be marked in bold letters and attached to canned goods by rubber bands. After use, the index cards can be placed in an envelope, thereby constituting the next shopping list.

Simplicity is usually the best approach to marking appliance dials. One or two temperatures are all that may be needed to mark an oven. If 325° is the most common oven temperature, with practice and honest feedback, 350° may be reliably estimated from the known 325° mark. Many manufacturers will supply tactually marked dials or overlays for their products.

Index cards with large print labels are also useful for labeling colors of clothing, canned goods, medicines, and other items. One can simply use a hole punch, add a rubber band, and attach the index card to the item. Examples of large-print labels are shown in Figure 16.14.

Clothing can be identified in a number of ways. Braille tags can be sewn into clothing in a nonvisual spot away from the skin. Some persons use different

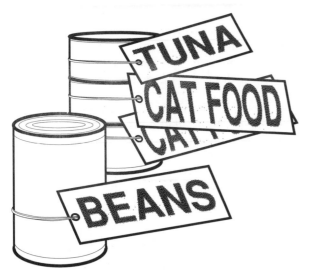

Figure 16.14 Large-print labels for food identification.

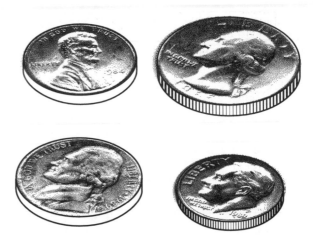

Figure 16.15 The edges of coins make identification easy.

sizes of buttons in different locations to distinguish between similar items. One way to keep socks in pairs is to use plastic disks with star-shaped cutouts in different shapes in which the socks are always kept when not being worn. They can remain attached through washing and drying and are stored that way. When the socks are being worn, the disks are kept in a spot where they are easy to locate. The disks can be attached to the socks as they are put into the laundry hamper. The shapes allow easy identification. Some persons use different sizes of safety pins to distinguish colors.

Closets can be organized into sections of "go together" clothes or outfits can be grouped together on the same hanger. Using the "simpler is better" approach, clothing details such as textures, buttons, or other distinguishing features can suffice for many persons.

The purchase of a new stove precipitated a referral to the vision rehabilitation specialist. M. P. had a severe loss of vision but was trying to be independent. An avid baker, she needed to accurately set oven temperatures. With the application of Hi-Marks she could feel, and at times even see, the location for her most common settings.

Personal Management

Money management. Coin identification is taught by tactually exploring the rim or edges of coins with a thumbnail. Pennies and nickels, the two least valuable coins, have smooth edges; dimes and quarters have a milled or ridged edge. The size differences between smooth and ridged coins make correct identification simple (see Figure 16.15).

Coin purses with separate channels for each denomination of coin are helpful in organizing change. The 35-mm film canisters or prescription bottles in various sizes can be used to keep coins separated (Flax et al., 1993).

Paper money can be organized by folding the different denominations in various ways. One dollar bills may be left unfolded; the fives may be folded in half so that they are almost a square; the tens might be folded in half the long, narrow way; and a twenty can be folded like a ten dollar bill and then folded over a second time. These methods are illustrated in Figure 16.16. Another common way to handle paper money is to put the different denominations in different compartments of a wallet or purse. Still another method to simplify the identification of bills is to limit the paper money to just ones and fives and keep them in separate compartments or pockets.

Using checks for purchases or paying bills is often the only option. A number of approaches can be effective, including the use of large-print checks, raised-line checks, or one of the many available check templates. One can contact the bank for information on the availability of accessible checks. Some persons use bold line markers to highlight the lines on personal checks. Large-print check registers can make financial recording easier for persons with low vision. Black plastic check templates have window cutouts to match the information fields. The Keitzer Check Guide is made of thicker plastic that makes a wider border to restrict the writing.

Credit cards are, of course, a convenient way to make purchases. The card can also function as a signature guide, as it underlines the signature line on

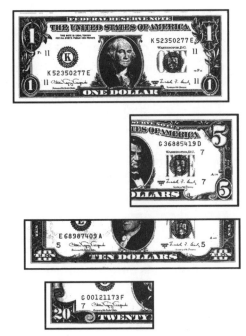

Figure 16.16 Paper money folded for quick identification.

the receipt. One should ask the clerk to place the card under the signature space to make signing easy.

Telling time. Large-print, braille, and talking watches are all available from the catalog suppliers (see Figure 16.17). Some persons adapt existing equipment by tactual or large-print means.

Grooming and hygiene. Techniques for shaving can be discussed and practiced, initially using a razor without the blade or an electric shaver. Using an

electric shaver relies simply on touch. If someone has been familiar with shaving and is comfortable with a specific type of shaver, that should be the type with which to practice. Magnifying mirrors, some with lights and up to five power of magnification, help with makeup and shaving. Many persons simply dispense toothpaste onto a finger or directly into their mouths if they are the only ones to use that particular tube of toothpaste.

Medication identification. Affixing rubber bands around the bottles easily identifies similar prescription bottles (see Figure 16.18). Large-print index cards can also be used to identify medications. A 7-day pillbox can help manage medication use.

Food Preparation

Food preparation is a process that includes numerous and varied activities and skills that must be mastered in sequence. Menu development, shopping, reading recipes, identification of similar appearing ingredients, peeling, chopping, slicing and dicing, accurately pouring and measuring, setting oven and stove-top temperatures, timing, and safely handling hot utensils are all part of the overall task.

Menu development. Reading large-print, braille, or cassette recorded cookbooks can help develop menu

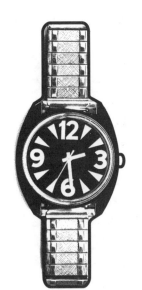

Figure 16.17 A large-print watch.

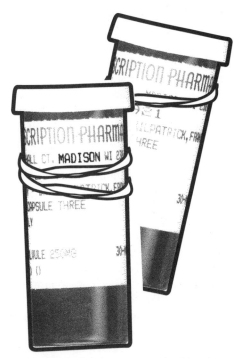

Figure 16.18 Medications are marked by the number of rubber bands.

items. Recipes may be put in large print, braille, or on cassette tapes, and cookbooks are available in the same formats.

Shopping. Shopping is easier when items to be included in a weekly menu are listed in advance. Index-card labels for canned goods can be used in addition to a standard shopping list. Store personnel will usually provide shopping assistance, or optical aids can be employed.

Product identification. Canned goods are identified by shapes, label designs, and often by their sound when shaken. Some persons use large-print labels on 3-inch by 5-inch index cards with a hole punched in a corner attached to the can by a rubber band. Others mark the cabinet and place all like items behind that label. Small bins can be used to contain just one item, mushroom soup, for instance. Light-colored squares of flexible magnetic sheets can be written on with bold permanent pens in large print or written in braille. These magnetic sheets can be affixed and easily reused. Some persons with low vision can recognize certain brands of products by their familiar red and white stripes, for instance, but cannot read the print label. The labels can then be recycled into a "shopping list" envelope after the item has been used. Spice containers, while appearing similar, can often be identified by smell, large print, or tactual labels.

Peeling, chopping, slicing, and dicing. Rinsing vegetables may make it easier to feel the peeled and unpeeled sections of foods. A dual-colored cutting board—dark on one side and light on the other—or two different cutting boards can provide color contrast. A cutting board with a funnel-shaped end allows for easier transfer and placement of chopped foods. It is essential for the kitchen to have sufficient task lighting or under-the-counter lights. Knives with adjustable slicing width guides make uniform slices in meats, breads, vegetables, and other foods an easy task.

Pouring and measuring liquids. Liquid level indicators make an audible signal when the poured liquid reaches the twin electrodes. Pouring and measuring can be practiced using cold water over a sink. Pouring colored liquids into a clear glass can be made easier if a contrasting background color is used. Consider a dark wall or backsplash to pour milk or a white background for pouring dark liquids into clear glass cups. White coffee cups provide better contrast for pouring black coffee. By hooking an index finger over the edge or lip of the glass, one can determine when the level of the liquid reaches that point. The client can practice over a sink or a cafeteria tray to build confidence.

Individual measuring cups are recommended and can be marked tactually or in large print. Large-print designations are available on some measuring spoons. Others can be marked with permanent bold line pens or by filing grooves into the handles.

Cooking timers. Large-print, audible, and braille timers are available (see Figure 16.19). Some may be marked with additional embellishments to ensure accuracy.

Safety issues. Large oven mitts protect arms when removing hot dishware from ovens. Every kitchen should have an operable fire extinguisher in a handy location.

Leisure Time Activities

Social and peer support groups. Local peer support groups for persons with visual impairments are available in many communities. One can contact a local information and referral agency or the state services for the blind or a local private agency for the blind. The Lighthouse National Center on Aging and Vision is a leader in information on peer support groups.

Table games. Playing cards are available in various large-print sizes, raised-line print, and in both standard and jumbo dot braille. Cribbage boards with raised borders around the pegging holes allow easy

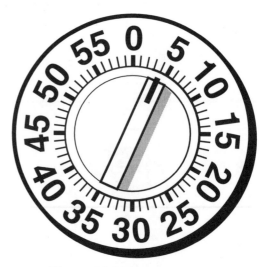

Figure 16.19 Large-print timer.

counting of points. Checkerboards that have indented squares and use round red and square black checkers make the game accessible for totally blind players. Braille dice are produced with raised dots on indented sides, and large-print dice are simply made larger. Large-print and braille bingo cards allow persons to continue playing these games. Other board games are available from the catalog suppliers. Many persons also tactually mark in braille (or other means) selected pieces of their favorite board games.

Case Study: Playing Cards

S. S. always had a close relationship with her granddaughter, but low vision severely affected her ability to continue card playing. After she purchased a deck of large-print cards, she was able to continue regular card games with her granddaughter. Even as she was losing more vision, she was able to learn the 15 braille symbols needed for playing cards. A rehabilitation teacher from the state agency for the blind developed a series of lessons whereby she practiced both reading and writing braille. After she became proficient at writing braille using a slate and stylus, she put the braille symbols on a deck of large-print cards. Her vision was often good enough for her to identify the cards in good light, and with sufficient time, but she did not want to slow down a heated game of war with her granddaughter.

Techniques for threading a sewing needle. Using wire loop needle threaders is an almost automatic way to thread sewing needles. The threader is first put into the eye of a needle using the sense of touch. As it is difficult to put the limp thread through this loop, it should first be wrapped around a toothpick. This rigid arrangement can easily be put through the loop. After that, it is quite simple to withdraw the wire loop, pulling the thread through the eye of the needle. The wire loop needle threader may also be used for putting fishhooks onto fishing line. Chimney-like needle threaders also work quite well. To use this tool, one places the eye of the needle down into the chimney, places the thread adjacent to the chimney, pushes the slide or button that pushes a wire rod through the tower picking up the thread, and pushes it through the eye. Spread eye needles are flexible needles that have a long eye that runs nearly the entire length of the needle. Self-threading needles have a notch just above the eye. To thread this type of needle, one places the sharp end in a bar of soap or a cork, locates the notch in the top, places the thread in the notch, and firmly pops it into the eye.

Community Resources

Community programs and resources play an important role in the service plan for persons with severe vision loss. Federally mandated Older Americans Act services include transportation, nutrition (both home delivered and in congregate settings), and benefits counseling, which are available to all persons more than 60 years of age. These and other in-home support services are administered through the local aging unit or Area Agency on Aging.

Senior centers often provide a rich array of services for older persons, including exercise therapy, craft classes, computer users groups, reading clubs, travel opportunities, a nutrition program, and recreation, as well as peer support groups.

The American Foundation for the Blind and the Lighthouse National Center for Vision and Aging, consumer groups, and special interest groups in support of specific eye conditions can provide a wealth of information and referral to local services.

The Library for the Blind and Physically Handicapped provides talking books on records, cassettes, or in braille for persons unable to read standard-print books. Accessible reading materials are mailed to persons and are returned postage free. Applications and eligibility criteria are available from your local library or the state or private agency for the blind.

Summary

Acquired visual deficits can be caused by health conditions such as diabetes and stroke, normal aging, and injuries to the eye. These deficits affect vision generally or can produce limitations affecting central or peripheral vision, with different functional consequences. Evaluating the functional needs of persons with low vision requires a thorough consideration of the person's living environment and lifestyle. Many adaptive devices and techniques can be used to help persons adapt to the functional challenges of vision loss. ◆

Study Questions

1. What is the definition of legal blindness?

2. What is the definition of severe visual impairment?

3. How do age-related macular degeneration and glaucoma differ in the type of functional vision loss they cause? Who will be expected to have more problems walking in areas of uneven pave-

ment? Who may have difficulty seeing small print or setting a thermostat dial?

4. When should a client be referred to a peer support group?

5. What is the general rule for positioning while using the sighted guide technique?

6. What is the activity of daily living task that carries the most personal significance for the client with a severe vision loss?

7. Who usually has a greater problem in low-light situations—clients with glaucoma or those with diabetic retinopathy?

8. What type of scriptwriting aids should be presented initially to a client with a less severe vision loss? With a very severe loss?

9. What are some of the practical means of controlling glare?

10. What is the general rule for positioning a light source for reading purposes?

References

Ashcroft, S. C., & Henderson, F. (1963). *Programmed Instruction in Braille*. Pittsburgh, PA: Stanwix House.

Carroll, T. J. (1961). *Blindness: What it is, what it does, and how to live with it*. Boston: Little Brown.

Flax, M., Golembiewski, D., & McCaulley, B. (1993). *Coping with low vision*. San Diego, CA: Singular Publishing Group.

Golembiewski, D. (1998). Asking the right questions. *RE:view, Rehabilitation and Education for Blindness and Visual Impairment, 30*(1), 29–30.

Hill, E., & Ponder, P. (1976). *Orientation and mobility techniques: A guide for the practitioner*. New York: American Foundation for the Blind Press.

Jose, R. T. (Ed.). (1983). *Understanding low vision*. New York: American Foundation for the Blind.

Kirchner, C., & Schmeidler, E. (1997). Prevalence and employment of people in the United States who are blind or visually impaired. *Journal of Visual Impairment and Blindness, 91*(5), 508–511.

Nelson, K. A., & Dimitrova, E. (1993). Severe visual impairment in the United States and in each state, 1990. *Journal of Visual Impairment and Blindness, 85*(5), 80–85.

Ponchillia, P., & Ponchillia, S. (1996). *Foundations of rehabilitation teaching with persons who are blind or visually impaired*. New York: American Foundation for the Blind Press.

Tuttle, D., & Tuttle, N. (1996). *Self-esteem and adjusting with blindness*. Springfield, IL: Charles C. Thomas.

Appendix
Assessment for Vision Rehabilitation Services (Adapted from Golembiewski, 1998)

Are you able to accurately tell time by reading your watch or wall clock?

Yes __ No __ > If "No" due to vision loss, check if help is needed. _____

Can you tell a nickel from a quarter and a $1 bill from a $10 bill?

Yes __ No __ > If "No" due to vision loss, check if help is needed. _____

Can you set the correct temperature on a thermostat or oven?

Yes __ No __ > If "No" due to vision loss, check if help is needed. _____

Are you able to write letters, a grocery list, or sign your name?

Yes __ No __ > If "No" due to vision loss, check if help is needed. _____

Can you handle your own household cleaning if you wish?

Yes __ No __ > If "No" due to vision loss, check if help is needed. _____

Can you continue with your favorite craft or leisure activities?

Yes __ No __ > If "No" due to vision loss, check if help is needed. _____

Are you able to adjust to very bright or very dim light?

Yes __ No __ > If "No" due to vision loss, check if help is needed. _____

Are you able to prepare your own meals if you wish?

Yes __ No __ > If "No" due to vision loss, check if help is needed. _____

Are you able to identify and properly take your medications?

Yes __ No __ > If "No" due to vision loss, check if help is needed. _____

Can you handle your own shopping?

Yes __ No __ > If "No" due to vision loss, check if help is needed. _____

Are you able to identify traffic signals from across the street?

Yes __ No __ > If "No" due to vision loss, check if help is needed. _____

Are you able to read your mail, your recipes, or the newspaper?

Yes __ No __ > If "No" due to vision loss, check if help is needed. _____

Are you able to identify friends from across the room or table?

Yes __ No __ > If "No" due to vision loss, check if help is needed. _____

Are you able to follow the action or see characters on TV?

Yes __ No __ > If "No" due to vision loss, check if help is needed. _____

Do any magnifiers you use for your reading work well enough?

Yes __ No __ > If "No" due to vision loss, check if help is needed. _____

When did you last go to an eye doctor for a checkup? _____

When did you last have your eyeglass prescription changed? _____

Do your eyeglasses work well enough to read, watch TV, or see in the distance?

No _____ Yes _____

Has anyone from services for the visually impaired or blind been out to see you?

No _____ Yes _____ When _____ Who _____

Do you want someone to contact you to help you with any of the above?

Yes _____ Not Yet _____

Referral Source _____

Date _____

Phone _____

Comments:

17

Addressing the Sexual Needs of Persons With Disabilities

Maureen Freda

Maureen Freda, MS, OTR/L, is Rehabilitation Program Director, Holy Cross Rehabilitation and Nursing Center, Burtonsville, Maryland.

Key Terms

counseling

functional effects on sexual activity

sexology

sexual activity

sexual orientation

sexual response cycle

sexual rights

Objectives

On completing this chapter, the reader will be able to

1. Describe the occupational therapy practitioner's role in dealing with the sexual needs of clients.

2. Describe common barriers to meeting these needs.

3. Identify the skills and knowledge needed by occupational therapy practitioners in addressing issues related to sexuality and sexual function.

4. Describe the effects of specific disabilities, disorders, and diseases on sexual function.

5. Identify practical strategies for dealing with the effects of disability on sexual function.

$\mathbf{S}$exuality is part of our daily living. It is intangible. It is a fundamental part of our personalities and how we see ourselves as men and women. "Adult sexuality is an essential component of our identity and self-image" (Freda, 1998, p. 364; Neistadt, 1986). We frequently see evidence of sexual, sensual, or flirtatious behavior in social interactions between persons. We are inundated with sexual images in the media. Sex, desirability, and sexual attractiveness are everywhere in our daily lives: songs on the radio, magazine articles, television shows, movies, news, advertisements, music videos, novels, and billboards.

We are all sexual beings. Sexual activity is the way in which we share this part of ourselves with a significant other person. "Sexual activity is our most intimate way of expressing and receiving affection" (Neistadt & Freda, 1987, p. ix). "As a human being, one is sexual from birth to death. Although acute, chronic, or disabling conditions and aging may necessitate certain adaptations in the way one expresses sexuality, one does not cease to be a sexual being" (Spica, 1989, p. 58). The perceived importance of sex and sexual activity is highly individual. Some put a very high value on this aspect of a relationship; for others it may take a "back seat" to companionship and friendship. Whatever the case, neither age nor disability changes the basic sexual nature of the person (Freda & Rubinsky, 1991).

The importance of sexuality to perceived well-being, quality of life, and even physical health has been demonstrated in many studies (McCabe, 1997; Ventegodt, 1998). Among other findings, these have shown that sexual activity may reduce the risk of heart disease in men (Davey Smith, Frankel, & Yarnell, 1997) and may increase life satisfaction in elders (Spector & Fremoth, 1996). Other studies have shown that satisfactory adjustment to disability is also accompanied by greater satisfaction with and participation in sexual activity (Bianchi, 1997; Kreuter, Sullivan, & Siosteen, 1996).

The importance of sexuality and sexual function to well-being makes it vital for occupational therapy practitioners to include this aspect of daily life in their intervention planning for persons with disabilities. Whereas physical disability may challenge "the usual way we think about sexuality" (Spica, 1989, p. 56), intervention plans that fail to consider this aspect of everyday living are incomplete. Through knowledge, the provision of information, and practi-cal problem solving, therapy practitioners can make important contributions to clients with disabilities. See Figure 17.1.

Understanding Sexuality Counseling Within Current Views of Occupational Therapy Intervention

As viewed within the current framework for occupational therapy services, practitioners provide four major categories of intervention: remediation, compensation, disability prevention, and health promotion. The provision of information regarding sexual function falls mainly within the categories of compensatory and health promotion strategies, with some intervention recommendations focusing on disability prevention. Many conditions require a modification of the manner in which sexual activities are performed or can benefit from modifications in the environment. These are compensatory strategies. Similarly, some devices that might be recommended also represent compensatory approaches or may assist in promoting safe performance of the activity. In this context, the concept is broader than that implied in the common expression "safe sex." Enabling participation in activities that express sexuality in a manner satisfying to the client is also a means of promoting overall health and well-being.

Counseling and Information Giving From a Functional Perspective

Occupational therapy practitioners are not trained to provide intense psychological counseling on any topic. Their role lies in the functional domain. Their profession is firmly rooted in function and meaning—this makes occupational therapy practitioners uniquely qualified to deal with the sexual issues that arise as they relate to disability. Occupational therapy practitioners routinely deal with persons who have had their lives disrupted by a chronic illness or disability. Their treatment interventions are geared toward returning persons to productive and meaningful lives; they assist persons in returning to an appropriate role within their family and their community. They are concerned with their clients' functional independence in all aspects of life. This should include

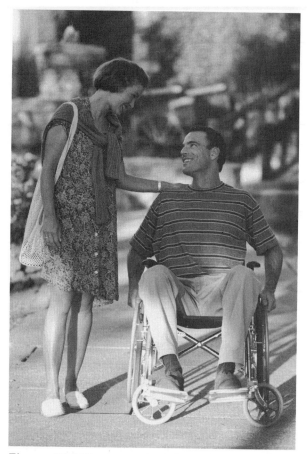

Figure 17.1 The expression of sexuality is a natural part of daily living for all persons, regardless of age or disability status. (Image © PhotoDisc, Inc.)

available, and, in some instances, the practitioner may choose to use a combination of approaches through a group or an individual education session. Knowing what is comfortable for and most acceptable to the client will determine the appropriate choice. The information must be presented at a level that is appropriate for the specific client. That is, the information must be understandable, provided at an appropriate educational level with familiar vocabulary, and presented in a manner that is straightforward yet responsive to individual needs.

During a counseling or education session it is important to stay within the comfort zone of the client. If a person is embarrassed, anxious, or concerned about privacy or other issues, he or she will not be able to benefit from the information. It is best to begin in a very basic and simple way, check with the client frequently to determine the level of comfort with and understanding of the material, and confirm the usefulness of the information to the client. The practitioner may ask at this point if the information being given is what the client needs or had expected. Effective counseling and educational intervention require that the practitioner be able to change approaches quickly to meet the informational needs of the client. A warm, yet professional tone should be maintained throughout the session.

The Occupational Therapy Practitioner as a Nonjudgmental Information Giver

As occupational therapy practitioners, our role is to give needed information and suggestions in a nonjudgmental fashion. This role can sometimes be difficult when practitioners are speaking about sexual issues. As sexual beings, we each have attitudes and values that have been shaped by our family members and personal experiences. It is important to acknowledge these attitudes but to put them aside during counseling sessions.

Clients come in different shapes, sizes, and colors; they come from various cultures and have differing sexual orientations. It is certainly possible that practitioners will encounter a client whose sexual orientation or sexual practices diverge from their own or, in some cases, even conflict with their own values and beliefs. Professionals must learn to put aside their own biases to give their clients the appropriate information while maintaining a solid therapeutic relationship.

supporting their return to an active, healthy sexual life as well.

Occupational therapy practitioners can counsel, educate, or advise clients from a functional perspective. Their knowledge of the functional effects of disability gives them a foundation that allows them to provide clients with practical suggestions for managing sexual activity. Occupational therapy practitioners have the skills that allow them to provide suggestions for alternative positions and adaptations needed to participate successfully in sexual activity. This suggestion may be as simple as helping a couple to start thinking about changing a favorite position to better accommodate the disability. Occupational therapy practitioners can use their knowledge of adaptation to help clients and their partners see the possibilities.

The occupational therapy practitioner can share sexual information by several different means. He or she can discuss the issues verbally, provide written material, make appropriate videos

It is extremely important that practitioners who are involved in discussing sexual issues with clients are comfortable with the topic of sexuality and have an open mind. They must first be comfortable with their own sexuality and then recognize that different viewpoints are not wrong, just different. Eckland and McBride (1997) suggested that the first step in increasing the practitioner's comfort level in these discussions is to be aware of values and beliefs about sexuality through values clarification and discussion with colleagues. They also remind practitioners to keep in mind that their values are their own and do not belong to the client; nor should practitioners try to impose those values on them. See Figure 17.2.

Because of the effective therapeutic relationship that often develops between the practitioner and the client, clients frequently turn to practitioners rather than to other team members when they have questions about sexual functioning and activity. "Generally, it is the professional who has a good interpersonal relationship with the patient who is cast in the role of counselor" (Neistadt & Freda, 1987, p. 10).

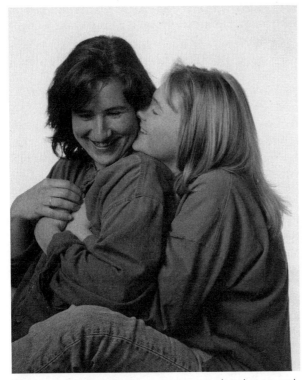

Figure 17.2 Practitioners must recognize that sexual expression takes many forms and should avoid imposing their values or lifestyle preferences on their clients. (Image © PhotoDisc, Inc.)

Barriers To Meeting the Sexual Information Needs of Clients With a Disability

Two major obstacles can interfere with providing effective intervention regarding sexual function. These are inhibitions residing within the professional community and boundaries set by the clients themselves.

As mentioned, many persons, including health professionals, are uncomfortable with the subject of sex. This discomfort alone is enough to prevent many health professionals from ever introducing the topic with a person in their care who has a disability. Some will assume it is the responsibility of someone else; they will not deliberately ignore the need, but they truly believe that another member of the team will handle the situation. In some cases the health professional who is uncomfortable with sexuality will assume that the client is also uneasy. As a result, no communication occurs.

Ageism (or prejudices against older persons) can be a barrier. Some health professionals will not address the issue of sexuality with the geriatric population because they assume that someone that old will not be interested in sex. They often make this assumption before they have any idea what role sexual activity has played throughout that person's lifetime. In making such assumptions, they perpetuate a common misunderstanding and may be revealing their own attitudes or prejudices about the sexual interests, needs, and capabilities of persons during the later years of their lives. See Figure 17.3.

Another barrier occurs when the health professional believes that the client would be so concerned about the disability that he or she would not be interested in sexual issues. Additionally, the health professional may assume that because of the severe functional limitations of the disability, sexual activity would be impossible or too much trouble for the person. Again, this assumption is inappropriate and probably incorrect.

Ignorance can also be a problem. Many health professionals simply do not know what the possibilities are for sexual activity within the framework of a particular disability.

Personal bias may also come into play with some persons. A health professional may have a personal belief that it is somehow wrong or inappropriate for a person with a particular physical or developmental disability to engage in sexual activity. This belief may prevent the health professional

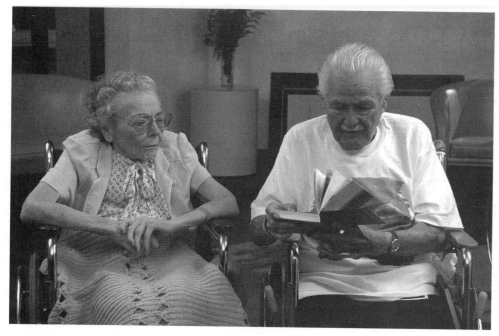

Figure 17.3 One common and incorrect assumption is that older persons do not need to express their sexuality. This assumption represents a type of barrier to effective intervention that practitioners should strive to avoid. (Image © PhotoDisc, Inc.)

from offering information on sexuality. "We are entitled to our own values and beliefs about sexuality. The danger lies in permitting these values (particularly those rooted in misconceptions) to interfere with our client's ability to meet their sexual health needs" (Eckland & McBride, 1997). Ideally, the practitioner should recognize and hold beliefs consistent with those embodied in the Valencia Declaration on Sexual Rights (see Box 17.1). This document identifies rights and principles for all persons to be able to express their sexuality. The presence of disease and disability should not compromise the sexual rights of clients seen in occupational therapy.

Client Barriers

Clients themselves often put up barriers to receiving information about sexuality or sexual activity. Sometimes an older persons with a disability may be embarrassed to bring up the subject of sexual activity. Sometimes, too, it is uncomfortable for an older person to discuss such personal issues with a younger person (the occupational therapy practitioner or other health professional may be a young person and the client much older, or vice versa). Often, persons from a different generation have been brought up to keep certain topics private and find it difficult to discuss them freely with virtual strangers.

Cultural barriers can also exist, wherein persons from certain cultures may not believe in sharing

their concerns about sexual activity with anyone. Additionally, once a conversation about sexual activity has started, the occupational therapy practitioner must be aware of any cultural taboos regarding sex, so that he or she does not offend the person with an inappropriate (from a cultural perspective) suggestion.

Clients may be depressed immediately after a disabling condition or during a flare-up of a chronic condition; their depression may hinder them from discussing sexual issues at that time. They may be feeling fearful. They may be afraid of a reoccurrence, or they may be afraid of being hurt during sex. Each of these factors may inhibit a person from discussing sexual issues with a health professional. Furthermore, clients may have had previous negative or harmful misconceptions about sexuality and disability, adding to their fear and discomfort regarding their own situation.

Knowledge Needed To Address Issues of Sexual Function Related to Disability

The occupational therapy practitioner must have a solid knowledge base regarding the diagnoses of persons seen in his or her practice environment (see Box 17.2). Before attempting any functional sexual counseling or education, the practitioner must thoroughly understand the disability or disease process

Box 17.1

Valencia Declaration on Sexual Rights

The 13th annual World Congress on Sexology (the scientific study of sex) held in Valencia, Spain, adopted a declaration on sexual rights. The declaration declared that sexual health is a basic and fundamental human right and that human sexuality is essential to the well-being of individuals, couples, families, and society. It concluded that respect for sexual rights should be promoted through all means. These rights are as follows:

- **The right to freedom,** which excludes all forms of sexual coercion, exploitation, and abuse at any time and in all situations in life. The struggle against violence is a social priority. All children should be desired and loved.
- **The right to autonomy, integrity, and safety of the body,** which encompasses control and enjoyment of our own bodies, free from torture, mutilation, and violence of any sort.
- **The right to sexual equity and equality,** which refers to freedom from all forms of discrimination, paying due respect to sexual diversity, regardless of sex, gender, age, race, social class, religion, and sexual orientation.

- **The right to sexual health,** including availability of all sufficient resources for development of research and the necessary knowledge of HIV/AIDS and sexually transmitted diseases, as well as the further development of resources for research, diagnosis, and treatment.
- **The right to wide, objective, and factual information on human sexuality** to allow decision making regarding sexual life.
- **The right to a comprehensive sexuality education** from birth and throughout the life cycle. All social institutions should be involved in this process.
- **The right to associate freely,** including the possibility to marry or not, to divorce, and to establish other types of sexual associations.
- **The right to make free and responsible choices regarding reproductive life,** the number and spacing of children, and the access to means of fertility regulation.
- **The right to privacy,** which implies the capability of making autonomous decisions about sexual life within a context of personal and social ethics as rational and satisfactory experience of sexuality is a requirement for human development.

affecting the person. To apply the principles of normal sexual functioning, the practitioner must realize what differences exist as a result of the specific disability or disease process. These disabilities include central nervous system disorders (i.e., spinal cord, brain, peripheral nerve disorders); cardiovascular disorders (i.e., heart attacks, bypass grafts); pulmonary disorders (i.e., chronic obstructive pulmonary disease, emphysema, asthma); musculoskeletal or orthopedic disorders (i.e., arthritis, joint replacements, back problems, amputations); and developmental disorders.

Knowledge of Anatomy and Physiology

To adequately address issues of sexual function related to disability, practitioners must understand male and female sexual anatomy and then be able to apply this information to their foundational knowledge of disability and diseases processes. Before a practitioner enters into a conversation about sexuality and disability, he or she must have this understanding about the normal sexual system and how it works. It would be difficult for a practitioner to discuss the changes caused by a specific disability if he or she did not fully understand the functioning of a normal system. This knowledge base includes the male and female genitalia and reproductive organs, human anatomy, normal physiology, and neuroanatomy.

The body's physiologic response during sexual activity, as identified by Masters and Johnson (1966), is an extremely important aspect of normal function for occupational therapy practitioners to understand so that they can assist persons with a disability. It is critical to know the difference between the normal physiologic effects of sexual activity and changes that occur for other reasons that could be problem-

---

Box 17.2
Preparing for Effective Sexuality Intervention

Practitioners need special skills and knowledge to provide sexuality education and counseling to their clients. To be effective, practitioners should have training in sexuality that addresses these four components.

1. **Knowledge.** Practitioners need a sound and comprehensive information base about human sexuality, including human development, relationships, personal skills, sexual behavior, sexual health, marital and family dynamics; and society and culture. Practitioners should have self-knowledge of their limitations. They should know when and where to refer clients with special problems and needs.

2. **Attitudes.** Practitioners should have an awareness and understanding of their own sexuality in order to increase their comfort level in addressing the sexual concerns of others. They should demonstrate an acceptance of the diversity of values, beliefs, and lifestyles in the communities they serve.

3. **Skill.** Practitioners should have communication and counseling skills to address sensitive and controversial subjects. Training should include opportunities for practice, and initial efforts should be supervised by more experienced practitioners.

4. **Personal Characteristics and Motivation.** Effective sexuality education and counseling require personal qualities such as emotional stability, patience, flexibility, and a sense of humor. Practitioners should possess the maturity and self-control to avoid imposing personal viewpoints and values on clients. They should have the motivation and commitment to address the sexual health needs of all clients needing such intervention.

---

atic. An example would be an autonomic response after sexual arousal in a higher level tetraplegic that causes a dangerous elevation in blood pressure.

Masters and Johnson (1966) identified four phases in a sexual response cycle for men and women.

1. Excitement—breathing, pulse, and blood pressure begin to increase; muscle tension increases; breast and genital tissues start to swell; vaginal lubrication in women and erection in men take place

2. Plateau—the physical changes continue

3. Orgasm—men ejaculate; women experience contractions in their vagina and uterus; heart rate, breathing, blood pressure, and muscle tension all reach a peak

4. Resolution—all the physiologic changes return to their pre-excitement levels

Additionally, the practitioner must have information on sexually transmitted diseases, including recommended measures of prevention such as hygiene, discretion in partner selection, and the use of protective barriers, such as male and female condoms.

Interpersonal Communication Skills

Dealing with the topic of sex can be a challenge and is a sensitive and private matter. Practitioners must have excellent interpersonal skills and be able to have very open communication with their clients. The practitioner may be cast in several different roles: facilitator, educator, counselor, and sometimes confidante. Each of these roles requires effective communication skills and the ability to maintain a trusting therapeutic relationship.

Providing effective sexuality education and counseling is a challenging endeavor, requiring good listening skills, compassion, and the ability to maintain a delicate balance between sensitivity and assertiveness. The occupational therapy practitioner must know when to listen and when to offer suggestions; when to push a bit and when to back off; when to offer comfort and when to point out potential problems. Being able to read the eyes and other nonverbal messages sent by the person is a necessary skill for successful counseling sessions. The practitioner must be able to recognize when the person has heard enough during a specific session and when the person wants and needs more information but may not quite know how to ask for it. The occupational therapy practitioner must always be alert to unspoken questions that are very important to the client.

It is the practitioner's responsibility to create the appropriate environment for the counseling session—one that is both comfortable and professional. The practitioner's empathy should be evident, while maintaining enough professional distance to provide the necessary information in the most therapeutic manner. The most critical point to keep in mind as a practitioner is to provide the most appropriate, accurate information in a manner that is comfortable and nonthreatening for the person.

The Functional Effects of Disability and Suggested Approaches During Sexual Activity

In the following sections, a brief review of the concerns, limitations, and recommended compensatory strategies for different kinds of conditions is presented. This review is not meant to be exhaustive. Rather, it provides an overview of the issues and strategies that would exemplify interactions with clients with various conditions. Before beginning intervention sessions with clients, the therapist should be fully informed about all aspects of the specific condition, as well as other health problems that may affect sexual activity. Inexperienced practitioners can benefit from role-playing, extensive reviews of the literature, and discussions with more experienced colleagues. It is also advisable to coordinate plans for sexual counseling with other members of the care team to ensure that information provided to the client is consistent with the overall plan of care.

Joint Inflammation

Persons who suffer from diseases or conditions resulting in joint inflammation frequently have symptoms that include pain, stiffness, fatigue, and decreased range of motion. Any of these symptoms can be a detriment to sexual activity. Kraaimaat, Bakker, Janssen, and Bijlsma (1996) stated that pain and limited range of motion may "interfere with sexual pleasure by distracting patients from pleasurable sensations, sexual thoughts, and fantasies" (p.121). The most common barriers to the enjoyment of sexual activity are the fear of causing severe pain and anxiety about the possibility of hurting the affected joint. Certainly the same principles that apply to other daily living tasks apply to sexual activity. Occupational therapy practitioners should include the topics of energy conservation and joint protection techniques when discussing how to ap-

proach sexual activity. Specific suggestions include the following.

- Recommend that the client use joint protection techniques when deciding on positions for sexual activity. Positions that stress the affected joints should be avoided.

- If there is a pain relief regimen, suggest that the client time the sexual activity when the pain relief is at its maximum to enjoy the activity a bit more. This may include medication, heat treatments, or both.

- If pain and stiffness are worse at the beginning of the day (as is typically the case with some types of joint inflammation), recommend that the client delay sexual activity until the stiffness has disappeared and joints move more freely. Conversely, if pain, swelling, and stiffness are problems later in the day, the client should arrange to have sexual activity earlier in the day.

- Recommend that clients use positions that take advantage of unaffected joints for support and motion (i.e., if the shoulders and elbows are affected, the person should not use the superior position, but should allow his or her partner to assume that position).

- Recommend using sidelying as a position because it may be fairly nonstressful for most joints.

- Suggest the use of pillows to assist in finding a comfortable position.

- When mobility is a problem on a given day, advise trying to enjoy sexual activities other than intercourse that may be less stressful on the body, such as oral sex or mutual masturbation.

- Suggest experimentation with assistive devices, such as a hand-held dildo (strapped on or with a built up-handle) or vibrator, if the person's hands are severely affected.

Spinal Cord Injury

Persons with a spinal cord injury (SCI) may have tetraplegia, paraplegia, or some other combination of motor loss, sensory loss, or both because of an incomplete injury. Persons with lesions above the T-4 level may experience autonomic dysreflexia in response to sexual stimulation. Both the person with SCI and his or her partner should be educated about this phenomenon and the actions to be taken to relieve it.

Although sexual functioning varies among persons with SCI (even those with the same level of injury), men with a cervical lesion are more likely to retain the ability for erections and women with cervical lesions are more likely to retain the ability for vaginal lubrication. Ejaculation capabilities are most frequently seen in men with lesions at the thoracic level. Additionally, reflexogenic erections and lubrication can occur if the reflex arc is left intact, as is frequently seen in persons with an injury at the cervical level (Smith & Bodner, 1993). Although persons with an SCI may not experience orgasms in the same manner as they did before the injury, many report some feeling of pleasure, a buildup of excitement, or any number of bodily reactions (i.e., muscle spasms, flushing) (Mooney, Cole, & Chilgren, 1975). The fertility of women with SCI is not permanently affected. If a man with an SCI is found to have viable sperm but cannot ejaculate, he may elect to have an electro-ejaculation procedure to collect sperm, followed by an insemination of his partner (Freda, 1998). Functional problems associated with SCI include mobility loss, sensory loss, bowel and bladder problems (including the use of catheters), spasticity, erectile dysfunction, and loss of vaginal lubrication in women. Specific suggestions are as follows.

- The partner should concentrate touching and fondling to the intact areas of sensation on the person's body.
- If the partner is touching a body part without sensation, he or she should either tell the person what area is being touched or be sure the area is within the visual field of the person so that enjoyment can occur on a level other than touch.
- The person and his or her partner should experiment to find new "erogenous" areas (frequently this occurs at the level of the last intact dermotone or surface area of sensation) (Neistadt & Freda, 1987).
- The person with the SCI should let his or her partner know the functional limitations currently present (i.e., where sensation is absent, whether erections are possible, if there are mobility deficits).
- If a man with an SCI has an external catheter, there are two possible solutions: (a) the man may secure the tubing to the shaft of the penis and engage in sexual activities, or (b) if the man with the SCI knows when he has to urinate, he may experiment with taking the catheter off for short periods of time and engaging in sexual activities during these intervals (Neistadt & Freda, 1987).
- If the person with an SCI is on an intermittent catheterization schedule, he or she should adjust the timing of the sexual activity accordingly.

- If an erection is not possible for the man with an SCI, there are several options:
  a. Engage in sexual activities other than intercourse, such as oral sex or manual stimulation.
  b. Make use of a vibrator or dildo, if penetration is important to the couple.
  c. Use vacuum devices that can facilitate a short-term erection (a urologist must be consulted for this).
  d. Consider surgical implants that can mimic an erection or a partial erection (consult a urologist).
  e. Explore the possible benefit of pharmacological agents that can cause an erection (consult a urologist).
- If a woman with an SCI has an indwelling catheter, the tube can be taped to the abdomen and the collection bag can be positioned away from the body. It is safe to engage in intercourse or digital stimulation while the tube is in place (Neistadt & Freda, 1987).
- For a woman with an SCI who has decreased or absent vaginal lubrication, lubricating jelly or other water-soluble agents can assist with lubrication or the male partner may want to use a lubricated condom (Neistadt & Freda, 1987).
- A person with tetraplegia might use a vibrator or another assistive device strapped onto his or her hand for manual stimulation; he or she may also use the heel of the hand or the side of the hand.
- If a reflexogenic erection is possible, it can be achieved by direct manual stimulation of the testicles, penis, and surrounding area. A *reflexogenic erection* is one achieved by manual stimulation of the nerves in the perineal region.
- Clients should be advised to use positions that take advantage of the movement and control that exists. The positions could include the following:
  a. The person with an SCI could take the position on the bottom.
  b. The person with an SCI may long sit in the bed, supported against the wall or the headboard and pillows while the partner sits on his or her lap.
  c. The person with an SCI can sit in the wheelchair or another chair while the partner sits on his or her lap.
  d. Sidelying may be a viable option.

Traumatic Brain Injury

Serious brain injuries occur most frequently to young persons (primarily men) at a time when they are beginning to explore and develop their sexuality. In addition to the physical problems (such as paralysis or movement disorders) that often accompany serious brain injury, there are also important cognitive and interpersonal effects. Depending on the site of the injury, brain injury can reduce sexual drive or increase its inappropriate expression by reducing inhibitions. This effect occurs when there is damage to the limbic areas of the brain.

Because of the complexity of the brain, the structures affected can result in vastly different physical, cognitive, and emotional consequences. Therefore, each person with traumatic brain injury must be carefully evaluated, and appropriate sexuality counseling should be provided based on an individual profile of the client. A recent study by Kreuter and others (Kreuter, Dahllof, Gudjonsson, Sullivan, & Siosteen, 1998) found that many persons with traumatic brain injury living in the community after rehabilitation experienced sexual problems. These problems included an inability to achieve an erection, the inability to achieve orgasm, decreased sexual desire, and a reduced frequency of sexual intercourse. Factors related to satisfactory sexual adjustment included better physical independence and the absence of sexual dysfunction. The researchers concluded that improved efforts at sexual counseling could improve these outcomes.

Stroke (Including Cognitive Deficits)

Persons who have had a stroke (cerebral vascular accident) may have a hemiplegia or hemiparesis, sensory loss, bowel and bladder problems, proprioceptive deficits, visual problems, communication disorders, swallowing problems, perceptual problems, and cognitive deficits. Fertility is not usually affected by a stroke; however, some decrease in *libido* (sexual drive or interest) has been reported. A decrease in ejaculatory function and erection may also be experienced by men (Monga, Lawson, & Inglis, 1986; Zasler, 1991). Persons after stroke may also be depressed and suffer moderate to severe fatigue. Because many persons who have a stroke are older, they may already have other health problems that may be intensified by the stroke. Sometimes, the normal consequences of aging may also be magnified by the stroke (Freda & Rubinsky, 1991).

Specific suggestions for sexual activity include the following.

- If *receptive aphasia* (the inability to understand spoken language) is present, the partner may want to physically guide the person with a stroke to the part of the body that the partner wishes to be touched.

- If *expressive aphasia* (the inability to use spoken language) is present, the couple may want to try incorporating a specific sexual activity communication board into their routine.

- The partner should observe the facial expressions and body language of the person with a communication problem to gauge whether there is a positive or negative response to a specific activity or position.

- If a functional communication problem exists, sexual partners should use familiar hand signals or develop a "safe" routine to decrease fear of the unknown.

- If there is a visual field loss, the partner should initiate the sexual activity within the intact visual field so that the person with a stroke can fully enjoy the activity.

- If there are severe visual problems, the couple may enjoy the use of verbal sharing and fantasies (Freda & Rubinsky, 1991).

- If there is a severe hemiplegia with a sensory loss, the partner will want to concentrate touching and fondling on the intact or uninvolved side of the body.

- If there is a motor loss, the couple should experiment with positions that allow the uninvolved side of the body to be active (i.e., lie comfortably and safely on the involved side, allowing the uninvolved side to be free for touching and fondling).

- Depending on the severity of the motor loss, the unaffected partner may want to take a more active role and be in the superior or more supporting position (Freda & Rubinsky, 1991).

- If fatigue is present, couples should plan sexual activity at a time of day when most of the person's energy has not already been expended. Energy conservation techniques are useful as general recommendations after stroke to enable the person to participate in many types of valued activities.

- If the person has difficulty focusing attention for an appropriate amount of time, the sexual activity should be planned for a quiet time of the day when there are few or no distractions; attention cues and assistance should be incorporated into the sexual activity.

- The partner may want to verbally take the person through the desired steps of a specific sexual activity when a cognitive sequencing deficit is present (Freda & Rubinsky, 1991).

- A person with a short-term memory deficit may wish to use a memory log if that strategy has worked in other daily life tasks (Freda & Rubinsky, 1991).

- The person with multiple cognitive issues should start out with simple, familiar activities for short periods of time (Freda & Rubinsky, 1991).

- If achieving or maintaining an erection is difficult, the person should consult his urologist to discuss the use of a vacuum device, a penile implant, or drug therapy.

Upper-Extremity Amputations

Upper-extremity amputations can occur as a result of trauma or disease, or they may be congenital in origin. Upper-extremity amputations should not affect sexual functioning or fertility physiologically. Certainly a person with an upper-extremity amputation may experience a change in his or her body image and self-esteem. These changes can sometimes result in psychological consequences, such as depression, that can affect sexual interest and drive. Depression is more likely to be a problem if the amputation was traumatic and recent. Specific functional suggestions for resuming sexual activity include the following.

- The person with a unilateral amputation could use the amputated side for support (depending on the level of the amputation) and use the intact hand and arm for stimulating the partner.

- The stump may be used for sexual touching and stimulation if it is not tender or painful.

- A man with bilateral amputations may still use a superior kneeling position (kneeling precludes the need for upper-extremity support) for intercourse.

- Oral sex is usually a viable option for either a man or a woman with one or both arms amputated.

- A woman with bilateral amputations could take the bottom position with her partner on top, as long as the partner is aware of how much weight is on the woman, because she may not be able to "push" her partner off.

- Another option for a woman with bilateral amputations is to sit on her partner's lap, either in a chair or on the bed in long sitting for intercourse.

- A man with bilateral amputations could long sit on a bed or sit in a chair with his partner sitting on top for intercourse.

- Sexual aids attached to a prosthesis or to the stump may also be incorporated.

Low Vision

Low or impaired vision may occur from cataracts, macular degeneration, diabetic retinopathy, retinal detachment, retinitis pigmentosa, or neurological disorders. Specific compensatory strategies for persons with low vision follow.

- All the senses should be emphasized by incorporating taste, smell, and hearing into the sexual activity.

- The partner must become aware of the exact visual acuity or field of vision (i. e., is the central vision impaired or the peripheral vision) and should keep much of the activity within the intact field of vision to maximize the pleasure of the person with low vision.

- Strategies that have worked in other daily life tasks may work in the sexual area as well (i.e., specific lighting, specific distances).

- The partner may want to talk about what he or she is about to do or is actually doing to increase the total experience for the person with low vision, as well as not surprising him or her with a touch or stimulation that is unexpected.

- The partner may physically guide the person with low vision to a desired part of the body.

- The person with low vision may want to use specific optical aids that have been helpful for other activities as appropriate and comfortable.

- A person with blurred vision may need some assistance in localizing touch to a specific part of the body; once guided to the desired spot, the person should have no difficulty.

Summary

Sex counseling and education from a functional perspective is an appropriate role for an occupational therapy practitioner to assume with clients who have a disability. It is an important and challenging responsibility, but one that the occupational therapy practitioner can handle with the proper prerequisite knowledge and competencies. Given the health-promoting benefits of being able to express sexuality, assisting clients to realize their fullest potential and participation in this aspect of life is a goal worth attaining. A lis of useful resources for information on sexuality follows the references. ◆

Study Questions

1. Why is it appropriate for an occupational therapy practitioner to deal with questions related to sexuality after a disability?

2. What is the occupational therapy practitioner's role in dealing with issues related to sexuality and disability?

3. What is the prerequisite knowledge needed for an occupational therapy practitioner to effectively deal with issues related to sexuality and disability?

4. What barriers exist within a health care environment that prevent adequate attention from being given to the issues of sexuality and disability?

5. What barriers exist within a person with a disability that often prevents him or her from asking questions related to sexuality and disability?

6. What are some specific strategies a person with a spinal cord injury might use for sexual activity?

7. What are some specific strategies a person with low vision might use for sexual activity?

References

Bianchi, T. L. (1997). Aspects of sexuality after burn injury: Outcomes in men. *Journal of Burn Care and Rehabilitation, 18*(2), 183–186.

Davey Smith, G., Frankel, S., & Yarnell, J. (1997). Sex and death: Are they related? Findings from the Caerphilly Cohort Study. *British Medical Journal, 315*(7123), 1641–1644.

Eckland, M., & McBride, K. (1997). Sexual health care: The role of the nurse. *Canadian Nurse, 93*(7), 34–37.

Freda, M. (1998). Sexuality and disability. In M. E. Neistadt & E. Crepeau (Eds.), *Willard and Spackman's occupational therapy* (pp. 364–369). Philadelphia: Lippincott.

Freda, M., & Rubinsky, H. (1991). Sexual function in the stroke survivor. *Physical Medicine and Rehabilitation Clinics of North America, 2*, 634–658.

Kraaimaat, F. W., Bakker, A. H., Janssen, E., & Bijlsma, J. W. J. (1996). Intrusiveness of rheumatoid arthritis on sexuality in male and female patients living with a spouse. *Arthritis Care and Research, 9*(2), 120–125.

Kreuter, M., Dahllof, A. G., Gudjonsson, G., Sullivan, M., & Siosteen, A. (1998). Sexual adjustment and its predictors after traumatic brain injury. *Brain Injury, 12*(5), 349–368.

Kreuter, M., Sullivan, M., & Siosteen, A. (1996). Sexual adjustment and quality of relationship in spinal paraplegia: A controlled study. *Archives of Physical Medicine and Rehabilitation, 77*(6), 541–548.

Masters, W. H., & Johnson, V. E. (1966). *Human sexual response.* Boston: Little, Brown.

McCabe, M. P. (1997). Intimacy and quality of life among sexually dysfunctional men and women. *Journal of Sex and Marital Therapy, 23*(4), 276–290.

Monga, T. N., Lawson, J. S., & Inglis, J. (1986). Sexual dysfunction in stroke patients. *Archives of Physical Medicine and Rehabilitation, 67*, 19–22.

Mooney, T., Cole, T., & Chilgren, R. (1975). *Sexual options for paraplegics and quadriplegics.* Boston: Little, Brown.

Neistadt, M. E. (1986). Sexuality counseling for adults with disabilities: A module for an occupational therapy curriculum. *American Journal of Occupational Therapy, 40*, 542–545.

Neistadt, M. E., & Freda, M. (1987). *Choices: A guide to sex counseling with physically disabled adults.* Malabar, FL: Robert Krieger.

Smith, E. M., & Bodner, D. R. (1993). Sexual dysfunction after spinal cord injury. *Urology Clinics of North America, 20*, 535–542.

Spector, I. P., & Fremeth, S. M. (1996). Sexual behaviors and attitudes of geriatric residents in long-term care facilities. *Journal of Sex and Marital Therapy, 22*(4), 235–246.

Spica, M. M. (1989). Sexual counseling standards for the spinal cord-injured. *Journal of Neuroscience Nursing, 21*(1), 56–60.

Ventegodt, S. (1998). Sex and the quality of life in Denmark. *Archives of Sexual Behavior, 27*(3), 295–307.

Zasler, N. (1991). Sexuality in neurologic disability: An overview. *Sexuality and Disability, 9*(1), 11–27.

Additional Resources

AUSTRALIA
Australian Association of Sex Educators, Counselors, and Therapists (AASERT)
P.O. Box 346
Lane Cove, NSW 2066

CANADA
International Academy of Sex Research (IASR)
Clarke Institute of Psychiatry
Child and Family Studies Centre
250 College Street
Toronto, Ontario M5T IR8
CANADA

Sex Information and Education Council of Canada (SIECCAN)
850 Coxwell Avenue
East York, Ontario M4C 5RI
CANADA

GREAT BRITAIN
Family Planning Association (FPA)
27/35 Mortimer Street
London W1N 7RJ
ENGLAND

Sex Education Forum, National Childrens Bureau
8 Wakely Street
London EC1V 7QE
ENGLAND

UNITED STATES
American Association of Sex Educators, Counselors, and
Therapists (AASECT)
P.O. Box 238
Mt. Vernon, IA 52314
Web site: www.aasect.org

The Kinsey Institute for Research in Sex, Gender, and
Reproduction
313 Morrison Hall
Indiana University
Bloomington, IN 47404
Web site: www.indiana.edu/~kinsey

Sexuality Information and Education Council of the
United States (SIECUS)
130 W. 42nd Street, Suite 350
New York, NY 10036-7802
Web site: www.siecus.org

Society for the Scientific Study of Sex (SSSS)
P.O. Box 208
Mt. Vernon, IA 52314
Web site: http://www.ssc.wisc.edu/ssss/

18

Using Assistive Technologies To Enable Self-Care and Daily Living

Roger O. Smith
Margie Benge
Marian Hall

Roger O. Smith, PhD, OT, FAOTA, is Director of Occupational Therapy, University of Wisconsin–Milwaukee, and Honorary Researcher, Waisman Center for Mental Retardation and Human Development, University of Wisconsin–Madison.

Margie Benge, OTR, is Director, Triangle Therapy Services, Eaton, Ohio.

Marian Hall, MBA, OT, is Program Manager, Stapely in Germantown and Sacred Heart Manor, Genesis ElderCare Rehab Services, Kenneth Square, Pennsylvania.

Key Terms

abandonment

Abledata

assistive technology device

assistive technology service

ATP

compliance

consumer

environment-adjusted score

environment-free score

functional independence

open market

prescription

RESNA

supplier

Objectives

On completing this chapter, the reader will be able to

1. Describe the prevalence of assistive technology and the historical use of assistive technology in occupational therapy.

2. Explain how assistive technology directly affects self-care function through the use of self-care devices and indirectly with devices that improve the self-care environment or skills needed to do self-care tasks.

3. Illustrate how assistive technology fits in as a key occupational therapy intervention approach, but in the context of other approaches.

4. Describe key steps in the assistive technology intervention process and the importance of each step.

5. Provide examples of the role of the assistive technology consumer in the delivery of assistive technology service.

6. Describe issues related to assistive technology intervention and the significance of each.

7. Illustrate the various mechanisms of service delivery of assistive technology related to self-care devices.

In 1778 Benjamin Franklin said, "Man is a tool-making animal" (cited in *The Oxford Dictionary of Quotations*, 1980, p. 218). While his gender-specific language is more than 200 years old and outdated, his observation about the unique relationship between humans and tools is timeless. This is fortunate. Today, tools used as assistive technologies enable persons with disabilities to maximize their self-care independence and efficiency.

The vast number of assistive technologies available today reflects the prominent contribution they make to independent living. It is important that occupational therapy practitioners take a central role in helping to link these technologies to the persons who will benefit from them. Abledata, the national database of assistive and rehabilitation technologies, includes more than 17,000 products. Of these, a large percentage is classified as self-care. Table 18.1 highlights more than 7,500 products that relate to self-care. These products are the assistive technologies addressed in this chapter.

This chapter, unlike many others in this book, does not focus on a disability or an impairment area. It focuses on an intervention strategy. Although it provides information about some self-care tools, it is beyond its scope to review and discuss the pros and cons of the multitude of technologies available. Thus, this chapter highlights concepts, many of which have evolved out of core philosophies of occupational therapy practice.

Legislation in the United States is recognizing assistive technology as a cost-effective intervention to assist persons with disabilities. The terms assistive technology devices and assistive technology services are now included in many federal agencies and their regulations. The Federal Rehabilitation Act of 1973 (as amended), especially with the 1986 additions of rehabilitation engineering services; the Education for All Handicapped Children Act of 1975 (Pub. L. 94–142), updated in 1991 as IDEA (Individuals With Disabilities Education Act; Pub. L. 101–476); the Developmental Disabilities Act; and the Older Americans Act all incorporate requirements for assistive technology. Two federal laws in the United States, however, have had a specific effect in increasing the awareness of the benefits of assistive technologies for helping persons accommodate to their disabilities. These are the Technology Assistance Act of 1988 (Tech Act; Pub. L. 100–407) and the Americans With Disabilities Act of 1990 (ADA; Pub. L. 101–336). The Tech Act provides federal funds to increase assistive technology resources available to persons with disabilities and partially measure their success on "consumer responsiveness." The ADA provides basic civil rights protection for persons with disabilities and recognizes the important role assistive technology plays in equal access and overall integration into society.

As the number of older persons in the population increases, the need for assistive technologies is greater. Assistive technologies help persons who must contend with functional limitations resulting from normal aging, as well as persons with disabilities who require functional support to gain and maintain independence.

A Swedish study (Parker & Thorslund, 1991) found that technical devices are essential to the independence of persons who are aging. The researchers surveyed a rural municipality with a population of about 20,000 people. They identified those persons 75 years of age and older who required technical aids or who had major functional limitations. The 57 persons randomly selected for this study had a total of 422 technical aids in their homes. Each person used an average of slightly more than seven devices. Twenty-nine percent of

Table 18.1 Self-Care Assistive Devices By Category

Assistive Device Category	Number of Product Listings in Abledata
Personal care	4,628
Home management	1,228
Wheeled mobility	1,993
Seating	1,429
Communication	2,525
Walking	872
Orthotics	886
Prosthetics	64
Architectural elements	1,690
Control	939

Note. Self-care products cataloged in Abledata have more than doubled in the past 5 years. This is an average increase of more than 1,000 products per year.

these devices were used for mobility, 20% for personal hygiene, 20% for communication, and 16% for environmental adaptations. Five percent were ortheses or prostheses, and 11% were other functional devices. The study concluded that it is essential for occupational therapy practitioners to be familiar with assistive technologies that aid self-care independence.

The use of assistive technology is often an inexpensive and quick method for a person with a disability to compensate for impairments and to achieve independence in self-care activities. Effective use of an assistive device, however, involves more than pulling it off a storage shelf and handing it to the client. The appropriate device must be carefully selected on the basis of functional need, environmental setting, and available resources. This selection includes decisions about whether the device is really necessary and how long it will be needed. Many steps, considerations, and decisions have to be made when providing even the simplest assistive technologies.

When principles for making correct decisions about assistive technology are not followed, the consequences can be costly. Poor outcomes can result from providing unnecessary or inappropriate equipment, providing the right equipment but not teaching the client how or why to use it, or failing to recommend a device because of lack of knowledge about its existence. When these problems occur, useful devices may never reach consumers who need them, or they may be purchased and delivered but never used. In the end, functional abilities are unnecessarily limited, and secondary disability can result.

In the best situations, decisions are made in consultation with the consumer, and delivery of the assistive technology results in successful long-term use of the device. Whereas the process of making sound decisions about assistive technology is often intuitive to experts, the goal of this chapter is to provide principles and guidance to enable good assistive technology decisions for practitioners regardless of their level of experience.

Overview of Assistive Technologies for Self-Care and Daily Living

The variety of assistive technologies for self-care and daily living is far reaching. Devices range from low technologies, such as a swivel spoon to enable eating independence, to futuristic and high technologies, such as a robot that feeds someone who is totally dependent. The terms low technology and high technology represent one way to think about the range of assistive technologies. Many ways can be used to classify self-care technologies, however. Technology can be minimal or maximal, custom or commercial, appliances or tools (Smith, 1991). A helpful way to review the scope of these technologies is by the functions they perform.

Practitioners may be aware of many persons who use assistive devices, and they may have helped to select quite a few of them. Often, however, the range of technology encountered in a specific area of practice is narrow. To provide a broad look at assistive technology used in self-care and daily living, this section provides a cross section of examples. The number of technologies that occupational therapy practitioners track, just for self-care independence goals, is surprising.

Self-Care Devices

Increasing eating and drinking independence is one purpose for using assistive technologies. Special forks, knives, spoons, bibs, dishes, cups, glasses, and straws can help a person with a mild motor impairment to eat independently or make it easier. Feeding evaluation kits are available to help practitioners think through the lower tech alternatives. Mealtime aids, a higher tech intervention, can help someone who has severe impairments (see Figure 18.1).

For enabling self-reliance in cleanliness, hygiene, and appearance, there are products that address dental care, eye glasses, hair care, nail care, and shaving. We take toileting and bathing for granted in our daily lives, but they require special methods and devices for many persons with disabilities. Toileting technologies include catheters and accessories, ostomy supplies, and devices dealing with incontinence, commodes, toilets, and urinals. For bathing, brushes and scrubbing devices, devices for seating, and equipment for helping to move in and out of tubs or showers are available.

Products for assisting in dressing and undressing independence include adaptive clothing for all ages and needs, along with shoes, helmets, dressing devices, shoe aids, stocking aids, and button aids (see Figure 18.2). Although smoking is clearly identified as a hazardous personal care activity, devices are available to help persons be more independent in smoking activities. Health care professionals, such as occupational therapy practitioners, are often placed in an ethical quandary when considering helping clients become more independent in smoking. This

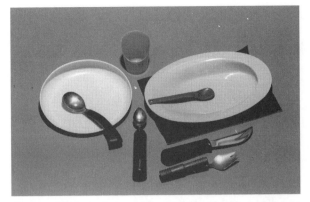

Figure 18.1 Assistive technology eating devices are available for many eating tasks, including drinking, using utensils, and picking up food from a plate. Some utensils are weighted, some swivel, and other are designed with built-up handles.

chapter emphasizes that the role of an occupational therapy practitioner is to help a consumer make good decisions. This role may mean obtaining and providing an assistive device for smoking if that is the consumer's decision. As a professional, one may express values for healthy living but may not impose them on others. It is important for the practitioner to provide consultation, professional opinions, and assistance in identifying alternatives.

Some assistive devices for self-care enable reaching, carrying, holding, dispensing, and transferring objects. A number of these devices are attached to wheelchairs and to walkers as generic carrying devices like pouches and baskets. Other products

hold specific objects, such as telephones or drinking glasses (Figure 18.3).

A variety of self-care assistive technologies pertain to a person taking care of his or her own health. Arm supports and health devices, such as scales, thermometers, medication storage systems, and restraint devices, fall into this category. Other devices in this category have specific uses, such as special sexual devices for persons with disabilities, or products to assist in child care activities, such as diaper changing.

Home-Care Products

A second category of assistive technologies includes products that allow a person to be independent while at home. These products include a wide variety of kitchen appliances and cooking tools for food preparation. Housekeeping items are also a part of home management, as is specifically designed furniture, including beds, tables, chairs, and steps.

Seating and Mobility

A third major classification includes devices for mobility and devices for seating and positioning. Wheeled mobility devices include manual and powered wheelchairs. Wheelchair accessories, wheelchair alternatives, transporters, carts, and stretchers are related devices. For walking mobility there are canes, crutches, walkers, and standing equipment. Additionally, seating systems include support de-

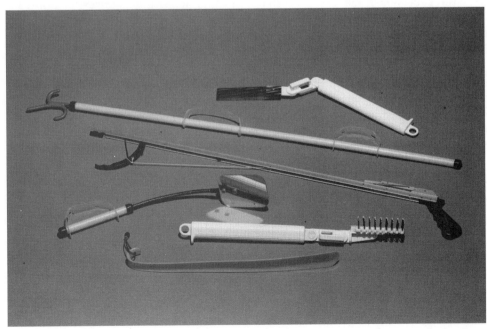

Figure 18.2 Assistive devices for donning and doffing clothing aid in tasks such as reaching and pulling clothing over body parts and in fine-motor manipulation of fasteners.

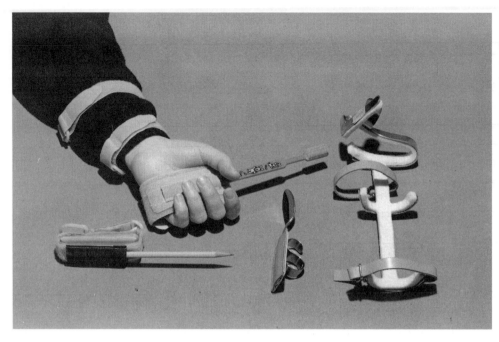

Figure 18.3 Orthotic devices often support weak or painful motion and can be extremely helpful for holding items or stabilizing joints.

vices for parts of the body, seat cushions, car seats, and seating monitors for keeping track of pressure points to prevent decubitus ulcers.

Communication

An important part of self-care is being able to communicate. Mouthwands, headwands, reading aids, book holders, writing utensils, writing guides, typing systems, telephone adaptations, and communication systems for those who are nonvocal and have speech impairments are types of assistive technology allowing a person to communicate his or her needs. A specific type of assistive device is signaling equipment. Many types of signaling products are designed for emergency situations. Advancements have been made in this area over the past several years, including monitors for persons who wander. These products are triggered by emergencies and are designed to notify help. Centralized communication systems linked by radio can track the situation.

Orthotics and Prosthetics

Orthotics and prosthetics are not often considered self-care devices, but they are critical in self-care management for two reasons. First, independence or optimal efficiency may not be possible for a person with disabilities without the assistance of some orthotic or prosthetic device. Sometimes these prostheses and orthoses are used in conjunction with other assistive technology to optimize independence

and efficiency. Additionally, persons who have prosthetic or orthotic devices have special needs pertaining to the maintenance and care of this equipment. Orthoses and prostheses become extensions of the body and require special techniques and considerations for donning and doffing, laundering, or cleaning.

Architecture

Self-care is frequently dependent on architectural design. For example, narrow doorways can prevent self-care activities in the bathroom. As suggested in the earlier chapter on self-care environments, it is prudent for occupational therapy practitioners to consider architectural assistive technologies to enable independent living activities. Assistive technologies pertaining to architectural elements include door handles, door locks, hinges, special windows, floor materials, fixtures in the bathroom, public restroom accommodations, kitchen fixtures, and storage needs. Lighting, safety, and security devices, as well as vertical lifts enable personal care management and independent living.

Environmental Control

Finally, controlling the environment is important. Switching lights off and on, managing room temperature and humidity, and controlling consumer products in the home can be essential activities for independence (see Figure 18.4). Assistive technolo-

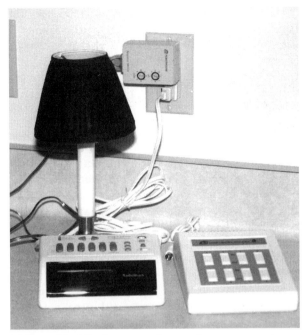

Figure 18.4 Environmental control systems can be very complex or simply plug into the house wall electrical outlet. Here, two similarly functioning devices can control more than 100 different household units, but they have a major difference. One is programmed via computer and has additional flexibility.

gies can include specific switches, remote switches, or switch interfaces that allow a person with a disability to maintain a safe environment.

This quick overview shows the wide range of assistive technologies for daily living that are available for consumers. Often, it is not apparent that if a practitioner fails to provide information about a product or a set of products from this array of possibilities, the consumer may not reach his or her functional potential. Although consumers need to take responsibility for obtaining information about the products they purchase, the health care professional in rehabilitation has corresponding obligation to remain fully informed about the availability and features of assistive devices. Occupational therapy practitioners must ensure that a person needing assistive technology is provided with all the information necessary to make the best decisions.

It is reassuring to know that resources are available to help occupational therapy practitioners meet this responsibility. The next section of this chapter reviews the process of choosing the most appropriate assistive technology. Charts, forms, and checklists can help occupational therapy practitioners with this task.

Intervention Approaches, Including Assistive Technology

Assistive technologies are not interventions in and of themselves. They are tools and must be integrated into the overall intervention plan to optimize the daily living independence and efficiency of a person. Providing a piece of equipment is not an outcome. It is a part of a strategy that should be a part of a clearly identified goal. The goal should be clear to all parties involved, including the client, the reimbursement agency, and the practitioner.

Assistive technology can be used with the entire range of intervention options available to practitioners in occupational therapy to help persons with disabilities overcome self-care problems. Within the category of remediation, technology can assist with resolving the impairments causing self-care deficits or with developing new skills. Within compensation strategies, devices help adapt tasks, modify the environment, or are used by trained caregivers in the home setting. Devices such as cushions and positioning devices help prevent disability. Other devices can assist in promoting the health of consumers by enabling improved time management or engagement in valued occupations. Examples within this spectrum of intervention possibilities will be useful to show how assistive technologies are applied in practice.

First, one optimal strategy is to reduce the impairments that result in the self-care deficits. For example, if a person is extremely weak and is dependent for self-care, solving the weakness problem would solve the self-care deficit. No assistive technology is required with this first approach. Remediating the impairments alleviates the need for any further intervention. As we know, however, total remediation of an impairment is not always possible.

A second category of intervention for a person with a disability is compensation. For example, a person with hemiplegia secondary to stroke, may not be able to perform standard tasks bilaterally. Activities such as tying shoes may require new techniques, such as one-handed tying. This alters the task.

Another compensatory method is to use assistive technology. Assistive technology can modify tasks to make them easier and more efficient. A simple example is a rocker knife, which can make cutting food during meals an easier task for someone who cannot use one hand.

An example of this type of approach involves a person who has trouble with closures and fasteners during dressing. One effective method may be to get rid of the fasteners so that they are not needed. Pullover shirts can be worn to avoid buttons, and pants with elastic waistbands can be worn to avoid zippers and buckles. Similarly, if someone cannot use his or her oven because of its design or location, the task can be changed by simply using a more accessible microwave oven instead.

Sometimes, what a person can do alone with the assistance of technology can be supplemented with human personal assistance. Preparing table settings, providing occasional verbal cues and reminders, putting on orthoses, and placing a bath bench can each facilitate independent activities. While this approach seems least independent, it can allow a person to make the most use of assistive technology and to maximize activities or parts of activities that can be performed independently. Figure 18.5 provides an example of each of these methods through the self-care activity of tying shoelaces.

It is very important to understand that there are several methods for approaching solutions to self-care problems. Technology represents an approach to self-care problems that must be viewed in concert with other intervention strategies. Technology should always be considered, but only as one of several possible approaches that might be used to solve problems related to daily living skills.

The multiple intervention approach is not unique to occupational therapy. There are advantages to recognizing that problems often have multiple solutions and that sometimes a combination of approaches may provide a beneficial answer. Smith and Sainfort (1989) recommended a model for fitting technology into work environments, using a human factors engineering perspective. The model proposes that four components—the physical environment, the task itself, the organizational structure in which the work takes place, and the technology—interact with each other and with the person's skills

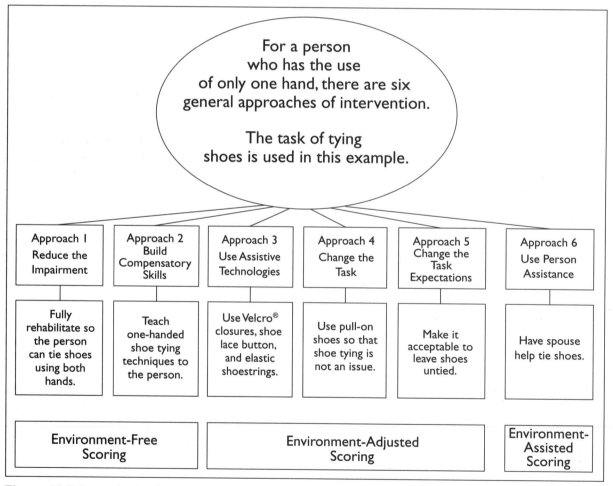

Figure 18.5 Six methods of approaching the self-care activity of tying shoelaces highlights their differences and how they might relate.

and personal attributes to explain outcomes. These components comprise an overall system that determines a worker's level of stress and productivity. Although not discussed in detail here, the idea of balancing intervention approaches is a sensible one to consider in the context of self-care interventions.

History of Self-Care and Technology

Occupational therapy has been applying assistive devices to self-care activities for many decades. Hundreds of articles have been written in journals, and dozens of textbooks and monographs have been published dealing with this topic. Generally speaking, these publications have highlighted do-it-yourself approaches, described existing commercial devices, or focused on product comparisons.

Do-It-Yourself Self-Care Devices

One of the best sources of information about the do-it-yourself fabrication of assistive devices to improve self-care independence is in the *American Journal of Occupational Therapy*. A wide range of devices has been described in this journal over the past several decades. In addition to journal articles, texts and monographs contain fabrication notes and construction ideas for self-care assistive devices. Many include dozens of products with fabrication diagrams and directions and cover topics related to daily living, learning and communicating, working, playing, and materials methods. Other documents are more focused, addressing specific categories of devices or diagnoses.

Publications focusing on do-it-yourself techniques are often viewed as fugitive literature. Many of the documents are published in small print runs and are not cited in mainstream bibliographical sources. They quickly go out of print. Do-it-yourself journal articles do not tend to be referenced in other literature. Often, commercially available devices supersede them.

Many books exist that describe available devices and specific applications. Comprehensive bibliographies with annotations are available in various assistive technology sourcebooks and on disability-related web sites.

Commercial Self-Care Devices

The computer age and electronic databases have improved our ability to stay current and go beyond hard copy books, which quickly go out of date. By using modern electronic database formats, information on an assistive technology can be updated more easily and maintained more comprehensively. Abledata is a key database developed more than a decade ago with support from the U.S. Department of Education. At that time, persons working through a library or other program could access the national computer system using a modem. In the early 1990s, access to Abledata information was extended beyond the central database. A microcomputer desktop version of the database was developed and distributed to persons and programs throughout the country. This desktop version included visual images of devices and other enhancements to facilitate comparisons. Currently, a version of the database is available on the Internet and is maintained through the National Institute for Disability and Rehabilitation Research of the U.S. Department of Education.

Assistive devices have moved from a small set of mostly custom-fabricated devices to the thousands of devices available today in the commercial market. Abledata organizes these devices with a thesaurus of terms. By providing combinations of more keywords to direct a search, the database provides a more focused list. For example, entering the keyword "spoons" provides a list of more than 100 products. By adding the keywords "pediatric" and "swivel," a user can narrow the resulting list to include only those products that might be suitable for a child with limited voluntary movement. The resulting list includes specific brand names, prices, and the addresses of distributors and manufacturers. Products listed may be commercially available, one-of-a-kind or prototype devices, custom adaptations of commercially available products, or do-it-yourself devices. By comparing the information available on devices and products, a suitable recommendation can be made.

Product Comparisons

In the early 1990s, the National Rehabilitation Hospital coordinated several product evaluation projects and published reports for self-care assistive devices, including bath aids, canes, crutches, walkers, patient lifts, transfer aids, scooters, wheelchair cushions, and toilet aids (Irvine & Siegel, 1990; National Rehabilitation Hospital & ECRI, 1992). Such product comparison reports provide a useful consumer guide for the devices reviewed. For example, a volume titled *Independence in the Bathroom* contains 173 pages of toilet and bath aids reviews. The reviews identify product features and specifications such as type of seat (hard or padded), shape, dimensions, inclusion of lid, adjustability of support legs, type of tip on the support legs, pail capacity, and other information.

Also, consumer magazines, such as *Consumer Reports*, are beginning to describe and rate features that are important to persons with disabilities, particularly the aging population. The terminology used, however, is not medical. Nonstigmatizing language such as "ease of use," "comfort," and "safety and security" are the types of relevant descriptors.

Product evaluation and comparison volumes are valuable resources for practitioners. Unfortunately, so many types of technologies now exist that it is becoming impractical to maintain up-to-date and exhaustive evaluative reports for available products.

Historical Summary

Several advances in self-care and independent living assistive technologies have been made over the years. Those changes have affected the role of occupational therapy practitioners. The literature highlights how there has been a slow shift from a do-it-yourself assistive technology orientation to a commercial product orientation. While once occupational therapy practitioners needed to learn how to identify self-care problems, design assistive devices, and fabricate them, today there is a much more pressing need to know what commercial products are available and to understand how to select the most appropriate device. An occupational therapy practitioner's ability to design, create, and modify devices is still an important part of his or her expertise. The need to effectively manage the large volume of available information, however, is an additional required skill for rehabilitation providers.

The move from primarily custom-made to more widely available commercial products has also had a major effect on occupational therapy practice. The wider availability of mass-market self-care products helps promote this consumer empowerment. Years ago, practitioners and other professionals working with persons with disabilities had a prescriptive role in selecting assistive devices. Consumers were usually thought of as "patients" and did not often have an active role in the process of selecting an assistive device. Today, however, the situation has changed. The view of the user has shifted from "patient" to "client" to "consumer." Consumers make their own decisions and need accurate information. Occupational therapy practitioners are in an ideal position to help persons with disabilities develop consumer skills related to assistive technology.

The contributions of occupational therapy in the delivery of assistive technologies have shifted over the years as well. Many of the most helpful self-care and independent living devices for persons with disabilities were developed for and are available as mass market consumer products, sold in department stores or from mail order catalogs. As consumers choose their assistive devices, occupational therapy practitioners have become a key resource: They provide information, instruction, and recommendations. Subsequent parts of this chapter further discuss this new role for occupational therapy practitioners.

Selecting Assistive Technology for Self-Care and Independent Living

The process of selecting the most appropriate assistive technology with a person is based on matching individual needs to the particular features of assistive devices. The context in which the device is to be used (both the task and the environment) is critical. The number of steps required for matching technology to individual needs varies from many (Rodgers, 1985) to a relatively simpler process. Basically, the process of selecting technology is as follows: (a) understanding the potential of technology; (b) evaluating the person within the relevant environments; (c) evaluating technology intervention alternatives; (d) selecting the most appropriate system; (e) acquiring the technology; (f) training in the use, maintenance, and repair of the technology; and (g) monitoring and revising the system as appropriate (Smith, 1991). If these steps are kept in mind, decision-making errors can be minimized. The following techniques and considerations address this overall framework.

Evaluating the Person's Needs and Performance

It is important to begin the process of selecting the most appropriate technology by comprehensively reviewing a person's self-care and independent living skills and the environments in which technologies might be added. This evaluation should include several components (Enders, n. d.). First, all of the activities a person performs need to be carefully evaluated to determine the person's degree of independence without the assistive technology. Assistive technology is only helpful for tasks in which the person is not already independent. Second, it is essential to determine the person's self-care priorities and how independent the person wants to be in each of the specific self-care activities. If a person does not share the practitioner's values about increased independence or efficiency in self-care tasks, then assistive technology is a useless intervention. Third, the helpfulness of assistance for each activity must be examined in terms of the type of assistance provided (e.g., assistive device, attendance, set-up) and the amount of time it takes. Independence and time are a trade-off. Being able to do a task completely by oneself may not be worthwhile if the cost in time is too burdensome. Last, self-care activities must be viewed across all daily activities. Practitioners must not assume that, for example, hygiene and appearance self-care tasks are limited only to morning. In reality, hygiene appearance activities are performed throughout the day in work or community settings. Persons without disabilities carry combs and brushes with them and are able to use them in various locations throughout the day. Persons with disabilities, therefore, should not be limited to using combs or brushes only during the morning routine. The same is true for going to the toilet or getting a drink of water. To summarize, the person's level of independence, his or her priorities, the benefits of the technology, and the frequency of its use must all be considered. Without evaluating all four, it is difficult to select self-care assistive technology.

The instrument used to assess the person's level of independence in self-care activities must be acceptable from an occupational therapy frame of reference. In regard to assistive technology, this means it must first be able to assess a person without the technology. Then it needs to reassess function with the assistive technology to make comparisons and to ascertain the effect of the assistive technology. Thus, the assessment should be capable of measuring both the need and the outcome. It is also important that the functional assessment avoid penalizing function because a person uses assistive technology. Some assessment scoring systems inherently build assistive technology into the scale. This method of scoring results in a definition that makes it impossible to be independent if one uses a device because the outcome score is less than maximum.

OT FACT (Smith, 1992) is a computerized, comprehensive, functional assessment that includes questions about self-care and independent living. Important features of OT FACT include its value as a self-care and independent living assessment and its philosophy and recommended protocol for assessing the effect of assistive technology. OT FACT measures the effect of assistive technology on the overall level of function by using a double-scoring

protocol (Rust & Smith, 1992). OT FACT distinguishes among environment-free scoring, environment-adjusted scoring, and environment-assisted scoring. Environment-free scoring measures how a person performs activities without any assistance or outside intervention and reflects only intrinsic abilities. This scoring is then repeated as necessary to observe the person's abilities over time to evaluate changes in performance. As intrinsic scores are assessed, the parallel environment-adjusted scores are observed. Environment adjustments involve assistive technology and interventions, such as adapting the task. Environment-assisted scoring then includes assistance from an attendant, cueing from a spouse, or hand-over-hand facilitated functional movement. In this way, OT FACT helps monitor the specific needs of a person and not only measures the effect of occupational therapy interventions on the person's intrinsic performance but also reflects the ability of the solutions to supplement a person's intrinsic attributes and skills. Figure 18.6 shows OT FACT headings scored as environment-free scoring and environment-adjusted scoring for a man with a high spinal cord injury using assistive technology.

Identifying Assistive Technology Options

The second step in the selection of assistive technology is to identify the available options for the person based on the assessed needs. This step requires information on the technologies available through commercial and other sources, as well as the ability to determine the quality of the information. Decision making is facilitated if one is able to use the information to reduce the number of possible alternatives.

Locating Information on Assistive Technology

Although many information-searching methods are available, there is no single, unassailable method. No flowcharts or formulas exist to sequence questions or to define the most appropriate answer. Several computerized expert systems that apply artificial intelligence techniques to help locate information are being studied. But state-of-the-art methods are still based on problem solving and intuitive logic and depend heavily on combining skill, luck, imagination, and curiosity. This is true whether one pages through catalogs, examines files, uses the library, or accesses an electronic database. This process is complex. The multitude of technologies on the market today and the constant changes in all the manufacturers' product lines make it virtually impossible

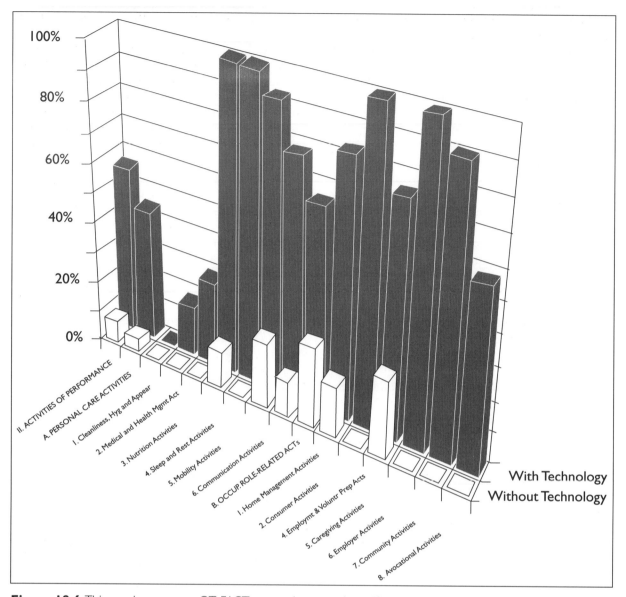

Figure 18.6 This graph compares OT FACT categories scored specifically to compare the functional effect of assistive technology for a man with a high spinal cord injury.

for any one person to know about all the available technologies. In fact, as much as 30% of product information changes each year. Many occupational therapy practitioners feel something is wrong if they cannot immediately provide all of the information needed to help someone with technology needs. Few practitioners, however, can truly do this, even in a focused technology specialty. The key is to know how to use appropriate information resources to obtain the most up-to-date information.

To locate the most helpful information on an assistive technology topic, the search must be focused. A broad request to an information source (e.g., reference librarian, an expert in the field, an electronic database) such as, "Please give me everything you have on X, Y, Z," usually results in a general overview of the range of information available on this broadly defined topic. Or, dangerously, an information specialist may arbitrarily define the topic and provide an entirely wrong set of information. If the information seeker is not aware of how this information was collected and provided, he or she may mistakenly assume that it is the best available. A third response to an information request that is too general is to acquire everything on the topic. Acquiring too much information may not be very helpful because combing through it could be time consuming and confusing.

With assistive technology, well-targeted questions are not always easy to formulate. Therefore, it is helpful to have a complete needs assessment before trying to find the right assistive technology product. Table 18.2 provides a framework of questions that should be answered before trying to find the appropriate assistive technologies.

Bias is a critical factor to remember when a vendor provides information about products. Vendors frequently make user decisions (consciously or unconsciously) on the basis of business decisions, such as what products are in stock at the time, which manufacturers have established accounts, or even which product gives the highest profit margin. Although there are many ethical assistive technology product vendors, they cannot avoid the subtle bias that comes from knowing their own products the best. Even if they suspect there might be another, better, product that they do not stock, it is easier for them to highlight their own. An occupational therapy practitioner must remain open-minded to alternative vendors and products and recognize that information supplied by vendors about their own products may contain bias.

As obvious as it seems, it is important to remember that assistive technologies do not work the same way for every person or in different environments. For example, a grab bar may be a good solution in a

Table 18.2 Helpful Questions to Think Through Before Selecting Assistive Technology

Person and Task Considerations	Product Considerations
What are the major tasks the user wants to accomplish?	What are the motor requirements (range of motion, strength) required for use of this product?
What are the user's functional abilities and inabilities?	Is the product used independently by the consumer or with the help of an attendant?
Motor (i.e., grasp, endurance, range of motion)	What are the size dimensions and environmental requirements of the product?
Sensory (i.e., visual, auditory, tactile)	What safety features are required for using this product?
Cognitive (i.e., knowledge, memory, ability to learn)	What are the power requirements for using this product?
Psychosocial (i.e., willingness to try something new, gadget tolerance, frustration level)	What materials are used, and are they strong enough for the intended use?
Will the level of disability change?	What is the weight of the device?
Is the person independent or attendant assisted?	Is the device portable, or does it require permanent installation?
Will the person need extensive training to use the equipment?	How difficult is the device to clean and repair?
Is the equipment intended for long- or short-term use?	What is the process for getting the device cleaned or repaired?
Are there environmental restrictions such as space or wiring?	What is the warranty?
Is a portable product required?	Are other products needed in conjunction with this product for complete system function?
Will the user need accessories and other options in the future?	What is the reputation of the distributor and the manufacturer of this product?
What are cleaning, maintenance, and repair requirements?	Will this product soon be obsolete?
What resources are available for providing cleaning, maintenance, or repair for the product?	Are there other effective alternatives besides this product?
What are the health and safety considerations?	
What funding is available, and are there budget limitations for purchase?	
What funding is available, and what are the budget limitations for future repair?	

clinical simulation, but in a particular home it may not work in the client's bathtub. When funding is not available to perform evaluations or site visits to the home or workplace, the consumers themselves or a friend or family member should be enlisted to measure the environment. Remembering to consider needs specific to each person and particular environment can avoid unfortunate situations (see Box 18.1).

Evaluating the Quality of Available Information Resources

Before an information resource is used, its content must be scrutinized. The words used to "advertise" an information book (e.g., a guide, directory) or a database usually provide a strong indication of its developers' knowledge. Phrases like "the most comprehensive," "the only up-to-date resource," "a single information resource for all of your needs," or "the complete directory available for the first time,"

Box 18.1

The Perils of Considering Assistive Technology Outside the Real Environment

An occupational therapy department always ordered a particular bath bench for everyone. In principle, it was ideal for a wide variety of persons. However, in this particular department there was no real bathtub to set it up for trial use. When one of the therapists moved to another hospital where there was a real bathtub setting, the usual bath bench was only rarely used. After some investigation, the therapist discovered why. It was never ordered for wheelchair users because the legs in the highest position of the seat were 4 in. below the standard wheelchair seat height with a seat cushion. None of the wheelchair users who received the bench had ever complained at the old hospital—they just did not use it. This is a real problem. Funding for a device is usually available only once in a given number of years. After being purchased, many assistive technologies cannot be returned, and there is no way to obtain a second round of funding.

---

are marketing tools and selling tactics. Information resource developers who are truly knowledgeable and ethical about the quality of their information systems rarely make these claims. They know that any information resource is just repackaged information about other programs or products. To have information available in a directory or database, the developer has to locate, abstract, enter, and edit it. This process usually takes 6 to 12 months. It is not possible for a single source to have all of the information available on even one assistive technology specialty.

The number of entries in a specific resource also provides critical information on how complete it is. A total listing of a few hundred products, facilities, or publications is not a comprehensive guide for assistive technologies for self-care and independent living. Some directories claiming to be comprehensive have relatively few listings.

Some information systems claim to match technology to disabilities. For these systems it is critical to know what decision-making process is used. Although computerized decision aids, called expert systems, will be one of the major advances made in the next 10 years, expert systems are now tentative and futuristic. Occupational therapy practitioners should not take for granted that any information system claiming to locate the products necessary for a person is thorough in its evaluation and analysis of the available products. For example, every self-care activity requires a certain degree of strength, range of motion, and motivation. It is necessary to identify how these factors were included in the process of selecting devices. The knowledge base and credibility of the person classifying the products must be taken into consideration. It is increasingly important for occupational therapy practitioners to be able to recognize the strengths and weaknesses of expert systems that claim to identify appropriate self-care assistive technologies.

The assistive technology field changes rapidly. As mentioned earlier, as many as 30% of assistive technology products have information that has changed within a 12-month period (i.e., new manufacturer phone number or address, new price, new product features, obsolete products). Therefore, it is important to know how old the information is in a resource guide or database and how often it is updated. The high frequency of information turnover also makes it prudent to know the lag time between when the information is collected and when it is received. If the lag time of a collection of data is more than 1 year, it is likely that a large percentage of the information will no longer be up to date. It is also helpful to know whether the update just adds more products or whether it edits the existing product entries.

Finally, it is helpful to know how the producer of the information system addresses quality control issues. Quality control usually includes technical procedures, such as standards or policies, for assigning search vocabulary or indexed keywords. Quality searches require consistency in keyword coding. Systems without careful, consistent coding may identify some key products or information, but similar items coded in a different way would not be found. At the very least, it is important to be aware that this problem can exist and to take it into consideration when planning an information search. If comprehensive information is being sought, several searches using different search strategies might be required.

Refining the Alternatives

Catalogs, databases, and other information resources all help to identify assistive technology alternatives. A few specific tools are provided here to help guide the search process.

A self-care device worksheet (see Figure 18.7) provides a way of formulating a problem-solving approach to help identify assistive device needs. Additionally, it may be helpful for an experienced practitioner to examine the elements on this worksheet periodically to refine assistive device searching skills. Sometimes experienced practitioners can fall into unproductive habits. Reconsidering that the esthetics or durability of a device might be a particularly important feature for a person can be helpful. This worksheet is intended to stimulate thinking regarding individualized needs for clients and to provide a helpful way of taking notes to document these needs.

Once a search of the assistive device alternatives has been made, it is helpful to compare one device to another. For example, five or six bath benches might be selected from a database of information and provided to a consumer to help think through the advantages and disadvantages of each. The assistive device comparison checklist (Figure 18.8) is a way for the practitioner and the consumer to talk through the various options to make a decision. Choosing an assistive device means working with the client or family members in the decision-making process. This step works best when an overview of the entire search and selection process is reviewed with the person who needs to use the products, before starting the search. Once alterna-

tives are identified, the user and the practitioner can compare the options. Ownership of the assistive technology device must transfer from the occupational therapy practitioner, who has the idea that a device might solve a functional problem, to the consumer. The consumer needs to own the device not only physically but also psychologically. If the consumer does not recognize the need for and help choose the particular device, then most likely the equipment should not even be purchased.

Trial Use

When possible, the potential device should be tried before its final purchase. Some devices can be designated for trial use and training within an occupational therapy department. Cooperative agreements can often be set up so that practitioners working independently can borrow products from other occupational therapy programs or agencies. Equipment vendors often stock items that can be borrowed on trial if proper hygiene precautions are followed. Vendors will frequently even arrange a loan from a manufacturer's representative or from the company directly if the product is not in stock. Consumers can sometimes order a device directly through a vendor with an option to return it if it does not work, with the exception of bathing and toileting aids. However, this arrangement may take weeks, which can delay assistive technology device decisions and risks the cost of return shipping.

Occupational therapy practitioners can also use available resources to simulate the item being contemplated as closely as possible or can use a similar product. This simulation might identify potential problems before the final decision is made. Sometimes this means trying a product similar to the one being targeted, accompanied by a discussion of how the actual targeted device differs from the particular one being examined.

Infection control measures always need to be considered before a client uses an item involving personal hygiene contact. Items that are stocked in a department for repeated use should be cleaned and, if necessary, sterilized routinely. Some items considered expendable cannot be returned, cleaned, or reused if personal contact is made. Sometimes disposable covers can be kept on items while a client is simulating an activity. If questions arise regarding correct hygienic procedures, the infection control department of any hospital is a good resource. In today's hospitals, special procedures have been developed for cleaning devices, especially when blood-borne pathogens are involved.

ADL Problem Identified: _____

Proposed Assistive Device: _____
Consideration Factors: (Note any factors that need to be considered.)

Cost:
    Insurance coverage?
    Client's remaining cost?
    Client's budget?
    Other funding options (church, community
       service clubs, diagnostic associations)?	

Psychological Factors:
    How does client feel about using device?
    Considerations they want to be aware of?
    How will device fit into client's body image?	

Physical Factors: (Identify any special needs
for using the device in the following:)
    Range of motion
    Muscle strength
    Sensation
    Cognition
    Perception	

Esthetics: (Note any client preferences for:)
    Color
    Materials
    Style
    General appearance	

Size:
    Where will the item be used?
    Where will the item be stored?
    Will it need to be portable or transported?	

Durability:
    Length of time of proposed use
    Frequency of use
    How hard is client on equipment?	

Maintenance:
    Hygiene considerations
    Replacement parts
    Assistance requirements	

Availability:
    When is item needed?
    Is trial use recommended?	

Operation:
    Will device significantly improve
      client's performance?
    What is the method for retrieval or
      donning or doffing?
    Is assistance available if needed?	

Miscellaneous Discussion: Does client have a personal preference for purchase source? Are family or friends able to assist with any construction?	

Figure 18.7 Self-care device worksheet.

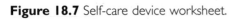

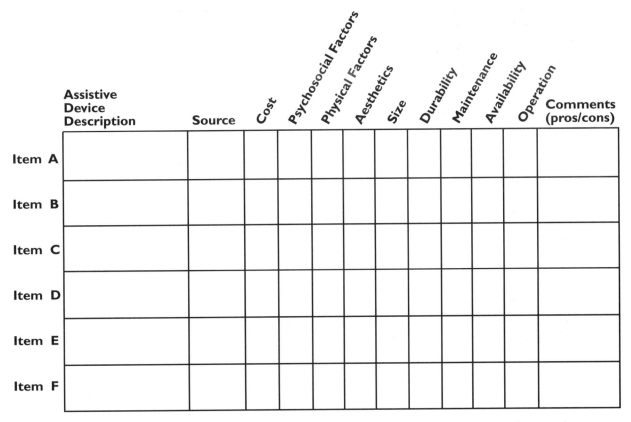

	Assistive Device Description	Source	Cost	Psychosocial Factors	Physical Factors	Aesthetics	Size	Durability	Maintenance	Availability	Operation	Comments (pros/cons)
Item A												
Item B												
Item C												
Item D												
Item E												
Item F												

Figure 18.8 Assistive technology comparison checklist. Use this chart to determine whether client needs are met in the listed areas.

Every occupational therapy practitioner has observed low- and high-technology systems left unused. Home health practitioners routinely find equipment stored away in closets, and clients frequently are not even aware of what they have. To avoid this problem, the consumer and his or her family members must be involved in the product-selection process. One way of doing this is to participate in a trial use of the item. Usually after completing a trial, the client and the family members are equipped to make a decision with the guidance and opinions of the practitioner. An item may be rejected for multiple reasons, and it is important to identify them. Whether the practitioner thinks the item is successful or not is of little consequence. If the client perceives the technology negatively in any way, it is highly probable that the equipment will not be used.

Training

Once the assistive technology decision has been made, training should begin immediately. If the item has been ordered, it may take some time to obtain. Simulated training can often be substituted. It is critical for the user to understand the device thoroughly to use it successfully.

Training should be directed to the user, but it should not stop there. Others in the environment who will be using or dealing with the device also require training. For example, a particular person may use an eating utensil, but it may be washed by family members. Both the consumer and the family members need specific information on relevant aspects of use and maintenance.

Training should always be done with respect to where the client will use the device. Occupational therapy does not usually occur in the person's home environment or in the other environments where the self-care technology might be used. Some self-care tasks may be done differently in the hospital, at home, at school, or at work. Training should consider all of these settings.

The consumer of the self-care technology may need to teach others how it works. Thus, the occupational therapy practitioner may need to help the consumer feel comfortable and skillful as a trainer. The consumer is often the best conveyor of information and training to others who need to learn

349

about a device. It can be very beneficial to have the client actually train another practitioner or family member in the use of the device under the supervision of the occupational therapy practitioner. In this format, if the client has difficulties, the occupational therapy practitioner can help point out missing information or suggest other methods of explaining the features of the equipment.

To optimize therapy's efficiency, it is sometimes helpful to design assignments that the client completes at home independently. On return, the client and practitioner can discuss how the task went. Some of the more complex assistive technologies cannot be learned through quick instruction. Augmentative communication devices and their interface technologies often require extensive training. Thus, it can be very helpful to take the assistive device into the natural environments in which it is used and report back on its success. Sometimes devices require practice, which can be done outside of therapy sessions. The client can then report on how the practice sessions have been going. Training is extremely important for many devices, but it is frequently overlooked. Self-care and independent living devices rarely come with owner's manuals.

Training is not always a one-time occurrence. Sometimes training needs to be reinforced or updated, depending on the particular needs of a person. This may seem logical enough; however, if a practitioner does not set up a follow-up system, it is often overlooked.

Owner's Manual

Much self-care technology is too simple to have an accompanying owner's manual from the manufacturer. It may be complex enough, though, to be confusing to someone who has never seen such a device before. Assistive technologies frequently require special care and maintenance. For example, many devices are made with plastics that can only sustain low levels of heat. Microwave ovens, automatic dishwashers, hot environments, dryers, and car dashboards can easily exceed the plastic's heat tolerance. These kinds of details may seem obvious to an occupational therapy practitioner, but if they are not explained carefully to the consumer, the device may be inadvertently damaged.

It sometimes makes sense for a practitioner to actually write an "owner's manual." Creativity and careful thinking are the keys for writing owner's manuals—they do not need to be restricted to a written format. Making a home video of the consumer using, cleaning, and storing the product is a type of

owner's manual. Audiotaped messages can supplement written instructions. When written instructions are provided, illustrations or pictures are helpful.

Some of the topics that should be included in the owner's manual are proper use, maintenance, precautions, and replacement procedures. Educational research indicates that information targeted to the general public should be geared to a grade-school reading level. It is important for occupational therapy practitioners to be sensitive to this and customize the owner's manual to the particular educational, social, and cultural needs of the client. In any case, wording should be concise. The client and family members should review the instructions before taking the device and should demonstrate that they understand the manual.

Follow-Up

After a person uses a self-care or independent living device, a follow-up procedure is almost always helpful. Follow-up is most effective when it is scheduled during the time that the person is initially given a device. If ongoing therapy is provided, it is easy to reevaluate the use of the equipment periodically. This reevaluation may not be the case if a person lives a great distance from the occupational therapy practitioner, or if funding is not available for follow-up visits. A follow-up schedule might be set up at 6-week, 3-month, 6-month, and 1-year intervals. The success of a system can usually be evaluated, and any modifications, tune-ups, or replacements can be made during those times.

If it is not possible to schedule follow-up sessions with the client, many creative options are available. These include the following: (a) making periodic phone calls to get feedback and to provide support to the client at home, (b) involving other health care professionals if continuing service is provided by someone else—another service provider can give feedback to the initial occupational therapy practitioner on specific issues, (c) tapping an involved case worker or an ongoing advocacy person to provide feedback, and (d) instructing the client to report any problems to the occupational therapy practitioner (if the client is capable). Self-responsibility is an important characteristic, with or without a disability. Telling the client that it is his or her responsibility to stay in contact with the occupational therapy practitioner is often very successful. But practitioners should not use this as an easy way out, and other follow-up mechanisms are often necessary. Although follow-up is the key to maintaining a high quality of service, funding may constrain it.

Occupational therapy practitioners must continually innovate and press for fundable ways to provide these important services.

Funding

Lack of adequate funding can be a major obstacle to improving functional performance through assistive technology. Funding sometimes depends on the setting in which the occupational therapy practitioner practices. Occupational therapy practitioners who charge their time directly to third-party reimbursers (i.e., inpatient and outpatient clinics, home health services) can sometimes bundle inexpensive assistive technologies into the cost of their services. Occupational therapy practitioners who do not charge their services to third-party reimbursers (i.e., practitioners working in school systems) may have a more difficult time acquiring devices for their clients. Although it is beyond the scope of this chapter to discuss fully different funding options and methods for obtaining resources, a few comments are prudent.

Practitioners should know how much assistive technology costs. Costs should always be one of the variables considered when recommending a particular device. The best procedure is to make sure the client and family members are aware of the various costs of the devices so they can factor this in when making their decision. Clients should never be surprised when they receive the bill for assistive technology.

Many federal laws have opened doors for paying for assistive technologies. Even funding agencies that have not yet agreed to pay for assistive technologies may someday concede that assistive technologies are a cost-effective way of improving or maintaining the functional abilities of persons with disabilities.

Another important concept to consider when searching for funds for assistive technology is that any funding agency will only provide payment for specified reasons related to its mission. Medical insurance providers must believe that a particular device is necessary because of the medical needs of a person. Educational funding providers need to believe that self-care devices are important for the education of a student within their system. Vocational funding providers need to believe that the self-care devices may affect the vocational readiness or success of a person seeking or trying to maintain employment. Occupational therapy practitioners may have to write letters of justification to these various funding agencies and orient the wording describing the specific needs for the assistive device to reflect each agency's function.

Funding assistive technologies for self-care and independent living is not a simple issue. It is intricately tied to the mechanisms of service delivery and society's perception of the importance of assistive technology (La Buda, 1988; Rein, 1988). The current funding situation is extremely complex. For many years, it was assumed that health insurance would pay for all rehabilitative and assistive technology. However, health insurance was initially designed to pay for health needs, not for the equipment needed to help someone become independent. In affluent times, third-party payers began funding equipment in the "gray area." Today's economic situation, together with the escalation of costs associated with equipment and the amount of equipment now available, threatens the easy access of funding for assistive technology. How to make insurers pay for assistive technology sometimes seems like the issue, but medical insurers never meant to pay for self-care and independent living assistive technology. There are no easy answers.

Issues Surrounding the Application of Self-Care Assistive Technology

Consumer Empowerment

The role of the consumer in selecting devices cannot be overemphasized. Occupational therapy practitioners in medical settings have historically thought of assistive technologies from an orthotic or prosthetic perspective, with the practitioner or physician prescribing a device for the person with a disability. This conceptual model must vanish. Over the past 20 years, it has become more and more evident from many clinical and scholarly observations that for successful assistive technology use the consumer must "buy in" to the device. The role of a practitioner, therefore, is not to do an evaluation and select a device for a person with a disability but to serve as a resource for helping a consumer do a needs assessment of his or her own disabilities and functional abilities. The practitioner then provides options and suggestions for ways of overcoming barriers to optimal function. Many ways exist for occupational therapy practitioners to include consumers in the process of obtaining and integrating assistive technologies into their lives (Enders, n. d.).

While the client's disabilities and impairments are being assessed, a technology needs assessment

351

can be done as a joint effort between the occupational therapy practitioner and the client. Identifying the particular functional problems and impairments that contribute to the overall dependence of a person (or, conversely, identifying what is needed to assist a person in becoming independent) can be identified by the team. Once the needs have been identified, they can be prioritized, and goals can be set. Again, a team composed of the occupational therapy practitioner and the client works best. When a client is not cognitively or emotionally ready to be involved in this process, the client's family members can act as advocates.

When goals for independence and living have been developed and prioritized, brainstorming with the client helps to identify the full range of possible solutions. Alternatives identified earlier in the chapter can be discussed with the client: (a) remedy the impairment, (b) learn skills to compensate for the impairment, (c) use assistive technologies, (d) change the task so that the person no longer needs to perform it, (e) use assistance for tasks or task components, or (f) use combinations of the above. An action plan can then be developed based on the alternative(s) selected. The occupational therapy practitioner should realistically prioritize the steps in the mutually agreed on plan. If there is a question about the feasibility or availability of resources or skills, the practitioner and client should agree on a back-up plan in case the first choice does not work. The client should also be involved in the training and follow-up methods needed for integrating the technology (see Box 18.2).

Independence Versus Efficiency Trade-Off

A critical trade-off is often made when using an assistive device for self-care or independent living. Many times, assistive devices allow someone to be independent in self-care. This independence can be an important benefit. The cost of a device may be relatively low, and if it actually helps somebody who might otherwise require personal assistance in self-care activities, substantial savings can result. A frequent problem, however, is that even though an assistive device may make someone more independent, it may now take 10, 20, or even 50 times longer to perform the activity independently than if someone simply assisted. Early morning activities are a common example of this paradox between independence and efficiency. Although assistive technology may enable someone to be totally independent in dressing, cleanliness, hygiene, and appearance-related activities, if he or she has a severe motor disability, it might take 3 to 4 hr to perform all these functions independently. A personal assistant could help the person achieve these tasks within 30 to 60 min. Fatigue is also a critical consideration. Independence may result in ineffective functioning during later parts of the day.

From a societal perspective, this situation is a very difficult trade-off. Society can choose to fund the assistive technology, the wages of the personal assistant, or both. This places the decision-makers in an awkward position. Assuming that the assistive technology costs nothing, there is an implicit comparison between the cost of having someone provide assistance to the person with a disability and the lost time no longer available for the person if he or she performs the task independently. Personal preferences are vital. Some persons highly value their independence, whereas others value their time more. Figure 18.9 portrays this problem as a cost-benefit formula.

Prescription or Open-Market Purchase

The issue of consumerism reveals an important paradox. If indeed some assistive technologies and devices are available to consumers in mass market outlets, then why should they not all be available on the open market? Why involve occupational therapy practitioners? A total open-market system might not be any better than the prescriptive system from which we are slowly evolving. When buying laundry detergent or apples from a grocery store, consumers expect to have access to all the information they need to make good purchasing decisions. For a person with rheumatoid arthritis who is purchasing a device, however, this may not be possible. A particular assistive device could be medically contraindicated and might actually stress joints improperly. Depending on how the catalog or department store happens to be marketing the device, a purchase might be made that aggravates the condition. Additionally, assistive technology products are not always easily understood. Consumers purchasing assistive devices often do not have the information they need about options and features and the advantages and disadvantages of each. Figure 18.10 provides examples of some assistive devices.

Occupational therapy practitioners play an important role as an information resource. Additionally, a person requiring an assistive technology device for one aspect of self-care commonly has other activity difficulties that might benefit from another type of assistive technology or intervention. An occupa-

Box 18.2
Consumer Viewpoint on Assistive Devices

C. H. is a woman 38 years of age who has been diagnosed with amyotrophic lateral sclerosis (ALS) for 10 years. She uses a powered wheelchair and requires maximum assistance for all self-care. She has worked with occupational therapy and used a variety of assistive devices as her status has changed over the years.

C. H. As a patient, I didn't know what was out there or what I needed, but I did know what I couldn't do. My first step was to learn what was on the market. Once I did that, trial use was the only way to really find out what would work.

OT Would you have been comfortable purchasing an item without trying it?

C. H. No! I have done that, and it can be a waste of money.

OT Have assistive devices been ordered that you have not used?

C. H. Yes. Mostly things I had not tried. I didn't feel good about paying for something I didn't end up using.

OT How do you feel about having more than one option?

C. H. It's really important to have more than one choice. Sometimes you are not ready for something even though you really need it. Knowing what is out there and being presented with choices helps with that. Pushing someone into a certain device is not a good approach to me, although I realize some people do need to be pushed. It was important for me to be believed when I said I wasn't ready for something and not be pushed. If I had ordered something I was not ready to accept, I probably wouldn't use it.

OT What importance do you place on esthetics?

C. H. It used to be more important to me than it is now, but I like to look as normal as I can. I like things to look as nonmedical as possible. As weak as my neck is, I don't want my head strapped unless I have to.

OT Is cost something of a factor?

C. H. It should always be considered. My insurance is good, so it has not been a factor for me as much as for some people.

OT Has the specific company selected to purchase equipment been important to you?

C. H. Not really. I wanted recommendations from therapists who knew the companies, so I could use someone reputable. I wanted good follow-up if I had any problems and someone easy to contact and help with maintenance if it was needed.

OT What psychological factors do you think are important?

C. H. I needed mental preparation for depending on an assistive device. I found that if I was not ready in my mind, I wasn't likely to use a device. When I was ready, I'd usually think, "Why didn't I do this a long time ago?"

OT How can a therapist assist with this process?

C. H. I don't think they can, other than to provide options and be patient. It is a personal thing that needs to be dealt with in your own mind. It takes time. A good approach for me is to know what my options are. Then when I'm ready, I can pursue getting something. When I first looked at computers to assist me, it was another year before I decided I was ready to get one. When you have to depend on something, you're admitting you've lost something.

OT What do you see as an occupational therapist's role?

C. H. To work with me as a partner. No one wants to be told what to do, but we don't always know what we need. So I see the occupational therapist as a resource and someone who can help me find what will work best for me. And the only way they can do that is to work together with me.

OT How do you feel about homemade equipment verus manufactured equipment?

C. H. Homemade items are usually a lot cheaper and that can be a factor. It doesn't matter to me as long as it does the job. I have known people that can make things for me, but you lose the option of trial use before something is made.

OT If you were not cognitively able to make your decisions regarding obtaining equipment, who would you want taking this role?

C. H. Definitely my family!

Five years later and with more experience living with ALS resulting in quadriplegia, C. H. reports how assistive technology has an interesting characteristic to self-care—privacy.

C. H. The thing I like most about my e-mail is I have privacy again. It is wonderful.

Formula for Optimizing Independence:

Val of Indep + AT Cost + Cost AW – LT Available = Overall Cost

---

Figure 18.9 Simple cost-benefit comparison between self-care independence and time efficiency. Note. Val of Indep = value of being independent, AT Cost = assistive technology device cost, Cost AW = costs of a human assistant's time (e.g., an attendant's wages), LT Available = Lost time available to the person with the disability, Overall Cost = resulting overall cost. Inefficient use of assistive technology may be more costly than having a paid assistant perform the task for the person with a disability. The time it takes a person to be independent in a task is a cost that must be figured in. If one cancels out the assistive technology device cost and the value of being independent, this cost-benefit problem reduces to being simply a comparison between the cost of a human assistant's time versus the lost time available to the person with the disability. Ideally this trade off is not necessary. If a person is efficient in the use of assistive technology, then the costs reduce to being only the cost of the assistive technology. Obviously this is the optimal target.

tional therapy practitioner can provide an overall perspective by asking about other needs and suggesting additional solutions. An important ingredient in this process is for occupational therapy practitioners to have the background and expertise to serve as this resource.

Compliance: An Outmoded Concept

Years ago, from the medical prescriptive model, the word compliance was used as a measure of successful integration of assistive technology into the lives of persons with a disability. It was thought that assistive devices ended up sitting in closets because users did not comply with the direction of health care providers. This issue is important enough to be

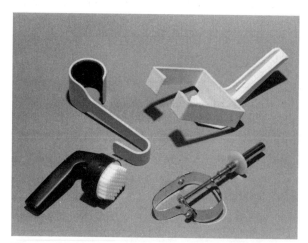

Figure 18.10 The usefulness of assistive technology devices is not always apparent. Trained professionals can often provide important information. Here are a few devices with functions that are not easy to see (door handle aid, suppository inserter, milk carton handle, and portable faucet handle extension).

highlighted here. User selection of and satisfaction with assistive technology indicate its successful integration. Evaluating how well a client complies with the instructions of some professional is an outmoded idea for the application of assistive technology. If a user does not comply with using an assistive technology, it is likely that the consumer was not adequately involved in the selection process.

Rogers and Holm (1992) suggested that more attention be paid to the issue of successful use of assistive technology devices by persons with arthritis. They reported that whereas the literature has definitional inconsistencies with terms and difficulties generalizing across cultures and populations, it does provide information to theorize a predictive model. Rogers and Holm proposed a predictive model that includes the consumer's perspective. Because of the consumer-oriented movement, we will likely see more models that include predictive variables, such as the extent of consumer involvement in device selection and the consumer's stated need for the technology.

Vendor Roles

Occupational therapy departments have sometimes taken on the responsibility of being direct vendors of assistive technology products, particularly in the area of self-care. It made sense for occupational therapy practitioners working in inpatient or outpatient rehabilitation to be able to go to the closet and select a self-care device for use by a person currently receiving services. Consequently a stock of inventory was developed, and occupational therapy practitioners became vendors. Some advantages and disadvantages are found in this approach, and therapy practitioners should weigh the convenience of stocking items with the costs of doing so in comparison to having a preferred supplier or relying on the open market.

Occupational therapy vendor. An advantage of being a vendor of self-care devices is the convenience of being able to provide a device to the client on the spot. When an occupational therapy program is able to vend a product directly, third-party reimbursers sometimes pay for it more readily, as it is incorporated into the occupational therapy costs. Disadvantages of this approach include higher prices because of the occupational therapy department's overhead (i.e., purchasing, managing the inventory, billing). It is also difficult to stock a wide variety of items (e.g., numerous types of wheelchair seat cushions are available, yet very few occupational therapy departments can maintain an inventory of more than a few of them). Consumers often perceive occupational therapy practitioners who have taken this vendor role as salespersons and feel obligated to purchase the practitioner's recommendation when it is handed to them for use in a therapy session. When occupational therapy practitioners are vendors themselves, they fall into the trap of vendors and tend to recommend the items that they know best, which are the ones in stock. This bias limits the consumer's options.

Use of a preferred equipment supplier. Another option is the use of a durable medical equipment dealer or an equipment supplier who has a business in the community. Sometimes focusing on one particular supplier is advantageous because the occupational therapy practitioner can become familiar with the inventory. Another advantage is that occupational therapy practitioners have no direct responsibility for financing the equipment. Consumers then assume some responsibility for purchasing the device from the supplier, which may lead to greater integration of the device into the person's life. A third advantage is that the consumer becomes familiar with the process of obtaining equipment from a vendor in the community and may be more willing to use this system again in the future.

Of course there are some disadvantages to this approach. It is less convenient than buying from an occupational therapy practitioner, and it can be physically difficult for a consumer to get to different locations as needed. Also, there are some fraudulent businesses that have only the bottom-line dollar in mind, as opposed to the needs of persons with disabilities, and take advantage of consumers.

Open-market suppliers. A third vending option is for occupational therapy practitioners to stay out of product acquisition entirely and leave all the procedures for acquiring the device up to the consumer. This option sometimes can be done when a practitioner provides a variety of catalogs to the consumer, who then makes his or her own decisions. It can also be done in large metropolitan areas where many different vendors are available and where a practitioner only has to provide a list of them to the consumer, who can hunt around to find the device from the vendor of his or her choice.

An advantage of this option is that the consumer becomes totally responsible for self-care and decision making. This is likely to lead to a high level of product use because the consumer will have already made a substantial commitment by purchasing the device on his or her own. One disadvantage is that the consumer assumes all financial responsibility. Additionally, consumers are sometimes overwhelmed by the process and simply stop it. Thus, they fail to purchase the assistive technology device even if it may help them. And when dealing with many different companies with extremely good marketing and advertising departments, a consumer can be potentially talked into different, inappropriate items.

In this option, the consumer is responsible for evaluating the vendor. He or she may only be concerned about the purchase cost of the device and buy an item from a fly-by-night operation or from a vendor who provides no services whatsoever. Also, if a client needs something but has to depend on caregivers for its acquisition, there may be a problem if the caregivers do not understand the particular needs of the device or do not take the time to obtain it.

As we have seen, there are many vending options for assistive technologies. None of these options is perfect, but perhaps if all three were made available to the consumer, he or she could choose from the advantages and disadvantages of each. Perhaps the key component that allows any of these systems to work is the role the occupational therapy practitioner takes. If the occupational therapy practitioner serves as a resource for persons with disabilities in self-care and independent living assistive devices, avoids vendor bias, and provides recommendations and options based on decisions made jointly with the consumer, any one of these models can turn out to be of major benefit.

Purchase, Adapt, or Fabricate?

If assistive technology has been decided on as a component of a person's intervention to optimize independence and efficiency, buying a device may not be the best answer. Another approach is to take a mass market or special assistive technology device and further adapt it for the particular needs of a person. A standard table utensil might only require a built-up handle. With the help of a technician or an engineer, an occupational therapy practitioner can design and fabricate assistive technologies from scratch that exactly match the particular needs of the person when other approaches do not work.

Cost is an obvious variable when deciding to purchase, adapt, or fabricate. Unfortunately, cost is not a simple variable. There are two types of costs involved in this discussion: (a) the assistive technology or the parts and materials and (b) the time of the person who designs, adapts, or fabricates the device. These costs need to be examined on a case-by-case basis. In some circumstances, many human resources are available for design and fabrication, but few resources are available for purchasing materials or parts. Examples are a school system, veterans' administration hospital, or community agency. In these situations the professional's time is already paid for, but supplies and equipment are additional lines in the budget that are not directly reimbursed.

Some settings can pay for materials and parts, but they cannot withstand personnel costs associated with the equipment's design, adaptation, and fabrication. Examples are occupational therapy departments in hospitals, home health agencies, or other medical programs in which the time spent with assistive device design and fabrication would be charged to third-party payers for reimbursement. When this cost is compared with the off-the-shelf price of an assistive device, it often becomes much more prudent simply to purchase the equipment.

A second obvious consideration in the decision to purchase, adapt, or fabricate is whether a mass market device is available, whether a device is available but needs to be adapted, or whether no device exists. Practitioners must be aware of what assistive technologies are already available. It is pointless to design a device if one already exists. Once again, this awareness emphasizes the importance of knowing (or being able to learn) what assistive devices are available.

Some commercially available devices are simply better made and may come with a warranty. The qualitative difference between a do-it-yourself product versus a purchased commercial product must also be considered.

Family Members, Friends, and Consumers as Experts

One of the most important resources available to occupational therapy practitioners is commonly missed. Many persons begin to develop assistive technology solutions on their own before encountering an occupational therapy practitioner. It is extremely important for the occupational therapy practitioner to know what assistive technology solutions have already been integrated into the person's lifestyle or what strategies are already being developed. In these circumstances, the role of the occupational therapy practitioner can be that of an advocate and adviser. Many consumers and their family members and friends have power equipment, innovative ideas, and much untapped ingenuity that need to be part of the assistive technology formula.

Special Needs in Long-Term Care

Clients in long-term-care hospitals, nursing homes, day-care programs, and community-based residential facilities are somewhat unique in their technology needs because they may not have consistent support available to them. In addition, the support personnel they encounter may have little education about assistive technologies and how they are used. Occupational therapy practitioners for assistive technology consumers in these types of settings should help integrate the devices into the long-term-care agency. The residential team must know how to use the assistive technology appropriately so that disuse does not occur by default. Even worse than disuse, it has been observed that assistive technologies that are highly valued by the consumers are sometimes withheld as punishment, or teams may unthinkingly withdraw the use of technology. Occasionally consumers in these facilities are not capable of being their own advocates because of cognitive or emotional limitations. Therefore, it becomes important for occupational therapy practitioners to examine the environment in which the assistive technology will be used and to ensure that support personnel understand its importance and application.

Impoverished Settings

Access to assistive devices is not equal for all person of different socioeconomic status. Dealing with disability in developing countries, impoverished inner cities, or rural areas often requires unique interventions. In many cases, potential users of assistive technology have limited access to medical care, even less access to rehabilitative care, and no money to purchase devices. It is important for occupational therapy practitioners to understand the situation and to apply special, creative, and innovative technology solutions for persons who do not have access to the resources available to many settings.

Low-cost construction of assistive devices or second-hand strategies may be useful. For example, fabricating wheelchair-accessible work surfaces using tri-wall cardboard or surplus materials may be possible when accessible furniture cannot be purchased. Or self-fastening closures on clothing or a wash mitt may need to be added instead of ordering finished items from catalogs. The occupational therapy practitioner may need to use professional expertise and innovation in applying skills in splint making, sewing, and other fabrication technologies.

Social policies that prevent the appropriate application of self-care and independent living assistive technology are often important. They also may be the most difficult to remedy (Enders, 1988; Enders & Heumann, 1988). Although occupational therapy practitioners should be innovative in the application of assistive technology, they must also be aware of the need to advocate for change.

Training Preservice Students

The field of assistive technology has changed dramatically over the past several decades and will continue to do so. This dynamic state of information change constantly challenges classroom teaching and fieldwork education. An issue that has not yet been adequately addressed by occupational therapy curricula is how self-care and independent living assistive technologies are best taught. Should there be an entire course in these assistive technologies? Should the information become part of an overall assistive technology course or should it be part of a set of technology courses? Or should it be integrated across all of the core disability-oriented courses in the curricula? Although there are no clear best methods for teaching self-care and independent living assistive technologies, two options seem to make sense. First, self-care and independent living assistive technologies need to be taught across the preservice training curricula. Technology needs to be discussed as an intervention option as each type of disability area is covered. This means technology

should be deliberately taught during fieldwork education. Second, additional elective and independent study opportunities should be made available for the students who desire more depth in this area. The complexity of assistive technologies is increasing, and the occupational therapy profession must take great care to assure that new students receive adequate information pertaining to assistive technology.

Teaming With Other Professionals

The role of occupational therapy in self-care and independent living assistive technology seems quite evident. Occupational therapy practitioners must assess the self-care needs of persons with disabilities comprehensively and help in the matching process so that consumers of technologies can make their best decisions. But occupational therapy practitioners cannot perform this function by themselves. The consumer and his or her family members need to be core team members of the process. Additionally, other professionals are immensely valuable members of the assistive technology team. For example, performance in self-care activities depends highly on mobility, and physical therapists have substantial information about the self-care technologies pertaining to walking and other mobility activities. Speech and language pathologists have extensive training and expertise in augmentative communication methods. Nurses know more than most occupational therapy practitioners about the particular self-care activities dealing with bodily functions, including bowel and bladder activities, and milieu self-care activities, such as sleeping. Additionally, technicians can help adjust, adapt, troubleshoot, and even fabricate assistive technologies for particular needs and for complex cases. Engineers are particularly qualified for design when it is necessary to invent and fabricate a piece of equipment not commercially available. This sampling of the roles of team members highlights the fact that occupational therapy practitioners must function as members of a multidisciplinary team when applying assistive technologies.

The Future of Assistive Technology in Self-Care

Higher electronic-based technologies will continue to advance and provide new opportunities for self-care management. Persons with severe disabilities may find more and more resources, such as using robots for their own cost-effective self-care management. Of course, the need will continue for improvement and for better applications of the low-technology solutions. With thoughtful research, occupational therapy practitioners can apply technology more wisely and efficiently. The occupational therapy practitioner will increasingly be a key source of information. Identifying and clarifying problems, pointing out what self-care technology solutions are available, and describing how the technology can be obtained will be vital to helping consumers make good decisions (see Mann & Lane, 1991).

Practitioners cannot maintain a complete knowledge base of all of the assistive technologies available. The number of products and their different features is increasing at an exponential rate. In the future, we may find larger clinics hiring assistive technology specialists. If every clinic had one resource person with a focused knowledge base, all staff members would not feel pressured to stay abreast of the latest technology developments. Funding assistive technologies in self-care will continue to be important. Although awareness of the need for assistive technology is increasing, the future direction of social policies (and thus, the availability of resources to support it) is unknown.

The growing interest in and emphasis on outcomes in health care and rehabilitation may influence future societal decisions about services that can or should be provided to persons with disabilities. It will be necessary for occupational therapy practitioners, whose models of practice blend traditional remediation and compensatory approaches within person-environment models of care, to demonstrate that many methods contribute to positive outcomes. ◆

Study Questions

1. How many assistive technology devices are available today and how prolifically are they used?

2. How has occupational therapy incorporated assistive technology in practice over the years?

3. What populations benefit from assistive technology devices and how widely used are assistive technology devices?

4. What are examples of assistive technology devices for each category of devices?

5. What is the relationship of assistive technology interventions compared with other intervention approaches?

6. What are comparative advantages of "make-it-yourself" assistive technology devices and those commercially available?

7. How do the concepts of patient, client, and consumer relate to assistive technology?

8. What does independence mean relative to assistive technology usage?

9. How does OT FACT draw out the effect of assistive technology?

10. How fast is the assistive technology field changing and what are strategies for accessing current expertise in practice?

11. What does an assistive technology owner's manual look like?

12. How is the funding of assistive technology unique?

13. How might consumer and practitioner viewpoints of assistive technology differ?

14. What are primary mechanisms for a consumer to acquire assistive technology devices and services?

15. What is the independence versus efficiency trade-off?

16. What are some of the unique challenges to service delivery of assistive technology and ideas for meeting these challenges?

References

Enders, A. (n.d.). *Spinal Cord Research Foundation briefing paper: Rehabilitation/technology: Daily living.* Unpublished manuscript.

Enders, A. (1988). Technology to assist physical function and aid independent living. In *Proceedings of ICAART 88, the 1988 RESNA Conference* (pp. 568–571). Washington, DC: RESNA.

Enders, A., & Heumann, J. (1988). How adults with disabilities get the everyday technology they need. *Proceedings of ICAART 88, the 1988 RESNA Conference* (pp. 580–583). Washington, DC: RESNA.

Irvine, B., & Siegel, J. D. (1990). Product comparison and evaluation: Canes, crutches, and walkers. *Request evaluating assistive technology.* Washington, DC: ECRI.

La Buda, D. R. (1988). Assistive technology for older adults: Funding resources and delivery systems. *Proceedings of ICAART 88, the 1988 RESNA Conference* (pp. 572–575). Washington, DC: RESNA.

Mann, W. C., & Lane, J. P. (1991). *Assistive technology for persons with disabilities: The role of occupational therapy.*

Rockville, MD: American Occupational Therapy Association.

National Rehabilitation Hospital & ECRI. (1992). Independence in the bathroom. *Request evaluating assistive technology.* Washington, DC: Author.

The Oxford Dictionary of Quotations (3rd ed.). (1980). London: Oxford University Press.

Parker, M. G., & Thorslund, M. (1991). The use of technical aids among community-based elderly. *American Journal of Occupational Therapy, 45,* 712–718.

Rein, J. (1988). Technology to assist physical function and aid independent living for children ages 0 to 21. *Proceedings of ICAART 88, the 1988 RESNA Conference* (pp. 567–579). Washington, DC: RESNA.

Rodgers, B. L. (1985). *A holistic perspective: An introduction. A future perspective on the holistic use of technology for people with disabilities.* Madison, WI: Trace Research and Development Center.

Rogers, J. C., & Holm, M. B. (1992). Assistive technology device use in patients with rheumatic disease: A literature review. *American Journal of Occupational Therapy, 46,* 120–127.

Rust, K. L., & Smith, R. O. (1992). Use of functional outcome measure to assess covariate dimensions of function. *Confronting our future.* Chicago: AAPMR, ACRM.

Smith, M. J., & Sainfort, P. C. (1989). A balance theory of job design for stress reduction. *International Journal of Industrial Ergonomics, 4,* 67–79.

Smith, R. O. (1991). Technological approaches to performance enhancement. In C. Baum & C. Christiansen (Eds.), *Occupational therapy: Overcoming human performance deficits* (pp. 747–786). Thorofare, NJ: Slack.

Smith, R. O. (1992). *OT FACT* [Computer program]. Rockville, MD: American Occupational Therapy Association.

19

Self-Care in Context: Enabling Functional Person–Environment Fit

Pearl Sarah Bates

Pearl Sarah Bates, MA, OTR, is an occupational therapist residing in San Francisco, California.

The author thanks Karen Mae Kaeter, Jean Cole Spencer, Margaretta Newell, June Long, Harlan Tjader, Thea Sheldon, Bill Quinn, and Johnnie Hyde for their generous assistance in the preparation of this chapter. The author also thanks her professors in the Occupational Therapy Departments of the University of Minnesota and Texas Woman's University for teaching the principles expressed herein. Finally, the author thanks her patients for teaching her about the importance of the self-care environment and why it needs to be made negotiable for all.

Key Terms

negotiability

press

self-care environment

sensory environment

social press

Objectives

On completing this chapter, the reader will be able to

1. List and explain the major implications of at least two laws affecting the self-care environment.

2. List factors to consider when recommending changes in someone's self-care environment.

3. Define the term negotiability.

As a relatively new practitioner, I once explained to a client who used a wheelchair that her bathroom could indeed be made accessible—it was only necessary to replace the in-cabinet sink with a pedestal or wall-mounted sink and add a sliding door in one wall. The client said nothing. Over the course of a week, however, it became apparent that she was not motivated for therapy, but she denied it when questioned. Eventually the client's daughter came privately to the clinic and explained the situation. "You see, mom has never felt comfortable with you since you told her to put in a different sink. She just got that bathroom redecorated after years of waiting, and she was really offended that you just told her to get rid of her new sink."

"But she can't get into the bathroom the way it is," I protested. "She may never get into it again."

"I know," replied the daughter. "But she doesn't care about that."

"You mean, she'll take bed baths for the rest of her life and use a bedside commode, just to avoid changing her bathroom?"

"Yes," replied the client's daughter. "That's exactly what I mean."

"So what I really need to do is help her order a bedside commode and tell her she doesn't have to redo the bathroom after all."

"Now you understand," replied the daughter.

The moral of this story is that we as occupational therapy practitioners must not assume that our clients have the same values and beliefs that we do. Just because an occupational therapy practitioner believes that functional independence should be the client's goal, that does not mean the client necessarily agrees. For some persons, the appearance of the home may be far more important than the ability to use it functionally. It is their absolute right to hold such beliefs. In evaluating and adapting the self-care environment, as in all occupational therapy interventions, our role is not to remake our clients according to *our* standards: Our role is to help them live according to their own.

Definitions

This chapter describes the self-care environment. Before proceeding, it is useful to consider the following definitions, which provide a foundation for understanding the concepts to be presented later.

Self

The self encompasses all that a person is, including one's beliefs about selfhood. These beliefs differ among cultures, religions, philosophies, scientific theories, and individual self-concepts. They range from the belief that one is simply a living body, of which mind and emotion are manifestations of biochemical processes, to the view that a "self" is an immaterial soul temporarily inhabiting a relatively unimportant material body. Because of this range of beliefs about the self, self-care activities can vary from bathing and dressing to prayer and meditation.

Care

The concept of care encompasses both attitude and action. The attitude of care is one of loving concern. In this context, self-care activities are the actions that preserve our bodily health and personal well-being and are not limited to specific activities of daily living (ADL). At the physical level, self-care activities consist of the maintenance of bodily temperature, hydration, nutrition, elimination of wastes, and prevention of injury. Care of the self includes related activities, such as grooming, which raise and improve our social and psychological well-being. The higher-level or instrumental activities of daily living are activities that support, make possible, and lend meaning to basic self-care tasks. These include household management, laundry, shopping, banking and money management, use of the telephone, reading of the newspaper, health maintenance, religious practices, recreational and creative pursuits, familial and social relationships, and community mobility.

While these distinctions seem clear-cut, they are not. Often difficult choices have to be made between long-term and immediate well-being, between comfort and sometimes painful healing processes. The client, his or her family members, and staff members may not always agree on the strategies to improve the well-being of the client. Determining what actually constitutes self-care for a given client in a given environment requires good judgment on the part of the occupational therapy practitioner.

Environment

The self-care environment is the complex, ever-changing, natural, built, physical, psychosocial, cultural, economic, and political setting in which the person cares for his or her own well-being. Because we must always do what is needed to maintain life and health, we are in the self-care environment all the time we are alive.

Our self-care is influenced by all aspects of our environment—natural, built, and social. Research indicates that the performance of basic and instrumental activities of daily living varies depending on the environment in which they are performed (Brown, Moore, Hemman, & Yunek, 1996; Nygard, Bernspang, Fisher, & Winblad, 1994; Park, Fisher, & Velozo, 1994; Schmitt, Kruse, & Olbrich, 1994). For this reason, self-care skills are best evaluated in the setting in which they are to be used. The environment in which treatment takes place influences functional self-care outcomes for populations as diverse as geriatric clients with dementia and recovering alcoholics (Landefeld, Palmer, Kresevic, Fortinsky, & Kowal, 1995; Timko, 1996).

Not only does the environment influence our self-care activities, but our self-care activities affect the environment in which we perform them. Persons with special needs are part of the self-care environments of their family members and caregivers. Some self-care products are dangerous to the natural environment, such as sprays that damage the ozone layer. Our wastes, unless properly treated or composted, become biological pollutants. Like all people, persons with special needs must make difficult choices between their personal needs and the needs of others. These difficult choices extend beyond the home to the global environment—planet Earth is a self-care environment for all living things, including humans.

Intervening in this system of client-in-environment, of client-attempting-to-care-for-self-in-environment, is a complex task. How can the practitioner be conscious of the full environment, take into account the client's individuality, and figure out how these two interact and how to intervene so as to improve the client's situation? We can answer this question by saying that there are no answers; however, increased awareness on the part of the practitioner lead to better working solutions. Thus, this chapter identifies issues in the self-care environment to heighten the practitioner's awareness so that he or she can apply creative problem-solving ability to improving the interactive fit between the self-care environment and the person with special needs.

Negotiability Versus Access

A Case Study in Environmental Negotiability

A woman in a sports wheelchair enters the cafeteria line at a nationally known rehabilitation center. She reaches a tray on a low shelf and balances it carefully on her lap as she wheels to the short-order area. The ventilation fan over the grill is so loud that she cannot make herself heard. Her head is below the level of the top of the counter. The cook cannot see her until he comes over to take the order of a standing person. When her order is ready, the cook sets it atop the 4-ft-high counter: there is a wheelchair-level counter in front of the high counter, but it is out of the cook's reach. With difficulty, the woman reaches her food and proceeds to the beverage area.

The canned sodas are in a refrigerated case on a standard 30-in.-high counter. She can reach only the lower two shelves. Her preferred selection is on the highest shelf. She looks around for assistance, but no one is in sight, so she gives in and takes the beverage container that is within reach, even though her own brand is a mere 12 in. away.

The counters are not continuous from one area to another. To get from the beverage counter to the checkout, she has to balance her tray, unevenly weighted with her plate and beverage can, on her knees while propelling her chair. She must then lift the tray from her knees to the checkout counter, pay her bill, lift the tray back onto her knees, and negotiate the ¼-in. ridge from linoleum to the carpeted dining area without spilling. Because she is a complete paraplegic, she is unable to adjust her legs to keep the tray in balance. By a quick grab with her hand, she saves the sliding tray. She has a choice of two types of tables: large round ones, which are accessible, and small square ones, which do not provide enough leg room for her wheelchair footrests. Dining alone, she would prefer a small table rather than sitting conspicuously alone at a table for eight, but she has no choice. At last she reaches her table and places the tray on it. Because of her slow progress, her meal is cold by the time she begins to eat.

In the United States, laws ranging from the Education for all Handicapped Children Act (1975) to the Americans With Disabilities Act, Accessibility Guidelines for Buildings and Facilities (1991) mandate that public spaces be made accessible to persons with disabilities. To the occupational therapy practitioner, functional independence is an equally familiar concept. To determine the effects of the environment on self-care, there is the need for a third concept that joins the ideas of access and independence. Negotiability refers to "the ability to access a feature of the environment and use it for its intended purpose, with only one's usual adaptive equipment" (Noris-Baker & Willems, 1978). This definition should be amended with the phrase "in a manner acceptable to the person." The need for a concept of negotiability is made clear by the preceding example. The cafeteria is accessible, but it is only marginally negotiable.

Evaluation

The occupational therapy practitioner may be called on to discern what the client's usual self-care environment is, and whether the client can become capable enough to return there. If so, how should the environment be adapted?

Before the home visit, the practitioner should conduct a thorough interview with the client (and with as many household members as possible) to become acquainted with the client's usual range of self-care activities. A simple, nonthreatening way to conduct such an interview is to ask the interviewee to review a typical day at home. This should be done with as much detail as possible, beginning with waking up and proceeding through getting up, the morning routine, and so on through the day. As each event is recalled and described, the practitioner should ask, "And what do you do after that?" until the pattern of the day emerges.

In evaluating the home environment, the practitioner will find that a home visit is well worth the time involved, as major differences in performance are found between clinic and home settings (Brown et al., 1996; Nikolaus et al., 1995; Nygard et al., 1994; Park et al., 1994; Rogers, Holm, & Stone, 1997).

Negotiability Rating

A thorough home visit should include a negotiability assessment. A negotiability rating differs from most self-care or ADL assessments in that it rates the person's performance in the environment, using adaptive equipment. Most self-care instruments focus solely on the person's ability to perform without specifying context.

The negotiability assessment begins with a careful inventory of all features of the home environment, starting with the approach to the door.

Table 19.1 Sample Negotiability Calculation

Number of environmental features:	76
Number negotiable:	42
Calculation:	$(42 \div 76) \times 100$
Negotiable environment = 55.26%	

The practitioner then retraces this path with the client. During the assessment, the client is asked to try to use each environmental feature for its intended purpose, with only his or her usual adaptive equipment. These activities include opening and passing through the front door, obtaining water from the sink, and transferring on and off the toilet. The client is asked to try each feature, regardless of whether he or she usually does so. Any environmental feature that cannot be used by the client should be noted, with descriptions and measurements (if appropriate) of factors that limited the function. For example, an observation note might read: "Cupboard not negotiable—client cannot reach in (6 in. above top of comfortable reach, 3 in. above maximal reach)." Once the list has been completed, the negotiability rating can be obtained by computing the proportion of the features negotiable by the user. This is a simple percentage calculation (see Table 19.1). This calculation is useful for documenting measurable changes that result from occupational therapy intervention. For example, if the practitioner provides adaptive equipment making two more features negotiable and recommends environmental adaptations that would make four more features negotiable, the rating would increase (see Table 19.2).

Table 19.2 Changes in Negotiability As the Result of Occupational Therapy Intervention

Environmental features:	76
Original number negotiable:	42
Number added by occupational therapy intervention:	6
Number currently negotiable:	48
New rating: $(48 \div 76) \times 100 = 63.42\%$	
Original rating = 55.26%	
Improvement = 8.24%	

It must be stressed that negotiability represents the interplay of the person, the environment, and the adaptive equipment. Negotiability cannot be assessed in general terms; it can only be assessed for the individual person in his or her own environment. Its strength as a concept, therefore, is that it is sensitive to changes in all three areas.

A negotiability rating is not a self-care scale in the ordinary sense. It does not rate the person's ability to perform in general. It rates only the person's ability to perform in a given environment with given equipment. It is not an activity-analyzed rating system. In other words, the units being rated are not units of performance, they are units of the environment. An environmental feature is negotiable—or not—for a given person, with given equipment. For an item to be negotiable, the person must be able to perform all logically related tasks or task components. That is, to negotiate a door, one unlocks a lock, turns a doorknob, opens the door, passes through a door frame, and closes and locks the door.

In rating negotiability, environmental features are left in their usual positions. They may be moved later as part of the intervention. In other words, if the person could possibly sit on a chair, but the chair is in an inaccessible corner, then the chair is not negotiable unless the person can reposition it un-aided. Negotiability is not rated in terms of levels of assistance required, as self-care skills often are. If a person requires minimal assistance to open a door, that person is still unable to negotiate the door independently. Ratings of relative degrees are useful to show progress in treatment settings, but to determine the person's ability to go home and function independently, the expected standard must be full independent performance. A person who needs minimal assistance to perform his or her self-care cannot be left alone in the environment any more than can a person who needs maximal assistance. For this reason, negotiability, the scale that measures the person's relationship to the self-care environment, is an "all or nothing" scale—either one can perform independently or one cannot. As a person's performance skills improve through occupational therapy intervention, his or her negotiability rating in a given setting should also improve.

To obtain an accurate rating, it is important to make an inventory of the individual environment. The list of features in Table 19.3 is provided merely to draw the reader's attention to areas of the self-care environment that may be neglected.

Although assistive technology issues are dealt with in a separate chapter, they are mentioned here because the practitioner must consider their effect on negotiability when assessing a client in his or her environment. Equipment or device factors bearing directly on negotiability include the size and weight of the devices, the presence of operating noises, the type and position of controls, the type and position of signage, and the type and position of feedback systems (whether visual, auditory, or tactile).

Human factors bearing directly on negotiability include a person's physical size, strength, coordination, endurance, sensation, perception, cognition, mode of mobility, nature of impairment, learned skills, emotional status, living arrangements, and personal values. Person-related factors that influence negotiability are dealt with in detail in other chapters of this book.

Table 19.3 Environmental Features and Associated Functions

Environmental Feature	Associated Function
Floor surface (each type)	Traverse floor
Light switches	Turn on and off
Doorways	Open door, traverse, close door
Chairs (each style)	Transfer onto, sit on, perform relevant functional tasks while sitting, and transfer or arise from chair
Table, desks, counters, workbenches	Approach surface and perform appropriate tasks (e.g., eat at table, work at desk or counter)
Storage (shelves, etc.)	Place and retrieve items
Windows	Approach, open, close, operate blinds or drapes, look out each window
Appliances	Approach appliance and perform all aspects of operating it
Outdoors, yard	Work in garden, operate grill, eat at picnic table

The environmental factors that have an effect on negotiability—and, consequently, on self-care performance—include structural characteristics, surface characteristics, type and location of fixtures and furnishings, lighting, acoustics, temperature, environmental press, and social press.

- *Structural characteristics of the environment* refer to the natural and built aspects of the environment, that is, buildings, sidewalks, hills, trees, and other relatively permanent environmental features.

- *Surface characteristics* include texture, firmness, appearance, and wear characteristics.

- *Fixtures* are portions of the environment that are not structural in nature but are relatively permanent. Often these facilitate self-care activities. Fixtures include toilets, bathtubs, light fixtures, and built-in cabinets.

- *Furnishings* include nonpermanent environmental features added to a structure for the physical and emotional comfort of the inhabitants.

- *Lighting* refers to natural and artificial sources of light. Both the quality and the amount of light are important.

- *Acoustics* refers to the behavior of sound waves in the environment and their effect on human auditory perception.

- *Temperature* refers to the thermal comfort (hot or cold) of the environment.

- *[Environmental] press* (Murray, 1938, et passim) is defined as the "kind of effect an object or situation is exerting or could exert upon the subject . . . which usually appears in the guise of a threat of harm or promise of benefit to the organism." Thus, press refers not to the way the person feels about the environment (i.e., loves it, hates it) but rather to the potential effect of environmental factors on the organism's ability to maintain itself, that is, perform its self-care skills. Therefore, the presence of obtainable nutritious food is a positive press, whereas the presence of food that is out of reach, as in the nonnegotiable cafeteria line, is a negative press. It should be self-evident that the press of an environment for able-bodied persons who are cognitively and emotionally intact may be very different from the press of that same environment on a person with impairments in any of these areas.

This is a separate issue from the person's perceptions of the press (i.e., what he or she believes is positive or negative in the environment). For example, a person with recent paralysis may feel that the world outside the rehabilitation facility "is just not prepared for wheelchairs to be all over the place" (Bates, Spencer, Young, & Rintala, 1993).

- *Social press* refers to the presence or absence of another human and how this circumstance influences the performance of the person. This includes the emotional effects of that person's presence (or absence), as well as his or her potential to physically further or hinder the self-care process.

Our self-care skills are influenced by our relationships with those around us. We may imitate their styles or rebel against them. We are also influenced by the responses of others to the ways in which we perform our own self-care. As children, we are taught self-care by our parents. During this process, we absorb all sorts of largely unstated expectations as to what to eat and how to feed ourselves, what to wear, and how to perform our hygiene and grooming. Children are, sometimes harshly, socialized by peers in school, who may be quick to make fun of those who appear to dress "funny," to eat "weird" food, to be dirty or too fussily clean and neat. The social environment seriously affects self-care practices from adolescence onward. Some elderly clients who are retired from their jobs may be relieved to have simpler social environments in which to function. But there are other persons whose self-concept requires formal dress even in old age and ill health. It is therefore essential to communicate with the client and determine that person's definition of "self" and what constitutes "care" for him or her.

In its broadest sense, social press includes all the cultural and societal forces acting on the person's self-care performance. These include tradition, law, economic status, religion, and the unwritten but powerful force of social approval or disapproval. The ultimate punishment for failure to meet social standards is exclusion from the group. Therefore, social press is often the single most powerful environmental force acting on a person's self-care standards and on the person's decisions regarding the self-care environment. This helps to explain studies that have shown that social acceptability is an important criterion in the acceptance and use of assistive technology.

The Home Environment

The most obvious setting for the performance of self-care tasks is the home. This is fortunate, because we can adapt these environments to our own needs and wishes. Despite the great gains being made in the accessibility of public spaces (within the United States) with the implementation of the Americans With Disabilities Act (1990), public spaces can never be as well-tailored to the person as private spaces are. This is not only because of discrimination but also because of the differing needs of different persons. An environment fitted solely to the needs of a wheelchair user would be inaccessible to a walking person, and a Braille signage system would be unreadable by the sighted.

Space and Layout in the Home

A well-laid-out floor plan facilitates self-care, whereas a poor one inhibits performance. Seven general principles to be observed in designing or arranging floor plans are cited in Table 19.4 and discussed in greater detail below.

1. *Allow enough space for ease of mobility, but no more.* Excess space forces a person to travel greater distances between tasks and raises the cost of construction, maintenance, heating, and cooling. For example, a "strip" style kitchen, with two facing counters, can be quite negotiable. Both counters can be reached with minimal repositioning of a wheelchair or with few steps for the person who walks with difficulty.

2. *Arrange the layout so that sequential tasks can be performed with little or no travel in between.* A bathroom off the bedroom requires less travel than one located down the hall. A kitchen with a pass-through to the dining room eliminates many steps. Of course, the pass-through should be at a reachable level for the wheelchair user.

3. *Place built-in controls (e.g., light switches, thermostats) where they are easily reachable or where they provide the least inconvenience.* A person who has difficulty getting out of bed should be able to reach the con-

Table 19.4 Principles for Layout of the Self-Care Environment

---

1. Allow enough space for ease of mobility, but no excess.
2. Limit travel between sequential tasks.
3. Position built-in controls where most often used.
4. Limit changes in level.
5. Limit interior doors.
6. Be aware of lighting, acoustics, and temperature.
7. Build in safety features.

---

trols from the bed, or a remote control system should be provided.

4. *Limit the number of changes in floor level.* Level change refers to steps, ramps, and elevators, as well as changes in floor surface, such as from linoleum to raised carpeting. All level changes require extra effort and sometimes present risks to persons with motor, sensory, or perceptual deficits. For some wheelchair users, a small step is passable. Nonetheless, doing a "wheelie" almost guarantees that whatever items are carried will fall to the floor. In the case of the laundry, this is inconvenient but in other instances, such as if a plate of hot food is spilled on one's lap, the outcome could be serious.

Steps present a great risk to the person with sensory or perceptual deficits who may trip or fall because the step cannot be seen. Brightly colored strips can be added to mark the edges of steps for those with residual vision. Textured strips can be used for the blind. The safest approach is to eliminate the step altogether.

Ramps are useful for wheelchair users. A grade no steeper than 1 in 8 over a 20-ft run is sufficient for most wheelchair users (Sanford, Story, & Jones, 1997). Nonetheless, a ramp is less negotiable than a level floor. Going over a ramp while using any sort of mobility aid requires effort. The prosthetic feet of the amputee often do not allow for dorsiflexion or plantar flexion sufficient to allow walking up or down a graded surface. A person with perceptual deficits is at greater risk on a ramp than on stairs, because he or she may not notice the grade at all, and thus may fall.

Home elevators and stair lifts allow entry to an otherwise inaccessible top floor in an existing home. However, in designing a new space, one should remember that a stair lift necessitates two transfers. An elevator requires travel across a troublesome opening, because there are spaces in the floor where a caster or a crutch tip can get caught. Reliance on mechanical devices also leaves one vulnerable to power failure. This is especially important when planning for fire and earthquake safety. A second mode of exit must be planned for the person who could be trapped upstairs.

5. *Limit the number of interior doors.* Everything from fire codes to the need for privacy and warmth requires the use of doors. Within existing constraints, however, one should eliminate as many doors as possible. Opening and closing doors is always a challenge for the wheelchair or walker user. Many doors have sills to trip over. Doors narrow the available opening in doorways by

approximately 2 in., often enough to prevent the passage of a wheelchair. The turning of doorknobs is a risk for the arthritic hand. For the person with cognitive deficits, doors also present the risk of getting locked in or out.

Careful layout will limit the need for privacy doors. If a person's private bedroom has a private bath and closet, there is no need for a door on either the bathroom or the closet. Curtains can be used to screen either of these spaces if desired.

6. *Plan for the sensory environment.* The effect of the environment on the human sensory system can mean the difference between dependence and independence in self-care. Lighting, acoustics, and temperature each play a part in environmental negotiability.

Adequate lighting, without glare, is essential to the performance of many self-care tasks, including grooming, cooking, and money management (Cate, Baker, & Gilbert, 1995; Lampert & Lapolice, 1995; Rosenthal, 1995). In addition, the ability to see out a window may greatly enhance a person's sense of well-being. Windows should be low enough for all to see out, and the controls for the windows and drapes should be within reach.

A person with diminished vision, relying on auditory discrimination for spatial orientation, may be rendered virtually incapable of function in a noisy environment. A person with auditory-processing deficits may be unable to discern what is said in an echoing room. This factor affects functional communication, including use of the telephone.

Temperature affects muscle tone, which increases with the cold. This has a functional effect on all persons with spasticity, including those with cerebral palsy, traumatic brain injury, stroke, and spinal cord injury. Sudden blasts of cold air, as from an air conditioning system, can cause spasms that temporarily diminish upper extremity control. The author, as a clinical practitioner, once accompanied a group of seven persons with quadriplegia to a restaurant. All went well until the restaurant's air conditioning system started up. Suddenly, one after another, the seven began to spasm and jerk their arms about, out of control. It became impossible to continue with dinner. At first, some were embarrassed; then someone commented that this was a good way to diet, and everybody collapsed in a fit of giggles. The manager was politely asked to turn down the air conditioning, and dinner proceeded without further mishap.

7. *Consider safety when laying out the floor plan.* Starting at the front door, one should make sure there are safety peepholes at the eye levels of all inhabitants. Wheelchair users and children are especially vulnerable to intruders when they are home alone. Built-in electronic door controls are useful for those unable to physically open or close a door.

Environments should be planned to assure safe exits from bedrooms during fires or emergencies. A slide makes a workable fire escape from an upstairs window. At the same time, one does not wish to invite break-ins. It is difficult to balance these two concerns, and decisions must be made based on the relative risks in a given setting. A city home may be more liable to a break-in, whereas a cabin in the woods is at greater risk from fire.

Fixtures

When determining the basic layout of a home environment, one must take built-in fixtures into account. The most important fact to consider is that they take up space. It is necessary to calculate the turning space for a wheelchair with the fixtures in place, rather than in an empty room without fixtures. A 60-in.-diameter space is needed to turn a wheelchair, a 34-in. width is needed to travel comfortably in a straight line, and a 48-in. width is needed to transfer (i.e., there should be 48 in. between a bed and a wall or 48 in. of clear space directly in front of a toilet).

Bathroom fixtures. A common mistake in the layout of wheelchair-accessible bathrooms is the failure to account for the floor space taken up by the toilet. An adult wheelchair measures approximately 48 in. from front to back. This means that at least that much clear space must be allotted to allow the privacy door of a bathroom stall to close behind the back wheels. Many bathrooms labeled with the universal symbol of accessibility fail to meet the accessibility standards required by law. This misleading signage is a source of much frustration for wheelchair users. The ADA "standard" for toilet stalls requires a 60-in. by 60-in. space, with the toilet in the opposite corner from the door to allow for transfers (ADA, 1991, p. 35501). Any other layout will make it impossible to get into position for a transfer. An alternative stall approved by the ADA allows for transferring only if the person backs into the stall.

Lengthened oval pedestal sinks are practicable for the wheelchair user. Exposed pipes should be covered with insulating foam to prevent burns to limbs without sensation. Wheelchair users have difficulty using cabinet-style sinks because there is no way to face the mirror, to lean over to spit out toothpaste, or to perform other morning routines. If space permits, a roll-in shower is preferable for wheelchair bathing; however, it is important to position the faucets within reach of the bather. It is easier for someone with limited hand function to hang something on a hook than on a rail. Also, the presence of towel bars invites their misuse as grab rails, sometimes with disastrous results. Roll-in showers are large and tend to be chilly. A heat lamp and a long shower curtain may be useful in this regard. A second choice is a standard shower with a tub transfer bench. The least preferred option is a bathtub with a tub transfer bench. Bathtubs are difficult to use because of the need to lift paralyzed legs over the edge of the tub to get onto the bench. Sliding glass doors on bathtubs are also problematic, so it is preferable to hang a shower curtain.

Regardless of the type of shower selected, the objective is to leave enough room to position the wheelchair for a transfer. A common problem is the location of the toilet, which is often placed adjacent to the tub to save floor space or construction costs. Although this practice may represent both sound plumbing and sound economics, it is not very workable for the bathroom of any person requiring a tub bench. This includes not only wheelchair users but also anyone too weak or too unsteady to lower himself or herself into the tub, such as persons with stroke, Parkinson's disease, cerebral palsy, and other conditions. Enough space must be allowed for the person to sit on the edge of the bench, swing his or her legs around safely, and then lift them into the tub.

Kitchen fixtures. The selection and positioning of kitchen features are strongly influenced by the type of impairments to be accommodated. For geriatric clients, the availability of microwave ovens increases independence in cooking, frequency of cooking, and variety of diet (Kondo, Mann, Tomita, & Ottenbacher, 1997).

Efficiency expert Lillian Gilbreth (1927; Gilbreth, Thomas, & Clymer, 1959) determined that the most efficient kitchens are organized so that they form a triangular path from stove to refrigerator to sink. This arrangement requires much less walking than a straight-line kitchen, where all the appliances are on one wall. The triangle formation can be created in a number of ways, but not all work equally well for all persons with impairments.

For the person who can walk but uses a walker, crutches, or two canes, the problem is how to carry items from one place to another. For such a person, it is best to set up a triangle with a continuous countertop connecting the three points. This arrangement enables the person to slide heavy items over the counter on a hot pad or wheeled trivet. For the wheelchair user with good upper-extremity strength, a narrow facing setup, with the oven and refrigerator on one wall and the sink on the other, may work well. Such persons have the strength to lift a pan or bowl across the space. Depending on the width of the passageway, it may not be necessary to move one's wheels to do so. For all persons, as much storage space as possible should be located between hip and shoulder levels to avoid the poor body mechanics of bending or overhead reaching.

Appliance height is another key factor. Standard counters are too high for the wheelchair user but too low for a tall standing person with a back injury. Appliances that require stooping, such as most ovens and dishwashers, are problems for both groups. If at all possible, ovens should be set up on counters between the shoulder and elbow height of the user. The wheelchair user will need a kneehole under this counter and a clear countertop right beside the oven or microwave oven on which to set hot food dishes. Side-opening doors, rather than swing-down doors, also enhance access. Oven racks that pull out easily and are stable in the forward position are extremely helpful as well.

The stovetop should be separate from the oven and placed at an accessible height. The kneehole for the stovetop should be shallow and should *not* extend under the burners. Kneeholes under the burners present a risk because the food could boil over and spill through the burner onto the knees of the cook. Clear counter space beside the stovetop is needed for placing hot pans.

Another important factor is the negotiability of appliance controls (Steinfold et al., 1979). In most cases, stove controls should be in front of the burners so that there is no need to reach over hot burners to turn off the stove (see Figure 19.1). There is one exception to this recommendation: Recessed controls may be preferable for a person with poor gait control or visual impairments, who could bump the stove and inadvertently turn on a burner. If they are not recessed, the controls should sit flat on the stovetop, not in a vertical layout on the front. For a person with sensory deficits, larger dials with high-contrast letters may be helpful, whereas dials with tactile feedback, that is, they "click" in at each

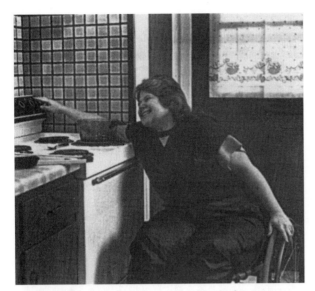

Figure 19.1 Stove controls should be in front to minimize the risk of burns.

heat level, can aid the blind person. A raised bump should mark the "off" setting for such a dial.

If the dishwasher can be raised, it should be positioned so that the open door is just over the lap height of the wheelchair user. This position enables the person to get close enough to reach in. A dishwasher with a front-opening door and pullout racks is the easiest to use in this position (see Figure 19.2).

Refrigerator selection depends on individual needs. Wheelchair users should avoid the freezer-

on-top style, unless it is a small apartment-size model. Side-by-side and bottom freezer models are more accessible (see Figure 19.3). For the person who cannot stoop, freezer-on-top and side-by-side models are the best choices. If financially feasible, features such as exterior water or ice dispensers can be useful to the person who has difficulty opening refrigerator doors. If a separate freezer is selected, the front-opening models are much more accessible than the top-opening chest freezers. Some clear counter space should be available next to the refrigerator or freezer, on the opening side of the door, so that the person can set down the items removed from storage.

Sinks should be at a comfortable working height for the person, usually 2 to 4 in. below elbow height. Because a wheelchair sink must accommodate a 27- to 29-in. kneehole, a shallow sink will fit best. Sufficient space must be left underneath for insulation to prevent hot water pipes from burning the user's knees (see Figure 19.4). The same sink will not provide optimal working conditions for both a wheelchair user and a standing person. If a kitchen is shared, a decision must be made either to build two sinks or to let one person be the sink's primary user. As each person should have his or her own "work-triangle," the building of two sinks is far less costly than purchasing two stoves or refrigerators, so it may be a reasonable option for some families.

For the person with arthritis, poor hand control, or weakness, the lever-type single faucet con-

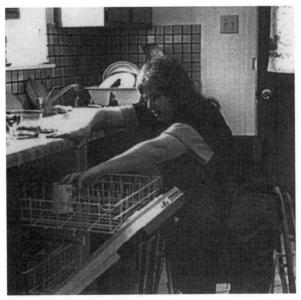

Figure 19.2 This dishwasher is virtually inaccessible.

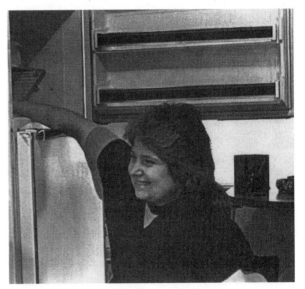

Figure 19.3 The refrigerator with freezer on top is a poor design for the wheelchair user.

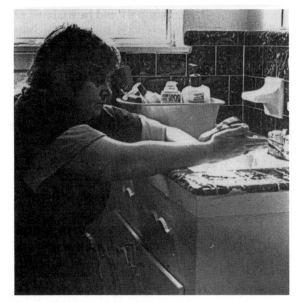

Figure 19.4 A cabinet-style sink is extremely awkward for the wheelchair user.

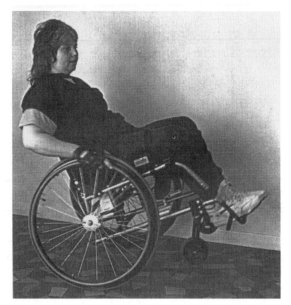

Figure 19.5 A tile floor is a great surface on which to tip back into a wheelie and relax.

trol is best. Conversely, for a person lacking coordination, adjustment of the lever-type control can be extremely difficult. Such a person could better control water temperature by using separate hot and cold faucets. Dual controls are also easier for the visually impaired person to operate.

Counters for wheelchair users should be lower than those for standing persons. The height should be selected for the person, if at all possible, as wheelchair heights and comfortable working levels vary. In general, a kneehole should allow 27 in. to 29 in. of floor-to-undersurface space. Kneeholes should be deep enough to allow the person to pull all the way into the counter: 19 in. minimum depth and 30 in. minimum width.

Because cupboard doors present access problems for the wheelchair user, it is better to have as few doors and drawers as possible. Open shelves and pull-out racks require less reaching, bending, and maneuvering.

Surfaces

The general principle for persons with mobility impairments is that surfaces should be firm and smooth, but they should still provide enough traction for good control and enough cushioning to prevent tissue breakdown. For the wheelchair, walker, crutch, or cane user, a smooth, uncarpeted floor, such as linoleum, hardwood, or tile, is by far the easiest to negotiate (see Figure 19.5). Anyone

who has ever attempted to propel a wheelchair through 2-in. deep pile carpet will appreciate this point. Any carpets that are used should be relatively firm and flat, such as indoor-outdoor carpeting. They should be firmly nailed down, with no protruding nail heads to puncture wheelchair tires, and their edges should be neatly covered with metal or plastic edging strips. Loose area rugs should not be used where there are persons with sensory, cognitive, or motoric mobility impairments in the environment.

For the wheelchair user, especially the novice, wall coverings should be sturdy and resistant to chipping. Nonglare surfaces are preferable for persons with visual impairment. Decorative mirrors and stark white laminated plastic should be avoided. The surfaces of built-in features such as countertops should also be nonglare, as well as being easily cleanable for those with weak hands or who have poor leverage for scrubbing. Counters that are easy to maintain are essential for wheelchair users, who are unable to position themselves for scrubbing. Solid color laminates (not white) are probably a better choice than decorative tiles or porous wooden butcher-block countertops.

Furniture

When purchasing furniture, consumers with a disability should consider function and quality of construction as well as appearance and comfort. Some functional considerations are as follows.

- *Ease or difficulty of transfers onto and off of beds, chairs, and couches.* As the old saying goes, "a lot of things are easier to get into than out of." This is especially true of waterbeds and overstuffed couches, which should be avoided. A firm surface that is level with the top of the wheelchair cushion provides the best support for both directions of transfer.

  The presence or absence of bed rails influences the simple process of getting out of bed. Bed rails, while useful for safety and repositioning, may be designed to prevent the person in the bed from lowering them. This makes it difficult to get out of bed unaided. (Persons with dementia, who do not understand that bed rails make it hard to get out of a bed, sometimes accomplish this difficult task)

  If a bed is too high, the person may have difficulty getting his or her feet on the floor for a transfer. If it is too low, it may be difficult to do an uphill transfer into a wheelchair or rise to standing. The best approach is to observe the principle that one should limit level changes. Level transfers are easiest in the long run. Most hospital beds are too high to allow for such transfers, unless the wheels are removed. Many regular beds are too high or too low as well. Bed heights are not standardized as table heights are. Bed heights can be adjusted either by using furniture leg extenders or by having carpenters shorten the lengths of legs. Chairs can be dealt with in the same manner.

- *Quality of positioning or postural support.* The supporting surface should be firm or structured enough to provide a solid base of support for functional activities. Many persons sit on the edge of the bed to dress. For such a purpose, the bed must be of the correct height, roughly 18 to 25 in. and should be firm enough so that the person can lean against it or sit on it in a stable manner. The person with poor balance may have to dress in bed. It is easier to dress on a wide bed than on a narrow one, because most persons who dress in bed must roll from side to side to pull up their trousers or pants. Although bed rails may be of assistance in this process, they often limit independent movement from the bed. A person with a spinal cord injury of C-7 or below can push to a sitting position on a firm mattress and, consequently, can dress independently. This cannot be accomplished on a soft mattress. A quadriplegic at the C-5 or C-6 level will be likely to require an electric bed to attain a sitting position to reach his or her feet to don slacks, socks, and shoes (Smith, 1988).

- *Interface pressures between the person's skin and the supporting surface.* Surface pressures must be distributed so as to limit the risk of decubitus ulcers (Krouskop, 1992, et passim). A medical sheepskin between mattress and sheet may help. If an egg crate mattress is used, it should be placed with the flat surface up for best results. A well-baffled waterbed can provide pressure relief without making transfers too difficult. Specialized pressure-relief beds, such as the air-fluidized beds, are very costly, but they can be essential for high-level quadriplegics with a tendency to a breakdown of the skin.

- *Texture of the supporting surface.* Shearing of fragile skin may occur if one slides across a rough bedspread or couch. Yet there must be sufficient friction to keep the person from sliding off the seat. Many persons with mobility impairments select satin sheets to ease turning in bed. However, some persons find that such sheets do not provide enough traction for pushing to a sitting position.

- *Allowance for position changes.* Is the chair, bed, or couch adjustable or does it provide only one position? Not all persons require these features, but they are very important for those who do. Powered beds are important for persons whose personal care is performed, all or in part, by others. The ability to raise the bed to an appropriate working height can prevent the caregiver from developing back strain.

  Chairs with powered assists can help weak persons to rise to their feet. Care must be taken in selecting these chairs, however, for if the assist is too fast, an unsteady person could be thrown forward into a fall. Before purchasing such a chair, one should make sure that the assist stops lifting when the button is released. The recliner chair is advantageous for persons on home dialysis. Tables that can be adjusted for height are useful if persons with different positioning needs may be using the same space at different times.

- *Functional considerations.* Does the item of furniture facilitate or inhibit the independent functioning of the person or persons in question? Can the person not only access the piece of furniture but also perform whatever functional tasks are generally performed using that item? Can he or she actually write at the desk; sleep, dress, and engage in sexual activity in the bed; watch television from the couch; and so forth?

  Tables and desks must be the correct height and, for wheelchair users, have adequate knee space. Shelves should be at a level that the person can reach. Persons with lower-extremity amputations, or anyone with a knee or back injury, should avoid low shelves. Conversely, high shelves are

373

out of reach for the wheelchair user. In general, no shelves should be placed so high that anyone's neck is hyperextended. Because shelves lack the front board to hold contents in place, they are potentially messier than drawers. For this reason, fewer items can be neatly placed on a shelf than can be put in a drawer with an equivalent surface area. More total square ft of shelf space must thus be allotted than if drawers were to be used to store the same items. However, shelves provide more usable storage for the same amount of floor space than do drawers.

- *Safety*. Furnishings that limit the risk of falls or other injuries should be selected. Loose scatter rugs are accidents waiting to happen. A thick rubber mat should be used if cushioning for the feet is desired at a sink or counter. Bath mats should have nonskid bottoms. They should be used only for bathing and should be hung on the side of the tub at other times to decrease any chance of slipping.

- *Selection of furniture*. The person who will use the furniture should be present when it is selected. That person must be the final judge of its esthetic acceptability. Increasingly, persons with disabilities have become informed consumers and active advocates on their own behalf. This movement is completely in concert with the occupational therapy principle of functional independence. Table 19.5 presents some factors to consider when selecting furniture.

Atypical Self-Care Environments

A practitioner may have clients from varying social and economic circumstances. The homeless person living outdoors in a city may lack facilities for personal hygiene and yet may possess a range of self-

Table 19.5 Considerations in Selecting Furniture for Persons With Disabilities

1. Ease of transfers
2. Postural support
3. Risk of skin abrasions or ulcers
4. Surface texture that aids or inhibits position or movement
5. Adjustability
6. Effect on function
7. Safety factors
8. Consumer involvement

care competencies that are unknown to the average housed person. He or she may know, for example, which churches serve free meals, which sleeping locations are ignored by the police, and other information necessary for survival and well-being on the street. Practitioners practicing in remote areas may have clients who use outhouses instead of indoor plumbing and whose drinking water must be hauled from a pump or lake. In such cases, although the general principles cited above still apply, the practitioner may have to figure out creative solutions for the immediate circumstances. For example, a taller wooden seat can be built in the outhouse or a commode can be set up in the cabin.

Out on the Town

Given adequate financial and other resources, the home environment can be made fairly negotiable for a person with relatively stable abilities and impairments. The public self-care environment is far less user friendly. Whereas legislation and increased public awareness have resulted in some improvements, many attempts to make public spaces more accessible and negotiable have been ill conceived or unsuccessful.

So-Called Public Toilets

A major problem in public access is the failure of either the lawmakers or the builders to thoroughly think through functional considerations. The two methods of wheelchair-toilet transfer illustrated in the text of the ADA (1990) are both unnecessarily difficult and risky. The easiest and safest transfer—a 45° angle approach—is not shown. Many of the bathroom layouts recommended by law are marginally accessible at best. A quick examination of wheelchair bathrooms in restaurants reveals that the symbol of accessibility is not based on an awareness of the actual requirements for their use by persons with disabilities (McClain et al., 1993). Thus, a wheelchair-accessible sink may be provided, but the paper towel dispenser is across the room and situated 5 ft from the floor.

Level transfers are far easier than uphill or downhill ones. Toilets in accessible stalls should be at least 19 in. high. This height will also be helpful for persons who can walk but have difficulty getting up. The doors must swing toward the outside, not into the stall. There must be enough room outside the stall to maneuver into the door, as well as enough room inside to shut the door. An adult wheelchair measures at least 48 in. from front to back. The standard toilet stall recommended by the ADA (1990) accommodates a wheelchair of this dimension; however, the alternative stall does not.

For a person on a self-catheterization program, a toilet stall should provide a small shelf on which to place the cath kit. One also needs 48 in. of clear space directly in front of the toilet to drain the catheter into the toilet.

Eating Out

Second only to difficulties with bathrooms are the difficulties encountered when attempting to eat in public (McClain et al., 1993) (see Figures 19.6 and 19.7). Fast food restaurants are notorious for high counters. Bars are filled with tall stools and high tables. Restaurants with built-in booths may have no place to sit in a wheelchair or to transfer out of one. It requires real assertiveness to order popcorn in a crowded, noisy cinema lobby when one's head is below the level of the counter. Then carrying the popcorn through the double doors into the movie becomes an adventure in itself. In addition to the obvious self-care problem of obtaining nutrition, these situations present problems in social well-being as well. It is difficult and embarrassing to take a date out for dinner when one cannot use the salad bar. Salad bars are virtually unreachable from a wheelchair because of the height and angle of the bins.

For persons with a limited ability to self-feed, the social aspects of the self-care environment may

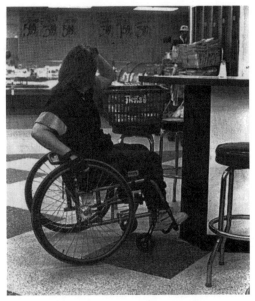

Figure 19.7 This snack bar is only for those who can climb.

be challenging indeed. To be forced to ask someone to feed you in public can lower anybody's self-esteem. An even more difficult situation involves the use of a feeding tube; for someone in this circumstance, going out for lunch with friends moves into the realm of the impossible.

Obtaining Beverages

Maintaining adequate hydration can also become a challenge. Although wheelchair users can operate the coin slot of beverage vending machines, they are generally unable to reach the dollar-bill slot. Even if the slot for the bill can be reached, it is difficult for most persons, in a position of full shoulder flexion, to align the bill correctly so that the machine will accept it. Most water fountains are too high, and those positioned for wheelchair users are often too low or lack kneeholes. Water coolers with paper cups are a better option.

Shopping

Obtaining food to cook and eat at home can also present problems (Spencer, Krefting, & Mattingly, 1993). Some grocery stores provide power scooters with grocery baskets on the front. These vehicles are especially useful for persons who can briefly stand up to obtain items from high shelves but lack the balance or endurance to walk all around the store. Simply pushing a grocery cart may provide enough stability for a walker user who has fairly

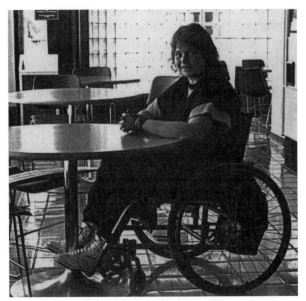

Figure 19.6 A pedestal table and tile floor make this snack bar easily negotiable.

good balance, provided there is a safe place to leave one's own walker while shopping.

Shopping from a wheelchair presents a great challenge (see Figure 19.8). Because the person cannot push a grocery cart, purchases must be limited to what can be carried in a basket on the lap or in a backpack slung behind the chair. Many items are simply out of reach. One person described the experience.

> It seems like they are just trying to make you feel as helpless and weak and useless as possible. You're always having to ask for help when you don't want to. It's "Excuse me ma'am, would you mind doing me a favor?" all the time. I'd rather do things for myself, but I have to do my shopping somehow, and they have so much of the stuff out of reach. I just hate it.

For the person with sensory or perceptual deficits, the overwhelming amount of visual stimuli can make the grocery store a very difficult environment. Waxed linoleum floors may create glare, further challenging the person with limited vision. For such persons, it is best to use a single store and memorize the layout. An alternative is to make a simple map of the store, marking the locations of the items most often purchased. The person can then photocopy a number of the maps and use one instead of a grocery list as a guide around the store. This system also works well for clients with post-traumatic brain injury or others who easily become disoriented in the high-sensory-stimuli environment of the store.

For persons who rely on wheelchairs, crutches, or walkers for mobility, transporting groceries to the car is another hurdle. Some stores do provide carry-out services, but the problem then develops when the person arrives home. A wheelchair user has difficulty getting groceries out of the trunk because so much leverage is required to lift large bags. Thus, only small quantities of items can be transported at a time, or willing neighbors must be recruited to help. A large wheelchair backpack with a relatively rigid frame may be useful; however, the person should be careful to avoid twisting and injuring his or her back while attempting to lift such a pack. It is better to remove items from the pack than to lift the full pack from the back of the chair. A person who walks but has limited ability to carry items may want to use a cart.

The purchases must still be put away in the cupboards and refrigerator once the person arrives home. Typically, because of the transportation difficulties, the person obtains only a small supply of groceries at a time, so he or she must repeat this procedure more frequently than an able-bodied person.

Some grocery stores have a delivery service, but the cost is often too great for persons on fixed incomes. Nevertheless, these services are very useful to those who can afford them. A chore service may also provide shopping services or may provide someone to accompany the person to the store. If the person lives with other family members, delegating the shopping to someone else may be the best solution.

Health and Appearance

Some self-care activities are directed not only toward survival but also toward health and appearance. Many persons join health clubs to work out, buy clothes to improve their appearance, wear makeup, shave, and style their hair.

Beauty shops and barbershops present a real problem for wheelchair users because many find it impossible to transfer into the chair. A haircut can be given in the wheelchair, but this has several disadvantages. The wheelchair inevitably collects hair

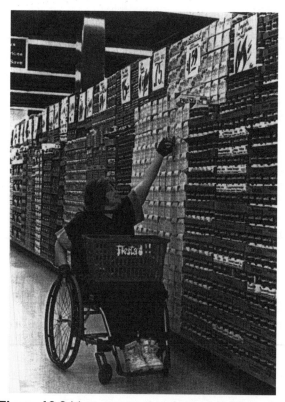

Figure 19.8 Most supermarket shelves have items out of reach of the wheelchair user.

clippings even when a drape is used, and the stylist cannot optimally position the person to cut the hair.

Wheelchair users must also contend with the fitting rooms in clothing stores. Newly constructed clothing or department stores often have dressing rooms with benches; this allows the person to transfer to the bench to change clothes and view the mirror. The new ADA regulations call for a bench 24 in. wide and 48 in. long. Although benches of this length aid some persons, they are not long enough for most adults to lie on, and then many persons are still unable to try on clothes before buying them. Trying on clothes is an option only for those who can dress or undress themselves completely in a wheelchair—and then only when the dressing room is large enough to accommodate the chair.

Another factor to be considered is maintaining personal safety while shopping. When a wheelchair user attempts to get into a car along with shopping bags, he or she is at risk for a holdup. It is thus wise to carry mace or some other personal safety device and to have a car phone to call for help. A cellular phone is preferable to a citizens' band radio because anyone can answer the call with the latter. The range of the cellular phone should extend to the area of the person's daily travels, as well as long distance if the person is traveling out of town.

Using Self-Service Laundries

Self-service laundries present major challenges to persons with disabilities. Whether at home or at a public self-service laundry, a person in a wheelchair is likely to be frustrated by a top-loading washer. The last sock will inevitably be just 2 in. out of reach. The use of a long-handled reacher is essential in this situation, so the wheelchair user must bring one along with the laundry. In most cases the folding tables in a self-service laundry are designed for the standing user—above the level of a wheelchair user's head. Factors such as these combine to make the use of a self-service laundry virtually impossible for the wheelchair user. Potential solutions are either to use a laundry service or to have a household member do the laundry. Clean, dry clothes can be brought home, where the wheelchair user can contribute by folding or putting them away.

Health Maintenance

Preventive health care is an important aspect of caring for the self. We are taught from childhood to have regular physical and dental checkups. Annual gynecological examinations begin in adulthood, and mammograms are started at 35 years of age. It is an odd paradox that the self-care settings of the health care system are among the least accessible in the public environment. The ADA (1990) devotes less than a page and a half of its accessibility guidelines to medical care facilities, and physicians' offices are not even mentioned. Facilities such as chemical dependency treatment centers, maternity hospitals, and burn units are often not accessible to wheelchair users (Gans, Mann, & Becker, 1993; Jones & Tamari, 1997; Kirby, O'Keefe, Neal, Bentram, & Edlich, 1996; Moore, 1997; Shuman & Bebeau, 1994; Tyas & Rush, 1993).

Even rehabilitation hospitals, which are designed for persons with physical and cognitive limitations, can be inaccessible, although the patient rooms in such hospitals or units are generally designed better than those in other types of hospitals. The rooms usually have closets with lowered rails and larger bathrooms with roll-in showers. However, these rooms are often set up for nursing care, not for self-care. Thus, the shower is large so that the nurse can roll the patient into it with ease, after the patient has been undressed and the nurse has procured the towels and soap. The nurse can then transfer the patient to the shower chair and proceed.

If the patient tries to shower independently in such a bathroom, however, the fact that it is not user friendly becomes obvious. The towels are stored in a high cabinet down the hall. There is no place to hang one's clothes after removing them. There is no place to put shampoo bottles and cream rinses except on the floor. This problem applies to both wheelchair users and walking patients who cannot bend safely. The towel hooks are frequently not within reach of the shower. Patients in rehabilitation are often taught to undress in bed for safety reasons. However, the clothes that have been removed must be put on the floor or on the bedside table—neither of which is an acceptable solution. A hamper placed beside the bed would solve this self-care problem.

Travel

Traveling is a particular challenge for the person with special self-care needs. In an unfamiliar setting, the person is constantly faced with unexpected conditions and may require forms of assistance that are not needed at home (Monnot, 1988). In some cases, the person may want to carry an information card to avoid having to repeat his or her special requirements (see Figure 19.9).

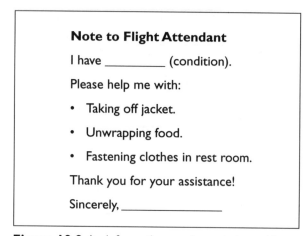

Note to Flight Attendant

I have _____ (condition).

Please help me with:

- Taking off jacket.

- Unwrapping food.

- Fastening clothes in rest room.

Thank you for your assistance!

Sincerely, _____

Figure 19.9 An information card may help avoid repetitive explanations.

Many persons with mobility impairments find it easiest to travel in their own vehicles. A van or a recreational vehicle is often more convenient than a car. The person can, in a sense, take his or her own negotiable home along for the trip. In the United States and Canada, there is a growing number of accessible campgrounds. A van, however, can be parked in virtually any campground. If the interior conversion has been well planned, the person's own self-care needs can be met in the vehicle. The van lift selected should be one that takes up as little of the van's interior floor space as possible. Good privacy curtains are a must. One such curtain can be drawn behind the driver's seat to obscure the view in through the windshield of the vehicle when it is parked. It is possible to sleep and dress, perform self-catheterization, or use a commode in the van. A folding commode should be obtained, if possible. Also, the person could purchase disposable bags with chemical inserts for solidifying liquid wastes and eliminating odors. These are available from medical supply houses.

A fold-down table can be used to prepare uncooked meals. The person can also transfer out of the van and cook and eat at a picnic table, using a lightweight backpacker's stove to prepare the food. It is wise to call the park in advance and ask such detailed questions as the following: "Has anyone with (my condition) ever stayed there, and if so, how did it work out?" For persons using a wheelchair inside a van, a narrow folding-frame chair is best. If one is quite strong, the simplest approach may be to eliminate the chair and scoot about inside the van, having a mattress down on the floor for comfort.

Travelers with disabilities soon learn to call or write to hotels in advance, specifying their needs

(Molnar, 1991). Simply to inquire whether a facility is accessible is insufficient. Much like the wheelchair symbol posted on the bathroom door, the label accessible hotel room is often deceptive. The person must explain in detail how much negotiating room is needed between the wall and the bed—a minimum of 32 in. is required but 48 in. is preferable for transferring into the bed. Often, the luxury suite of a hotel has larger dimensions and can be used more easily than the accessible suite. If so, this room should be made available at the regular price. The closet should have both low and standard rails, and the bed should be firm and of the appropriate height. When the person calls, he or she should be prepared to provide the hotel manager with the dimensions of the wheelchair and ask if the chair will fit into the bathroom.

Hotel rooms should be safe for the user with sensory deficits. There should be a fire exit plan for the person with mobility impairments—ideally, the room should be on the ground floor. If the neighborhood is relatively safe, sliding glass doors leading directly to the courtyard provide good egress. A member of the hotel staff should be designated to assist persons who cannot transfer quickly or who have sensory deficits and may need direction in an unfamiliar setting. There should be flashing fire alarms for the hearing impaired and braille labels on hot and cold faucets for the blind. The latter is especially important in geographical areas where the right or left, hot or cold convention may not be followed. A TTY phone should be available for persons with hearing impairments.

The bathroom should have a tub transfer bench (the kind that extends over the edge of the tub), not simply a shower chair. The controls and towel hooks should be reachable from the tub bench.

Sliding glass doors on the tub make it inaccessible to the person who needs a tub bench. Grab rails should extend down most of the length of the tub. There should be a pedestal sink or a sink that has a counter with a kneehole. The toilet should be 19 in. high and have 48 in. of clear space to one side, with enough room to get into position for a side to side 45-in. angle transfer and to close the door for privacy. The layouts of bathrooms in foreign countries are often different from those in the United States. For example, in some areas of Mexico, the toilet stalls are at a level 4 to 6 in. above the floor level, presumably to accommodate plumbing. This renders them totally unusable for the wheelchair user and other persons who are unable to negotiate the step.

Hotel restaurants and bars should be fully accessible to the mobility impaired and should provide braille menus. If the restaurant is not accessible, room service should be provided at no extra charge. This should be established in writing in advance.

Another factor to be taken into account when traveling is sightseeing. Before visiting any historic buildings or scenic locations, the person should call to find out whether accessible bathrooms and water fountains are available. Some historic landmarks have been exempted from the access laws. These determinations are made by the local historical societies, based on whether the adaptations would significantly detract from the accurate historical preservation of the site. When planning a trip, it is wise to contact other persons who have made the same trip or who live in the area for additional information.

Recommendations for Change in the Self-Care Environment

For each environmental feature that is found not to be negotiable, determine whether the client wishes to be able to negotiate this item. Question closely in this regard. Persons will sometimes deny interest in an activity because they believe it is not an option, so "why want what you can't have?" In other cases, the person genuinely has no interest in performing a given activity. If the disability is new to the person and his or her family members and household, exploration of changing life roles and activities will be an important process in rehabilitation (Jongbloed, 1994; Quigley, 1995).

If the person does wish to be able to negotiate a given environmental feature, attempt to discern what is limiting the negotiability of that feature—is it the environmental feature, the need for adaptive equipment, or the person's status? Consider what would be involved in making changes to each area. After eliminating the medically, physically, or financially impossible, proceed to implement the remaining options. Select the area or areas of intervention that seem likely to yield the best results for the least outlay of resources. That is, if one could either purchase a stove with the controls in front or purchase a self-standing power wheelchair to allow the person to reach the existing controls, the price differential makes the choice a simple one. The new stove costs several hundred dollars, whereas the self-standing chair costs thousands of dollars.

Options for Change

What follows are some suggestions for meeting the needs of persons with disabilities, not an exhaustive compendium. Creative problem solving is the practitioner's best asset, for no existing solution may meet the needs of some clients. The local Center for Independent Living is an excellent resource for those wishing to move into or build a negotiable home. The following are familiar concepts that have worked well in the past, arranged roughly from the least to the most costly.

1. *Rearrange existing furniture.*
   - Eliminate unnecessary items.
   - If transfers from a wheelchair are rare, eliminate at least one chair from the living room and dining room.
   - Discard throw rugs.
   - Rearrange items on kitchen shelves so that the most commonly used items are in front.
   - Switch rooms—if necessary, a large living room can replace an unreachable bedroom.

2. *Adapt existing furniture and fixtures.*
   - Add leg extenders to low chairs and beds.
   - Cut legs from high chairs and beds.
   - Put plywood under the mattress or couch cushions to add firmness.
   - Add a locking raiser to the toilet seat.
   - Purchase grab rails and install them in the bathroom—make sure they are mounted into the stud and never use a towel rack for a grab rail. Towel racks are held in place only by short screws inserted into the plaster and thus pull out easily.
   - Add lumbar cushions to chairs.
   - Add a foam wedge to the bed for positioning.
   - Remove interior doors (this adds approximately 2 in. of available space to a doorway).
   - Remove cabinet doors to create open shelves.
   - Remove lower doors from cabinet-style sinks to allow knee room.
   - Remove sliding glass shower doors and replace them with a shower curtain.
   - Lower closet rails.

3. *Purchase new furniture and fixtures.*
   - Purchase a commode for over-the-toilet or bedside use.
   - Replace the standard toilet with a higher style model.
   - Obtain a tub transfer bench or a shower chair, depending on the transfer skills of the client.
   - Obtain a refrigerator with side-by-side doors or a bottom freezer for the wheelchair user or a top freezer for the person who is unable to bend.
   - Obtain an environmental control system or have it installed.
   - Purchase or rent an electric bed.

4. *Move to an accessible environment.* When contemplating the cost and inconvenience of making architectural changes to a person's home, especially a rented home, one might explore the feasibility of moving to a setting that has already been adapted. This, of course, depends on the availability of such housing.

As with the purchase of furniture, the person with special self-care needs should carefully inspect the apartment in person before moving in. A building designed for the elderly may not meet the needs of a young person with a disability, and vice versa. The person should not assume that the accessible label means it will work for all persons. He or she should rate the apartment for negotiability, as outlined above, before moving in.

5. *Make architectural changes.*
   - Widen doorways.
   - Add ramps, stair lifts, or elevators.
   - Replace carpets with tile, wood, flagstones, or linoleum.
   - Install lower counters with kneeholes in the kitchen.
   - Obtain side-opening standard or microwave ovens and place them on a new lowered counter.
   - Have a shallow sink positioned in a lowered counter.
   - Replace drawers with built-in shelves for the wheelchair user.

6. *Custom build.* Considering the cost and inconvenience involved in architectural changes, even to an owned home, it may be preferable to build a new home to one's own specifications. If this is done, the recommendations at the beginning of this chapter regarding layout and environmental surfaces should be considered.

Factors Affecting Decisions To Change the Environment

While it is not possible to know what is best in each case, it is possible to identify the factors that should be considered to improve the negotiability of a self-care environment. The following list may be of help.

- *Which factor is easiest to change?* This could be the environment, the equipment, or the abilities of the person—or some combination thereof.

- *What will the available funding sources pay for?* This is not necessarily the least expensive option in an ultimate sense, but if the funding sources will pay for one thing and not another, this may be the determining factor in the decision. Contact the

insurer or the government agency to determine this in advance. So-called *retrofitters* (professionals who adapt existing structures) may charge as much as the funding source allots rather than charging what the same job would cost if done by a regular carpenter. However, some funding sources may mandate use of a retrofitter instead of a general contractor. It is also worthwhile to check out community resources. Victims of violent crimes are sometimes eligible for grants. Some religious and charitable organizations provide funds. A rehabilitation social worker can furnish information about local sources of funding.

- *Is the expected result worth the effort and cost?* Is it worthwhile to purchase a $30,000 wheelchair to be able to stand up and slice carrots? Would the purchase of a low table be a more realistic solution?

- *What is the effect of this environmental adaptation on the other persons who share the same environment?* Some adaptations, such as changing bed heights, have little effect on others, whereas other changes radically affect other persons' accessibility. Kitchens generally work well for either wheelchair level or standing cooks, but not both. Unless one has the space and money for two sinks and two stove tops, someone's access will be limited. Thus, it is important to decide who will be doing the most cooking and dish washing in the kitchen.

- *Legal requirements and building codes.* These requirements vary considerably from place to place, so before beginning a construction project of any kind, it is necessary to contact the local authorities and obtain any needed permits. ◆

Study Questions

1. What effects does hospitalization have on self-care? How can occupational therapy influence these effects?

2. What is the relationship of a person's self-concept to his or her self-care practice and self-care environment?

3. How does a disabled member of the household affect the self-care environment of other household members? How do the household members affect the self-care environment of the person with a disability?

4. How does the self-care environment affect the natural environment? How does the natural environment affect the self-care environment?

5. In which aspects of the self-care environment are occupational therapy interventions most and least likely to be effective? Why or why not?

6. How might a self-care environment differ for the following: a woman, a man, a child, a teenager, an adult, an elder, or someone of a different culture?

7. Using the information given in this chapter, draw a floor plan for an apartment for a wheelchair user. Include fixtures and furnishings. Write a brief justification of your choices.

8. Perform a negotiability rating of your home. List all features and then rate for negotiability in at least two of the following modes: (a) wheelchair, (b) walker, (c) crutches, (d) cane, (e) blindfolded, and (f) unimpaired. Actually attempt all activities— do not guess or project.

References

Appendix to Part 1191—Americans with Disabilities Act (ADA): Accessibility Guidelines for Buildings and Facilities. 56 Fed. Reg. 35455–35542 (1991).

Bates, P. S., Spencer, J. C., Young, M. E., & Rintala, D. H. (1993). Assistive technology and the newly disabled adult: Adaptation to wheelchair use. *American Journal of Occupational Therapy, 47*(11), 1014–1021.

Brown, C., Moore, W. P., Hemman, D., & Yunek, A. (1996). Influence of instrumental activities of daily living assessment method on judgments of independence. *American Journal of Occupational Therapy, 50*(3), 202–206.

Cate, Y., Baker, S. S., & Gilbert, M. P. (1995). Occupational therapy and the person with diabetes and vision impairment. *American Journal of Occupational Therapy, 49*(9), 905–911.

Education for all Handicapped Children Act. (1975). U.S.C., Title 20, § 1232, 1401, 1405, 1406, 1411 *et seq.*, 1453.

Gans, B. M., Mann, N. R., & Becker, B. E. (1993). Delivery of care to the physically challenged. *Archives of Physical Medicine and Rehabilitation, 74*(12 Spec. No.), S15.

Gilbreth, L. E. M. (1927). *The home-maker and her job.* New York: D. Appleton & Company.

Gilbreth, L. E. M., Thomas, O. M., & Clymer, E. (1959). *Management in the home: Happier living through saving time and energy* (Rev. and enlarged ed.). New York: Dodd Mead.

Jones, K. E., & Tamari, I. E. (1997). Making our offices universally accessible: Guidelines for physicians. *Canadian Medical Association Journal, 156*(5), 647–656.

Jongbloed, L. (1994). Adaptation to a stroke: The experience of one couple. *American Journal of Occupational Therapy, 48*(11), 1006–1013.

Kirby, D. L., O'Keefe, J. S., Neal, J. G., Bentram, D. J., & Edlich, R. F. (1996). Does the architectural design of burn centers comply with the Americans with Disabilities Act? *Journal of Burn Care and Rehabilitation, 17*(6), 156–160.

Kondo, T., Mann, W. C., Tomita, M., & Ottenbacher, K. J. (1997). The use of microwave ovens by elderly persons with disabilities. *American Journal of Occupational Therapy, 51,* 739–747.

Krouskop, T. A. (1992). *Selecting a support surface.* Unpublished paper, Baylor College of Medicine, Houston.

Lampert, J., & Lapolice, D. J. (1995). Functional considerations in evaluation and treatment of the client with low vision. *American Journal of Occupational Therapy, 49,* 885–890.

Landefeld, C. S., Palmer, R. M., Kresevic, D. M., Fortinsky, R. H., & Kowal, J. (1995). A randomized trial of care in a hospital medical unit especially designed to improve the functional outcomes of acutely ill older patients. *New England Journal of Medicine, 332*(20), 1338–1344.

McClain, L., Beringer, D., Kuhnert, H., Priest, J., Wilkes, E., Wilkinson, S., & Wyrick, L. (1993). Restaurant wheelchair accessibility. *American Journal of Occupational Therapy, 47,* 619–623.

Molnar, M. (1991). Questions to ask before hitting the vacation trail. *Mainstream, 15*(6), 11–13.

Monnot, M. (1988). *From rage to courage: The road to dignity walk.* Northfield, MN: St. Denis Press.

Moore, G. (1997). Improving health access: It's about attitude. *Nursing British Columbia, 29*(3), 27–30.

Murray, H. A. (1938). *Explorations in personality.* New York: Oxford University Press.

Nikolaus, T., Detterbeck, H., Gartner, U., Gnielka, M., Lempp-Gast, I., Renk, C., Suck-Rohrig, U., Oster, P., & Schlierf, G. (1995). Diagnostic house call within the scope of inpatient geriatric assessment. *Zeitschrift fur Gerontologie und Geriatrie, 28*(1), 14–18.

Noris-Baker, C., & Willems, E. P. (1978). Environmental negotiability as a direct measurement of behavior-environment relationships: Some implications for theory and practice. In A. D. Seidel & S. Danford (Eds.), *Proceedings of the tenth annual conference of the Environmental Design Research Association.* Houston, TX: Environmental Design Research Association.

Nygard, L., Bernspang, B., Fisher, A. G., & Winblad, B. (1994). Comparing motor and process ability of persons with suspected dementia in home and clinic settings. *American Journal of Occupational Therapy, 48,* 689–696.

Park, S., Fisher, A. G., & Velozo, C. A. (1994). Using the assessment of motor and process skills to compare occupational performance between clinic and home settings. *American Journal of Occupational Therapy, 48,* 697–709.

Quigley, M. C. (1995). Impact of spinal cord injury on the life roles of women. *American Journal of Occupational Therapy, 49*, 780–786.

Rogers, J. C., Holm, M. B., & Stone, R. G. (1997). Evaluation of daily living tasks: The home care advantage. *American Journal of Occupational Therapy, 51*, 410–422.

Rosenthal, S. B. (1995). Living with low vision: A personal and professional perspective. *American Journal of Occupational Therapy, 49*, 861–864.

Sanford, J. A., Story, M. F., & Jones, M. L. (1997). An analysis of the effects of ramp slope on people with mobility impairments. *Assistive Technology, 9*(1), 22–33.

Schmitt, E., Kruse, A., & Olbrich, E. (1994). Formen der Selbstandigkeit und Wohnumwelt—Ein empirischer Beitrag aus der Studie "Moglichkeiten und Grenzen der selbstandigen Lebensfuhrung im Alter" [Forms of independence and the residential environment—An empirical contribution from the study "Possibilities and limits of independent living for elderly patients"]. *Zeitschrift fur Gerontologie, 27*(6), 390–398.

Shuman, S. K., & Bebeau, M. J. (1994). Ethical and legal issues in special patient care. *Dental Clinics of North America, 38*(3), 553–575.

Smith, R. (1988). Quality assurance in equipment ordering for the spinal cord-injured patient. *American Journal of Occupational Therapy, 42*, 36–39.

Spencer, J., Krefting, L., & Mattingly, C. (1993). Incorporation of ethnographic methods in occupational therapy assessment. *American Journal of Occupational Therapy, 47*, 303–309.

Steinfold, E., Schroeder, S., Duncan, J., Faste, R., Chollet, D., Bishop, M., Wirth, P., & Cardell, P. (1979). *Access to the Built Environment: A review of the literature.* Washington, DC: U.S. Government Printing Office.

Timko, C. (1996). Physical characteristics of residential psychiatric and substance abuse programs: Organizational determinants and patients' outcomes. *American Journal of Community Psychology, 24*(1), 173–192.

Tyas, S., & Rush, B. (1993). The treatment of disabled persons with alcohol and drug problems: Results of a survey of addiction services. *Journal of Studies on Alcohol, 54*(3), 275–282.

20

Therapeutic Partnerships: Caregiving in the Home Setting

Margaret A. Perkinson
Patricia LaVesser

Margaret A. Perkinson, PhD, is Instructor, Program in Occupational Therapy, Washington University School of Medicine, St. Louis, Missouri.

Patricia LaVesser, MAT, OTR, is Instructor, Program in Occupational Therapy, Washington University Medical School, St. Louis, Missouri, and Doctoral Student, Washington University's George Warren Brown School of Social Work.

The authors thank Dr. Carolyn Baum, Vicky Mlady, and David Rockemann for their thoughtful comments and assistance with this chapter.

Key Terms

ethnographic approach

explanatory model of illness

family caregiver

family-centered care

personal care attendant

Objectives

On completing this chapter, the reader will be able to

1. Understand the scope of the caregiving services currently provided by family members.

2. Describe the characteristics of a family-centered approach to occupational therapy practice.

3. Define an explanatory model of illness.

4. Identify the family caregiver's values, needs, and priorities as part of the occupational therapy evaluation process for any client.

5. Describe the contributions that a family caregiver can make to the planning and implementation of treatment.

6. Identify the three stages of a caregiving career and the ways in which the occupational therapist can work with the family caregiver at each stage.

7. Recognize the occupational therapist's role in working with a person to develop the instrumental activities of daily living skill of attendant care manager.

Family caregivers frequently play a pivotal role in developing strategies for self-care for persons with disabilities. In addition to assisting with the actual tasks of self-care, family caregivers often act as gatekeepers to the health and social service system for relatives requiring more extensive assistance with activities of daily living (ADL). For persons too impaired to manage health decisions alone, the family caregiver is usually the person who interprets the illness, decides how symptoms should be managed, and eventually decides when and how professional health care providers should become involved. This chapter explores ways that occupational therapy practitioners can best work with family caregivers in accomplishing self-maintenance tasks for persons with disabilities. It also explores issues related to the use of personal care attendants.

The Importance of Family Caregiving

Family caregivers are the major source of care for persons with disabilities. It has been estimated that family members provide at least 80% of the care received by older adults (Doty, 1995). Whereas most recipients of home care are elderly, more than one third are persons under 60 years of age (Marks, 1996). Family members provide home care to persons with a variety of physical or mental disabilities or chronic conditions, ranging from cerebral palsy and Down syndrome to cancer, AIDS, diabetes, dementia, arthritis, multiple sclerosis, and heart disease.

The role of the family in caregiving is especially important now for a number of reasons. Shorter hospital stays result in persons being discharged to the community at an earlier point in their recovery, placing greater responsibility on the family members to provide posthospital care. Increased rates of survival for serious injuries and conditions that were previously fatal, the AIDS epidemic, and policies favoring deinstitutionalization are additional factors that contribute to the increase in home care (Baum & LaVesser, 1994). Perhaps most important to the rise in family caregiving is the rapidly growing number of older adults in our population. Less than 100 years ago, persons more than 65 years of age represented only 4% of the U.S. population. By 1990, their number had grown to 32 million, or 12.6%; and by 2050, persons more than 65 years of age are projected to reach 79 million, or 20.6% of the total population (U.S. Bureau of Census, 1992). Persons more than 85 years of age represent the fastest growing segment of the population, and this age group is expected to double by 2020 (U.S. Bureau of Census, 1992). Aging does not inevitably lead to disability, and the majority of older adults do not require help with ADL (Zedlewski, 1990). Nevertheless, functional impairment does tend to increase over time because of underlying disease states (Kunkel & Applebaum, 1992).

The need for assistance with ADL rises rapidly with age: Fewer than 3% of persons less than 65 years of age require help with ADL, compared with 9.3% of persons 65 to 69 years of age, 10.9% of persons 70 to 74 years of age, 18.9% of persons 75 to 79 years of age, 23.6% of persons 80 to 84 years of age, and 45.4% of persons 85 years of age and older (U.S. Bureau of the Census, 1990). Most adults with impairments live in the community (Day, 1985), and they are able to do so because of the informal care they receive from family members (Doty, 1995).

Research on family caregiving shows that maintaining persons with disabilities in the community is difficult (Pruchno, 1999; Schulz & Quittner, 1998). The general consensus is that family caregiving is disruptive and stressful, and it has considerable negative effects on the mental and physical health of the care provider (Wright, Clipp, & George, 1993). Caregivers as a group do not receive sufficient support from family members and friends, and health and social service providers generally do not offset this need for assistance (Aneshensel, Pearlin, Mullan, Zarit, & Whitlatch, 1995). How can occupational therapy practitioners more effectively aid family caregivers in providing care to persons with disabilities?

The Relationship Between Occupational Therapy Practitioners and Family Caregivers

Occupational therapy practitioners may view family caregivers in several ways. Unfortunately, family members are all too frequently perceived as barriers who get in the way of treatment (Clark, Corcoran, & Gitlin, 1994; Gitlin, 1993). Some practitioners may focus only on the edical needs of the person with the disability and forget his or her psychosocial needs and the relevance of family members to the situation. This may lead to problems, especially with compliance, and may even cause the therapeutic relationship to end.

Occupational therapy practitioners may also view family members as clients in need of help themselves. Family caregivers typically experience a major amount of stress, and that stress often leads to physical and mental distress. Signs of depression, such as emotional exhaustion, listlessness, inability to sleep (or sleeping too much), loss of appetite, loss of interest in favorite activities, and feelings of guilt or sadness, are signals that the family member requires some form of intervention (Morris & Gainer, 1997). Suggestions for coping with stress and using approaches, such as time management techniques and the use of respite care, may be helpful for family members who are nearing caregiving burnout.

Whereas the "family caregiver as client" approach is useful in certain situations, it still defines the relationship between the occupational therapy practitioner and family member as one between the "expert" and the person in need. This type of relationship implies an imbalance of power, in which the client is expected to submit to the authority of the expert (Lawlor & Mattingly, 1998; Perkinson, 1992). The client is, by definition, assigned to a dependent status and encouraged to rely on experts to define his or her problem, to evaluate its cause, and to determine its treatment. The client is expected to comply with the plan proposed by the expert, with little opportunity for active input into solutions. Such a relationship frequently leads to *unilateral dependency* (Estes & Binney, 1991), in which clients give up the responsibility of active involvement in decision making and passively accept the expert's advice (or orders).

A different model of care, based on a philosophy of "helping people to help themselves," emphasizes the development of self-reliance and empowerment. Advocates of this model encourage persons to take a more active role in resolving their problems and needs. The goal is to encourage persons to discover and develop their strengths and talents and to improve their possibilities of success in dealing with current situations (Perkinson, 1992).

Occupational therapy practitioners using this model would approach family caregivers (and their care receivers, to the extent that this is possible) as partners in care and would work to develop a collaborative therapeutic relationship (see Figure 20.1). The therapeutic alliance is based on mutual understanding, respect, and cooperation between the practitioner and the family member and patient

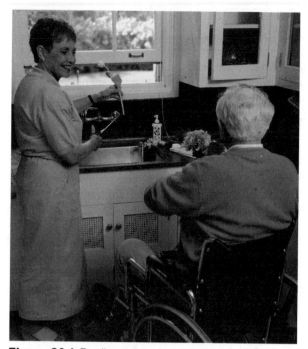

Figure 20.1 Family-centered caregiving is a philosophy that encourages partnerships between practitioners and family members. It recognizes that family members bring important knowledge and are essential to the caregiving process. (Photo © PhotoDisc, Inc.)

(Brown, 1998). The trend toward a family-centered partnership approach has evolved throughout the field, from pediatric to geriatric occupational therapy (Baum, 1991; Case-Smith & Nastro, 1993; Hasselkus, 1991). It is the fundamental intervention model promoted in Part H of the Education of the Handicapped Act Amendments of 1986 (Schultz-Krohn, 1997).

Family-centered care acknowledges that family members know their relative (i.e., child, spouse, elderly parent) in ways that the practitioner does not and that they are well qualified to make decisions regarding their relative's care (Law, 1997). Unlike health care professionals who come and go, family members are a permanent and vital part of the care receiver's life (Weinstein, 1997). With family-centered care, the focus is on the care recipient as part of a family (rather than on the care recipient alone). The practitioner provides information, knowledge, and options to the family members and then respects the decisions made by the family members, rather than using his or her own professional expertise to control and direct intervention (Allen & Petr, 1998). In a collaborative relationship, the family members and practitioner are both involved in the evaluation, problem-solving, and decision-making processes. The family members have major input in deciding the extent, type, and priorities of therapy.

The traditional practitioner-as-expert thinking that is supported by a strict medical model is hard to give up. Consider the following case.

> Carrie, a 12-month-old girl, is diagnosed with cerebral palsy, moderate right hemiplegia. She was referred for early intervention services, including occupational therapy. Carrie lives with her mother, father, and three older siblings in a one-story ranch style house on a farm owned and operated by her parents and grandparents.
>
> Even with years of parenting experience, her mother was having tremendous difficulty dealing with Carrie's needs and emerging developmental delays. At the time of referral, Carrie was not using her right hand at all, was demonstrating asymmetrical posture, and used scooting in a sitting position as her primary means of mobility. Her drooling and difficulty handling table foods made mealtimes difficult. The occupational practitioner assigned to the case quickly established a home program emphasizing neurodevelopmental treatment techniques to address the identified motor difficulties. Although she could find time in her schedule to see Carrie only once a week, the practitioner spent considerable time teaching the home program she had designed to Carrie's mother. As progress was beginning to be made, the occupational practitioner was greatly surprised when the mother informed her that she was no longer in need of occupational therapy services through the early intervention agency. Instead, she was going to drive 50 miles round-trip to the nearest Children's Hospital to have Carrie receive outpatient occupational therapy services two times per week.
>
> An interview with the family members at this time revealed some interesting information. It was learned that although the occupational practitioner had always been professional and friendly, she was always rushed and never seemed to ask Carrie's mother for her opinion of what was needed. The home program instructions were always written out and reviewed, but they were more complicated and took more time than the mother thought she could handle. She reported feeling very inadequate and guilty that she couldn't get everything done, frustrated with her attempts, and angry with the practitioner for not being aware of these difficulties. When routinely asked, "How are you doing with the exercises?" she felt chastised for not having done more. She also had mixed feelings about the direction that therapy was taking. While she agreed that motor skill development

> was important, she was really worried that Carrie was not getting enough nutrition because of her feeding difficulties, and she really just wanted to have a pleasant mealtime with the entire family. Finally, she believed that more therapy on a regular schedule was desirable and that she could handle the drive better than she could handle being a surrogate practitioner to her daughter.

If the occupational practitioner had approached this case from a family-centered perspective, the results may have been different. On the very first visit, a family member interview could have been completed during which family member strengths, needs, and goals were identified and prioritized. Collaborating with the family members on an ongoing basis most likely would have moved things along on a different course, resulting in both progress on Carrie's part and satisfaction on the part of the family members.

A truly collaborative partnership represents a fundamental shift in the way therapy is defined and delivered. Lawlor and Mattingly (1998) outlined some of the challenges this model presents, such as understanding issues confronting the care receiver and family members from the family members' point of view and sharing decision-making power. The following section suggests ways to deal with some of these issues and achieve an effective partnership with family caregivers.

How To Work as Partners With Family Caregivers

An effective partnership between caregivers and practitioners depends, first of all, on a shared view and understanding of the illness or disability of the care receiver and how it should be treated (Hasselkus, 1988; LeNavenec & Vonhof, 1996). The first step toward achieving this understanding is to identify what anthropologists call the *explanatory model* of illness that the caregiver holds. Explanatory models are sets of beliefs and knowledge that persons use to explain sickness and treatment. These models provide a way of thinking about illness that guides choices among various therapies (Kleinman, 1988; Krefting & Krefting, 1995). An explanatory model can include beliefs about the cause of an illness, how long it will last, how serious it is, and the possibility of a cure; the appropriate treatment and what represents a legitimate source of help for the illness; and the expected outcome.

The views and beliefs of an explanatory model form the basis for decision making in regard to the illness. The model influences whether the person thinks there is a problem to begin with. It also guides decisions regarding treatment and help seeking and also defines legitimate sources of help and caregiving goals.

Persons understand information given to them (messages) about health care within the context of their own beliefs. One might think of these messages (e.g., suggestions from the practitioner) as being "filtered" through a person's explanatory model. Those aspects of the message that are most compatible with the family caregiver's model are the parts of the message that are most likely to be "heard." Elements of the health message that conflict with the model are more likely to be tuned out or dismissed. Practitioners need to recognize this. For example, if a family caregiver of a cardiac patient views the heart to be like a machine that has been "fixed" as a result of bypass surgery, he or she may feel that the heart problem has been resolved and treatment is over. The caregiver may not understand the need for ongoing attention to lifestyle changes, such as modification of diet or maintenance of a permanent exercise plan.

To develop a collaborative partnership with the family caregiver, the practitioner must identify the caregiver's explanatory model or set of health beliefs and recognize potential points of conflict or differences in understanding or perception between the caregiver's explanatory model and that held by the practitioner. In conducting the initial evaluation with the family caregiver, the practitioner might include questions to elicit the family member's explanatory model (and that of the care receiver, when appropriate). Such questions might include the following: What do you think caused the care receiver's problem? Why do you think this illness happened at this particular time? How serious do you think this illness or condition is? What worries you the most about this illness or condition? What kind of treatment would you like your family member to receive? What are the most important results you expect to achieve? (Kleinman, 1980; Krefting & Krefting, 1995).

In addition to identifying and understanding the caregiver's explanatory model, the evaluation should also determine the meaning of the caregiving role to the family member. This would include how the caregiver makes sense of caregiving experiences (what motivates him or her, what is the significance of caregiving to him or her), what influences how daily care is provided, what is most burdensome and most satisfying about caregiving, and what are the major concerns (Gubrium &

Sankar, 1990; Hasselkus, 1988, 1989). The evaluation should include a joint evaluation by the caregiver and practitioner of the problems and resources of the caregiving situation. The joint evaluation should provide the basis for a collaborative effort to develop goals and procedures acceptable to all involved.

The Canadian Occupational Performance Measure (COPM; Law et al., 1994) is one useful assessment tool. It is an interview-based rating scale that asks the care receiver or family member to identify problem areas and priorities for intervention. The Functional Behavior Profile (Baum, Edwards, & Morrow-Howell, 1993) is another excellent tool for enlisting a caregiver's input. It asks caregivers to report the frequency of various behaviors that they have observed during recent interactions with the care receiver and provides valuable information for case planning.

The practitioner may wish to add to traditional assessment techniques using a more ethnographic approach to gathering information on the caregiving situation. Ethnographic methods offer ways to understand the family caregiver's perspective and techniques for achieving a joint evaluation of the situation and the care receiver's needs (Gitlin, Corcoran, & Leinsmiller-Eckhardt, 1995; Hasselkus, 1990, 1997). When using an ethnographic approach, one attempts to understand another way of life as it is viewed by another person (in this case, the family caregiver). An ethnographic interview focuses on values, meanings, beliefs, and how the person providing the information (informant) makes sense of his or her situation. The interview is conducted in a nonjudgmental manner, that is, the practitioner suspends his or her own beliefs and values as to the appropriate course of treatment in an attempt to discover what actually goes on (Gitlin et al., 1995). The ethnographic interview is semistructured, consisting of open-ended questions and appropriate probes, in which the practitioner attempts to elicit and understand the informant's (i.e., family caregiver's or, when appropriate, care receiver's) story or point of view.

Weinstein (1997) has designed a semistructured interview for family members or principal caregivers. Its purpose is to discover their level of knowledge of and comfort with their role. It also identifies their opinions, personal goals, and needs. She asks them to describe their perception of the care receiver's problem, a typical day at home, the effect of the situation on themselves and other members of the family, and what they would personally like from her as the occupational therapy practitioner. Such an interview can lay the groundwork for establishing the collaborative partnership that is central to the philosophy of family-centered care.

As the practitioner takes the time to understand the caregiver's perspective (including the meaning ascribed to caregiving, how care is provided in the home, and what is perceived as problematic), he or she is also developing rapport with the family caregiver. This lays the foundation for a future discussion, in which the practitioner can share his or her own perspectives on the caregiving situation (Hasselkus, 1997). After identifying the caregiver's views and understanding of the care receiver's condition and needs, the practitioner may want to discuss any differences in perspectives that could lead to misunderstandings or points of disagreement. Respect for the other's point of view is always maintained during this process.

Often the explanatory model (including values, beliefs, and goals) of the family caregiver is not the same as that held by the practitioner. Medical anthropologists have developed a therapeutic approach to enhance cross-cultural communication between patients and health care providers (Berlin & Fowkes, 1983) that could be relevant here. Structured around the acronym LEARN (listen, explain, acknowledge, recommend, and negotiate), this set of guidelines should help practitioners and family caregivers who may initially have different points of view to "get on the same wavelength" and take the first step toward developing a therapeutic alliance. As discussed above, the practitioner should begin by listening with sympathy and understanding to the caregiver's perception of the illness and caregiving situation. Once he or she understands the family caregiver's perspective and has developed a good rapport with that caregiver, the practitioner should share his or her own point of view, explaining his or her perceptions of the problem. Once both viewpoints have been discussed, both parties should acknowledge and review the areas in which they agree and work to resolve major conceptual conflicts. The next step is to recommend a treatment plan, with both sides fully involved as partners in deciding what to do. Underlying the entire process is negotiation between the two parties to reach a treatment plan that is agreeable to all and that takes the family caregiver's perspective as well as the practitioner's into account.

The ethnographic approach and the LEARN guidelines are techniques that can help practitioners develop treatment strategies with the family caregiver that fit the values and beliefs of the family members but that are still rooted in the theory and practice of occupational therapy. Viewing the family caregiver as a partner and taking the values and beliefs of the family members into account will increase the likelihood that the jointly developed treatment plan will be successfully integrated into family member routines (Corcoran & Gitlin, 1992; Gitlin, 1993). In acknowledging the family caregiver as a partner who has much to contribute, the practitioner acts as an "enabler" and encourages the family members to assume and maintain responsibility for long-term care (see Figure 20.2)

What the Family Caregiver Can Contribute

The family caregiver has much to contribute as a partner in the planning and execution of the treatment process. As a mediator between the care receiver and practitioner, the family caregiver can communicate the care receiver's needs and concerns to the practitioner (and assist the care receiver

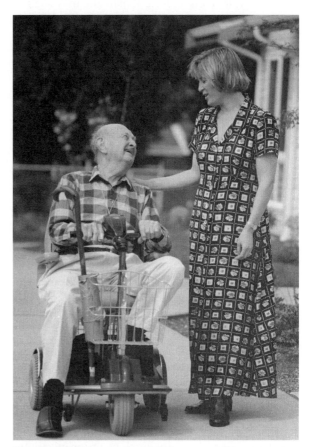

Figure 20.2 Occupational therapy practitioners can advise family caregivers on strategies to promote the well-being of their loved ones while avoiding burnout. (Photo © PhotoDisc, Inc.)

in voicing his or her own concerns) and communicate or clarify treatment plans and goals to the care receiver. The family caregiver typically has a wealth of information that will help practitioner better understand the care receiver, his or her needs, and how best to address them.

Usually, family caregivers are attuned to nuances of behavior and physical states of the care receiver. The care receiver knows what is normal or typical of the care receiver and can thus help the therapy practitioner define realistic treatments goals. The family caregiver can also advise practitioner of important changes in the care receiver's health status. He or she also has knowledge of the receiver's ability to conduct everyday activities (including self-maintenance activities) that may affect treatment plans.

The family caregiver can give the practitioner tips on interacting with the care receiver and on interpreting care receiver's reaction to the practitioner and to treatment suggestions. That caregiver can often sense how receptive the care receiver is likely to be a given treatment plan and may suggest ways to present the plan to maximize the likelihood that the care receiver will accept it. This suggestion might involved having the caregiver present the plan to the care receiver or, to the extent possible, enlisting the care receiver in contributing to the development of the plan so that he or she would be more invested in it.

The caregiver knows how the care receiver will usually react to stressful demands (i.e., how well the person responds to pain or stress). The family caregiver can alert the practitioner to the care receiver's general mood, level of sociability, and interaction style—whether he or she is talkative, quiet, a loner, generally receptive to other's suggestions, distrustful, skeptical, and so forth. The caregiver can also identify the care receiver's typical style of help seeking (e.g., asks for help only in emergencies, never seeks help, seeks and accepts help only from certain persons) and receptivity to trying new activities or modifying old routines.

The family caregiver can share important background information about the care receiver so that the practitioner can know him or her as a person and better understand the care receiver's behavior and moods. Information in such areas as the care receiver's past occupation, hobbies, interests, major life events, memberships in clubs or organizations, and travels will help the practitioner interact with him or her on a more personal level. The family caregiver can suggest various topics of interest to the care receiver (sports, television shows, local events) that may help the practitioner break the ice and develop rapport.

The family caregiver can alert the practitioner to special concerns or idiosyncrasies of the care receiver, for example, whether the care receiver is an extremely modest person and finds it disturbing to have an attendant assist with the more intimate activities of personal maintenance such as toileting or bathing. The family caregiver can also inform the practitioner of any fears the care receiver may have, such as being in a confined area or being left alone with someone (such as an attendant) that he or she does not know. The caregiver can inform the practitioner of any special techniques that work to soothe or comfort the care receiver when he or she is upset, such as certain types of music, massage, diverting attention, talking about a favorite activity or relative. The family caregiver can identify what generally works to bring the care receiver out of a depression or slump, and what makes him or her happy.

The family caregiver can suggest ways to motivate the care receiver, for example, what to say to prompt him or her to cooperate with therapies or self-maintenance activities (e.g., "your daughter would be happy if you would do X"). The family caregiver can assist in motivating the care receiver by encouraging him or her to cooperate with the treatment plan.

Any treatment plan for self-maintenance activities should incorporate the care receiver's various preferences regarding ADL tasks. The family caregiver can help to identify the care receiver's attitudes and preferences regarding various aspects of ADL. For example, the care receiver may place great value on maintaining his or her appearance. He or she may have definite preferences in regard to elements of grooming, such as hairstyle; style of clothing; amount and type of makeup; use of perfume, cologne, or lotions; and the like.

Attitudes regarding bathing may include a preference for showers instead of tub baths, for timing of bathing, and for the use of favorite bathing accessories (e.g., bath oils, loofah mitts, back scrubbers). The care receiver may have definite feelings about receiving assistance with bathing. The family caregiver may be able to identify who would be an acceptable bathing assistant and who would not (e.g., some care receivers may prefer attendants of the same sex).

Family caregivers can also identify food preferences and dislikes and general eating habits (e.g., whether the care receiver likes to snack throughout the day, prefers to eat a large breakfast and smaller meals later in the day). For care receivers who are unable to prepare their own meals, the family caregiver plays an essential role in maintaining a proper diet. Caregivers can identify favorite types of exercise and how motivated the care receiver is to maintain an exercise and diet program. The family caregiver may also assist with the exercise program, such as helping with range of motion exercises, or accompanying the care receiver on a walking program. Persons often are more motivated to continue an exercise program when they have a buddy to accompany and encourage them.

Occupation is a critical factor in determining quality of life, no matter how ill or disabled a care receiver may be (Baum, 1995). With their knowledge of the care receiver's past history and preferences, family members can play a vital role in identifying meaningful tasks and engaging the care receiver in those activities.

These are just a few suggestions on how family caregivers can contribute to the joint evaluation, development, and enactment of a treatment plan. They can help to identify the care receiver's abilities and limits, what frustrates the care receiver, and what gives him or her satisfaction. This helps in setting realistic, appropriate, and challenging goals. Identifying the care receiver's preferences and incorporating those preferences into the treatment plan should greatly improve the quality of life of the care receiver and the probability that he or she will find that plan acceptable. As the plan is carried out, the family caregiver can assist in its evaluation and modification by giving feedback to the practitioner on what is working and what should be changed.

What Family Caregivers Need

As research on family caregiving has expanded to include longitudinal studies, researchers have begun to develop the outlines of various stages of the caregiving career (Aneshensel et al., 1995). Each stage is characterized by different challenges and different needs on the part of both care receiver and caregiver. The family-centered treatment plan should take into account these stage-related needs. As a partner in the treatment process, there are many ways in which the practitioner can assist the family caregiver in meeting his or her own needs and those of the care receiver.

The Role Acquisition Stage

This stage occurs at the onset of the care receiver's illness, or when the family member first assumes the role of caregiver. During this stage, both the care receiver and the caregiver must learn to adjust to the new situation and plan for the future. The family caregiver typically has little knowledge of the illness (unless it tends to run in the family or the family caregiver has had experience in the health care field). The practitioner can assist by providing information to help the care receiver and family members understand the illness, its possible causes, the various options for treatment, and what typically lies ahead. The initial stage of a major illness represents a major life transition for both care receiver and caregiver and often requires considerable adjustments in life goals, relationships, daily activities, and routines. Emotional support is essential at this stage, and the practitioner may consider linking the family members to appropriate counseling services, if necessary. Interaction with family caregivers of persons with similar conditions or illnesses through support groups or peer counseling programs can be especially helpful. Peer caregivers can share their strategies for dealing with issues of everyday life (including dealing with ADL tasks) and can provide encouragement rooted in empathy (Perkinson, 1995).

Much of the assistance that the practitioner can provide at this stage is preventative in nature, taking steps to avoid future problems. He or she can identify potential legal and financial issues, such as the possible need for obtaining a durable power of attorney for management of assets and health care, and find help in dealing with these concerns. Other issues include the writing of advance directives and wills, as well as making financial arrangements to anticipate increased medical costs (Baum, 1991; Overman & Stoudemire, 1988).

The Role Enactment Stage

This stage is of longer duration, encompassing most of the caregiving career. It includes the delivery of home care and, in some cases, the decision for institutional placement. During this stage the caregiver requires continued education regarding the nature of the illness trajectory. He or she may also benefit from training in direct care skills, especially those relating to self-maintenance tasks, such as techniques to safely transfer or bathe the care receiver, learning to cue various self-care tasks, and setting up routines to promote the highest level of performance (Baum, 1991). When appropriate, behavior management techniques may be especially helpful in dealing with disruptive behaviors (Zarit & Teri, 1991).

In some cases, as, for example, in the advanced stages of dementia, family caregivers may benefit from instruction in communication techniques. A growing literature offers suggestions on ways to preserve the sense of identity and personhood for persons with severe cognitive impairments and to communicate more effectively with these persons (Perkinson, 1999; Sabat & Hare, 1992).

The practitioner can instruct the caregiver on the use of relevant assistive devices. He or she can do a home evaluation and suggest various environmental interventions to make the home safer (Gallagher-Thompson, 1994; Heagerty & Eskenazi, 1994).

The family caregiver may benefit from instruction in stress management and time management. He or she may need help in setting limits, developing realistic standards, and prioritizing goals (Aneshensel et al., 1995). The caregiver may also require help in dealing with changing family dynamics. Disagreements often emerge over differences in perceptions of the illness and methods for managing it. Conflicts may arise in determining who will assume tasks previously done by the care receiver and how the additional work required in providing care will be shared. The family caregiver may also need guidance on how to explain the illness to family members and friends in such a way that they maintain continued supportive relations (Fortinsky & Hathaway, 1990).

Often family caregivers are unaware of available community resources and how to access them (Morris & Gainer, 1997). Practitioners should develop a resource file to identify relevant resources and sources of payment. Such resources would include programs offering training and support, such as classes in caregiving and health education, support groups, e-mail discussion groups, and 24-hour hot lines. The practitioner can identify a number of useful health newsletters, web sites, and publications on caregiving, such as *The 36-Hour Day* (Mace & Rabins, 1994).

The practitioner can provide advice to family caregivers regarding in-home services that offer help with self-maintenance tasks, such as home health aides who help with bathing, dressing, grooming, and transfers. Homemakers can help with household chores. Nutritionists can instruct the caregiver about special nutritional needs, and agencies pro-

viding home-delivered meals can assist with meeting those needs. Physical therapists and exercise or rehabilitation programs can assist in developing and maintaining an exercise regimen.

Family caregivers must recognize the stressful nature of their role and take active steps to prevent caregiving burnout. The practitioner can assist in this by encouraging self-care and identifying community sources of respite, such as adult or child day-care programs and extended overnight respite programs offered by some nursing homes, or by encouraging the delivery of respite through the caregiver's informal support systems of family members and friends (see Figure 20.3).

In addition to learning how to access community services and programs and appropriate sources of payment for these services, caregivers can also benefit from instructions on how to work effectively with health providers. The following section offers suggestions on working with personal care attendants, a type of health provider especially relevant for care receivers requiring assistance with ADL.

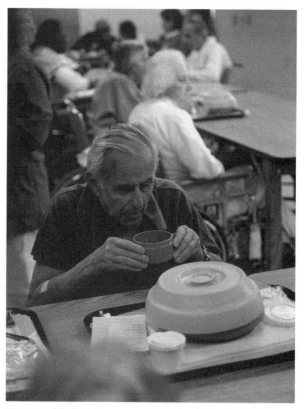

Figure 20.3 When caregiving burdens become too great for family members, therapy practitioners can assist in exploring institutional options or can recommend temporary respite care. (Photo © PhotoDisc, Inc.)

Suggestions for Working With Personal Care Attendants

A *personal care attendant* is a paid employee who provides in-home assistance with essential ADL to a person with a severe disability who is functionally dependent (Hutchins, Thornock, Lindgre, & Parks, 1978). Attendant care is a service associated with the independent living movement, which began in the early 1970s (DeJong & Wenker, 1983). The concept of independent living focuses on allowing persons with disabilities to live as they choose in their communities rather than confining them to institutions.

The relationship between persons with disabilities and attendants has been described as an employer–employee relationship (Lindley, 1995). Lack of management skills on the part of new employers is described as one of the most common problems encountered by the person with a disability in dealing with a personal care attendant. An occupational therapy practitioner can play a crucial role in assisting that person and his or her family caregiver with the development of the instrumental activities of daily living skill of attendant manager.

Necessary management skills related to personal care attendants include the ability to communicate expectations in terms of standards of performance, provide appropriate and timely feedback, and terminate employment when necessary (Opie & Miller, 1989). Early in the course of rehabilitation, the occupational therapy practitioner should help both the care receiver and the family caregiver begin the process of acquiring these skills by clarifying the care receiver's needs and expectations regarding relationships, work, and family members. It is important to encourage the care receiver to become assertive and to discuss the personal care needs necessary to achieve independence. What is important to the person with the disability? What does he or she want from the attendant? Should he or she struggle for more than an hour getting dressed alone? If so, how much energy will be left for the rest of the day? Some will find it very important to be independent. Others may find that the challenge of work and the pleasures of family or other relationships are enhanced when they receive assistance from a person whom they have personally chosen and trained to help with self-care and other daily requirements.

Recruitment and selection of attendants can be facilitated through the use of carefully defined sets of tasks. Initial organization is a key step in the process (Ulicny & Jones, 1985). Personal care chores should be defined, as well as the time of day the assistance is needed. A person who needs to leave for work early in the morning, for example, might need a personal care attendant to provide the bare minimum in the morning—perhaps, washing, dressing, and tooth brushing. More time-consuming tasks like bowel care and showering could be left for the evening when time is not at a premium. Housekeeping and environmental management tasks can be sorted and consolidated into specific time slots. Meals may be prepared ahead of time, cleaning tasks interspersed with cooking, and laundry started in the morning and finished in the evening.

Ulicny and Jones (1985) proposed the use of performance checklists to outline certain job tasks for the attendant. Specific work routines are outlined to identify the frequency of the task, the materials needed to support the task, and the setup. Checklists provide specific instructions and help the employer monitor, evaluate, and provide feedback on the attendant's performance. Once training is completed, checklists can be used for continued supervision. The process of developing a checklist is straightforward. First, those personal care tasks that require assistance are defined. Then the identified tasks are analyzed and procedures developed to support the tasks. The resulting task and procedure lists become the checklist. Checklists can be used in the interview process so that the prospective employee knows what will be expected of him or her.

Another suggestion for potential employers of attendants is to write a contract (De Graff, 1988). The contract can outline all of the tasks to be performed in great detail and identify the expectations of both the attendant and the employers. Items such as hourly rate, the rate for portions of an hour worked, if and what the attendant will be paid if work is cancelled, expectations if the attendant cancels, and any other potential problems can be included.

Occupational therapy practitioners should make family members and care receivers aware of the many community resources available to assist in the effective employment and management of attendants. Independent living centers may help to recruit and interview them. A nearby college may have a service program for students with disabilities, or even a personal care attendant pool. The local National Spinal Cord Injury Association chapter, local rehabilitation center, or public library may also provide assistance. Finally, hiring through a home health agency may provide convenience, extra reliability, and a higher level of training in exchange for some control, especially in terms of choice of providers.

Residential Options for Family Care Providers

If the demands of caregiving exceed the abilities and resources of family care providers even with the help of in-home and community services, the practitioner can identify various residential options for placement of the care receiver. These might include assisted-living facilities, group homes, board and care facilities, continuing-care retirement communities, hospice, or nursing homes. The practitioner can review the pros and cons of each option and suggest the level of care most appropriate for the care receiver. He or she can also offer suggestions on criteria to use in evaluating and selecting a residential facility.

Placement of a loved one in an institutional setting represents a difficult transition for the family caregiver as well as the care receiver. Many family members prefer to continue their involvement in their relative's care but are not sure what they could do or would be allowed to do (Perkinson, in press). There is growing evidence that family involvement in nursing home care is linked to lower levels of depression among family caregivers and higher life satisfaction among care receivers (Bowers, 1988; Brody, Dempsey, & Pruchno, 1990). Practitioners can assist family caregivers at this stage of the caregiving career by helping them learn to negotiate the nursing home system. Practitioners can identify daily routines within the facility, suggest how to voice concerns effectively within the nursing home, and outline strategies to help the care receiver adjust to life in this new setting (Perkinson, Rockemann, & Mahan, 1996). Although family members of nursing home residents are generally not encouraged to assist in the more physically demanding tasks of self-care, such as toileting, transferring, or bathing, for fear of hurting either themselves or their relative, help with ADL tasks such as grooming and feeding is usually quite welcome. In addition to help with these kinds of self-care tasks, family members often continue their caregiving role within the nursing home by acting as advocates for their relative and offering companionship (Perkinson, in press).

Role Disengagement

The death of the care receiver signals the final stage of the caregiving career, in which the family member must deal with bereavement and loss. The family member undergoes a period of adjustment in which he or she must come to terms with the end of the caregiving role. Caregiving in the later stages of an illness is often all-consuming. Caregivers frequently cut out social activities and neglect friendships in an attempt to maintain the ever-growing needs of the care receiver. When the care receiver dies, the caregiver often finds himself or herself socially isolated. In addition to emotional support, the caregiver may need help in developing new activities for a life that was formerly structured by the caregiver role (Aneshensel et al., 1995; Mullan, 1992). The practitioner can assist with these needs and help the family member with the transition to a new phase of life (see Table 20.1).

Some Final Thoughts

There are limits to the delivery of family-centered care. Some families may not be comfortable with the new role of full participation in decision making, preferring to remain in the more passive role traditionally assigned them by the health care system (Weinstein, 1997). With family-centered care, family caregivers should be able to select their own level of involvement. This involvement may vary according to the age of the care receiver, the type of services available, the caregivers' comfort level with their own opinions, and their experiences as providers of care. They should not be pressured into taking on more than they can handle. Some family members may lack the necessary skills or knowledge to be partners in the therapeutic relationship. Some practice environments may simply not support the implementation of a family-centered model.

To overcome these obstacles, a number of strategies can be put into place. One possibility is to make a personal commitment as a practitioner to change your own approach to intervention. Weinstein (1997) also suggested becoming better educated in the family-centered approach. In-service training on the topic can be scheduled to share ideas for increased collaboration with family members. Practitioners can also encourage family member participation in the treatment process through modeling appropriate behaviors and recognizing that family member resistance may have to be overcome gradually. To incorporate family-

Table 20.1 Stages and Needs of the Caregiving Career

Stage	Family Challenges	Practitioner Role
Role acquisition	Must adjust to new demands Must learn about illness and what lies ahead	Provide information and reassurance Help family anticipate future needs
Role enactment	May need training in direct care skills and behavioral management May need advice about institutional placement or community resources	Provide training as needed, such as use of assistive devices and transfers skills Provide information on placement options and resources
Disengagement	Adjustment to death of care receiver Adjustment to social isolation and burnout	Assist family with transition Make referrals to resources that can help with grief or readjustment

centered approaches into existing service delivery systems, these concepts should be taught in educational programs for occupational therapy practitioners. Expanding the family-centered model into practice with persons at all stages of the life cycle should be a priority.

Finally, practitioners should be mindful that the legal and ethical issues of care do not disappear when family-centered approaches are used. Personal safety issues must come before family member preference. And, of course, a health care professional cannot, and should not, endorse a family member's choice to use violence. Occupational therapy practitioners will always be challenged to balance the best interests of the care receiver, respect for the family as a unit, and their own professional expertise in any situation (Allen & Petr, 1998). ◆

Study Questions

1. List four reasons why there has been a notable rise in the number of families providing care to family members in recent years.

2. What is the difference between a medical model approach to working with caregivers and one that is family centered?

3. Imagine yourself in the role of caregiver to an elderly relative or a child with special needs. Describe your explanatory model of the illness. How might your model differ from someone else's model of the same illness?

4. Identify one assessment tool that would be useful in identifying a family caregiver's values, needs, and priorities to use in a collaborative approach to

intervention. Practice filling out this assessment with a peer or client.

5. A woman 35 years of age who was diagnosed with multiple sclerosis in her late 20s is referred to you for home health occupational therapy evaluation and intervention. She lives with her mother and father. At what stage of their caregiving career are her parents and how will you include them in your evaluation and treatment plan?

6. You have been working with a young man with spinal cord injury as an inpatient in a rehabilitation unit. He is ready for discharge to his home and needs to consider hiring a personal care attendant. Plan a treatment session during which you will address this need.

References

Allen, R. I., & Petr, C. G. (1998). Rethinking family-centered practice. *American Journal of Orthopsychiatry, 68*(1), 4–15.

Aneshensel, C. S., Pearlin, L. I., Mullan, J. T., Zarit, S. H., & Whitlatch, C. J. (1995). *Profiles in caregiving: The unexpected career.* San Diego, CA: Academic Press.

Baum, C. M. (1991). Addressing the needs of the cognitively impaired elderly from a family policy perspective. *American Journal of Occupational Therapy, 45,* 594–606.

Baum, C. M. (1995). The contribution of occupation to function in persons with Alzheimer's disease. *Journal of Occupational Science: Australia, 2*(2), 59–67.

Baum, C., Edwards, D. F., & Morrow-Howell, N. (1993). Identification and measurement of productive behaviors in senile dementia of the Alzheimer type. *Gerontologist, 33,* 403–408.

Baum, C. & LaVesser, P. (1994). Caregiver assistance: Using family members and attendants. In C. Christiansen (Ed.), *Ways of living: Self-care strategies for special needs* (pp. 453–482). Rockville, MD: American Occupational Therapy Association.

Berlin, E. A., & Fowkes, W. C. (1983). A teaching framework for cross-cultural health care. *Western Journal of Medicine, 139*, 934–938.

Bowers, B. J. (1988). Family perceptions of care in a nursing home. *Gerontologist, 28*(3), 361–368.

Brody, E., Dempsey, N., & Pruchno, R. (1990). Mental health of sons and daughters of the institutionalized aged. *Gerontologist, 30*, 212–219.

Brown, P. J. (1998). *Understanding and applying medical anthropology*. Mountain View, CA: Mayfield.

Case-Smith, J., & Nastro, M. A. (1993). The effect of occupational therapy intervention on mothers of children with cerebral palsy. *American Journal of Occupational Therapy, 47*, 811–817.

Clark, C. A., Corcoran, M., & Gitlin, L. N. (1994). An explanatory study of how occupational therapy practitioners develop therapeutic relationships with family caregivers. *American Journal of Occupational Therapy, 49*, 587–594.

Corcoran, M. A., & Gitlin, L. N. (1992). Dementia management: An occupational therapy home-based intervention for caregivers. *American Journal of Occupational Therapy, 46*, 801–808.

Day, A. T. (1985). Who cares? Demographic trends challenge family care for the elderly. *Population Trends and Public Policy, 9*, 1–17.

De Graff, A. (1988). *Home health aides: How to manage the people who help you*. Fort Collins, CO: Saratoga Access Publications.

DeJong, G., & Wenker, T. (1983). Attendant care. In N. M. Crewe & I. K. Zola (Eds.), *Independent living for physically disabled people* (pp. 157–170). San Francisco: Jossey-Bass.

Doty, P. (1995). Informal caregiving. In C. Evashwick (Ed.), *An integrated systems approach*. Albany, NY: Delman Publishers.

Estes, C., & Binney, E. (1991). The biomedicalization of aging: Dangers & dilemmas. In M. Minkler & C. Estes (Eds.), *Critical perspectives on aging: The political and moral economy of growing old*. Amityville, NY: Baywood.

Fortinsky, R. H., & Hathaway, T. J. (1990). Information and service needs among active and former family caregivers of persons with Alzheimer's disease. *Gerontological Society of America, 30*(5), 604–609.

Gallagher-Thompson, D. (1994). Direct services and interventions for caregivers: A review of extant programs and a look to the future. In M. H. Cantor (Ed.), *Family caregiving: Agenda for the future* (pp. 102–122). San Francisco: American Society for Aging.

Gitlin, L. N. (1993). Therapeutic dilemmas in the care of the elderly in rehabilitation. *Topics in Geriatric Rehabilitation, 9*, 11–20.

Gitlin, L. N., Corcoran, M., & Leinsmiller-Eckhardt, S. (1995). Understanding the family perspective: An ethnographic framework for providing occupational therapy in the home. *American Journal of Occupational Therapy, 49*(8), 802–809.

Gubrium, J. F., & Sankar, A. (1990). *The home care experience: Ethnography and policy*. Newbury Park, CA: Sage.

Hasselkus, B. R. (1988). Meaning of family caregiving: Perspectives on caregiver/professional relationships. *Gerontologist, 28*, 686–691.

Hasselkus, B. R. (1989). The meaning of daily activity in family caregiving for the elderly. *American Journal of Occupational Therapy, 43*, 649–656.

Hasselkus, B. R. (1990). Ethnographic interviewing: A tool for practice with family caregivers for the elderly. *Occupational Therapy Practice, 2*, 9–16.

Hasselkus, B. R. (1991). Ethical dilemmas in family caregiving for the elderly: Implications for occupational therapy. *American Journal of Occupational Therapy, 45*, 206–212.

Hasselkus, B. R. (1997). Everyday ethics in dementia care: Narratives of crossing the line. *Gerontologist, 37*(5), 640–649.

Heagerty, B., & Eskenazi, L. (1994). A practice and program perspective on family caregiving: Focus on solutions. In M. H. Cantor (Ed.), *Family caregiving: Agenda for the future* (pp. 35–48). San Francisco: American Society for Aging.

Hutchins, T. K., Thornock, M., Lindgre, B., & Parks, J. (1978). Profile in in-home attendant care workers. *American Rehabilitation, 4*(2), 18–22.

Kleinman, A. (1980). *Patients and healers in the context of culture*. Berkeley, CA: University of California Press.

Kleinman, A. (1988). *The illness narratives: Suffering, healing, and the human condition*. New York: Basic Books.

Krefting, L., & Krefting, D. (1995). Cultural influences on performance. In C. Christiansen & C. Baum (Eds.), *Occupational therapy: Overseeing human performance deficits*. Thorofare, NJ: Slack.

Kunkel, S. R., & Applebaum, R. A. (1992). Estimating the prevalence of long-term disability for an aging society. *Journal of Gerontology, 47*, S253–S260.

Law, M. (1997). *Client-centered occupational therapy*. Thorofare, NJ: Slack.

Law, M., Baptiste, S., Carswell, A., McColl, M. A., Polatajko, H., & Pollack, N. (1994). *Canadian occu-*

pational performance measure (2nd ed.). Toronto, ON: CAOT Publications.

Lawlor, M. S., & Mattingly, C. F. (1998). The complexities embedded in family-centered care. *American Journal of Occupational Therapy, 52,* 259–267.

Le Navenec, C., & Vonhof, T. (1996). *One day at a time: How families manage the experience of dementia.* Westport, CT: Greenwood.

Lindley, J. (1995). *Finding and keeping an attendant.* Puyallup, WA: Center for Independence.

Mace, N. L., & Rabins, P. V. (1994). *The 36-hour day* (2nd ed.). Baltimore: The Johns Hopkins University Press.

Marks, N. F. (1996). Caregiving across the lifespan: National prevalence and predictors. *Family Relations, 45,* 27–36.

Morris, A., & Gainer, F. (1997). Helping the caregiver: Occupational therapy opportunities. *OT Practice, 2,* 36–40.

Mullan, J. T. (1992). The bereaved caregiver: A prospective study of changes in well-being. *Gerontologist, 32*(5), 673–683.

Opie, N. D., & Miller, E. L. (1989). Personal care attendants and severely disabled adults: Attributions for relationship outcomes. *Archives of Psychiatric Nursing, 3,* 205–210.

Overman, W., & Stoudemire, A. (1988). Guidelines for legal and financial counseling of Alzheimer's disease patients and their families. *American Journal of Psychiatry, 145*(12), 1495–1500.

Perkinson, M. A. (1992). Maximizing personal efficacy in older adults: The empowerment of volunteers in a multipurpose senior center. *Physical and Occupational Therapy in Geriatrics, 10*(3), 57–72.

Perkinson, M. A. (1995). Socialization to the family caregiving role within a continuing care retirement community. *Medical Anthropology, 16,* 249–267.

Perkinson, M. A. (1999). Family and nursing home staff's perceptions of quality of life in dementia. In R. Rubinstein, M. Moss, & M. Kleban (Eds.), *The many dimensions of aging.* New York: Springer.

Perkinson, M. A. (in press). Defining family roles within a nursing home. In P. Stafford (Ed.), *Gray areas: An anthropology of the nursing home.* Santa Fe, NM: School for American Research.

Perkinson, M. A., Rockemann, D., & Mahan, L. (1996). *Families in nursing homes manual.* Washington, DC: AARP Andrus Foundation.

Pruchno, R. A. (1999). Caregiving research: Looking backward, looking forward. In R. Rubenstein, M. Moss, & M. Kleban (Eds.), *The many dimensions of aging.* New York: Springer.

Sabat, S. R., & Harre, R. (1992). The construction and deconstruction of self in Alzheimer's disease. *Aging and Society, 12,* 443–461.

Schulz, R., & Quittner, A. (1998). Caregiving for children and adults with chronic conditions. *Health Psychology, 17*(2), 107–111.

Schultz-Krohn, W. (1997). Early intervention: Meeting the unique needs of parent-child interaction. *Infants and Young Children 10*(1), 47–60.

Ulicny, G., & Jones, M. L. (1985). Enhancing the attendant management skills of persons with disabilities. *American Rehabilitation, 2*(2), 18–20.

U.S. Bureau of the Census (1990). *The need for personal assistance with everyday activities: Recipients and caregivers* (19). Washington, DC: U.S. Government Printing Office.

U.S. Bureau of the Census (1992). *Population projections of the United States, by age, race, sex, and Hispanic origin: 1992 to 2050* (1092). Washington, DC: U.S. Government Printing Office.

Weinstein, M. (1997). Bringing family-centered practices into home health. *OT Practice, 2*(7), 35–38.

Wright, L. K., Clipp, E. C., & George, L. K. (1993). Health consequences of caregiver stress. *Medicine, Exercise, Nutrition, and Health, 2,* 181–195.

Zarit, S. H., & Teri, L. (1991). Interventions and services for family caregivers. *Annual Review of Gerontology and Geriatrics, 11,* 287–310.

Zedlewski, E. A. (1990). *The needs of the elderly in the 21st century.* Washington, DC: Urban Institute Press.

Glossary

abandonment. A preferred term to describe the disuse of an assistive technology device and avoids the connotation of consumer misbehavior that compliance implies.

Abledata. An Internet and CD-ROM format directory, funded by the National Institute for Disability and Rehabilitation Research (NIDRR), that provides a searchable database of assistive technology and rehabilitation devices.

acquisition. Initial learning of a skill but not to a point of complete mastery.

activities of daily living (ADL). Activities or tasks that a person does every day to maintain personal independence.

adaptive strategies. Actions used by persons to accomplish certain tasks that organize life. These strategies may involve equipment or techniques or routines.

aesthetic anxiety. Fear of others whose characteristics are perceived as disturbing or unpleasant.

Alzheimer's disease. A progressive degenerative disease of uncertain causes that manifests itself in damage to the brain.

amputee center of excellence. A specialized amputee program that includes experienced physicians, prosthetists, therapists, nurses, and other clinicians who have several years of background experience and training with amputees. This type of center is recommended for complex upper-limb proximal levels and bilateral upper-extremity amputees because of the unique and complex nature of their many rehabilitation needs.

ankylosing spondylitis. A chronic systemic disease in which the primary sites of inflammation are the ligamentous, capsular, and tendinous insertions into the bone (the entheses) that primarily involves the sacroiliac, spinal apophyseal, and axial joints.

antecedents. Planned or unplanned events that are present or happen before a target response.

aphasia. The loss of ability to communicate orally, through signs, or in writing, or the inability to understand such communications; the loss of language usage ability.

assertive community treatment. Program offering case management services via an interdisciplinary team in the community to persons with psychiatric disabilities.

assessment. Specific tools used in the evaluation process.

assistive technology device. A commercial, fabricated, or adapted device used to assist in functional performance of the tasks required for everyday living.

assistive technology service. An agency or unit that provides information or other assistance regarding the need, acquisition, modification, or maintenance of assistive technology devices.

ataxia. Impaired voluntary muscular coordination.

ATP. Assistive technology practitioner with credentials as the nonspecialized foundation level of competence by RESNA.

augmentative communication. A system, which can be personal, technical or electronic, that enhances communication abilities.

autograft. A graft of tissue taken from a different area of the same person receiving the graft.

autonomic dysreflexia. A life-threatening sympathetic response of the nervous system that occurs in persons with spinal cord injuries at the T-7 level or above as a reaction to noxious stimulus. Can be caused by temperature extremes, bowel or bladder distension, catheter obstruction, skin irritation, or other factors.

ball-bearing forearm orthosis (BBFO). See mobile arm support.

baseline data. Test information gathered on the learner's performance of a target skill before instruction on that skill.

biscapular abduction. The motion of bringing both shoulders forward, and sliding the shoulder blades apart, which exerts pressure on the cable to open the terminal device.

body-powered prostheses. A prosthesis whereby shoulder or arm movements or both operate the terminal device or elbow or both by means of a shoulder harness and cable. It is also known as a conventional, or a standard upper-limb, prosthesis.

boutonnière deformity. A deformity caused by disruption of the extensor apparatus at the proximal interphalangeal joint level resulting in proximal interphalangeal joint flexion and distal interphalangeal joint hyperextension when active finger extension is attempted.

boutonnière precautions. Avoidance of composite active flexion of the fingers with deeper partial or full-thickness dorsal hand burns; instead, isolated metaphalangeal flexion is combined with interphalangeal joint extension to avoid stress to a possibly compromised extensor tendon mechanism. Passive proximal interphalangeal flexion is avoided, and protective splinting is used when the hand is at rest.

case management. A practice in which the service recipient is a partner, to the greatest extent possible, in evaluating needs; in obtaining services, treatments, and supports; and in preventing and managing crises. The focus of the partnership is recovery and self-management of mental illness and life. The person and the practitioner plan, coordinate, monitor, adjust, and advocate for services and supports directed toward the achievement of the person's personal goals for community living.

cerebral palsy. A disability resulting from a non-progressive lesion of the central nervous system originating before, during, or shortly after birth that manifests as a muscular incoordination. Intellectual, sensory, speech, seizure, and behavioral disorders may coexist with these motor deficits.

cognitive deficits. The loss or abnormality of mental processes, including thinking, attending, remembering, problem solving, learning, judging, and reflecting about one's thoughts.

cognitive rehabilitation. A remedial intervention approach that uses systematic, reductionistic, and mechanistic techniques to train and compensate for cognitive deficit.

community supports. Persons and institutions that support the integration of persons with psychiatric disorders into the community, including family members, mental health professionals, employers, and the like.

compassion. From the Latin, *com* (with) + *patior* (to feel). A quality among caregivers of feeling kindly when faced with another person's sufferings and responding willingly and helpfully to their needs.

compensation. Finding new ways to accomplish a task when performance capabilities are limited, through modifying the task or task environment.

competence. Being able to accomplish tasks or perform social roles in a manner that is acceptable to oneself and others.

compliance. An outdated term used to describe whether a person is using an assistive technology device according to prescription.

consequences. Planned or unplanned events that are presented or happen after a target response.

consumer. A person who requires assistive technology devices or services.

context. An everyday situation consisting of a person and the environment in which the person finds himself or herself. The environment has both physical objects, such as buildings and objects, and social dimensions, including other persons and attitudes.

correlation. The extent to which two or more variables or tests are related. An index of the degree to which two phenomena are related, expressed as a value from 0 to 1. The sign before a correlation coefficient indicates the direction of a relationship. Phenomena may be correlated directly or positively, that is when one changes, the other changes proportionally in the same direction. They may also be correlated negatively or inversely. In this case, they change in opposite directions; that is, as the value of one goes up, the value of the second goes down, or vice-versa.

counseling. Giving information to clients from a functional perspective related only to sexuality and disability.

counts fingers (CF) or finger counting (FC). An unreliable and seldom used designation of vision.

dermis. The corium, the layer of skin beneath the epidermis.

desensitization. The therapeutic process of lessening the sensitivity of the residual limb of a person with an amputation.

developmental disabilities. A severe, chronic disability of a person that is attributable to a mental or physical impairment or combination of mental and physical impairments; is manifested before the person attains age 22; is likely to continue indefinitely; results in substantial functional limitations in three or more of the following areas of major life activity: self-care, receptive and expressive language, learning, mobility, self-direction, capacity for independent living, or economic self-sufficiency; and reflects that person's need for a combination and sequence of special, interdisciplinary, or generic care, treatment, or other services that are individually planned and coordinated.

disability. The inability to engage in valued daily occupations as a result of physical, cognitive, or emotional impairment and limitations in the environment.

disability prevention. Those parts of the plan of care that promote safety or prevent health problems.

disablement. The condition of not being able to participate fully in life situations based on impairments, limitations in function, or restrictions imposed by the social and physical environment (context).

disarticulation. An amputation that occurs through the joint (wrist, elbow, or shoulder).

disease. A disorder as defined by medical science.

division of labor. A pattern of work roles linked to age and sex within a family and in the wider society.

donor site. Area from which the upper layer of the skin is taken for a skin graft.

dysarthria. A motor disorder that results in difficulty in motor speech mechanisms.

dysphagia. Difficulty with swallowing

ecological inventory. An assessment that provides information about the discrepancies between a person's abilities and the demands within a particular environment.

ectropion. The turning outward or eversion of the eyelids or lips because of skin contractures.

electric prostheses. Prostheses that are externally powered by a motor with batteries and are controlled in various ways, which may include an electromyograph signal, switch, or touch control.

enthesopathy. Pain amplified from tenderness at sites where tendons attach to bones.

environment-adjusted score. A functional performance measure that takes into account performance in the context of the environment, its adaptations, modifications of tasks, or use of assistive technology.

environment-free score. A functional performance measure that takes into account intrinsic abilities of a person with no environmental or task modifications or use of assistive technology.

epidermis. The outermost layer of the skin.

erythema. The redness of the skin produced by inflammation and capillary congestion.

eschar. Nonviable slough of necrotic tissue produced by a burn.

ethnographic approach. The attempt to understand another way of life from the informant's point of view. An ethnographic interview focuses on values, meanings, beliefs, and how the informant makes sense of his or her situation.

evaluation. An ongoing process of collecting and interpreting data necessary for planning intervention.

excoriation. An abrasion or separation of the epidermis usually caused by shearing or blunt trauma, often resulting in blisters or an open superficial wound.

existential anxiety. An unconscious fear about loss of physical capabilities that able-bodied persons often experience when in contact with person with disabilities.

explanatory model of illness. A set of beliefs and knowledge used to explain sickness and treatment and that provide a conceptual framework to give meaning to a particular illness experience and guide choices among various therapies.

family caregiver. Any family member providing unpaid care to a person who would not be able to care for himself or herself because of a physical, cognitive, or psychological impairment.

family-centered care. A term used to describe a constellation of beliefs, values, and treatment approaches that recognizes the role of family members as full collaborators on the health care team.

feasibility. The extent to which a test is practical for widespread use.

fibromyalgia syndrome. A chronic and painful disorder characterized by widespread discomfort and tenderness to palpation at anatomically defined "tender points" and is believed to be the result of a disturbance of the neuroendocrine, biorhythmic, and nociceptive systems.

flat affect. The lack of emotional response to situations or conditions.

fluency. Later learning of a skill with an emphasis on improving the speed, quality, and accuracy of performance.

Frankel scale. A method for classifying the completeness of a spinal cord injury. A complete transection will result in total loss of sensory and motor function below the level of the injury.

full-thickness burn. A burn that extends through and causes necrosis of all three layers of the skin.

functional effects on sexual activity. The effects of a disability that may impede sexual activity.

functional independence. The ability to perform required activities and tasks of daily living without the assistance of another person (usually an undeclared combination of environment-free and environment-adjusted constructs).

functional mobility. The use of wheeled devices, such as strollers, transport chairs, or wheelchairs, to give transportation to persons without independent ambulation.

functional skills. Skills that if not performed by the person in part or in full must be completed or performed by another; purposeful for a given person and valued by others.

functional training. A remedial intervention system that uses cognitive or behavioral strategies to train and compensate for disabilities in the day-to-day activities expected of the person (depending on culture, age, and gender).

functional use training. The staged process of instructing a person with an upper-extremity amputation in how to use his or her prosthesis in the activities of daily living.

generalization. Later learning of a skill under changing conditions (i.e., location, materials, people, time of day).

graduated guidance. A response-prompting method involving the presentation of physical prompts given as minimally as necessary and requiring moment-to-moment decisions by the instructor during instruction based on the learner's performance.

hand movement (HM). The ability to see movement or gross forms.

health promotion. Strategies aimed at enabling completion of valued tasks and finding fulfillment while conserving energy.

hemianopia. Blindness in half of the field of vision in one or both eyes.

hemiplegia. Paralysis of only one half of the body.

hemorrhage. Bleeding from the rupture of a blood vessel.

heterotopic ossification. Bone formation occurring at an abnormal location in the body.

humeral flexion. The motion of raising the humerus forward and exerting pressure (the pressure is applied to a cable on the prosthesis, enabling the terminal device to open).

hybrid prosthesis. A prosthesis with both a body-powered prosthetic component and an electric prosthetic component.

hyperpigmentation. Excessive darkening of skin color caused by overproduction of skin pigment, often accelerated by sun exposure.

hypertrophic scar. Excessive scar formation that rises above the level of the skin plane but does not extend beyond the original borders of the burn wound.

hypopigmentation. Lighter than normal skin color caused by underproduction of skin pigment.

ICIDH-2. *International Classification of Impairment, Disability, and Handicap,* Second Edition. A classification system for disability developed by the World Health Organization.

identity. The mental picture of a person as he or she appears to self and to others; individual characteristics that make a person unique.

illness. A person's actual experience of disorder or suffering, whether or not caused by an identifiable disease.

independent living movement. A philosophy in which persons are responsible for their decision making and performance of self-care and community activities within the limits of their capabilities.

infantilization. The tendency of some caregivers to treat an adult who needs help with self-care as if he or she were a baby; an inappropriate manner of talking to and providing services to person with impairments.

instrumental activities of daily living (IADL). More complex activities or tasks that a person does to maintain independence in the home and community.

juvenile rheumatoid arthritis. A different disease from adult rheumatoid arthritis; delineated into three major types and seven subtypes, defined by the symptoms present during the first 6 months after onset. The major types are systemic onset, polyarticular onset, and pauciarticular onset. All forms of JRA are systemic in nature and have an element of fatigue, fever, and malaise associated with the active disease.

keloid scar. Excessive scar formation that rises above the level of the skin plane and continues to extend, mushroom-like, beyond the original borders of the burn wound.

legal blindness. Having vision of 20/200 (20 over 200) or less (using the Snellen eye chart measurement) in the better eye with best standard eyeglass correction, or having a visual field that subtends an angle of 20° or less.

light perception (LP). The ability to perceive light only.

light projection (L. Proj.). The ability not only to see light but also to determine the direction of the source.

maintenance. Later learning of a skill with an emphasis on its routine use under fairly stable and unchanging conditions.

mobile arm support (MAS). An assistive device for support of the forearm, used when shoulder and elbow muscles are weak or paralyzed, to assist with feeding. Another term for this orthotic device is *ball-bearing forearm orthosis* (BBFO).

mood disorders. Disorders that range from sadness to grief to bipolar disorder, major depression, and anxiety.

narrative. The story within a person's personal life experience.

negotiability. The ability to access a feature of the environment and use it for its intended purpose, with only one's usual adaptive equipment.

no light perception (NLP). Total blindness.

occupational therapy diagnosis. A problem statement that succinctly describes the occupational status of a person and identifies the problems that are amenable to intervention.

open market. Items available for purchase from the mass commercial market.

osteoarthritis. The most common rheumatic disease, affecting both men and women equally during their middle age and beyond, with its prevalence increasing with age. The progression of osteoarthritis arthritis involves a two-stage process: (a) the articular cartilage wears down or deteriorates and (b) bone builds up around the margin of the joint, creating a lumpy, enlarged appearance. This process is frequently painless, with stiffness and limited range of motion as the primary problems, or inflammation and associated pain and swelling. Joints typically affected include the hands, spine, knees, hips, the metatarsophalangeal joint of the large toe, shoulders, and elbows.

osteolysis. Dissolution of the bone ends in involved joints.

osteophytes. Bony outgrowths.

paraplegia. Paralysis of the lower portion of the body and of both legs, resulting from injury to the spinal cord.

partial participation. Performance of a task or activity in part or in full that is made possible through one or more adaptations (i.e., personal assistance on difficult steps, changes in the sequence or rules, modification of task materials, the addition of adaptive devices).

partial-thickness burn. A burn injury extending through the epidermis and into the dermis.

performance failure. An inability of the body to perform activities that were once done automatically and taken for granted.

personal care attendant. A paid employee who provides in-home assistance with essential activities of daily living to a person with a severe disability who is functionally dependent.

personality disorders. Disorders that exaggerate traits of persons such as unstable emotional responses, self-absorption, and fearfulness.

plan of care. The goals and intervention strategies in addressing diagnoses and problems.

polyarticular. A disease involving many joints.

powered mobility. Motorized devices for mobility, such as wheelchairs or scooters, that allow a person mobility through switch-activited battery power and various steering mechanisms.

preprosthetic program. The therapy program that prepares a residual limb for a prosthesis. Ideally, this program begins when the sutures are removed. It consists of limb shaping, desensitization, range of motion exercises, muscle strengthening, proper hygiene of the limb, maximization of independence, and an orientation to prosthetic components.

prescription. Specific instructions or specifications regarding needed rehabilitation services or equipment.

press. The kind of effect an object or situation is exerting or could exert on the subject, which usually appears in the guise of a threat of harm or promise of benefit to the organism.

probe data. Test information gathered on the learner's performance of a target skill at planned intervals once instruction has been initiated on that skill.

psoriatic arthritis. A systemic disease in which psoriasis is associated with inflammatory arthritis.

psychiatric impairments and disorders. Disorders causing persons to be indifferent to social expectations; to lack self-esteem; to lack knowledge, motivation, or skills to carry out their daily occupations; or to systematically process demands from the environment.

psychiatric rehabilitation. Program emphasizing rehabilitation toward recovery rather than treatment for persons with psychiatric disabilities.

psychoeducational models. Educational approaches to change habits, routines, and skills; includes behavioral and cognitive approaches.

reciprocity. A system of exchanging goods and services between persons and groups that is a fundamental basis for social relations.

reliability. The consistency and precision with which an assessment measures a specific behavior or skill.

remediation. Strategies that focus on restoring or improving function within performance components, such as in sensation, cognition, or voluntary movement, and includes training.

RESNA. Rehabilitation Engineering and Assistive Technology Society of North America. An interdisciplinary association for the advancement of rehabilitation and assistive technologies.

resorption. Dissolution of the ends of the distal phalanges that causes shortening of the digits.

response latency. A brief period of time provided by the instructor after presenting the task request and stimuli and before giving assistance, which allows the learner to respond independently.

response prompts. Various types of assistance that are directed antecedent to the learner's behavior.

rheumatoid arthritis. A systemic disease with inflammation of the synovium (or sac), which provides lubrication for the joint, as a primary symptom, as well as exacerbations and remissions, and primarily affects the extremity joints and the neck.

routines. Behaviors that are repeated over time and organized into patterns and habits.

scar maturation. Progressive remodeling of a scar as demonstrated by a softening and flattening of scar texture and complete resolution of erythema, usually over a 12- to 18-month period after the initial burn injury or surgical reconstruction procedure.

schizophrenia. A pervasive and usually chronic disorder that affects performance in work, self-care, or interpersonal relations.

self-advocacy. The ability to express personal needs and work within a larger social or legal system to get those needs met.

self-care assessments. Instruments to assess the daily living needs of persons with psychiatric disabilities; includes direct observation and self-report.

self-care environment. The complex, ever-changing, natural, built, physical, psychosocial, cultural, economic, and political setting in which the person cares for her or his well-being.

self-care management. The administration of care and coordination of services for clients who require training or self-care management, including personal care, mobility, communication, and the performance of basic tasks such as housecleaning, child care, banking, and shopping.

self-care occupations. Those basic personal care activities such as eating, grooming, dressing, mobility, and personal hygiene.

self-care strategies. Methods to manage self-care needs.

self-efficacy. The belief that desired tasks can be accomplished successfully.

self-maintenance. The ability to handle tasks ranging from basic personal care, including dressing, eating, grooming, toileting, and getting around (mobility), to doing laundry, using the telephone, shopping, banking, and managing medications (used as a synonym for activities of daily living).

sensory environment. Illumination; quality of light; color; pattern and contrast; acoustics, including clutter and echo; textures and other surface qualities; and temperature.

severe visual impairment. A self- or proxy-reported inability to read standard newsprint.

sexology. The science or study of sexuality.

sexual activity. Activities aimed at giving or receiving sexual pleasure.

sexual orientation. A person's erotic, romantic, and affectional attraction to persons of the same sex (homosexuality), to the opposite sex (heterosexuality), or to both sexes (bisexuality).

sexual response cycle. The physiologic responses to sexual stimulation or excitement as described by Masters and Johnson (1966).

sexual rights. The rights of persons to have the information, education, skills, support, and services they need to make responsible decisions about their sexuality consistent with their own values.

sick role. A social attitude enabling persons who are ill to be excused temporarily from performing everyday roles during the time that they are recovering. The sick role involves giving up control over one's situation and status as a competent member of society until declared well by a medical authority.

sighted guide technique. The most comfortable, widely used, safe, and efficient way to assist a blind person in traveling. In this position, the blind person holds the arm of the guide just above the elbow. The blind person will be a half-step behind and to the side of the sighted guide. In this position, a blind person can safely follow the guide's body movements as they walk.

situational observation. Observation of a person's ability to perform a specific task within the environment in which the task usually occurs.

skin appendages. Epithelial-lined skin pockets containing oil glands and sweat glands from which a partial-thickness burn can reepithelialize.

social press. The effect of other humans on the self-care performance of the person, including the emotional effects of a person's presence or absence, as well as his or her potential to physically further or hinder the self-care process.

split-thickness skin graft. A skin graft containing the epidermis and the upper portion of the dermis.

stability. The consistency of a measure over time.

stages of learning. Phases through which one attains and masters a skill, beginning with acquisition and progressing through to maintenance, fluency, and generalization.

standardized. Instruments that have a well-defined procedure, norms (if applicable), and standards for administration.

stigma. Social prejudice that devalues persons with limiting conditions or disfigurements by viewing them as incapable of fulfilling roles and responsibilities.

stigma symbols. Aspects of appearance that others may unfairly use as evidence that someone is not a fully competent member of society.

stimulus prompts. A procedure for facilitating learning that involves a gradual change in the instructional stimuli from those that immediately control the student's responding to the target stimuli.

substance abuse and dependence. Regular or periodic intake of a substance (alcohol or other drugs) that may or does interfere with several aspects of function.

superficial burn. A burn injury that involves only the epidermis.

supplier. A distributor of assistive technology devices, sometimes called durable medical equipment (DME) dealer.

system of least prompts. A response-prompting procedure in which the instructor provides assistance based on the student responding in order of the least amount of assistance to the maximum amount of assistance required to ensure correct performance of the target behavior.

systemic lupus erythematosus. A systemic inflammatory disease characterized by small vessel vasculitis with a diverse clinical picture that occurs most often in women.

systemic sclerosis. The generalized or systemic form of a group of disorders that include sclerosis of the skin as a predominant feature.

terminal device. The end effector, or prehensor, located at the end of an arm prosthesis.

tetraplegia. Paralysis of all four extremities and the trunk caused by injury to the cervical portion of the spinal cord. Generally, the higher the injury, the less voluntary movement available for performing tasks of living.

time delay. A response-prompting procedure characterized by inserting a planned amount of time between a task stimulus that cues a student to perform a task and a response prompt that evokes the student's response.

topographical orientation. Understanding and remembering the relationship of one place to another; the ability to find the way from one place to another independently.

total active motion (TAM). A method of goniometry measuring simultaneous, composite, active range of motion of multiple, adjacent joints.

training data. Information gathered on the learner's performance during instruction when prompts and reinforcement are available.

transparent equipment. Adapted equipment not readily identifiable as an adaptive devise.

traumatic brain injury. Nonprogressive, persistent damage to the brain caused by a blow or the impact to the head of a high-speed acceleration or deceleration force.

unilateral neglect. A disturbance of a person's awareness of space on the side of the body opposite a stroke-causing lesion.

universal cuff. An elastic or plastic device to assist with eating; it fits around the palm and has a pocket for inserting the handle of a utensil.

validity. The extent to which one can have confidence in the results of an assessment.

Wanchik device. An orthosis to hold the wrist in a neutral position for holding writing implements.

Index